W9-AWK-823

MKSAP® 16

Medical Knowledge Self-Assessment Program®

General Internal Medicine

Welcome to the General Internal Medicine section of MKSAP 16!

Here, you will find updated information on routine care of the healthy patient; patient safety; professionalism and ethics; palliative care; chronic pain; acute and chronic cough; chronic fatigue; musculoskeletal pain; dyslipidemia; obesity; men's and women's health; eye, ear, nose, mouth, and throat disorders; mental and behavioral health; geriatric medicine; perioperative medicine; and many other clinical challenges. All of these topics are uniquely focused on the needs of both generalists and those who practice subspecialty internal medicine.

The publication of the 16th edition of Medical Knowledge Self-Assessment Program heralds a significant event, culminating 2 years of effort by dozens of leading subspecialists across the United States. Our authoring committees have strived to help internists succeed in Maintenance of Certification, right up to preparing for the MOC examination, and to get residents ready for the certifying examination. MKSAP 16 also helps you update your medical knowledge and elevates standards of self-learning by allowing you to assess your knowledge with 1,200 all-new multiple-choice questions, including 168 in General Internal Medicine.

MKSAP began more than 40 years ago. The American Board of Internal Medicine's examination blueprint and gaps between actual and preferred practices inform creation of the content. The questions, refined through rigorous face-to-face meetings, are among the best in medicine. A psychometric analysis of the items sharpens our educational focus on weaknesses in practice. To meet diverse learning styles, we offer MKSAP 16 online and in downloadable apps for PCs, tablets, laptops, and smartphones. We are also introducing the following:

High-Value Care Recommendations: The General Internal Medicine section starts with several recommendations based on the important concept of health care value (balancing clinical benefit with costs and harms) to address the needs of trainees, practicing physicians, and patients. These recommendations are part of a major initiative that has been undertaken by the American College of Physicians, in collaboration with other organizations.

Content for Hospitalists: This material, highlighted in blue and labeled with the familiar hospital icon (H), directly addresses the learning needs of the increasing number of physicians who work in the hospital setting. MKSAP 16 Digital will allow you to customize quizzes based on hospitalist-only questions to help you prepare for the Hospital Medicine Maintenance of Certification Examination.

We hope you enjoy and benefit from MKSAP 16. Please feel free to send us any comments to mksap_editors@acponline.org or visit us at the MKSAP Resource Site (mksap.acponline.org) to find out how we can help you study, earn CME, accumulate MOC points, and stay up to date. I know I speak on behalf of ACP staff members and our authoring committees when I say we are honored to have attracted your interest and participation.

Sincerely,

Patrick Alguire, MD, FACP
Editor-in-Chief
Senior Vice President
Medical Education Division
American College of Physicians

General Internal Medicine

Committee

Gary H. Tabas, MD, FACP, Editor[1]
Professor of Medicine
Division of General Internal Medicine
Department of Medicine
University of Pittsburgh School of Medicine
University of Pittsburgh Medical Center Presbyterian—
Shadyside
Pittsburgh, Pennsylvania

Jack Ende, MD, MACP, Associate Editor[1]
    Professor of Medicine
University of Pennsylvania
Chief, Department of Medicine
Penn Presbyterian Medical Center
Philadelphia, Pennsylvania

Paul B. Aronowitz, MD, FACP[1]
Adjunct Associate Professor of Medicine
Dartmouth Medical School
Associate Professor of Clinical Medicine
University of California, San Francisco
Program Director
Internal Medicine Residency Program
California Pacific Medical Center
San Francisco, California

Rosemarie L. Conigliaro, MD, FACP[1]
Professor of Medicine
Senior Assistant Dean for Curriculum
University of Kentucky College of Medicine
Lexington, Kentucky

Rosanne Granieri, MD, FACP[1]
Professor of Medicine
Division of General Internal Medicine
Department of Medicine
University of Pittsburgh School of Medicine
Pittsburgh, Pennsylvania

Eric H. Green, MD, MSc, FACP[1]
Associate Professor of Clinical Medicine
Drexel University College of Medicine
Philadelphia, Pennsylvania
Associate Program Director
Internal Medicine Residency Program
Mercy Catholic Medical Center
Darby, Pennsylvania

Scott Herrle, MD, MS[1]
Assistant Professor of Medicine
University of Pittsburgh School of Medicine
VA Pittsburgh Healthcare System
Pittsburgh, Pennsylvania

Christopher L. Knight, MD, FACP[2]
Associate Professor
Department of Medicine
University of Washington
Seattle, Washington

Megan McNamara, MD, MSc[1]
Assistant Professor of Medicine
Director of Student Assessment, Program Evaluation, and
the Center for the Advancement of Medical Learning
Case Western Reserve University School of Medicine
Cleveland, Ohio

Mohan Nadkarni, MD, FACP[1]
Professor of Medicine
Chief, Section of General Internal Medicine
University of Virginia Health System
Charlottesville, Virginia

Consulting Contributor

P. Preston Reynolds, MD, PhD, FACP[1]
Professor of Medicine
Division of General Medicine, Geriatrics and Palliative
Care
Center for Biomedical Ethics and Humanities
University of Virginia Health System
Charlottesville, Virginia

Editor-in-Chief

Patrick C. Alguire, MD, FACP[1]
Senior Vice President, Medical Education
American College of Physicians
Philadelphia, Pennsylvania

Deputy Editor-in-Chief

Philip A. Masters, MD, FACP[1]
Senior Medical Associate for Content Development
American College of Physicians
Philadelphia, Pennsylvania

Senior Medical Associate for Content Development

Cynthia D. Smith, MD, FACP[2]
American College of Physicians
Philadelphia, Pennsylvania

General Internal Medicine Clinical Editor

Michele Heisler, MD[1]

General Internal Medicine Reviewers

Stewart Babbott, MD, FACP[1]
Elizabeth A. Cerceo, MD, FACP[1]
John K. Chamberlain, MD, MACP[1]
Timi Edeki, MD[2]
Douglas Einstadter, MD, MPH, FACP[1]
Stephanie L. Elkins, MD[2]
Richard M. Hoffman, MD, MPH, FACP[2]
Medha Munshi, MD[2]
Asher Tulsky, MD, FACP[1]
Peter H. Wiernik, MD, FACP[2]

General Internal Medicine Reviewers Representing the American Society for Clinical Pharmacology & Therapeutics

John Thomas Callaghan, MD, PhD[2]
Anne N. Nafziger, MD, FACP[2]

General Internal Medicine ACP Editorial Staff

Becky Krumm[1], Senior Staff Editor
Sean McKinney[1], Director, Self-Assessment Programs
Margaret Wells[1], Managing Editor
John Haefele[1], Assistant Editor

ACP Principal Staff

Patrick C. Alguire, MD, FACP[1]
Senior Vice President, Medical Education

D. Theresa Kanya, MBA[1]
Vice President, Medical Education

Sean McKinney[1]
Director, Self-Assessment Programs

Margaret Wells[1]
Managing Editor

Valerie Dangovetsky[1]
Program Administrator

Becky Krumm[1]
Senior Staff Editor

Ellen McDonald, PhD[1]
Senior Staff Editor

Katie Idell[1]
Senior Staff Editor

Randy Hendrickson[1]
Production Administrator/Editor

Megan Zborowski[1]
Staff Editor

Linnea Donnarumma[1]
Assistant Editor

John Haefele[1]
Assistant Editor

Developed by the American College of Physicians

---

1. Has no relationships with any entity producing, marketing, re-selling, or distributing health care goods or services consumed by, or used on, patients.

2. Has disclosed relationships with entities producing, marketing, re-selling, or distributing health care goods or services consumed by, or used on, patients. See below.

Conflicts of Interest

The following committee members, reviewers, and ACP staff members have disclosed relationships with commercial companies:

John Thomas Callaghan, MD
Employment
Eli Lilly & Co. (Retiree)
Stock Options/Holdings
Eli Lilly, Abbott, Isis
Consultantship
Marcadia, Biogen Idec

Timi Edeki, MD
Employment
AstraZeneca
Stock Options/Holdings
Abbott Laboratories

Stephanie L. Elkins, MD
Speakers Bureau
Celgene, Cephalon Oncology, GlaxoSmithKline

Richard M. Hoffman, MD, MPH, FACP
Employment
Foundation for Informed Medical Decision Making
Research Grants/Contracts
NIH
Royalties
UpToDate

Christopher L. Knight, MD, FACP
Royalties
Oakstone Medical Publishing

Medha Munshi, MD
Consultantship
Novartis (spouse), Celgene (spouse), Millenium (spouse)

Anne N. Nafziger, MD, FACP
Consultantship
Bertino Consulting

Cynthia D. Smith, MD, FACP
Stock Options/Holdings
Merck and Company

Peter H. Wiernik, MD, FACP
Honoraria
Celgene

Acknowledgments

The American College of Physicians (ACP) gratefully acknowledges the special contributions to the development and production of the 16th edition of the Medical Knowledge Self-Assessment Program® (MKSAP® 16) made by the following people:

Graphic Services: Michael Ripca (Technical Administrator/Graphic Designer) and Willie-Fetchko Graphic Design (Graphic Designer).

Production/Systems: Dan Hoffmann (Director, Web Services & Systems Development), Neil Kohl (Senior Architect), and Scott Hurd (Senior Systems Analyst/Developer).

MKSAP 16 Digital: Under the direction of Steven Spadt, Vice President, ACP Digital Products & Services, the digital version of MKSAP 16 was developed within the ACP's Digital Product Development Department, led by Brian Sweigard (Director). Other members of the team included Sean O'Donnell (Senior Architect), Dan Barron (Senior Systems Analyst/Developer), Chris Forrest (Senior Software Developer/Design Lead), Jon Laing (Senior Web Application Developer), Brad Lord (Senior Web Developer), John McKnight (Senior Web Developer), and Nate Pershall (Senior Web Developer).

The College also wishes to acknowledge that many other persons, too numerous to mention, have contributed to the production of this program. Without their dedicated efforts, this program would not have been possible.

Introducing the MKSAP Resource Site (mksap.acponline.org)

The MKSAP Resource Site (mksap.acponline.org) is a continually updated site that provides links to MKSAP 16 online answer sheets for print subscribers; access to MKSAP 16 Digital, Board Basics® 3, and MKSAP 16 Updates; the latest details on Continuing Medical Education (CME) and Maintenance of Certification (MOC) in the United States, Canada, and Australia; errata; and other new information.

ABIM Maintenance of Certification

Check the MKSAP Resource Site (mksap.acponline.org) for the latest information on how MKSAP tests can be used to apply to the American Board of Internal Medicine for Maintenance of Certification (MOC) points.

RCPSC Maintenance of Certification

In Canada, MKSAP 16 is an Accredited Self-Assessment Program (Section 3) as defined by the Maintenance of Certification Program of The Royal College of Physicians and Surgeons of Canada (RCPSC) and approved by the Canadian Society of Internal Medicine on December 9, 2011. Approval of Part A sections of MKSAP 16 extends from July 31, 2012, until July 31, 2015. Approval of Part B sections of MKSAP 16 extends from December 31, 2012, to December 31, 2015. Fellows of the Royal College may earn three credits per hour for participating in MKSAP 16 under Section 3. MKSAP 16 will enable Fellows to earn up to 75% of their required 400 credits during the 5-year MOC cycle. A Fellow can achieve this 75% level by earning 100 of the maximum of 174 *AMA PRA Category 1 Credits*™ available in MKSAP 16. MKSAP 16 also meets multiple CanMEDS Roles for RCPSC MOC, including that of Medical Expert, Communicator, Collaborator, Manager, Health Advocate, Scholar, and Professional. For information on how to apply MKSAP 16 CME credits to RCPSC MOC, visit the MKSAP Resource Site at mksap.acponline.org.

The Royal Australasian College of Physicians CPD Program

In Australia, MKSAP 16 is a Category 3 program that may be used by Fellows of The Royal Australasian College of Physicians (RACP) to meet mandatory CPD points. Two CPD credits are awarded for each of the 174 *AMA PRA Category 1 Credits*™ available in MKSAP 16. More information about using MKSAP 16 for this purpose is available at the MKSAP Resource Site at mksap.acponline.org and at www.racp.edu.au. CPD credits earned through MKSAP 16 should be reported at the MyCPD site at www.racp.edu.au/mycpd.

Continuing Medical Education

The American College of Physicians is accredited by the Accreditation Council for Continuing Medical Education

(ACCME) to provide continuing medical education for physicians.

The American College of Physicians designates this enduring material, MKSAP 16, for a maximum of 174 *AMA PRA Category 1 Credits*™. Physicians should claim only the credit commensurate with the extent of their participation in the activity.

Up to 24 *AMA PRA Category 1 Credits*™ are available from December 31, 2012, to December 31, 2015, for the MKSAP 16 General Internal Medicine section.

Learning Objectives

The learning objectives of MKSAP 16 are to:
- Close gaps between actual care in your practice and preferred standards of care, based on best evidence
- Diagnose disease states that are less common and sometimes overlooked and confusing
- Improve management of comorbid conditions that can complicate patient care
- Determine when to refer patients for surgery or care by subspecialists
- Pass the ABIM Certification Examination
- Pass the ABIM Maintenance of Certification Examination

Target Audience

- General internists and primary care physicians
- Subspecialists who need to remain up-to-date in internal medicine
- Residents preparing for the certifying examination in internal medicine
- Physicians preparing for maintenance of certification in internal medicine (recertification)

Earn "Same-Day" CME Credits Online

For the first time, print subscribers can enter their answers online to earn CME credits in 24 hours or less. You can submit your answers using online answer sheets that are provided at mksap.acponline.org, where a record of your MKSAP 16 credits will be available. To earn CME credits, you need to answer all of the questions in a test and earn a score of at least 50% correct (number of correct answers divided by the total number of questions). Take any of the following approaches:

1. Use the printed answer sheet at the back of this book to record your answers. Go to mksap.acponline.org, access the appropriate online answer sheet, transcribe your answers, and submit your test for same-day CME credits. There is no additional fee for this service.

2. Go to mksap.acponline.org, access the appropriate online answer sheet, directly enter your answers, and submit your test for same-day CME credits. There is no additional fee for this service.

3. Pay a $10 processing fee per answer sheet and submit the printed answer sheet at the back of this book by mail or fax, as instructed on the answer sheet. Make sure you calculate your score and fax the answer sheet to 215-351-2799 or mail the answer sheet to Member and Customer Service, American College of Physicians, 190 N. Independence Mall West, Philadelphia, PA 19106-1572, using the courtesy envelope provided in your MKSAP 16 slipcase. You will need your 10-digit order number and 8-digit ACP ID number, which are printed on your packing slip. Please allow 4 to 6 weeks for your score report to be emailed back to you. Be sure to include your email address for a response.

If you do not have a 10-digit order number and 8-digit ACP ID number or if you need help creating a username and password to access the MKSAP 16 online answer sheets, go to mksap.acponline.org or email custserv@acponline.org.

Permission/Consent for Use of Figures Shown in MKSAP 16 General Internal Medicine Multiple-Choice Questions

The figures shown in Self-Assessment Test Item 29, Item 148, and Item 61 appear courtesy of Edward A. Jaeger, MD, Jefferson Medical College, Wills Eye Institute, Philadelphia, PA. The figure shown in Self-Assessment Test Item 163 is reprinted with permission from Physicians' Information and Education Resource (ACP PIER). Philadelphia, PA: American College of Physicians.

Disclosure Policy

It is the policy of the American College of Physicians (ACP) to ensure balance, independence, objectivity, and scientific rigor in all of its educational activities. To this end, and consistent with the policies of the ACP and the Accreditation Council for Continuing Medical Education (ACCME), contributors to all ACP continuing medical education activities are required to disclose all relevant financial relationships with any entity producing, marketing, re-selling, or distributing health care goods or services consumed by, or used on, patients. Contributors are required to use generic names in the discussion of therapeutic options and are required to identify any unapproved, off-label, or investigative use of commercial products or devices. Where a trade name is used, all available trade names for the same product type are also included. If trade-name products manufactured by companies with whom contributors have relationships are discussed, contributors are asked to provide evidence-based citations in support of the discussion. The information is reviewed by the committee responsible for producing this text. If necessary, adjustments to topics or contributors' roles in content development are made to balance the discussion. Further, all readers of this text are asked to evaluate the content for evidence of commercial bias and send any relevant comments to mksap_editors@acponline.org so that future decisions about content and contributors can be made in light of this information.

Resolution of Conflicts

To resolve all conflicts of interest and influences of vested interests, the ACP precluded members of the content-creation committee from deciding on any content issues that involved generic or trade-name products associated with proprietary entities with which these committee members had relationships. In addition, content was based on best evidence and updated clinical care guidelines, when such evidence and guidelines were available. Contributors' disclosure information can be found with the list of contributors' names and those of ACP principal staff listed in the beginning of this book.

Hospital-Based Medicine

For the convenience of subscribers who provide care in hospital settings, content that is specific to the hospital setting has been highlighted in blue. Hospital icons (🏥) highlight where the hospital-only content begins, continues over more than one page, and ends.

Educational Disclaimer

The editors and publisher of MKSAP 16 recognize that the development of new material offers many opportunities for error. Despite our best efforts, some errors may persist in print. Drug dosage schedules are, we believe, accurate and in accordance with current standards. Readers are advised, however, to ensure that the recommended dosages in MKSAP 16 concur with the information provided in the product information material. This is especially important in cases of new, infrequently used, or highly toxic drugs. Application of the information in MKSAP 16 remains the professional responsibility of the practitioner.

The primary purpose of MKSAP 16 is educational. Information presented, as well as publications, technologies, products, and/or services discussed, is intended to inform subscribers about the knowledge, techniques, and experiences of the contributors. A diversity of professional opinion exists, and the views of the contributors are their own and not those of the ACP. Inclusion of any material in the program does not constitute endorsement or recommendation by the ACP. The ACP does not warrant the safety, reliability, accuracy, completeness, or usefulness of and disclaims any and all liability for damages and claims that may result from the use of information, publications, technologies, products, and/or services discussed in this program.

Publisher's Information

Copyright © 2012 American College of Physicians. All rights reserved.

This publication is protected by copyright. No part of this publication may be reproduced, stored in a retrieval system, or transmitted in any form or by any means, electronic or mechanical, including photocopy, without the express consent of the ACP. MKSAP 16 is for individual use only. Only one account per subscription will be permitted for the purpose of earning CME credits and MOC points/credits and for other authorized uses of MKSAP 16.

Unauthorized Use of This Book Is Against the Law

Unauthorized reproduction of this publication is unlawful. The ACP prohibits reproduction of this publication or any of its parts in any form either for individual use or for distribution.

The ACP will consider granting an individual permission to reproduce only limited portions of this publication for his or her own exclusive use. Send requests in writing to MKSAP® Permissions, American College of Physicians, 190 N. Independence Mall West, Philadelphia, PA 19106-1572, or email your request to mksap_editors@acponline.org.

MKSAP 16 ISBN: 978-1-938245-00-8
(General Internal Medicine) ISBN: 978-1-938245-08-4

Printed in the United States of America.

For order information in the U.S. or Canada call 800-523-1546, extension 2600. All other countries call 215-351-2600. Fax inquiries to 215-351-2799 or email to custserv@acponline.org.

Errata and Norm Tables

Errata for MKSAP 16 will be available through the MKSAP Resource Site at mksap.acponline.org as new information becomes known to the editors.

MKSAP 16 Performance Interpretation Guidelines with Norm Tables, available July 31, 2013, will reflect the knowledge of physicians who have completed the self-assessment tests before the program was published. These physicians took the tests without being able to refer to the syllabus, answers, and critiques. For your convenience, the tables are available in a printable PDF file through the MKSAP Resource Site at mksap.acponline.org.

Table of Contents

Interpretation of the Medical Literature

Study Design 1
    Threats to Validity 1
    Experimental Studies 1
    Observational Studies 1
    Other Study Designs 3
Statistical Analysis 3
Sources of Evidence 4

Routine Care of the Healthy Patient

Important Health Care Initiatives and Trends 4
Screening 6
    Screening During the History and Physical
    Examination 8
    Periodic Health Examination 8
    Specific Screening Tests 8
Family History and Genetic Testing 11
    Taking a Family History 11
    Caveats to Genetic Testing 11
    Referral for Genetic Counseling 11
Immunization 12
    Vaccinations Recommended for All Adults 13
    Vaccinations Recommended for Some Adults 13
Lifestyle Risk Factors 16
    Behavioral Counseling 16
    Diet and Physical Activity 16
    Substance Use Disorders 17
    Sexual Behavior 18
    Domestic Violence 18

Patient Safety

Introduction 19
Principles of Patient Safety 19
Quality Improvement Models 19
    Measurement of Quality Improvement 20
Sources of Error 20
    Diagnostic Errors 20
    Medication Errors 20
    Transitions of Care 20
Health Information Technology and Patient Safety 22
National Patient Safety Goals 22

Professionalism and Ethics

Professionalism 22
Decision-Making and Informed Consent 24
    Informed Consent 24
    Assessing Decision-Making Capacity 24
    Advance Directives and Surrogate Decision-Making . 24
Withholding or Withdrawing Treatment 25
Physician-Assisted Suicide and Euthanasia 25
Confidentiality 25
Conflicts of Interest 26
Medical Error Disclosure 26
Sexual Contact between Physician and Patient 27
The Impaired Physician and Colleague Responsibility . . . 27

Palliative Care

Introduction 27
Deciding When Hospice Palliative Care Is Indicated 28
Assessment and Communication 29
Symptom Management 29
    Pain 29
    Constipation 30
    Fatigue 30
    Dyspnea 32
    Nausea 32
    Anorexia and Nutrition 32
    Depression 32
    Delirium 32
Bereavement and Grief 32

Common Symptoms

Overview 32
Chronic Noncancer Pain 33
    Assessment 33
    Management 34
Cough 36
    Acute Cough 37
    Subacute and Chronic Cough 37
    Cough in the Immunocompromised Patient 39
    Hemoptysis 39
Chronic Fatigue and Chronic Fatigue Syndrome 39
    Diagnosis and Evaluation of Chronic Fatigue 39
    Management of Chronic Fatigue and Chronic
    Fatigue Syndrome 40

Dizziness 40
    Vertigo 40
    Presyncope 43
    Dysequilibrium 43
    Nonspecific Dizziness 43
Insomnia 43
    Evaluation of Insomnia 44
    Management of Insomnia 44
Syncope 45
    Neurocardiogenic Syncope 45
    Orthostatic Hypotension 46
    Cardiac Causes of Syncope 46
    Diagnostic Evaluation of Syncope 46
    Risk Stratification and Management of Syncope 47
Chest Pain 47
    Differential Diagnosis 47
    Chest Pain and Decision to Hospitalize 49
Edema 50

Musculoskeletal Pain

Acute Low Back Pain 50
    Diagnosis and Evaluation 50
    Treatment 51
Neck Pain 52
    Diagnosis and Evaluation 52
    Treatment 53
Shoulder Pain 53
    Diagnosis and Evaluation 53
    Rotator Cuff Disorders 54
    Adhesive Capsulitis 55
    Acromioclavicular Joint Degeneration 56
Elbow Pain 56
    Diagnosis and Evaluation 56
    Epicondylitis 56
    Olecranon Bursitis 56
    Ulnar Nerve Entrapment 56
Wrist and Hand Pain 57
    Indications for Imaging 57
    Carpal Tunnel Syndrome 57
    Other Causes of Wrist and Hand Pain 57
Hip Pain 58
    Diagnosis and Evaluation 58
    Specific Causes of Hip Pain 58
Knee Pain 58
    Diagnosis and Evaluation 58
    Degenerative Joint Disease 59
    Trauma 59
    Patellofemoral Pain Syndrome 59
    Bursitis 60

    Iliotibial Band Syndrome 60
    Baker Cyst 61
Ankle and Foot Pain 61
    Ankle Sprains 61
    Hind Foot Pain 61
    Midfoot Pain 62
    Forefoot Pain 62

Dyslipidemia

Screening 62
Evaluation of Lipid Levels 62
    LDL Cholesterol 62
    Triglycerides 63
    HDL Cholesterol 64
    Nonstandard Lipid Risk Factors 64
Management of Dyslipidemias 64
    Therapeutic Lifestyle Changes 64
    Drug Therapy 64
    Combination Drug Therapy 65
    Management of Hypertriglyceridemia 66
    Management of Low HDL Cholesterol 67
Metabolic Syndrome 67
    Epidemiology and Pathophysiology 67
    Management of Metabolic Syndrome 67
Dyslipidemia Management in Older Patients 68
Dyslipidemia Management and Stroke Prevention 69
Aspirin as an Adjunct to Dyslipidemia Management 69

Obesity

Definition and Epidemiology 69
Screening and Evaluation 70
Treatment 71
    Lifestyle Modification 72
    Pharmacologic Therapy 72
    Surgery 73

Men's Health

Male Sexual Dysfunction 74
    Erectile Dysfunction 74
    Premature Ejaculation 76
    Decreased Libido 77
Androgen Deficiency 77
Benign Prostatic Hyperplasia 78
Acute Testicular and Scrotal Pain 78
    Testicular Torsion 79
    Epididymitis 79
Hydrocele and Varicocele 79
    Epididymal Cyst 79
    Varicocele 79

Acute and Chronic Prostatitis and Pelvic Pain 80
Hernia. 81

Women's Health

Female Sexual Dysfunction 81
    Approach to the Patient 81
    Classification of Female Sexual Disorders 81
Evaluation of a Breast Mass 82
    Clinical Presentation. 83
    Evaluation 83
Breast Pain. 84
    Clinical Presentation. 84
    Evaluation 84
    Treatment. 84
Contraception 84
    Oral Contraceptive Pills 84
    Long-Acting Contraceptives 86
    Intrauterine Devices 86
    Barrier Methods 86
    Emergency Contraception 86
    Sterilization 86
Preconception Counseling. 86
Menopause 87
    Overview 87
    Management of Vasomotor Symptoms 88
    Management of Urogenital Symptoms 89
Abnormal Uterine Bleeding. 90
    Clinical Presentation and Evaluation 90
    Management 90
Dysmenorrhea 90
Chronic Pelvic Pain 91
Vaginitis. 92
    Clinical Presentation and Evaluation 92
    Bacterial Vaginosis 92
    Trichomoniasis 92
    Vulvovaginal Candidiasis. 93

Eye Disorders

Red Eye. 93
    Clinical Evaluation 93
    Conjunctivitis 93
    Subconjunctival Hematoma 94
    Corneal Conditions 94
    Episcleritis and Scleritis 95
    Uveitis 95
    Blepharitis. 95
Macular Degeneration 96
    Pathophysiology and Clinical Presentation 96
    Treatment. 96

Glaucoma 96
    Primary Open Angle Glaucoma 96
    Acute Angle Closure Glaucoma 97
Cataract. 97
Dry Eye. 97
Excessive Tearing. 98
Retinal Detachment. 98
Retinal Vascular Occlusion. 99
    Central Retinal Vein Occlusion 99
    Central Retinal Artery Occlusion 99
Eye Emergencies 99

Ear, Nose, Mouth, and Throat Disorders

Evaluation of Hearing Loss 100
Tinnitus. 101
Otitis Media 102
Otitis Externa 102
Cerumen Impaction 103
Upper Respiratory Tract Infections 103
    Sinusitis 103
    Allergic Rhinitis 103
    Nonallergic Rhinitis 104
    Pharyngitis 104
Epistaxis 105
Oral Health 105
    Oral Infections and Ulcers 106
    Dental Infection 106
    Halitosis 106
    Tongue Syndromes. 106
    Burning Mouth Syndrome 106
Temporomandibular Disorders 106

Anorectal Disorders

Approach to the Patient with Anorectal Disorders 107
Hemorrhoids and Rectal Bleeding 107
Anal Fissure 108
Anorectal Abscess 108
Chronic Anorectal Pain 108
Pruritus Ani 108

Mental and Behavioral Health

Depression. 108
    Diagnosis of Depressive Disorders. 108
    Management of Depression 109
Anxiety Disorders 110
    Posttraumatic Stress Disorder 111
    Social Anxiety Disorder. 111
    Obsessive-Compulsive Disorder 111

Intermittent Explosive Disorder 112
Bipolar Disorder 112
Somatoform Disorders. 112
    Clinical Presentation and Evaluation 112
    Management 113
Eating Disorders 113
    Types of Eating Disorders. 113
    Medical Complications of Eating Disorders. 114
    Treatment of Eating Disorders 114
Schizophrenia 114
Attention-Deficit/Hyperactivity Disorder 115
Autism Spectrum Disorders 115
Difficult Patient Encounters. 116

Geriatric Medicine

Functional Assessment. 116
    Fall Prevention and Home Safety 117
    Mild Cognitive Impairment and Dementia 118
    Depression 119
    Hearing 119
    Vision. 119
    The Older Driver 120
Levels of Care 120
Polypharmacy 120
Urinary Incontinence. 121
    Epidemiology. 121
    Evaluation 121
    Treatment. 121
Pressure Ulcers 123
    Clinical Presentation. 123
    Prevention and Management 123

Perioperative Medicine

General Recommendations 124
    Perioperative Testing 124
    Perioperative Medication Management. 125
Cardiovascular Perioperative Management. 125
Pulmonary Perioperative Management. 128
Hematologic Perioperative Management 129
    Venous Thromboembolism Prophylaxis 129
    Perioperative Management of Warfarin Therapy . . . 129
    Perioperative Management of Antiplatelet
    Medications, Coagulopathies, and
    Thrombocytopenia. 130
    Perioperative Management of Anemia. 131
Perioperative Management of Endocrine Diseases 132
    Diabetes Mellitus 132
    Thyroid Disease 132
    Adrenal Insufficiency 132
Perioperative Management of Kidney Disease 133
Perioperative Management of Liver Disease 133
Perioperative Management of Neurologic Disease 134

Bibliography 134

Self-Assessment Test 141

Index 259

General Internal Medicine High-Value Care Recommendations

The American College of Physicians, in collaboration with multiple other organizations, is embarking on a national initiative to promote awareness about the importance of stewardship of health care resources. The goals are to improve health care outcomes by providing care of proven benefit and reducing costs by avoiding unnecessary and even harmful interventions. The initiative comprises several programs that integrate the important concept of health care value (balancing clinical benefit with costs and harms) for a given intervention into various educational materials to address the needs of trainees, practicing physicians, and patients.

To integrate discussion of high-value, cost-conscious care into MKSAP 16, we have created recommendations based on the medical knowledge content that we feel meet the below definition of high-value care and bring us closer to our goal of improving patient outcomes while conserving finite resources.

High-Value Care Recommendation: A recommendation to choose diagnostic and management strategies for patients in specific clinical situations that balances clinical benefit with cost and harms with the goal of improving patient outcomes.

Below are the High-Value Care Recommendations for the General Internal Medicine section of MKSAP 16.

- The value of the periodic health examination for healthy, asymptomatic adults is debatable and there is no consensus interval.
- The U.S. Preventive Services Task Force recommends against screening for the following conditions: carotid artery stenosis, COPD, hereditary hemochromatosis, and peripheral arterial disease.
- According to the U.S. Preventive Services Task Force, screening for coronary artery disease is not recommended in low-risk persons, and the evidence for screening high-risk persons is inconclusive, as is the evidence for screening using nontraditional risk factors, such as high-sensitivity C-reactive protein, homocysteine level, Lp(a) lipoprotein level, ankle-brachial index, carotid intima-media thickness, and coronary artery calcium score.
- The U.S. Preventive Services Task Force recommends against routine screening for hepatitis C virus infection in the general population.
- The U.S. Preventive Services Task Force recommends against screening for asymptomatic bacteriuria in men and nonpregnant women.
- Evidence for the benefits of screening mammography is lacking for women age 75 years and older.

- The American Cancer Society does not recommend using MRI for breast cancer screening in average-risk women and finds the evidence regarding breast self-examination to be insufficient.
- Owing to poor specificity, cervical cancer screening with human papillomavirus (HPV) DNA testing alone is not recommended, although clinicians can consider using HPV DNA testing along with cervical cytology in women age 30 years and older to help guide further investigation and decrease the frequency of testing (see Item 34).
- Owing to limitations of currently available screening tests and unclear benefits of screening, prostate cancer screening remains controversial (see Item 49).
- The American College of Physicians and the American Academy of Family Physicians both recommend that clinicians have individualized discussions with their patients regarding obtaining prostate-specific antigen (PSA) measurements and support obtaining PSA levels after such discussions in patients 50 years and older who have life expectancies of at least 10 years (see Item 49).
- Palliative care consultation programs are associated with significant hospital cost savings, with an adjusted net savings of $1696 in direct costs for patients discharged alive from the hospital and $4908 net savings for patients dying in the hospital as compared with patients who receive usual care (see Item 76).
- Evidence suggests that more aggressive care at the end of life—whether prolonged hospitalization, intensive care unit admission, or performance of procedures—does not improve either quality or duration of life (see Item 89).
- Feeding tubes are not recommended for terminal cancer.
- There is no specific role for diagnostic testing in the assessment and management of chronic noncancer pain because abnormalities that are identified may not be the source of the patient's pain (see Item 117).
- Routine antibiotic treatment of uncomplicated upper respiratory tract infections and acute bronchitis in nonelderly immunocompetent patients is not recommended (see Item 13).
- Patients with chronic fatigue for longer than 1 month rarely have abnormalities on either physical or laboratory evaluation; testing should thus be judicious and performed only when clearly indicated (see Item 7).
- Patients with chronic fatigue syndrome should have regular follow-up to monitor their symptoms, for support and validation, and to avoid unnecessary diagnostic and treatment interventions.

- Tests with the lowest likelihood of affecting diagnosis or management of syncope include head CT scan, carotid Doppler ultrasonography, electroencephalography, and cardiac enzyme levels; these studies may be indicated if symptoms point to specific etiologies but otherwise should be omitted from the work-up (see Item 86 and Item 156).
- Neurocardiogenic and orthostatic syncope both are generally benign in nature and do not require hospitalization (see Item 86).
- Patients with nonspecific low back pain and no symptoms or signs to suggest systemic illness should not routinely receive additional diagnostic testing (see Item 91).
- Mechanical neck pain outside of the setting of acute trauma rarely requires imaging, although plain films can be helpful in patients older than 50 years to exclude malignancy and to assess for osteoarthritic changes (see Item 37).
- A repeat lipid screening interval of 5 years is considered appropriate in low-risk patients, with a shorter interval in those with borderline results and a longer interval in those with consistently normal results.
- Several nontraditional risk factors may be related to cardiovascular outcomes, including levels of Lp(a) lipoprotein, small LDL particles, HDL subspecies, apolipoproteins B and A-1, and the total cholesterol/HDL cholesterol ratio; however, the U.S. Preventive Services Task Force and updated National Cholesterol Education Program Adult Treatment Panel III (ATP III) guidelines do not recommend measuring or treating any of these risk factors when managing lipid levels (see Item 66).
- The benefits of statin therapy are generally class specific, and there is no compelling evidence that newer agents are more effective than established statin medications, which may be more cost effective.
- Because the risk of significant liver or muscle damage is very low in patients on statin therapy, routine follow-up testing is not indicated and should be performed based on the development of symptoms or other clinical findings while on therapy (see Item 158).
- Cardiovascular primary prevention with statin therapy in older patients (ages 65-80 years) is controversial.
- Because many episodes of erectile dysfunction are transient, an extensive laboratory evaluation is not mandatory at presentation without symptoms or findings suggestive of an underlying systemic disorder or before implementing lifestyle modification or counseling therapy.
- In adult men, asymptomatic hydroceles and varicoceles can usually be diagnosed clinically and generally do not require advanced imaging or treatment.
- Intrauterine devices (IUDs) combine the highest contraceptive efficacy (typical failure rate <1%) with the lowest cost.

- Initial evaluation of women with dysmenorrhea includes a thorough history, with particular attention to sexual activity and risks for abuse or infection; unless pelvic pathology is suspected (previous radiation, trauma, infection, foreign body), treatment may be initiated without further evaluation (see Item 131).
- There is no role for antibiotic eye drops in the treatment of viral conjunctivitis (see Item 11).
- Treatment of allergic conjunctivitis includes oral antihistamines, topical antihistamines, and artificial tears; antibiotic treatment is not indicated.
- Imaging of the central nervous system is not considered part of a routine evaluation for bilateral hearing loss.
- For the diagnosis of sinusitis, imaging is rarely necessary in an average-risk patient; however, it should be considered in immunocompromised patients at risk for unusual organisms, such as fungal or pseudomonal sinusitis (see Item 107).
- Empiric antibiotic treatment for acute pharyngitis not based on a clinical decision tool (such as the Centor criteria) should be discouraged (see Item 161).
- In the management of epistaxis, unless the patient has severe bleeding or has an associated systemic disease, laboratory studies and imaging are usually not necessary (see Item 4).
- In patients with dental infections without cellulitis or systemic symptoms, antibiotic therapy is not necessary if dental intervention can be performed within several days.
- Visualizing a hemorrhoid or other source of rectal bleeding in a low-risk patient younger than 40 years without other symptoms to suggest inflammatory bowel disease or colon cancer may spare the patient further endoscopic evaluation (see Item 48).
- When a somatoform disorder is suspected, laboratory and other testing should be ordered logically to evaluate plausible medical diagnoses; extensive and elaborate testing to explore unsupported or very unlikely diagnoses should be avoided (see Item 85).
- Frequent, routine review to verify need for medication and appropriate dosing is an important aspect of optimal geriatric care (see Item 46).
- Interventions to prevent pressure ulcers are much more cost effective than the prolonged and intensive efforts required for treatment of existing ulcers (see Item 24).
- Comprehensive batteries of laboratory testing, chest radiographs, and electrocardiograms should not be routinely performed in the preoperative setting without specific indication as they may result in further testing, delay surgery, and add expense, and such testing rarely influences perioperative care (see Item 8).
- Preoperative tests should be based on known or suspected comorbidities and should only be ordered when a result will alter management (see Item 8).

- Comprehensive preoperative testing has not been shown to be helpful in cataract surgery and is not endorsed by any major specialty society or payor.
- Preoperative pulmonary function testing should be reserved for patients with unexplained dyspnea (see Item 47).
- Laboratory testing for underlying bleeding disorders and anemia should be reserved for patients in whom there is a reasonable probability of an abnormal test and is not required as a routine component of preoperative evaluation (see Item 8).
- Blood transfusion is reserved for patients with symptomatic anemia, a preoperative hemoglobin concentration below 6 g/dL, postoperative hemoglobin concentration below 7 g/dL, or patients with symptomatic cardiovascular disease and hemoglobin concentrations between 6 and 10 g/dL.

General Internal Medicine

Interpretation of the Medical Literature

Study Design

Threats to Validity

Investigators attempt to infer validity, or "truth," by comparing two groups of people in a well-designed study. Many factors can threaten a study's validity, including errors in measurement, data collection, selection of subjects, or analysis. *Internal validity* refers to the degree to which the investigators' conclusions (usually implying cause and effect) are supported by the study. *External validity* refers to the generalizability of the study. There is always some error in any research study. Error is typically shown in scientific publications by way of a confidence interval (CI), typically the 95% confidence interval, which signifies that the investigators can be 95% certain that the value derived from a study truly lies within that interval. If the CI is wide, the point estimate is said to have less certainty, or precision; this is often due to small sample size. A small sample size can also decrease the *power* of a study. Power is the probability of detecting a difference between two groups when a true difference exists. Random error due to chance alone can sometimes result in uneven distribution of patient characteristics, affecting study results. When error is not random, but is applied differentially to one group, it is called *bias*. Bias can occur in selection of patients, measurement, and analysis. Selection bias occurs when patients chosen for a study group have characteristics that can affect the results of the study. Bias can be minimized using carefully constructed research protocols that ensure that the comparison groups are selected, measured, and analyzed in the same way.

Another major challenge in interpreting studies is confounding. A confounder is a third factor that influences both exposure (treatment) and outcome. For example, the false conclusion that smokeless tobacco in the form of snuff poses a greater risk for developing coronary artery disease (CAD) than cigarette smoking could occur because being male (the confounder, which is associated with CAD) is more likely among snuff users than among cigarette smokers. A failure to recognize the presence of a confounder distorts the cause-effect relationship. Confounding can be minimized by using a randomized study design or with statistical techniques if randomization is not possible.

Experimental Studies

In an experimental study, patient selection, treatment, and analysis are determined from the outset to minimize error and bias. In addition, many experimental studies blind patients, treating physicians, and investigators to which treatment a patient is receiving in order to reduce bias, because knowledge of which treatment a patient receives can affect patient reporting and investigator assessment of outcomes. To minimize bias associated with measurement, assessors of clinical outcomes are typically blinded even if patients and treating physicians cannot be blinded.

Various types of study designs are compared in **Table 1**. In a randomized controlled trial (RCT), randomization is performed in an effort to distribute all potential prognostic factors equally across both the experimental and the control groups, minimizing confounding and bias. Although historically, most RCTs compared a new intervention with a placebo, RCTs can also compare a new therapy with an existing one. The objective of these trials, which are often used when the new therapy is less costly or easier to use, is typically to prove that the new therapy is "noninferior" to accepted therapies. These studies require careful attention to the power of the study; studies with small numbers of patients can mask a true difference.

Well-designed RCTs typically have a high degree of precision and internal validity. However, RCTs are typically conducted on patients with a narrow spectrum of disease and use treatment protocols that may be difficult to implement outside of a research setting. Therefore, many RCTs lack generalizability.

Two other experimental study designs are used when randomization of individual patients is unfeasible or unethical (for example, evaluating a new patient safety initiative). In a quasi-experimental study design, data can be compared in the same group of patients both before and after an intervention. In cluster-randomized studies, groups of patients are randomized, rather than individual patients.

Observational Studies

In an observational study, the investigator has no role in assigning individuals to interventions, but rather compares the effects of exposures or treatments among two or more observed groups. By their very nature, observational studies are more susceptible to bias and confounding than experimental studies. Strengths of observational studies, however, include their ability to include a broader spectrum of disease (and diseases or exposures that are rare) and that treatments

TABLE 1. Types of Study Designs

Study Design	Description	Strengths	Weaknesses	Key Threats to Validity
Experimental Studies				
Randomized controlled trial (RCT)	Patients receive one of two interventions, often one being a placebo	Strongest design for determining causation	Expensive, time-consuming, not practical for many clinical situations Limited follow-up duration Limited number of outcomes that can be assessed Limited generalizability	If randomization is ineffective If data are not analyzed according to initially assigned group If key individuals are aware of group assignment (not blinded) If follow-up is incomplete
Cluster-randomized trial	Patients grouped by clusters (e.g., nursing unit) rather than assigned randomly	Same as for RCTs Can be used if randomization of patients is not ethical or feasible	Same as for RCTs Challenging to analyze	Same as for RCTs If analysis does not account for clustering
Quasi-experimental design	Review of data collected before and after an intervention	Can be used if randomization of patients is not ethical or feasible	Patients not randomized	If no adjustment for possible confounding
Observational Studies				
Cohort study	Studies outcomes of groups using observed assignment	Able to detect associations, but these are not always cause-effect relationships Able to study multiple outcomes over a long period of time Large sample size	Requires complicated statistical techniques to minimize confounding Prospective designs can be expensive and take many years before results are available	Selection bias in cohort Bias in measurement of exposures and outcomes If important confounders not accounted for
Case-control study	Compares past exposures in patients with and without disease	Useful for rare diseases or exposures Inexpensive	High risk for bias High risk for confounding Cannot assess incidence/prevalence	Selection bias, especially in controls Measurement bias, especially recall bias

are administered in a "real-world" environment. Two types of observational studies are cohort studies and case-control studies. A cohort study compares the outcomes of groups with and without exposures or treatments not initiated by the investigator; for example, rates of lung cancer between smokers and nonsmokers. Cohorts are compared by following them forward in time (prospectively) or by looking backward in time (retrospectively); prospective design minimizes recall bias (inaccurate recall of past events).

A case-control study retrospectively compares the experience of patients who have a disease with those who do not have the disease. For example, patients with and without lung cancer can be compared with respect to their exposure to asbestos. Case-control studies are particularly useful to study rare diseases or diseases that occur many years after specific exposures. These studies are highly susceptible to

bias, especially recall bias, as patients with disease may be more likely to remember previous exposures. Careful attention is needed in both measurement of exposures and selection of controls.

Other observational study designs are limited in their ability to establish causality but may be useful as relatively inexpensive means of generating hypotheses for future research or for determining estimates of prevalence of a disease. A cross-sectional study assesses for both exposure and disease at the same time point (rather than prospectively or retrospectively). A case series is a report of clinical outcomes in a group of patients; the absence of a control group prevents any conclusions about the effectiveness of the treatment. Epidemiologic studies compare outcomes, in aggregate, of two different populations (countries, socioeconomic groups). These studies are potentially subject to the *ecologic fallacy*, erroneously assuming that population-level associations imply individual-level associations.

Other Study Designs

Systematic reviews summarize existing experimental or observational studies in a rigorous way. Systematic reviews are characterized by a focused clinical question, exhaustive review of the published literature, a systematic protocol for selecting articles and abstracting data (often utilizing independent reviewers), qualitative or quantitative combination of the results, and narrative summary of strengths and limitations of the analysis. Systematic reviews that quantitatively combine data are called meta-analyses. The strength of systematic reviews lies in combining the data from many small studies to minimize the impact of random error. Potential weaknesses, in addition to the weaknesses of the composite studies, include study identification and selection variability in the design of the included studies.

In general, meta-analyses are considered the highest quality sources of evidence, followed (in descending order) by qualitative systematic reviews, RCTs, cohort studies, and case-control studies. Within each category, however, quality may vary, so a well-designed prospective cohort study may be superior to a small RCT with a high rate of drop-out.

Comparative effectiveness research (CER) is intended to produce evidence that can help patients, physicians, and policy makers better understand the effectiveness, benefits, and harms of treatments or procedures. CER employs systematic reviews as well as new clinical trials to determine effectiveness in routine clinical practice.

KEY POINTS

- Internal validity refers to the degree to which the investigators' conclusions are supported by the study; external validity refers to the generalizability of the study.
- Bias occurs when systematic differences between groups affect the outcome of a study.
- Meta-analyses are considered the highest quality sources of evidence, followed (in descending order) by qualitative systematic reviews, RCTs, cohort studies, and case-control studies.

Statistical Analysis

Published studies of therapies typically express results in either relative or absolute terms (**Table 2**). Relative comparisons, such as relative risk, odds ratio, and hazard ratio, compare the ratio between rates of events (such as death or hospitalizations) in two groups. Absolute comparisons, such as absolute risk differences, express absolute differences in rates of disease or events in two groups. Relative risk differences may exaggerate the impact of an intervention, especially for relatively uncommon outcomes. For example, an intervention that reduces the rate of a disease from 20% to 10% and an intervention that reduces it from 2% to 1% each have a relative risk reduction (RRR) of 50%. However, the absolute risk reduction (ARR) for the first case is 10%, whereas the ARR for the second is 1%. The effect size, a measure of the general impact of an intervention, is best characterized by the number needed to treat (NNT), which is number of patients needed to receive a

TABLE 2.	Common Terms Used in the Interpretation of the Medical Literature for Therapeutics		
Term	**Definition**	**Calculation**	**Notes**
Absolute risk (AR)	The probability of an event occurring in a group during a specified time period	AR = patients with event in group / total patients in group	Also known as *event rate*; can be for benefits or harms. Often, an experimental event rate (EER) is compared with a control event rate (CER)
Relative risk (RR)	The ratio of the probability of developing a disease with a risk factor present to the probability of developing the disease without the risk factor present	RR = EER / CER	Used in cohort studies and randomized controlled trials Any two ARs can be substituted for EER and CER
Absolute risk reduction (ARR)	The difference in rates of events between experimental group (EER) and control group (CER)	ARR = | EER − CER |	Any two ARs can be substituted for EER and CER
Relative risk reduction (RRR)	The ratio of absolute risk reduction to the event rate among controls	RRR = | EER − CER | / CER	Any two ARs can be substituted for EER and CER
Number needed to treat (NNT)	Number of patients needed to receive a treatment for one additional patient to benefit	NNT = 1 / ARR	A good estimate of the effect size
Number needed to harm (NNH)	Number of patients needed to receive a treatment for one additional patient to be harmed	NNH = 1 / ARI	ARI = absolute risk increase and equals | EER − CER | when the event is an unfavorable outcome (e.g., drug side effect)

treatment for one additional patient to be expected to benefit from the intervention. NNT is the reciprocal of the ARR. In the example above, the NNT in the first case is 10 (1/0.10) and in the second case, 100 (1/0.01). Number needed to harm (NNH) is the reciprocal of the absolute risk increase (ARI), and reflects the number of patients that would need to be treated to expect one of them to be harmed by the intervention. Defining risk in absolute terms and calculating the NNT/NNH is the best way to understand the magnitude of difference in the sample (effect size).

A *P* value allows the reader to assess how likely any difference seen is due to chance alone. For example, a *P* value of less than 0.05 (corresponding to a less than 1 in 20 chance of getting the results found in the trial assuming there is no difference between the treatments) is often accepted as a cut-off for statistically significant results. *P* values are related to both the degree of difference found between groups and the number of patients in a study, so studies with many patients often produce highly statistically significant results. However, it is important to recognize that differences found to be statistically significant in large trials may not be clinically important. For example, a large study could find a statistically significant decrease in an event rate from 0.2% in the control group to 0.1% in the treatment group. However, the ARR would be 0.1%, yielding a NNT of 1000.

Many measures are used to define the properties of diagnostic tests (**Table 3**), including sensitivity, specificity, and predictive value. Understanding these characteristics for a given test is essential in knowing how effective and helpful a study will be in the diagnostic process. For example, the sensitivity is an indicator of the ability of a test to detect a disease if it is present, and the specificity reflects how effectively a test can exclude illness in a patient without the disease. Both sensitivity and specificity are properties of the test itself and do not vary with the prevalence of disease. The predictive value of a test, however, does vary according to the prevalence of the disease. For example, consider a test with 90% sensitivity and 90% specificity. In a population in which 80% of people have the disease (prevalence of 80%), positive test results will be true positives 97% of the time (positive predictive value [PPV]); however, negative test results will be true negatives only 69% of the time (negative predictive value [NPV]). Conversely, if only 8% of the population has the disease (prevalence of 8%), the PPV of the test is 44% and the NPV is 99%.

The Bayes theorem uses sensitivity, specificity, and the pretest probability of a disease to calculate the posttest probability of the disease. The likelihood ratio (LR) is the ratio of the probability of a particular test result (positive or negative) among patients with a disease to the probability of that same result among patients without the disease. The pretest odds of a disease multiplied by the LR equals the posttest odds of the disease. The posttest odds can be converted to a percentage to yield the more commonly used posttest probability.

KEY POINTS

- Defining risk in absolute terms and calculating number needed to treat/harm is the best way to understand the magnitude of difference in the sample (effect size).
- The positive predictive value of a test increases with increasing prevalence of the disease being tested for, whereas the negative predictive value increases with *decreasing* prevalence of the disease.

Sources of Evidence

The Cochrane collection offers a single source for systematic reviews (www.mrw.interscience.wiley.com/cochrane/); PubMed's clinical queries page offers assistance for common clinical searches (www.ncbi.nlm.nih.gov/pubmed/clinical), including searches for systematic reviews and other clinical study categories; and PubMed (www.ncbi.nlm.nih.gov/pubmed/) can be used for more comprehensive searches. Textbooks and review articles typically offer "predigested" evidence on a clinical topic, although they lack the formal rigor of a systematic review. Guidelines, in contrast, allow groups of experts to synthesize and interpret available evidence. The authors grade their recommendations based on the quality of the evidence reviewed. As guidelines are evidence-supported expert opinion, there are often differences between guidelines put out by different organizations. These differences may reflect the unconscious biases of the authors and sponsoring organization. The American College of Physicians (ACP) publishes clinical practice guidelines, guidance statements, and best practice advice based on reviews of available evidence (www.acponline.org/clinical_information/guidelines). A useful compilation of guidelines is also available at www.guidelines.gov. Critical evaluation tools and evidence-based medicine (EBM) calculators are available at www.cebm.net. Other EBM resources include ACP's PIER (http://pier.acponline.org), ACP Journal Club (www.acpjc.org), ACP JournalWise (www.journalwise.org), and Clinical Evidence (http://clinicalevidence.bmj.com).

Routine Care of the Healthy Patient

Important Health Care Initiatives and Trends

Many recent national initiatives attempt to improve quality and safety of patient care, standardize practice patterns, provide more transparency about hospital outcomes, and nudge heterogeneous health care systems into the electronic age (**Table 4**). In a health care system with many stakeholders with varying and sometimes conflicting goals, there is an

TABLE 3.	Common Terms Used in the Interpretation of the Medical Literature for Diagnostic Tests		
Term	**Definition**	**Calculation**	**Notes**
Prevalence (Prev)	Proportion of patients with disease in the population	$Prev = (TP + FN) / (TP + FP + FN + TN)$	
Sensitivity (Sn)	Proportion of patients with disease who have a positive test	$Sn = TP / (TP + FN)$	
Specificity (Sp)	Proportion of patients without disease who have a negative test	$Sp = TN / (FP + TN)$	
Positive predictive value (PPV)	Proportion of patients with a positive test who have disease	$PPV = TP / (TP + FP)$	Increases with *increasing* prevalence
Negative predictive value (NPV)	Proportion of patients with a negative test who do not have disease	$NPV = TN / (TN + FN)$	Increases with *decreasing* prevalence
Positive likelihood ratio (LR+)	The likelihood that a positive test result would be expected in a patient with the disease that a positive test result would be expected in a patient without a disease	$LR+ = Sn / (1 - Sp)$	
Negative likelihood ratio (LR−)	The likelihood that a negative test result would be expected in a patient with the disease compared with the likelihood that a negative test result would be expected in a patient without a disease	$LR- = (1 - Sn) / Sp$	
Pretest odds	The odds that a patient has the disease before the test is performed	$Pretest\ odds = \dfrac{pretest\ probability}{1 - pretest\ probability}$	
Posttest odds	The odds that a patient has the disease after a test is performed	$Posttest\ odds = pretest\ odds \times LR$	LR+ is used if result of test is positive; LR− is used if result of test is negative. A nomogram is available to calculate posttest probability using pretest probability and LR without having to convert pretest probability to odds (see www.cebm.net/index.aspx?o=1043)
Pretest probability	Proportion of patients with the disease before a test is performed	Pretest probability can be estimated from population prevalence, clinical risk calculators, or clinical experience if no evidence-based tools exist	
Posttest probability	Proportion of patients with the disease after a test is performed	$Posttest\ probability = \dfrac{posttest\ odds}{1 + posttest\ odds}$	

FN = false negative; FP = false positive; TN = true negative; TP = true positive.

increasing drive to stress value—health outcomes achieved per dollar spent—for the patient above all else.

Value in health care is defined by the outcomes achieved rather than by the volumes of procedures performed or services rendered. To determine value, the measurement of processes and their improvement is trumped by the measurement of clinical outcomes and the economic costs of attaining those outcomes. This measurement can be complex. For example, measurement of the outcome of care of a patient with cardiovascular disease should include the costs of treating comorbidities or contributory risk factors, such as hypertension, hyperlipidemia, and obesity, as well as the costs associated with potential adverse effects of treatments.

Frail elderly persons with limited life expectancies should have different outcome measures than younger adults. For example, seeking to achieve a hemoglobin A_{1c} level below 7% in an 80-year-old woman with multiple comorbidities who is recently diagnosed with diabetes mellitus would have less value (in terms of improved clinical outcomes, potential adverse effects, and economic costs) than achieving that clinical target in a young adult recently diagnosed with diabetes.

TABLE 4. Important Health Care Initiatives, Organizations, and Terms

Term	Definition	Additional Resources
Diabetes Recognition Program (DRP)	A voluntary NCQA program designed to provide clinicians with tools to support the delivery and recognition of consistent high quality care in diabetes	www.ncqa.org/tabid/139/Default.aspx
Electronic Health Record (EHR) incentive program	Medicare program to provide incentive payments to physicians and hospitals that demonstrate meaningful use of certified EHR technology	www.cms.gov/ehrincentiveprograms
Healthcare Effectiveness Data and Information Set (HEDIS)	Measures that are widely used across health systems (e.g., β-blocker use after myocardial infarction or breast cancer screening)	www.ncqa.org/tabid/187/default.aspx
Hospital Compare	U.S. Health and Human Services (HHS) Web site that compares Medicare data between hospitals	hospitalcompare.hhs.gov
Physician Quality Reporting System (PQRS [formerly PQRI])	The 2006 Tax Relief and Health Care Act required the establishment of a physician quality reporting system, including an incentive payment for eligible professionals who satisfactorily report data on quality measures for covered professional services furnished to Medicare beneficiaries	www.cms.gov/pqri
National Committee for Quality Assurance (NCQA)	Not-for-profit organization dedicated to improving health care quality	www.ncqa.org/tabid/675/Default.aspx
Accountable care organization (ACO)	A formally organized entity comprising physicians (primary care, specialists, subspecialists) and other health service professionals that is responsible through contracts with payers for providing a broad set of health care services to a specific population of people. A key goal of the ACO structure is to control growth of health care costs while maintaining or improving quality of care.	www.acponline.org/ppvl/policies/aco.pdf
Concierge medicine	Relationship between a patient and a physician in which the patient pays an annual fee for increased access to that physician	www.physiciansnews.com/business/204.kalogredis.html
Electronic prescribing	Computer-based electronic generation, transmission, and filling of a prescription, taking the place of paper and faxed prescriptions	www.ama-assn.org/ama/pub/physician-resources/health-informationtechnology/health-it-basics/eprescribing.page
Patient-centered medical home (PCMH)	Team-based model of care led by primary care physician providing continuous, coordinated care for the patient	www.acponline.org/running_practice/pcmh/
Pay for performance (P4P)	Payment to providers of health care based upon quality of care rather than just services provided	www.ahrq.gov/qual/pay4per.htm

In practice, many quality performance measures assess compliance with care processes rather than the outcomes of those processes. For example, all of the more than 70 Healthcare Effectiveness Data and Information Set (HEDIS) measures updated by the National Committee for Quality Assurance (NCQA) each year are process measures. None are outcome measurements. This method of quality improvement attempts to standardize the provision of care by different providers (for example, measurement of hemoglobin A_{1c} in patients with diabetes) but rarely measures the actual outcomes of that care (for example, risk of microvascular or macrovascular disease in diabetes). Performance measures stressing value will emphasize outcomes and the costs to achieve those outcomes more heavily than the processes utilized in care. Practicing physicians will need to be vigilant for the types of metrics by which they are measured, both responding to and influencing the development of specific process and outcome care measures.

Screening

Screening, which typically refers to the identification of a condition in the asymptomatic state, should be reserved for common conditions, with well-understood natural histories, that have significant negative consequences on society and for which early detection provides clinical benefits. Early detection and treatment of the condition should lead to increased survival or improved quality of life compared with identification at a later, symptomatic stage. The screening test needs to be acceptable to persons available for screening and should possess adequate sensitivity and specificity such that the frequency of false-positive and false-negative results is minimized.

Evaluating the effectiveness of screening tests in reducing morbidity and mortality is best accomplished with randomized controlled trials. Three types of bias are commonly observed in such studies. *Lead-time bias* occurs when a screening test leads to earlier identification of a condition, and an apparent improvement in 5-year survival, but does not actually result in improved mortality. *Length bias* occurs when the variable rate of progression of a disease is not accounted for. For example, a patient with a prolonged asymptomatic phase (for example, a slowly progressing cancer) has a greater likelihood of being identified in a screening study than a patient with a more rapidly progressing cancer. This results in an apparent—but not actual—survival benefit. *Overdiagnosis* in screening refers to the identification of cancers that are not destined to progress, thereby inflating survival statistics.

Balancing the benefits of screening with the potential to identify inaccurate or insignificant findings that lead to additional low yield, high cost, and low value testing; increased patient anxiety; and possible harm to patients requires an understanding of specific screening tests and their appropriate use. The American College of Physicians (ACP) has developed a number of clinical practice guidelines, guidance statements, and best practice statements to help understand the optimal use of specific screening tests. The U.S. Preventive Services Task Force (USPSTF) has systematically reviewed the available evidence and published evidence-based recommendations on screening for a wide range of conditions (www.uspreventiveservicestaskforce.org/recommendations.htm). **Table 5** summarizes these recommendations (see Geriatric Medicine for preventive care measures specific to the geriatric patient). A Web-based and mobile application for use at the point of care to individualize screening recommendations from the USPSTF is available (http://epss.ahrq.gov/PDA/index.jsp). Other organizations also publish focused guidelines for proper use of screening tests, and multiple clinical calculators and risk assessment tools are available to assess the need for specific screening tests.

TABLE 5. Summary of USPSTF Screening Recommendations

Condition	Recommendation
Depression	All adults, when appropriate support system available
Alcohol misuse	All adults
Obesity	All adults
Hypertension	All adults
Lipid disorders	All men ≥35 years of age; consider in men 20-35 years of age with increased cardiovascular risk. Women ≥45 years of age with increased cardiovascular risk; consider in women 20-45 years of age with increased cardiovascular risk.
Diabetes mellitus	All adults with sustained blood pressure >135/80 mm Hg
Osteoporosis	Women ≥65 years of age; any other woman whose fracture risk is ≥ that of a 65-year old white woman without additional risk factors.
Abdominal aortic aneurysm	One-time screening in all men 65-75 years of age who have ever smoked
HIV infection	All persons at increased risk of HIV infection
Hepatitis B virus infection	All pregnant women at the first prenatal visit
Chlamydial infection	All women ≤24 years of age who are sexually active; all women >24 years of age who are at increased risk of infection.
Gonorrhea	Sexually active women who are at increased risk of infection
Asymptomatic bacteriuria	Pregnant women at 12-16 weeks' gestation or at the first prenatal visit, whichever comes first.
Syphilis	High-risk persons and pregnant women
Breast cancer	Biennial screening mammography for average-risk women 50-74 years of age; initiation of screening between 40 and 49 years of age should be individualized.
Cervical cancer	Screen with Pap smear: initiate no sooner than 21 years of age; test every 3 years thereafter or, for women aged 30-65 years who want to lengthen the duration of screening, every 5 years if combined with HPV testing. Screening is not indicated in women following hysterectomy and without previous high-risk Pap smears. Screening may be discontinued at age 65 years in non–high-risk women with no recent abnormal Pap smears.
Colon cancer	All adults 50-75 years of age (see MKSAP 16 Gastroenterology and Hepatology)

HPV = human papillomavirus; USPSTF = U.S. Preventive Services Task Force.

Screening During the History and Physical Examination

The USPSTF recommends screening adults for depression when appropriate supports are available for accurate diagnosis, treatment, and follow up. There is little evidence to support one screening method over another, although evidence suggests that asking two questions ("Over the past 2 weeks, have you felt down, depressed, or hopeless?" and "Over the past 2 weeks, have you felt little interest or pleasure in doing things?") will detect almost all cases of significant depression and may be as effective as longer instruments. There is also evidence that asking only one question, "Have you felt sad or depressed much of the time during the past year?" is also effective. A positive response to any of these questions requires additional assessment to determine diagnosis and treatment.

Several organizations, including the USPSTF, the American Medical Association, the American Society of Addiction Medicine, and the Canadian Task Force on Preventive Health Care recommend screening and performing behavioral counseling interventions to reduce alcohol misuse by adults. The USPSTF recommends that all adults be asked about tobacco use. Although the USPSTF concludes that there is insufficient evidence to recommend screening for illicit substance use, they also conclude that there is little evidence of harms associated with either screening or subsequent behavioral interventions. Screening for alcohol misuse, smoking, and drug use is discussed further in Lifestyle Risk Factors.

Owing to the increasing rate of obesity in our society, the USPSTF recommends screening all adults for obesity and, for those determined to be obese, to offer intensive counseling and behavioral interventions to promote sustained weight loss.

The USPSTF recommends screening all adults age 18 years and older for hypertension but concludes that evidence is lacking regarding the optimal interval of screening. The Seventh Report of the Joint National Committee on Prevention, Detection, Evaluation, and Treatment of High Blood Pressure (JNC 7) recommends screening every 2 years for those with blood pressures of less than 120/80 mm Hg and every year for those with systolic blood pressures of 120 to 139 mm Hg and diastolic blood pressures of 80 to 89 mm Hg. According to JNC 7 guidelines, the mean of two or more seated clinic measurements should be used to make the diagnosis of hypertension. A recent study confirms the importance of using multiple measurements to make the diagnosis of hypertension and the potential error in using only one measurement.

Because of insufficient evidence, the USPSTF does not recommend for or against screening for glaucoma in adults or for either visual acuity or dementia in older adults. There was also insufficient evidence for the USPSTF to recommend for or against screening for family and intimate partner violence among children, women, and older adults.

Periodic Health Examination

Although most Americans view the periodic health examination as essential to high quality care, the value of the periodic health examination for healthy, asymptomatic adults is debatable and there is no consensus interval. At the very least, it appears that the periodic health examination improves the delivery of some preventive services and reduces patient worry. Executive periodic physical examinations, frequently performed on behalf of many corporations, remain controversial without clear evidence of benefit.

Specific Screening Tests

The USPSTF strongly recommends screening for dyslipidemia in certain populations based on age, sex, and cardiovascular risk factors (see Table 5). The National Cholesterol Education Program's Adult Treatment Program III recommends obtaining a fasting lipid profile once every 5 years in all adults over the age of 20 years with a normal initial lipid profile (see Dyslipidemia for specific lipid values).

The USPSTF recommends screening for type 2 diabetes in asymptomatic adults with a sustained blood pressure of greater than 135/80 mm Hg. In contrast, the American Diabetes Association recommends screening all adults age 45 years and older without risk factors and all adults with a BMI of equal to or greater than 25 who have one or more of the following risk factors: gestational diabetes, hypertension, hyperlipidemia, and family history of type 2 diabetes in a first-degree relative. Appropriate screening tests include a fasting plasma glucose level, hemoglobin A_{1c} level, or a 2-h, 75-g oral glucose tolerance test. The USPSTF concludes that there is insufficient evidence regarding screening for gestational diabetes.

The USPSTF recommends screening for osteoporosis in all women age 65 years or older and also in younger women with an elevated fracture risk. Although the USPSTF concludes that evidence is insufficient to recommend screening in men, ACP practice guidelines from 2008 recommend screening those men who are at increased risk. The USPSTF currently has no guidelines regarding screening for vitamin D deficiency.

According to the USPSTF, screening for abdominal aortic aneurysm (AAA) should be performed with abdominal ultrasonography on a one-time basis in all men between the ages of 65 and 75 years who have ever smoked (defined as 100 lifetime cigarettes). They make no recommendation for or against screening men who have never smoked and recommend against routine screening for AAA in women regardless of smoking history.

The USPSTF recommends against screening for the following conditions: carotid artery stenosis, COPD, hereditary hemochromatosis, and peripheral arterial disease. Screening for coronary artery disease is not recommended in low-risk persons, and the evidence for screening high-risk persons is inconclusive, as is the evidence for screening using nontraditional risk factors, such as high-sensitivity C-reactive protein level, homocysteine level, Lp(a) lipoprotein level, ankle-brachial index, carotid intima-media thickness, and coronary artery calcium score. Owing to insufficient evidence, the USPSTF does not recommend for or against screening for thyroid disease.

Screening for Infectious Diseases

The Centers for Disease Control and Prevention (CDC) recommend that all persons between the ages of 13 and 64 years be screened for HIV infection, whereas the USPSTF recommends screening only persons at increased risk of infection. In addition, the USPSTF recommends that all pregnant women be screened for HIV infection.

The USPSTF strongly recommends screening for hepatitis B virus infection in all pregnant women at their first prenatal visit but otherwise recommends against routine screening.

The USPSTF recommends against routine screening for hepatitis C virus infection in the general population and found insufficient evidence to recommend for or against screening in persons at increased risk. The CDC recommends screening persons at increased risk of infection (history of illicit injection drug use, history of receiving clotting factors before 1987 or blood products or organs before 1992, or on chronic hemodialysis at any time). Additionally, the CDC recommends one-time testing for baby boomers (born 1945-1965) regardless of risk factors, followed by a brief screening for alcohol use in those identified as having hepatitis C virus infection.

The USPSTF recommends screening for chlamydial infection in all women 24 years of age or younger who are sexually active and all women older than 24 years who are at increased risk of infection (history of sexually transmitted infection [STI], new or multiple sexual partners, inconsistent condom use, or exchanging sex for drugs or money). There is insufficient evidence to recommend for or against chlamydial infection screening in men.

According to the USPSTF, screening for gonorrhea infection should be limited to sexually active women who are at increased risk of infection (same risk factors as for chlamydial infection). The task force recommends against screening low-risk men and women and states that there is insufficient evidence for screening in all other groups.

Although the USPSTF recommends against screening for asymptomatic bacteriuria in men and nonpregnant women, it supports screening with urine culture for pregnant women at 12 to 16 weeks' gestation or at the first prenatal visit, whichever comes first. Syphilis screening is recommended in all high-risk persons and in all pregnant women but not in other persons.

Cancer Screening Tests

Breast Cancer Screening

Age is the most important risk factor for women developing breast cancer. A woman's individual risk of developing breast cancer can be determined using the breast cancer risk assessment tool (www.cancer.gov/bcrisktool), which is based on the Gail model.

Mammography, the most widely used method of screening for breast cancer, is the only available breast cancer screening modality that has been shown to reduce mortality, with the strongest evidence for its use being in average-risk women between the ages of 50 and 69 years. Screening mammography may be less effective for average-risk women between the ages of 40 and 49 years owing to the lower incidence of breast cancer and lower accuracy of mammography in this age group. Whereas two randomized controlled trials have demonstrated the benefits of screening mammography in average-risk women between the ages of 70 and 74 years, evidence for the benefits of screening mammography is lacking for women age 75 years and older.

The optimal frequency of mammography screening is unclear for all age groups. For average-risk women, the USPSTF recommends performing biennial screening mammography for women ages 50 to 74 years. This approach yields a median breast cancer reduction of 16.5% compared with no screening (number needed to invite [NNI] to screening to prevent one breast cancer death = 1339, ages 50-59 years; NNI = 377, ages 60-69 years). In contrast, the USPSTF states that initiation of screening between the ages of 40 and 49 years (NNI = 1904) should be individualized, taking into account both the patient's risk and the testing characteristics of mammography. The ACP provides similar recommendations for women in their 40s. A recent study supports these recommendations, finding that mammography performed every 2 years was effective in women with relatively high breast density or who possess additional risk factors for developing breast cancer. The American Cancer Society (ACS), American Medical Association, American College of Obstetricians and Gynecologists (ACOG), and the National Comprehensive Cancer Network (NCCN) all recommend beginning annual mammography at the age of 40 years. The ACS does not recommend using MRI for breast cancer screening in average-risk women and finds the evidence regarding breast self-examination to be insufficient. No mention is made of what age to stop annual screening mammography in the ACOG, ACS, or NCCN guidelines.

Women who are either *BRCA1* or *BRCA2* mutation carriers have a high risk of developing breast cancer by the age of 70 years (65% and 45%, respectively). Despite most patients having a family history of breast cancer, less than 10% of all women with breast cancer have an inherited genetic mutation. Features of the family history that should raise concern for an inherited syndrome include having multiple affected family members, young age at time of diagnosis, and the presence of multiple primary tumors. The USPSTF and NCCN both recommend referral to a geneticist if concern exists for an inherited syndrome. The ACS recommends screening with annual MRI alternating every

6 months with annual mammography for women with a greater than 25% lifetime risk of developing breast cancer beginning at the age of 30 years and continuing as long as the woman is in good health.

Based on the results of the Study of Tamoxifen and Raloxifene (STAR) trial, which demonstrated a 50% reduction in the incidence of hormone receptor–invasive breast cancer with the use of these agents, postmenopausal women with a ≥1.66 risk of developing breast cancer over the next 5 years based on the Gail model should be offered a 5-year course of either tamoxifen or raloxifene.

Cervical and Anal Cancer Screening

Screening with conventional cervical cytology (Pap smear) results in a 95% decrease in mortality from cervical cancer. **Table 6** summarizes the recommendations from major professional organizations. Owing to poor specificity, screening with human papillomavirus (HPV) DNA testing alone is not recommended, although clinicians can consider using HPV DNA testing along with cervical cytology in women age 30 years and older to help guide further investigation and decrease the frequency of testing.

If cervical cytology is interpreted as unsatisfactory, the test should be immediately repeated. When interpreted as atypical squamous cells of undetermined significance, acceptable options include referring for colposcopy, obtaining HPV DNA testing and then referring for colposcopy if positive, or repeating the Pap smear in 6 to 12 months. With any other abnormal result, the patient should be referred for colposcopy.

Although some experts recommend anal cytologic screening for anal cancer in high-risk persons (persons who practice receptive anal intercourse, have known anal HPV infection, or who have HIV infection), the USPSTF, ACS, and the CDC do not currently recommend such screening.

Prostate Cancer Screening

Owing to limitations of currently available screening tests and unclear benefits of screening, prostate cancer screening remains controversial. The two most commonly used methods of screening for prostate cancer include prostate-specific antigen (PSA) measurement and digital rectal examination (DRE), with the former being more sensitive.

The USPSTF has concluded that the harms of screening for prostate cancer outweigh the benefits in men of any age regardless of risk factors. In contrast, the ACS and American Urological Association (AUA) recommend offering both PSA measurement and DRE to men on an annual basis beginning at the age of 50 years. The ACP and American Academy of Family Physicians (AAFP) both recommend that clinicians have individualized discussions with their patients regarding obtaining PSA measurements and support obtaining PSA levels after such discussions in patients 50 years and older who have life expectancies of at least 10 years. Men should be informed about the gaps in the evidence and should be assisted in considering their personal preferences before deciding whether or not to be tested. The presence of benign prostatic hyperplasia symptoms should not increase the propensity to screen for prostate cancer with PSA testing.

Additional Cancer Screening Tests

The USPSTF recommends against routine screening for bladder, ovarian, and pancreatic cancers. The USPSTF concludes that the evidence is insufficient to recommend for or against screening for skin and oral cancer. The USPSTF recommends that fair-skinned persons aged 10 to 24 years be counseled about reducing their exposure to ultraviolet radiation to reduce the risk of skin cancer. Colon cancer screening is discussed in depth in MKSAP 16 Gastroenterology and Hepatology.

TABLE 6. Recommendations for Cervical Cancer Screening from Major Professional Organizations			
Professional Organization	**Age to Initiate Screening**	**Screening Interval**	**Age to Discontinue Screening**
American Cancer Society	21 y	Ages 21-29 y: cytology alone every 3 y Ages 30-65 y: cytology alone every 3 y, or cytology with HPV co-testing every 5 y	65 y if no recent abnormal Pap smears and no risk factors
U.S. Preventive Services Task Force	21 y	Every 3 y, or every 5 y with HPV co-testing for women ages 30-65 y	65 y if no recent abnormal Pap smears and no risk factors
American College of Obstetrics and Gynecology	21 y	Ages 21-29 y: cytology alone every 2 y Ages 30-65 y: cytology alone every 3 y if three consecutive Pap smears have been negative and no risk factors	65-70 y if three or more consecutive negative Pap smears, including no abnormal Pap smears within the past 10 years, and no risk factors

NOTE: Risk factors for cervical cancer: history of in utero diethylstilbestrol exposure, immunocompromise, HIV positivity.

HPV = human papillomavirus.

- The U.S. Preventive Services Task Force recommends periodic screening for alcohol misuse, smoking, obesity, and hypertension in all adults and for hyperlipidemia, osteoporosis (women), and abdominal aortic aneurysm (men, one-time screening) based on age and risk factors.

- The U.S. Preventive Services Task Force recommends pregnant women be screened for HIV infection, hepatitis B virus infection, syphilis, and asymptomatic bacteriuria.

- The U.S. Preventive Services Task Force recommends screening persons at increased risk for sexually transmitted infections for HIV infection, hepatitis C virus infection, chlamydial infection (women), and gonorrhea infection (women).

- The U.S. Preventive Services Task Force recommends periodic screening for breast cancer (women ≥50 years of age), cervical cancer, and colon cancer (50-75 years of age).

Family History and Genetic Testing

Taking a Family History

Family history has an important role in the practice of medicine; it can motivate behavior change, help prevent or predict disease, and improve health outcomes. As many common diseases have genetic contributions, obtaining a family history may identify patients who would benefit from genetic testing. For the clinician, the details of the family history help establish the risk (or pretest probability) of genetically associated disease in an individual patient, and forms the basis upon which clinical decisions regarding the need for additional testing may be made.

The definition of *family* may differ among patients, so clarification may be necessary. The accuracy of the information obtained may vary based on the method by which it is obtained (for example, through standardized form, computer, or in person) as well as on patient characteristics.

Key elements of a family history include number of relatives affected by a condition, relationship degree, gender, age at onset, ethnicity, and lineage (maternal or paternal). Additional demographic and environmental data may be needed, as these may modify risk. Available evidence suggests that patients are better at reporting information on first-degree relatives and are more accurate in reporting the absence than the presence of diseases. Older persons report more accurate family histories than younger persons; women and persons with higher educational levels report more information.

Barriers to obtaining an accurate family history include patient understanding, lack of available knowledge about family medical issues, desire to hide or protect, anxiety about subsequent testing or procedures, and fear of psychological harm. Provider barriers include limited clinic time, lack of tools to analyze and interpret data, and lack of understanding of the implications of the data, especially regarding necessity of further genetic testing.

Caveats to Genetic Testing

The advent of greater availability to the public of genetic tests through direct-to-consumer marketing of personal DNA analysis is likely to have an effect on the process of genetic testing and counseling. Current recommendations support the concept that knowledge of one's DNA is only one component of a complex process. As demand for genetic knowledge increases, primary care providers may be asked to weigh in on issues for which they were not specifically trained. The American College of Medical Genetics recommends that a knowledgeable health care provider be involved in the process of ordering and interpreting genetic tests, that the patient be informed about what the test can actually reveal, and that attention be paid to privacy issues as well as the potential psychological impact of knowing that one is a carrier of a genetic disease.

Specific components of genetic testing should include the following: ethical considerations, including patient autonomy regarding the decision to test and the amount of information the patient wishes to know (the right "not to know"); legal considerations, including informed consent and confidentiality; and issues of potential genetic discrimination by the employment or insurance sectors. In addition, religious and cultural considerations may come into play. Patients should be made aware that not all genetic testing and counseling is covered by insurance plans. Finally, providers may be faced with family members who do not wish to disclose information to others who may be affected, thus creating an ethical conflict for the provider.

Referral for Genetic Counseling

Controversy exists as to whether primary care providers have the training to provide adequate genetic counseling. However, the supply of trained genetic specialists may currently be inadequate for providing all recommended genetic counseling services. Different types of genetic tests require different levels of genetic counseling. In more routine testing, in which adequate physician training and patient education materials are available (for example, routine prenatal testing for α-fetoprotein and markers for inborn errors of metabolism), referral may not be necessary. Recommendations for referral for genetic counseling include situations in which patients, families, or providers require assistance in interpreting family and medical histories to assess chance of disease and whether genetic testing is an option, and to promote informed choices about further actions based on risk.

Specific indications for genetic testing include the following: to diagnose a condition in a person with signs and symptoms of a disease; to assess risk status for a family member who may be an asymptomatic carrier or at risk to develop a disease (for example, muscular dystrophy, cystic fibrosis, Huntington disease); concerns about cancer risk based on family history; an abnormal prenatal or newborn screening test that may indicate increased risk of a genetic disorder; concern about risk to a future pregnancy because of family history, maternal age, or a previous abnormal pregnancy outcome; maternal exposure to teratogens; or an ethnic background suggesting an increased risk for a genetic disease (for example, sickle cell disease, thalassemia, Tay-Sachs disease, or Fanconi anemia).

The genetic counseling process includes a complete genetic pedigree, usually of three generations; risk assessment; review of medical records; physical examination of the patient and/or relatives; laboratory testing as appropriate; a discussion of options and potential courses of action; and a thorough explanation of the potential consequences of the genetic testing process. Genetic counselors may also recommend to test or not to test and must always provide posttest counseling.

KEY POINT

- Recommendations regarding genetic testing include that a knowledgeable health care provider be involved in the process of ordering and interpreting genetic tests, that the patient be informed about what the test can actually reveal, and that attention be paid to privacy issues as well as the potential psychological impact of knowing that one is a carrier of a genetic disease.

Immunization

Immunization is a cornerstone of both pediatric and adult preventive care and a major component of public health policy. Vaccination, or the administration of live, attenuated virus or inactivated virus proteins, can protect a person from acquiring, having complications from, or dying of an infection. Vaccination also reduces transmission and spread of a disease in the population at large, thereby helping even unvaccinated persons. More than 24 different vaccines are currently available for clinical use. Recommendations for their use are updated frequently by the CDC's Advisory Committee on Immunization Practices (ACIP). Current recommendations are available at www.cdc.gov/vaccines/pubs/ACIP-list.htm. Although a few vaccinations are recommended for all adults, most are limited to persons of a specific age group or with certain comorbid illnesses (**Table 7**).

A comprehensive approach to vaccination requires information about previous vaccination as well as current health and comorbid conditions. Many recommendations have changed over time, and adults may need "catch-up" vaccinations. Clinicians should pay particular attention to previous vaccination for pertussis, pneumococcal disease, human papillomavirus, and herpes zoster, as recommendations regarding these vaccinations are newer or have recently changed. Unfortunately, patients may not remember previous vaccinations, and documentation of childhood vaccination may be difficult to obtain. Patient self-report should only be considered valid for influenza and pneumococcal vaccination. For all other vaccines, clinicians should either revaccinate for age-appropriate diseases or obtain serology to document immunity viruses.

TABLE 7. Summary of Recommendations for Vaccines for Adults[a]

Vaccine	Type	Indications
Influenza	Live, attenuated or inactivated	All adults
Tetanus, diphtheria, pertussis (Td, Tdap)	Inactivated	All adults. Booster every 10 y. One-time Tdap for all (see text)
Varicella	Live, attenuated	Persons born after 1980, HCWs, persons with ↑ risk of disseminated varicella without documented vaccination or immunity.
Herpes zoster	Live, attenuated	Adults ≥60 y
Pneumococcal disease	Inactivated	Adults ≥65 y; adults 19-64 y with risk factors (see Table 8)
Human papillomavirus	Inactivated	Females 11-26 y; males 11-21 y (permitted 21-26 y)
Measles, mumps, rubella	Live, attenuated	Adults born after 1957 without documented vaccination or immunity. One dose usually sufficient; second dose indicated in HCWs, international travelers, college students, and post-exposure.
Meningococcal disease	Inactivated	Adolescents; persons living in dormitories; persons with HIV or asplenia
Hepatitis A	Inactivated	Travelers to endemic areas, men who have sex with men, users of illicit drugs, persons with chronic liver disease.
Hepatitis B	Inactivated	Adults with increased risk of transmission, morbidity, or exposure (see Table 9)

HCW = health care worker.

[a]Full recommendations are available at www.cdc.gov/vaccines/pubs/ACIP-list.htm.

Vaccines with live, attenuated virus are generally contraindicated in patients with immunodeficiency, although most patients with HIV infection with a CD4 cell count above 200/microliter can receive these vaccines. Inactivated vaccines typically are contraindicated only when the patient has had an allergic reaction to the vaccine. In order to achieve a sustained immunologic response, most immunizations require a series of vaccinations. Manufacturer's guidelines for vaccines indicate the minimum interval between vaccinations, and good immunologic response is typically seen if longer intervals are used. Thus, in patients whose vaccination series was interrupted (for example, a patient who received only two of three injections in a series), the clinician can resume a vaccination series where it was interrupted. Restarting a vaccination sequence is rarely, if ever, required. Although most vaccines should not be given to a patient with a serious acute illness, a patient with mild or moderate disease (such as upper respiratory tract infection), even if associated with fever, can be vaccinated. Multiple vaccines can be given at the same time, although each should be administered at a different site.

Vaccinations Recommended for All Adults

Influenza
Influenza is a respiratory virus that spreads seasonally, with peak activity typically in the fall and winter. Because of antigenic drift, a different strain typically circulates each year, and immunity to the previous year's influenza (vaccine-induced or natural) is not protective of future infection. Vaccination has been shown to reduce incidence, morbidity, and mortality from influenza, and is thought to provide a public health benefit by reducing community spread of influenza. Two types of vaccination are used: a live, attenuated vaccine and an inactivated vaccine. Each is developed during the spring based on projections of the most likely strains to be responsible for the following winter's infections. The live, attenuated vaccine is administered as a single intranasal infusion and is approved for nonpregnant persons from 2 years to 49 years of age without medical conditions that predispose to influenza or its complications (see below). The inactivated vaccine is given as a single intramuscular injection and is approved for adults of any age. Both types are contraindicated in patients with a history of Guillain-Barré syndrome after influenza or severe egg allergy (for example, anaphylaxis), as the vaccine is produced in chicken eggs. Patients without a history of severe egg allergy can be vaccinated, although some patients should be observed for 30 minutes after inoculation. The inactivated vaccine often produces local reaction at the vaccine site and may induce a brief period of myalgia and low-grade fever. The live, attenuated vaccine frequently has side effects of rhinorrhea, headache, and cough. Between 10% and 78% of recipients of either vaccine will have a mild adverse effect.

Influenza vaccination is currently recommended for all adults, although in a time of scarcity, patients more likely to become infected by or develop serious complications from influenza should be prioritized. This includes patients older than 50 years and those younger than 50 years who have cardiovascular disease, pulmonary disease, or immunodeficiency. In addition, health care workers should be prioritized. Vaccination can start whenever the vaccine is available; mass vaccination events should be planned starting in the fall. Clinicians should continue offering vaccination until influenza activity fades in their community, typically in March or April.

Each season, vaccines contain influenza A (including H1N1) and influenza B.

Tetanus, Diphtheria, and Pertussis
Primary vaccination for tetanus and diphtheria (Td) with a three-shot series in childhood followed by booster vaccination every 10 years is highly effective in preventing these diseases. The incidence of adult pertussis has been rising, likely due in part to a declining immunity among adults. Therefore, all adults 19 years and older who have not received a dose of Tdap (tetanus and diphtheria combined with acellular pertussis) should be administered a dose regardless of the interval since their last tetanus and diphtheria toxoid–containing vaccine (although it may also be given in place of a scheduled decennial Td booster). Because recent data suggest that the actual burden of pertussis in persons older than 65 years may be at least 100 times greater than previously reported, pertussis vaccination with at least one dose of Tdap is particularly important in this patient population. Postpartum women, health care workers, and adults who have close contact with infants younger than 12 months (such as child-care workers and grandparents) should also receive a one-time booster of Tdap regardless of the timing of their last Td booster. As this is a relatively recent update, many adults currently coming due for their Td booster should more appropriately receive Tdap.

Vaccinations Recommended for Some Adults

Varicella and Herpes Zoster
The primary focus of varicella immunization is in pediatric care, and childhood vaccination has been recommended since 1996. Persons born before 1980 in the United States are considered likely to have immunity resulting from childhood exposure. Persons born after 1980, health care workers, and those born before 1980 who have a high risk for disseminated varicella should receive a two-dose varicella vaccination series unless they have serologic evidence of varicella immunity or physician-documented evidence of either varicella or varicella vaccination. Patient or parent self-report is not considered reliable. Childhood recommendations changed in 2007 from a single to a two-step varicella vaccination, and some persons may need a single catch-up immunization.

Because the varicella vaccine is a live, attenuated vaccine, vaccination should be done with caution in immunocompromised patients. Pregnant women should not be vaccinated. Women who become pregnant within 1 month of vaccination should be counseled that there is a low risk of birth defects.

A more concentrated version of the live attenuated virus is used for immunization again herpes zoster. In clinical trials, vaccinated patients had a much lower rate of both herpes zoster and postherpetic neuralgia. All adults aged 60 years and older should be vaccinated unless vaccination is contraindicated because of immunodeficiency, regardless of whether they have experienced previous episodes of zoster.

Pneumococcal Disease

Immunization with the 23-valent pneumococcal polysaccharide vaccine decreases the risk of invasive pneumococcal disease. A single dose is recommended for all persons aged 65 years or older and those 19 to 64 years with specific risk factors (**Table 8**); these risk factors were broadened in 2010 to include smokers and persons with asthma. Revaccination after 5 years is recommended in patients who have asplenia or immunocompromise, including kidney failure. Patients vaccinated before age 65 years should receive a booster at 65 years, or 5 years after their initial vaccination if they were initially vaccinated between the ages of 60 and 64 years. There is no current recommendation for additional boosters and no recommendation for a booster for those vaccinated after age 65 years. A 13-valent pneumococcal conjugate vaccine is also available. The ACIP has approved its use in patients 19 years of age and older with immunocompromising conditions, defined as functional or anatomic asplenia, HIV infection, cancer, advanced kidney disease, or other immunocompromising conditions; however, the recommended dosing regimen for these patients is not yet available. Although it is also FDA-approved for use in persons 50 years of age and older, the ACIP has not yet made a recommendation for its routine use in this patient population as an alternative to the polysaccharide vaccine.

Human Papillomavirus

Human papillomavirus (HPV) is the most common STI in the United States, and exposure to certain serotypes can lead to genital warts and cervical cancer. Vaccination against the most pathogenic serotypes has been shown to reduce infection with HPV as well as the development of precancerous cervical lesions and genital warts. The vaccine is an inactivated vaccine and is licensed for males and females between the ages of 9 and 26 years. Vaccination is recommended for all girls and boys starting at age 11 or 12 years. The CDC recommends catch-up vaccination of women to age 26 years and men to age 21 years but permits vaccination of men up to age 26 years. Both a bivalent and quadrivalent vaccine exist; both are licensed and recommended for females, but only the quadrivalent vaccine is recommended for males. Ideally, vaccination should begin before a person has sexual intercourse, but vaccination is still indicated in individuals who have had

TABLE 8. Indications for Pneumococcal Polysaccharide Vaccination in Adults 19 to 64 Years of Age[a]		
Patient Category	**Specific Indications**	**Dosing Interval**
Immunocompetent patients[b]	Chronic cardiovascular disease (including hypertension)	Single vaccination; single booster at age 65 y or 5 y after initial vaccination, whichever is later
	Chronic pulmonary disease (including asthma and COPD)	
	Diabetes mellitus	
	Chronic liver disease (including cirrhosis)	
	Alcoholism	
	Cigarette smoking	
	Cerebrospinal fluid leak	
	Cochlear implant	
Immunocompromised patients[c]	HIV infection	Two doses separated by 5 y
	Chronic kidney disease or nephrotic syndrome	
	Malignancy (leukemia, lymphoma, generalized malignancy)	
	Use of immunosuppressive treatment (corticosteroids, antirejection medication, radiation therapy)	
	Multiple myeloma	
	Congenital or acquired immunodeficiency	
Patients with asplenia[c]	Functional asplenia (sickle cell disease, other hemoglobinopathies)	Two doses separated by 5 y
	Anatomic asplenia (congenital, surgical, others)	

[a]Vaccination recommended for all adults aged 65 years or older.

[b]A 13-valent pneumococcal conjugate vaccine has been FDA approved for use in patients 50 years of age and older, although the ACIP has not made a recommendation for routine use in this patient population.

[c]A 13-valent pneumococcal conjugate vaccine has been approved by the ACIP for use in patients 19 years of age and older with immunocompromising conditions, defined as functional or anatomic asplenia, HIV infection, cancer, advanced kidney disease, or other immunocompromising conditions; however, the recommended dosing regimen for these patients is not yet available.

intercourse or even have evidence of HPV infection, as immunization can prevent infection with other serotypes. The vaccine is administered as a series of three injections.

Measles, Mumps, and Rubella

Measles, mumps, and rubella have been nearly eliminated in the United States after the introduction of universal childhood vaccination. Adults born before 1957 are considered immune to these diseases. Younger adults without either a documented history of immunization or documented immunity should receive a single dose of measles, mumps, and rubella (MMR) vaccine; this is especially important in women of reproductive age. Health care workers, persons exposed to measles or mumps, international travelers, and students in post-secondary education should receive a second vaccination. MMR is a live, attenuated vaccine that is contraindicated in severe immunodeficiency and pregnancy.

Meningococcal Disease

Vaccination against meningococcus is primarily recommended for adolescents. Unvaccinated adults living in college dormitories or who are in the military should receive a single dose, whereas those with asplenia, complement deficiencies, or HIV infection should receive two doses. Patients with asplenia and those with complement deficiencies should receive boosters every 5 years.

Hepatitis A

Universal vaccination of children against hepatitis A is currently recommended by the ACIP. As hepatitis A epidemics are typically spread by children, this strategy provides a combination of both individual and "herd" immunity and has decreased the extent of hepatitis A outbreaks among adults. Currently, hepatitis A vaccination is recommended for adults with increased likelihood of exposure, including travelers to endemic areas, men who have sex with men, and users of illicit drugs (both injected and noninjected drugs). Hepatitis A vaccination is also recommended for adults with chronic liver disease. The vaccination is not recommended for patients with chronic hepatitis B or C without evidence of liver dysfunction. Immunization typically consists of two injections separated by at least 6 months.

Hepatitis B

Hepatitis B is a vaccine-preventable disease with potential serious complications, and universal vaccination of children is currently recommended. In adults, vaccination is recommended for unvaccinated persons with increased risk of exposure from a sexual, percutaneous, or mucosal source; those planning travel to an endemic area; those with increased risk for morbidity; and any other person who requests vaccination (**Table 9**). Several vaccination strategies exist, all requiring at least three injections.

Special Considerations for Health Care Workers

Health care workers have additional vaccination requirements, both because of their potential exposures to disease and their ability to act as a vector to spread diseases to or between patients. All health care workers should be vaccinated against or have serologic evidence of immunity to hepatitis B, varicella, measles, mumps, and rubella; most employers routinely request or provide pre-employment screening and/or vaccination. In addition, health care workers should receive a one-time Tdap vaccination. Annual influenza vaccination is also recommended for all health care workers, and there have been efforts by some states to require these vaccinations.

TABLE 9. Indications for Adult Hepatitis B Vaccination	
Patient Category	**Specific Indications**
Increased risk of sexual transmission	More than one sex partners/6 months
	Men who have sex with men
	Evaluation or treatment for sexually transmitted infection
	Sex partner of a patient with hepatitis B
Increased risk of percutaneous or mucosal transmission	Current or recent injection drug user
	Close contact of a person with hepatitis B
	Resident or staff of long-term facility for developmentally disabled
	Health care worker or public-safety worker who may be exposed to blood or blood-contaminated fluids
	End-stage kidney disease
Increased risk of morbidity	HIV infection
	Chronic liver disease
	Diabetes mellitus (type 1 or 2) in ages 19-59 y (and at clinician's discretion for age ≥60 y)
Others	Travelers to countries with endemic hepatitis B
	Anyone who requests hepatitis B vaccination

- Annual influenza vaccination is recommended for all adults without contraindications.

- Herpes zoster vaccination is recommended for all adults older than 60 years without contraindications.

- Pneumococcal polysaccharide vaccination is recommended for all adults aged 65 years or older; younger persons who should receive the vaccine include those with specific risk factors, including smokers and those with asthma.

- All health care workers should be vaccinated against or have serologic evidence of immunity to hepatitis B, varicella, measles, mumps, and rubella, receive a one-time Tdap vaccination, and receive an annual influenza vaccination.

Lifestyle Risk Factors

Behavioral Counseling

Motivational interviewing describes a patient-centered counseling process whereby the provider engages the patient in behavior change and allows the patient to direct many aspects of the change process, exploring how behavior changes relate to their key goals and values. Many studies attest to the success of motivational interviewing for addressing dietary and lifestyle changes, substance abuse, and other behaviors known to be detrimental to patients' health. Many providers give patients information and advice in an effort to convince them to change behavior. In contrast, motivational interviewing uses patient-identified issues to initiate and continue the change process. Classic motivational interviewing teaches that patients may be ambivalent about making behavioral changes, and that the purpose of motivational interviewing is to encourage patients themselves to identify and voice reasons for making behavioral changes.

Components of motivational interviewing include using open-ended questions; inviting patients to consider how and why they might change behavior; eliciting patients' understanding of the problem or process and what they feel might be barriers to and facilitators of change; providing information and support; and accepting their current level of commitment to change. Key features of motivational interviewing are that the patient chooses the agenda, the provider is not in "control" and does not tell the patient what he or she should do, and the provider assesses the patient's sense of the importance of issues for him or her and level of confidence in making changes, which are usually small and incremental.

Motivational interviewing is one form of a *brief intervention*, which consists of delivering clear, concise advice designed to increase patients' awareness of an unhealthy behavior and its negative consequences. Brief interventions usually involve one or two counseling sessions of 10 to 30 minutes each, usually following a positive screen for unhealthy behaviors. Sessions as short as 5 minutes, referred to as *brief advice*, may also be effective. Brief interventions can easily be administered in a busy office setting, an emergency department, or other urgent-care or community-based settings. One framework for administering a brief intervention is the FRAMES (Feedback, Responsibility, Advice, Menu, Empathy, Self-efficacy) model, whereby clinicians provide *feedback* on risks, with an emphasis on the patient's *responsibility* to change behavior; clear *advice*, with a *menu* of change options; support and *empathy*; and facilitate the patient's *self-efficacy*. Brief interventions may be delivered by physicians, nurses, health educators, counselors, or via printed or computer-based information. Follow-up is critical to assess patient progress.

Diet and Physical Activity

Despite a large body of literature attesting to the benefits of counseling interventions for increasing physical activity, few studies have been performed in the primary care setting. Most studies that have demonstrated a benefit relied on specially trained health educators or nurses, counselors or psychologists, dietitians or nutritionists, or exercise instructors or physiologists; very few involved primary care providers.

A recent systematic review showed that medium- to high-intensity dietary behavioral counseling, with or without physical activity counseling, resulted in small but statistically significant improvements in adiposity, blood pressure, and cholesterol level, as well as moderate to large changes in self-reported dietary and physical activity behaviors. The evidence for changes in physiologic outcomes was strongest for high-intensity counseling interventions. Benefits beyond 1 year are limited and require continued high-intensity interventions, defined as frequent (monthly) contacts in person, by phone, or by e-mail. Several advisory groups recommend 150 minutes of leisure-time physical activity per week, usually broken into five 30-minute sessions weekly. Several national organizations recommend seeing a physician before embarking on an exercise program only if there is a history of heart disease or hypertension, musculoskeletal disorder, or if symptoms such as chest pain or dizziness have been experienced when trying to exercise in the past.

- Key features of motivational interviewing are that the patient chooses the agenda, the provider is not in "control" and does not tell the patient what he or she should do, and the provider assesses the patient's sense of the importance of issues for him or her and level of confidence in making changes, which are usually small and incremental.

- Physician evaluation before embarking on an exercise program is recommended only if there is a history of heart disease or hypertension, musculoskeletal disorder, or if symptoms such as chest pain or dizziness have been experienced when trying to exercise in the past.

Substance Use Disorders

Tobacco

Smoking is a leading cause of illness and death in the United States. Smoking is no longer viewed as a habit but as a chronic disease, and scientifically validated treatments are available for tobacco use and dependence. Thus, tobacco use assessment should be performed for all patients. Brief advice from a physician has been shown to increase tobacco cessation rates. Despite the availability of several FDA-approved medications for smoking cessation, the proportion of smokers who make quit attempts has increased very little, and many smokers who do attempt to quit do not take advantage of these new treatment options. In addition, innovative and more effective counseling strategies are needed, especially in adolescents and young adults.

Current recommendations are that all clinicians assess tobacco use at every visit, given the likely need for repeated quit attempts and the importance of reinforcing positive behaviors. Clinicians should encourage every patient to make a quit attempt and counsel the patient appropriately. One simple approach for use in the clinical setting is the 5 A's (Ask, Advise, Assess, Assist, and Arrange), wherein the clinician *asks* patients about their smoking status at every visit, *advises* them to quit, *assesses* their willingness/readiness to quit at this time, *assists* them with a quit plan, and *arranges* for follow-up. For smokers not ready to quit, motivational interviewing, with emphasis on nonconfrontational strategies and discussion of patient choices, has shown higher cessation rates than use of brief advice or usual care. High-intensity counseling (greater time and number of sessions) is more effective than low-intensity strategies; for clinicians with limited time, recommendations are to use adjunctive telephone counseling, as every state in the United States has telephone counseling quit line services. In addition, counseling that addresses practical problem-solving skills and social support has been shown to be more effective.

Combining counseling with medication use is more effective than either intervention alone. In addition, combinations of nicotine replacement therapy (available as nicotine gum, inhaler, lozenge, nasal spray, and patch) with bupropion have been shown to be more effective than either alone. Varenicline has been demonstrated to be more effective than bupropion, and combinations of varenicline with various nicotine replacement therapies have showed cessation rates higher than nicotine replacement or bupropion alone. Precautions for bupropion include contraindication in patients on monoamine oxidase inhibitors or with seizure or eating disorders; varenicline must be used with caution in patients with kidney impairment or on dialysis, and in patients with cardiovascular disorders; both drugs must be used with caution in patients with serious psychiatric illness, as they may cause neuropsychiatric symptoms such as personality changes, vivid dreams, or suicidal ideation. The specific method or medication chosen is less critical than that a cessation plan is agreed upon and arranged. The various options offer alternatives for patients with contraindications, side effects, or who have relapsed with one type of treatment.

Hospitalization provides a unique counseling opportunity for patients with smoking-related diseases, especially cardiovascular disease. Smoking cessation counseling that begins during hospitalization and continues after discharge increases the odds of long-term abstinence. The Joint Commission (formerly JCAHO) has instituted an accreditation requirement to provide tobacco cessation interventions for patients hospitalized for acute myocardial infarction, heart failure, and pneumonia.

Alcohol

Alcohol misuse includes "risky" or "hazardous" and "harmful" drinking patterns. *Hazardous drinking* is a pattern of alcohol consumption that increases the risk of harmful consequences. *Harmful drinking* refers to alcohol consumption resulting in negative psychological, physical, and social effects but without meeting criteria for dependence. *Alcohol dependence* is a cluster of behavioral, cognitive, and physiologic phenomena that may develop after repeated alcohol use, which includes a strong desire to consume alcohol, impaired control over its use, persistent drinking despite harmful consequences, increased tolerance, and physical withdrawal when use is discontinued. A standard alcoholic beverage is considered to be one 16-ounce beer, one 5-ounce glass of wine, or one shot (1.5 ounces) of spirits.

The USPSTF recommends screening and counseling for all adults for alcohol use and abuse, identifying quantity and frequency of drinking, adverse consequences, and patterns of use. The Alcohol Use Disorders Identification Test (AUDIT) is the most studied screening tool for detecting alcohol-related problems in primary care settings. It consists of ten questions and is easy to administer; a three-question version (the AUDIT-C) is more sensitive but less specific than the ten-question AUDIT (www.hepatitis.va.gov/provider/tools/audit-c.asp). The four-item CAGE questionnaire may also be used. (Have you ever felt you should Cut down on your drinking? Have people Annoyed you by criticizing your drinking? Have you ever felt bad or Guilty about your drinking? Have you ever had a drink first thing in the morning to steady your nerves or get rid of a hangover [Eye-opener]?) With a cutoff of two positive answers, the CAGE questionnaire is 77% to 95% sensitive and 79% to 97% specific for detecting alcohol abuse or dependence in primary care settings and indicates that further assessment is warranted. The AUDIT is more sensitive than the CAGE questionnaire in identifying hazardous drinking and alcohol dependence, whereas the CAGE is easier to deliver in a primary care setting. The TWEAK test, designed specifically for pregnant women, identifies a lower level of alcohol use, as any amount of alcohol may be considered hazardous to the fetus. Clinicians should choose a screening test appropriate to their practice, and provide counseling and intervention when patients screen positive.

Effective interventions for alcohol-use disorders include counseling regarding appropriate amounts and negative consequences, and agreeing on goals for reducing alcohol intake. Sessions may be performed by the provider or other members of the health care team and are most effective when combined with other assistance such as Alcoholics Anonymous or specialty referral. Frequent follow-up and reassessment are important.

No guidelines clearly delineate how often alcohol screening should be performed; however, all adults should be screened and all women who are pregnant or contemplating pregnancy should be advised of the known ill effects of alcohol on the fetus. Patients with a history of alcohol or other substance abuse are at higher risk for alcohol abuse or relapse and should be screened frequently. The effects of screening adolescents are not known.

Drugs

Unlike alcohol use, all illicit drug use may be considered harmful as any use carries a risk for health and legal ramifications, even amounts and patterns of use that do not meet criteria for drug dependence. Patients with drug abuse are more likely to experience anxiety, depression, psychosis, chronic back and other pain disorders, peptic ulcer disease, headache, chronic lung disease (usually from associated tobacco use), and alcohol-related illnesses, such as pancreatitis, hepatitis, and gastritis. Additional risks associated with illicit drug use include unsafe sexual practices, STIs, and intravenous injection–associated complications.

Prevalence of drug use (illicit and prescription) is much lower than for alcohol and depends on the clinical setting. Several screening instruments have been validated for drug use in the primary care setting. The Alcohol Smoking and Substance Involvement Screening Test (ASSIST) may be used for tobacco, alcohol, marijuana, cocaine, stimulants, sedatives, opioids, and several other agents. It has excellent sensitivity and specificity but is considered too long for use in the primary care setting. The 10-item Drug Abuse Screening Test (DAST-10) is similar to the AUDIT and used for assessing drug use. A single-item screening question, "How many times in the past year have you used an illegal drug or used prescription medications for nonmedical reasons?" was 100% sensitive and 74% specific in a single urban primary care practice for the detection of a current drug use disorder, similar to the longer DAST-10, and may be more appropriate in a busy primary care setting with time constraints. Currently no practice guidelines exist for screening patients for unhealthy drug use.

Once patients have been identified as using drugs, the same interventional techniques (brief interventions, motivational interviewing) may be used for counseling, although data are limited regarding outcomes of these interventions.

Challenges unique to this population include the high likelihood of drug dependence and polysubstance use; the legal ramifications of illicit drug use, and, in the case of prescription drug use, the distinction between appropriate and inappropriate use.

KEY POINTS

- All patients who smoke should be offered cessation assistance, including counseling and medical therapy.
- Smoking cessation counseling that begins during hospitalization and continues after discharge increases the odds of long-term abstinence.

Sexual Behavior

All sexually active adolescents are considered at increased risk for STIs, including chlamydial infection, hepatitis B and C, HIV, HPV, and herpes simplex virus. Adults considered at increased risk include those with multiple sexual partners, a current or previous (in the past year) STI, and all non-monogamous sexually active partners in communities with high rates of STIs. The USPSTF recommends that providers take a sexual history and perform risk assessment during periodic and other health-related visits, particularly in high-risk patients.

Once risk and behavioral factors have been identified, targeted counseling should be provided. Counseling issues may include numbers of partners, partner selection, what constitutes consensual sexual behavior, proper use of condoms and other contraceptives, and appropriate vaccines (HPV, hepatitis). Current USPSTF recommendations are to provide high-intensity counseling targeted to sexually active adolescents and adults at risk for STIs. "High-intensity" counseling refers to a single 4-hour session or a minimum of three 1-hour sessions, with longer duration or counseling up to 16 hours or 10 sessions; this intensity is unlikely to be achieved in the primary care setting. Evidence exists, however, that as little as one or two 20-minute sessions in a primary care office are effective for reducing STIs. Recommendations regarding counseling for low-risk adults and non–sexually active adolescents are lacking.

Domestic Violence

Domestic violence, which refers to intimate partner violence as well as child and elder abuse, is defined as intentional controlling or violent behavior by a person in an intimate relationship with the victim. Risk factors for intimate partner violence include low socioeconomic status, young age, psychiatric illness, alcohol or substance abuse, separated or divorced status, and history of childhood sexual or physical abuse. Risk factors specific for elder abuse include increasing age, non-white race, functional impairment, cognitive disability, low self-esteem, and lack of social support. Victims of domestic violence have a high rate of disability and somatic symptoms, such as chronic pain, headache, and abdominal pain, as well as vaginal and urinary tract infections, STIs, and depression. Providers are often unaware that their patients are victims of domestic violence, despite its pervasiveness in clinical practice. Domestic violence is associated with high-risk behaviors such as substance abuse and risky sexual behavior, eating disorders, and limited access to health care.

Recommendations for screening for domestic violence vary, as there is no gold standard screening test. However, a 2012 USPSTF systematic review concluded that screening instruments can accurately identify women experiencing intimate partner violence, and that screening may improve health outcomes in this population. Studies suggest that women (who constitute the majority of victims) are comfortable with questions from their health care providers regarding abuse. Patients with repeated traumas, even minor, should be asked about abuse. However, many providers may not feel comfortable asking, nor be versed in further counseling strategies and legal issues if their patient is a domestic violence victim. Health care providers' primary responsibilities are to assist with health, assess for safety, and maintain a supportive relationship. Improved health outcomes have been shown even if victims remain in the abusive relationship when their providers have given validation, support, empathy, and nonjudgmental, patient-centered discussions about available options and services. Many domestic violence victims are helped by the acknowledgment that violence is unacceptable, that they do have choices, and that they may proceed at their own pace.

KEY POINT

- Health care providers' primary responsibilities in caring for a patient who may be a victim of domestic violence are to assist with health, assess for safety, and maintain a supportive relationship.

Patient Safety

Introduction

Overall, patients in the United States receive only approximately 50% of recommended preventive care measures, while unnecessary procedures and tests continue to be performed, partially owing to payment systems that incentivize quantity over quality as well as to a culture that tends to demand more testing rather than less. The harms to patients from such excessive testing are being increasingly recognized and documented, such as recent reports of harm from radiation exposure from excessive imaging.

Principles of Patient Safety

In the report *To Err is Human: Building a Safer Health System*, the Institute of Medicine defined safety as "freedom from accidental injury." Since publication of this report in 2000, the patient safety movement has evolved to focus on systems of care and the potential to do harm to patients inherent in the structure of those systems. Emphasis is placed on creating systems of care that have built-in safety nets for avoiding patient harm. The construction of these systems has relied on the concept of the "Swiss cheese model" of medical errors (**Figure 1**). In this model, bad outcomes result when errors occur at several layers in the system. Efforts to improve patient safety also encourage the growth and discussion of patient safety, wherein participants feel they can openly discuss and address medical errors or concerns that an error may occur if the system is not changed.

Quality Improvement Models

Most health care quality improvement programs utilize the Model for Improvement, which emphasizes methods with specific and measurable results. The key to quality improvement using this model is to establish what is to be accomplished with a change, clarify how the results of a change will be measured, and determine what changes will be made that will lead to improvement. These changes are tested and implemented using the Plan-Do-Study-Act (PDSA) cycle (**Figure 2**).

Several important quality improvement models have gained popularity in the United States over the past decade. One is the "lean thinking" model developed by Toyota, which aims to optimize efficiency, value, and safety on a continuous basis. Other systems sometimes utilized are Six Sigma and the Malcolm Baldrige Model for Performance Excellence. Six Sigma is a disciplined, data-driven approach for identifying and removing the causes of defects (errors) and minimizing variability in patient care processes (aiming for six standard deviations between the mean and the "customer's" specification limit). A Six Sigma process is one in which there are only 3.4 errors per million events. For example, in

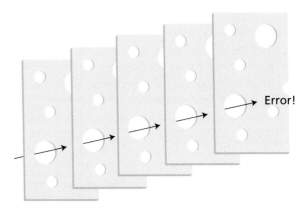

FIGURE 1. "Swiss cheese" model of error.

Adapted with permission from Reason J. Human error: models and management. BMJ. 2000;320(7237):768-770. [PMID: 10720363] Copyright 2000, BMJ Publishing Group Ltd.

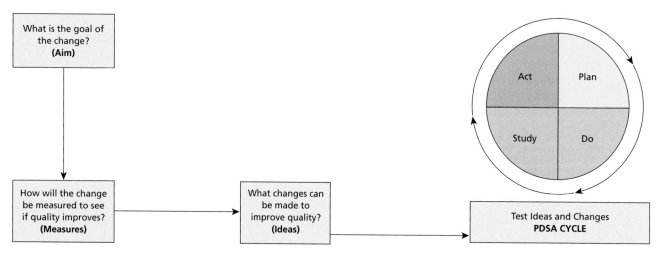

FIGURE 2. PDSA Model for Improvement.

assessing prescribing errors, 99.99966% of prescriptions would have no errors. The Baldrige model focuses on seven components: leadership, strategic planning, student and stakeholder focus, information and analysis, faculty and staff focus, educational and support process management, and organizational performance results.

Measurement of Quality Improvement

Quality improvement measurement began in 1996, when the Joint Commission (formerly JCAHO) implemented the ORYX initiative, a national program for the measurement of hospital quality. This movement gathered momentum in 2004, when the Joint Commission began requiring the collection and reporting of core measure sets (myocardial infarction, congestive heart failure, pneumonia, and pregnancy). A set of quality indicators have been developed to measure health care quality that make use of readily available hospital inpatient and outpatient administrative data. For example, prevention quality indicators identify numbers of hospital admissions that evidence suggests could have been avoided through access to high-quality outpatient care. Inpatient quality indicators assess quality of care inside hospitals as well as across geographic areas, including inpatient mortality for medical conditions and surgical procedures. Patient safety indicators measure potentially avoidable complications and iatrogenic events.

Sources of Error

Diagnostic Errors

A diagnostic error is defined as a diagnosis that is missed, delayed, or wrong; this error may or may not result in harm. Misdiagnosis-related harm is preventable harm resulting from a diagnostic error. Despite the fact that 40,000 to 80,000 deaths result from misdiagnosis annually in the United States

and that tort claims for diagnostic errors are twice as common as claims for medication errors, the science of diagnostic errors is in its infancy. Approximately 40% of malpractice payments in 2003 were related to diagnostic errors, with average payouts of $300,000/claim. The lack of attention to this important area is largely because of the complexity of most diagnostic errors. Diagnostic errors tend to result from a faulty cognitive approach (for example, settling on a diagnosis too soon or not re-examining new information adequately) or from systems-based issues (for example, communication breakdown or failure to obtain important data in a timely way). Suggestions to help avoid diagnostic errors are provided in **Table 10**.

Medication Errors

Between 500,000 and 1.5 million preventable adverse drug events occur each year in the United States, with an estimated 1 medication error daily for each hospitalized patient. Common medication errors by individual physicians include failure to recognize drug interactions among prescribed medications or to adjust dosing to account for impaired kidney or liver function or other conditions requiring dosing adjustments. The focus of efforts to reduce medication errors has been on computerized order entry, banning of abbreviations causing medication errors, bar code implementation in pharmacies, and medication reconciliation at the time of hospital admission and discharge.

Transitions of Care

Transitions of care between the inpatient and outpatient settings present unique challenges in patient safety. Forty percent of discharged patients will have pending studies of which patients and outpatient physicians are not aware despite the need for action on them. One in five patients discharged from the hospital will suffer an adverse event related to medical

TABLE 10. Twelve Tips for Avoiding Diagnostic Errors

Technique	Comments
(1) Understand heuristics[a]	*Availability heuristic:* Diagnosing based upon what is most easily available in the physician's mind (e.g., because of a patient recently seen) rather than what is most probable
	Anchoring heuristic: Settling on a diagnosis early in the diagnostic process despite data that refute the diagnosis or support another (premature closure)
	Representativeness heuristic: Application of pattern recognition (a patient's presentation fits a "typical" case, therefore it must be that case)
(2) Utilize "diagnostic timeouts"	Taking time to periodically review a case based on data but without assuming that the diagnosis is that which was previously reached
(3) Practice "worst-case scenario medicine"	Consider the most life-threatening diagnoses first: • Lessens chance of missing these diagnoses • Does not mandate testing for them, however
(4) Use systematic approach to common problems	For example, anatomic approach to abdominal pain beginning from exterior to interior
(5) Ask why	For example, when a patient presents with diabetic ketoacidosis or a COPD exacerbation, ask what prompted this acute exacerbation of a chronic condition
(6) Utilize the clinical examination	Decreases reliance on a single test and decreases chance of premature closure
(7) Use Bayesian theory	Utilize pre- and posttest probabilities • Helps avert premature closure based on a single test result
(8) Acknowledge the effect of the patient	How does the patient make the physician feel? • Physicians may avoid making bad diagnoses in patients they identify with • Physicians may discount important data in patients with whom they have difficult encounters
(9) Look for clinical findings that do not fit the diagnosis	Encourages a comprehensive approach and incorporates healthy skepticism
(10) Consider "zebras"	Resist temptation to lock onto common diagnoses at risk of missing the uncommon
(11) Slow down and reflect	Difficult to do in most health care systems, which stress the economy of "getting it right the first time"
(12) Admit mistakes	Awareness of one's own fallibility may lead to fewer diagnostic errors later

[a]Heuristics are shortcuts in reasoning used in discovery, learning, or problem solving.

Based on Trowbridge RL. Twelve tips for teaching avoidance of diagnostic errors. Med Teach. 2008;30(5):496-500. [PMID: 18576188]

H
CONT.

management within 3 weeks of hospital discharge, 66% of which are related to medications. Fourteen percent of elderly patients with medication discrepancies between prescribed outpatient and discharge medications are rehospitalized within 30 days, compared with 6% of those without medication discrepancies. Timely follow-up with a primary care physician after hospital discharge, particularly within 1 month, leads to lower rates of rehospitalization.

The key components of good transitions of care include effective hospitalist–to–primary care physician communication both during hospitalization and at the time of discharge (hand-off), pre-discharge patient education, medication reconciliation, and timely post-hospitalization follow-up. Despite the importance of the discharge summary, it often fails to arrive to the primary care physician in a timely fashion and frequently does not convey important information about diagnosis, medications, test results, follow-up plans, or pending studies. The quality of discharge summaries is improved with the use of standardized content (**Table 11**).

Medication reconciliation can be arduous and time-consuming. Information gathered at the time of hospitalization should include that provided by the patient, caregivers, primary care providers, and, when necessary, prescription information from the patient's outpatient pharmacy. This information should be entered on a standardized form or electronic record in the patient's medical chart. This form can then be compared with medications prescribed throughout the hospitalization and at the time of discharge. Medication reconciliation is a dynamic process that should occur throughout the hospital stay as new information is obtained or medications are altered or discontinued. Patients should receive a list of medications at the time of discharge and be informed of previous medications which have been discontinued or changed (and the reason for the change). When

TABLE 11. Suggested Content of a Standardized Discharge Summary

Dates of admission and discharge

Reason for hospitalization

Discharge diagnosis

Significant findings from admission work-up:

• History and physical examination

• Laboratory studies

• Imaging studies

• Other tests

Procedures performed

Results of procedures and significant testing

Condition at discharge

Discharge medications and reasons for any changes from admission medications

Follow-up issues

Pending studies and laboratory tests

Counseling provided to patient and family

Follow-up appointments/plans

H CONT. medication reconciliation efforts are led by pharmacists, the rate of adverse drug events at 30 days is 1% versus 11% in control patients. **H**

KEY POINTS

• Common medication errors include failure to recognize drug interactions among prescribed medications or to adjust dosing to account for impaired kidney or liver function.

• Medication reconciliation should occur throughout the hospital stay; patients should receive a list of medications at the time of discharge.

• Timely follow-up with a primary care physician after hospital discharge (≤1 month) leads to lower rates of rehospitalization.

Health Information Technology and Patient Safety

Health information technology comes in three general forms: computerized physician order entry (CPOE), electronic health record (EHR), and clinical decision support. Each of these technologies can be used in an inpatient or outpatient environment and can improve patient safety. Health information technology systems should allow information sharing and integration across the continuum of care.

CPOE refers to the direct entry of orders (for example, prescriptions, radiology) into a computer interface by a physician. CPOE eliminates medication error related to physician handwriting, ensuring that the medication, dose, and directions are exactly what is requested. CPOE improves efficiency by eliminating delays between order entry and order receipt.

A patient's EHR comprises a collection of clinical data (notes, reports) in a computerized format. The EHR should allow multiple users, including specialists, primary care physicians, and the patient, to maintain an accurate, dynamic health record.

Clinical decision support refers to the use of these technologies to supplement a practitioner's clinical reasoning. For example, a CPOE system can warn the ordering clinician about drug interactions, need for renal dosing, or potential contraindications to studies. An EHR interface can prompt physicians to order needed medications, screening tests, or chronic disease management.

Health information technology is not a panacea. The potential for new errors is present in all systems; for example, CPOE can allow multiple physicians to enter potentially conflicting orders simultaneously. Poorly designed systems can introduce even more errors.

National Patient Safety Goals

Each year, the Joint Commission publishes national patient safety guidelines (www.jointcommission.org/standards _information/npsgs.aspx). These guidelines span the continuum of care, including acute care hospitals, ambulatory practices, nursing homes, and free-standing surgical centers, although not every standard is applicable at every site. The goals are focused on those that have the highest impact for both quality and patient safety. Each goal provides specific objectives and metrics. For example, under the goal *Improve accuracy of patient identification* are objectives such as "Use at least two patient identifiers when providing care, treatment, and services." The Joint Commission also includes measurable elements of performance such as "Label containers used for blood and other specimens in the presence of the patient." These safety goals provide a frame for interdisciplinary collaboration around quality and safety and can provide concrete objectives and criteria for quality improvement projects.

Professionalism and Ethics

Professionalism

In exchange for the authority to train, license, certify, and credential physicians, the medical profession has an obligation to society to ensure that physicians uphold ethical and professional behaviors, including maintenance of clinical competence and the fulfillment of clinical and hospital responsibilities in a timely manner. This obligation requires that physicians honestly assess their knowledge and skills and pursue learning where gaps exist. It also creates the expectation that physicians will disclose errors to patients and others and perform duties and meet standards established by local medical and hospital staffs.

In the routine delivery of patient care, physicians must model exemplary interactions with trainees and colleagues, both physician and nonphysician. Teamwork and collaboration, with mutual respect and recognition of one another's contributions to the health care team, are fundamental in today's health care environment and fundamental to demonstrating professionalism with trainees.

As part of their contract with society, physicians must also advance the public good, which requires they serve as judicious stewards of public resources. The Charter on Medical Professionalism comprises three principles and ten commitments (**Table 12**). Three commitments link professionalism with the public's health: the commitment to improving quality of care, the commitment to improving access to care, and the commitment to a just distribution of finite resources.

Together, these commitments create an expectation that every physician advocate for and work to ensure that all persons have access to quality health care, and that medical care is delivered equitably across racial, ethnic, religious, and socioeconomic groups. A commitment to social justice requires physicians to guard the health of the public by eliminating unsafe and low-value services that generate expenses for care with potential harm and little to no benefit to the patient. The American College of Physicians' High-Value, Cost-Conscious Care initiative strives to promote this commitment by helping physicians assess the value and the costs of specific interventions.

TABLE 12.	Principles and Commitments of Professionalism
Principle or Commitment	**Comment**
Fundamental Principle	
Primacy of patient welfare	Altruism is a central trust factor in the physician-patient relationship. Market forces, societal pressures, and administrative exigencies must not compromise this principle.
Patient autonomy	Patients' decisions about their care must be paramount, as long as those decisions are in keeping with ethical practice and do not lead to demands for inappropriate care.
Social justice	Physicians should work actively to eliminate discrimination in health care, whether based on race, gender, socioeconomic status, ethnicity, religion, or any other social category.
Professional Commitment	
Competence	Physicians must be committed to lifelong learning and to maintaining the medical knowledge and clinical and team skills necessary for the provision of quality care.
Honesty with patients	Obtain informed consent for treatment or research. Report and analyze medical errors in order to maintain trust, improve care, and provide appropriate compensation to injured parties.
Patient confidentiality	Privacy of information is essential to patient trust and even more pressing with electronic medical records.
Appropriate patient relations	Given the inherent vulnerability and dependency of patients, physicians should never exploit patients for any sexual advantage, personal financial gain, or other private purpose.
Improve quality of care	Work collaboratively with other professionals to reduce medical errors, increase patient safety, minimize overuse of health care resources, and optimize the outcomes of care.
Improve access to care	Work to eliminate barriers to access based on education, laws, finances, geography, and social discrimination. Equity requires the promotion of public health and preventive medicine, as well as public advocacy, without concern for the self-interest of the physician or the profession.
Just distribution of resources	Work with other physicians, hospitals, and payers to develop guidelines for cost-effective care. Providing unnecessary services not only exposes one's patients to avoidable harm and expense but also diminishes the resources available for others.
Scientific knowledge	Uphold scientific standards, promote research, create new knowledge, and ensure its appropriate use.
Manage conflicts of interest	Medical professionals and their organizations have many opportunities to compromise their professional responsibilities by pursuing private gain or personal advantage. Such compromises are especially threatening with for-profit industries, including medical equipment manufacturers, insurance companies, and pharmaceutical firms. Physicians have an obligation to recognize, disclose to the general public, and deal with conflicts of interest that arise.
Professional responsibilities	Undergo self-assessment and external scrutiny of all aspects of one's performance. Participate in the processes of self-regulation, including remediation and discipline of members who have failed to meet professional standards.

- Physicians have a responsibility to guard the health of the public by eliminating unsafe and low-value services that generate expenses for care with potential harm and little to no benefit to the patient.

Decision-Making and Informed Consent

Decision-making is at the core of medicine. A common source of ethical challenges in practice is that while the authority for decision-making rests with the patient, the knowledge needed for informed decision-making is often in the hands of the clinician.

Informed Consent

Informed consent requires that the patient understand the nature of the decision being made or intervention being proposed, alternative options to the proposed intervention or decision, and the risks and benefits of each of the various alternatives. To obtain informed consent, the clinician explains the options and their risks and benefits to the patient and makes a recommendation if there is a preferred course of action. In addition, the clinician must assess the patient's understanding of the options and verify the patient's final decision. Although clinicians should make a recommendation if they feel that a particular choice is the most medically appropriate, they must not coerce or entice the patient into making that choice.

The greater the complexity of the decision, the greater the importance of detailed informed consent. Complexity can be characterized by three domains: the potential effect on the patient; the consensus within the medical community as to the appropriate action; and the number and uncertainty of possible outcomes. By convention, most invasive procedures such as surgery require written informed consent, which should reflect the outcome of the conversation described above. However, other complex decisions may also benefit from the principles of informed decision-making, even if an explicit signed consent document is not required. For example, deciding whether to obtain a screening mammography in a woman younger than 50 years is a complex decision by the criteria above, and the principles of informed consent apply even if one does not obtain a specific signed consent for the test in question. In a study of outpatient practices, it was shown that fewer than 10% of all clinical decisions made met standards for informed decision-making, and fewer than 1% of complex decisions were considered fully informed.

Assessing Decision-Making Capacity

The core components of decisional capacity are understanding the situation at hand, understanding the risks and benefits of the decision being made, and the ability to communicate a decision. Assessing understanding can be challenging, particularly in patients with underlying mental health disorders or cognitive deficits. A diagnosis of dementia or a mental illness does not necessarily mean that a patient is incapable of making health care decisions. The clinician must assess whether or not the patient's decision appears consistent with his or her values and goals of care. If it does, it can probably be accepted as valid. A decision that seems inconsistent is a prompt to further explore the patient's beliefs, values, and comprehension of the situation and the decision. A given decision does not have to be rational, however, nor need it reflect what most people would do in that situation. Patients who are able to understand the consequences may refuse life-saving therapy, even for reasons that may be difficult to understand, such as religious preferences, community beliefs, or other values. The decisional capacity of these patients should only be questioned if they are acting in a way that is inconsistent with their personal beliefs or those of their community.

Advance Directives and Surrogate Decision-Making

When patients lack the capacity to make a decision on their own, they may have provided guidance in the form of an advance directive. Advance directives fall into two broad categories: instructive directives and proxy directives. Advance directive documents may include both components, for example, a living will (instructive) and durable power of attorney for health care (proxy).

Instructive directives provide guidance about what the patient would want to have done in certain situations. These may be straightforward, such as a request not to receive cardiopulmonary resuscitation. They may also be complicated, such as instructions for what specific life-sustaining treatment the patient may or may not want if they are unable to communicate their wishes (for example, in a persistent vegetative state). Instructive directives are subject to interpretation, as they cannot capture all the nuances of a given clinical situation. Many U.S. states have legal guidelines and forms that address the scope of advance directives, but unfortunately the legal forms may be difficult for patients to read and understand.

Proxy directives designate a surrogate decision maker (also known as a durable power of attorney for health care). Ideally, before incapacity occurs, the patient will have designated a surrogate to make health care decisions. If not, the clinician must try to identify the legal next of kin who is empowered to act as a surrogate decision maker. This is typically determined by state law in the United States. Most jurisdictions also have a mechanism to appoint a legal guardian in situations in which the patient is incapable of making health care decisions and there is no designated surrogate or next of kin.

The role of the surrogate is to strive to make decisions based on what the patient would have wanted in that situation (the ethics concept of *substituted judgment*). A living will or instructive directive can help inform the surrogate's decisions. If the surrogate has no knowledge of what the patient would have wanted, either because this was never discussed or because the surrogate did not know the patient well, a secondary standard would be to make decisions the surrogate considers to be in the patient's best interest. If the surrogate's decisions seem inconsistent with the patient's values or previous directives, the clinician should proceed with extreme caution. Ethics consultations are helpful in reconciling conflicts.

> **KEY POINT**
> - The core components of decisional capacity are understanding the situation at hand, understanding the risks and benefits of the decision being made, and the ability to communicate a decision.

Withholding or Withdrawing Treatment

Although a primary goal of care is usually to sustain life, there are circumstances under which life-sustaining treatment should be withheld or withdrawn. The emotional implications may differ whether one withholds care (never starts a treatment) or withdraws care (stops a treatment previously started), but the two are equivalent from the standpoint of medical ethics.

The two most common reasons to withhold or withdraw treatment are that the patient or the surrogate has decided that the patient no longer wishes to receive such treatment, or that life-sustaining treatment no longer offers benefit to the patient. If the patient has decided that he or she no longer wishes treatment, the decision to withhold or withdraw is usually straightforward. In most cases, it is reasonable to continue efforts at relief of symptoms and discomfort, while stopping invasive or uncomfortable treatments that serve only to sustain life. In some circumstances, clinicians may disagree with the patient's decision to withhold or withdraw treatment, particularly if they feel that the patient's death is not imminent or inevitable. However, there is ample legal and ethical precedent for competent patients to refuse care. Unless the patient is a minor or lacks decisional capacity, the clinician should abide by the patient's wishes.

A scenario in which life-sustaining treatment no longer offers benefit to the patient who wants it can be more challenging. Although one is on solid ethical ground denying futile treatment, the precise definition of futility can be quite difficult. A treatment is futile either when it has a very low probability of producing any benefit whatsoever (quantitative futility), or when the amount or quality of benefit produced is so small as to be trivial (qualitative futility). If the physician feels that a specific intervention is unlikely to produce an outcome that the patient would find to be meaningfully beneficial, the intervention is likely futile. Although physicians have no ethical obligation to provide futile treatments, even if the

patient wants them, they may need to request ethical and legal consultations in such cases.

Populations that have historically faced discrimination by the health care system and may have greater mistrust of health care providers' intentions, such as blacks in the United States, are more likely to request aggressive end-of-life treatment. Physicians need to be sensitive to such cultural and historical factors that may shape patients' and their families' attitudes about end-of-life care.

> **KEY POINT**
> - Competent patients may refuse care even if the clinician believes that the patient's death is not imminent or inevitable; unless the patient is a minor or lacks decisional capacity, the clinician should abide by the patient's wishes.

Physician-Assisted Suicide and Euthanasia

The issue of when it is appropriate to provide a treatment that may hasten the death of a dying patient is a heavily debated area of medical ethics. Most agree by virtue of the principle of double effect that it is ethically permissible to give a terminally ill patient a treatment that may hasten death when the primary intent is therapeutic. A common example is high doses of opiate analgesics used to relieve pain or dyspnea in a patient who is dying.

The practice of prescribing medications or interventions with the primary intent of hastening a patient's death (physician aid in dying, physician-assisted suicide) remains intensely controversial. Although the American Medical Association and the American College of Physicians have both taken positions against the practice, it is legal in some states under specific circumstances.

Active administration of a drug to cause death (active euthanasia) is illegal in all states, regardless of consent. All requests for a hastened death should be carefully evaluated and responded to with empathy and compassion, regardless of the physician's ethical position on the specifics of the request.

> **KEY POINTS**
> - A terminally ill patient may be given a treatment that may hasten death when the primary intent is to provide therapy for another condition.
> - Active administration of a drug with the intent to cause death is illegal in all states, regardless of consent.

Confidentiality

Implicit in the physician-patient relationship is a commitment to confidentiality. Information disclosed by a patient to a physician should not be disclosed to anyone not directly involved in the patient's care (and therefore bound by a similar requirement for confidentiality). Patients may specify other persons, such as friends or family members, with whom they wish the physician to share information, but in the absence of specific permission, the physician should not disclose anything.

Confidentiality is not absolute, however. Situations in which there is an established risk of patients harming themselves or others may require the clinician to disclose confidential information. If the clinician believes that the patient poses a serious risk of harm to a specific person, he or she has a duty to warn that person. This is usually best handled with the assistance of law enforcement authorities, and it is also often helpful to get legal advice, if available. Another situation in which confidentiality may be sacrificed for the public welfare is for reportable communicable diseases, which are usually determined by local jurisdictions and public health departments.

Constraints on decisional capacity also have implications for confidentiality. If the patient is unable to make an important medical decision, then the person who is making that decision for him or her is entitled to be fully informed as to the aspects of the patient's condition that pertain to the decision. In the case of minor children, parents usually have a legal right to be informed about the child's condition, and the physician has an obligation to disclose any suspicion of abuse. Both ethics and law regarding confidentiality can be complicated for adolescents. Some U.S. states have laws specifically protecting adolescent confidentiality for certain medical issues such as reproductive health. When interviewing adolescents, the physician should perform at least some of the interview without the parents present and explicitly discuss with the patient what will and what will not be confidential, informed by an awareness of applicable local law.

KEY POINTS

- A physician may be required to disclose confidential information if the patient poses a serious risk of harm to self or others or has a reportable communicable disease.

- If a patient is unable to make an important medical decision, the person who is making that decision for him or her is entitled to be fully informed as to the aspects of the patient's condition that pertain to the decision.

Conflicts of Interest

The fiduciary nature of the physician-patient relationship dictates that the physician place the interests of the patient above his or her own. There are, however, numerous opportunities for conflicts of interest. A common area of conflict with the physician's own interests is that of financial relationships. At the most basic level, physician payment structures can generate conflicts of interest. In fee-for-service systems such as those prevalent in the United States, physician compensation often increases with the number and complexity of services provided. Moreover, if the physician has a financial interest in facilities used for diagnosis or treatment, he or she has an incentive to provide additional diagnostic or therapeutic services, or to provide those services in a manner that increases compensation (for example, intravenous instead of subcutaneous or oral medication administration). Although these relationships are regulated by federal law in the United States, regulation has not eliminated them or the associated financial incentives.

The relationships between physicians and companies in the health care industry that profit from physician decisions have also come under increasing scrutiny. The manufacturers of prescription drugs and medical devices devote considerable funds to marketing their products, using both direct and indirect approaches to influence physician behavior. A considerable amount of medical research is funded by companies that stand to gain from the results, which has led to concerns about bias in the content or publication of research papers. In addition, concern has been raised regarding whether experts whose research is heavily funded by industry can make impartial decisions when serving on panels to draft clinical practice guidelines. Many physicians also benefit indirectly from industry funding for continuing medical education programs. Both industry and accrediting organizations have developed standards to help manage these relationships. The Institute of Medicine has published recommendations for controlling conflicts of interest (**Table 13**).

Medical Error Disclosure

Research shows that patients expect disclosure of harmful medical errors. The National Quality Forum endorsed guidelines in 2006 that included three key components of error disclosure:

- Provide facts about the event (including an analysis of system failure, if available)

- Express regret for the unanticipated outcome

- Give a formal apology if the unanticipated outcome was caused by error or system failure

Apologizing for errors can be particularly difficult owing to concern that an apology or admission of responsibility may cause problems in subsequent malpractice litigation. A majority of U.S. states now have laws that offer at least limited protection for apologies or expressions of regret. Caution is indicated, however; whereas apologizing for errors is both ethically and interpersonally desirable, it is reasonable to obtain additional counsel on the legal implications.

TABLE 13. A Selection of Institute of Medicine Recommendations for Individual Physicians to Control Conflicts of Interest

Forgo all gifts or items of material value from pharmaceutical, medical device, and biotechnology companies, accepting only payment at fair market value for a legitimate service in specified situations.

Do not make educational presentations or publish scientific articles that are controlled by industry or contain substantial portions written by someone who is not identified as an author or who is not properly acknowledged.

Do not meet with pharmaceutical and medical device sales representatives except by documented appointment and at the physician's express invitation.

Do not accept drug samples except in certain situations for patients who lack financial access to medications.

Until institutions change their policies, physicians and trainees should voluntarily adopt these recommendations as standards for their own conduct.

Adapted with permission from Steinbrook R. Controlling conflict of interest—proposals from the Institute of Medicine. New Engl J Med. 2009;360(21):2160-2163. [PMID: 19403898] Copyright 2009, Massachusetts Medical Society.

Sexual Contact between Physician and Patient

The inherent asymmetry of power and trust in the physician-patient relationship makes it ethically unacceptable to maintain a sexual relationship with a patient, even if the patient initiates sexual contact.

Sexual relationships with former patients are also concerning. The greater the depth and duration of the previous professional physician-patient relationship, the more caution is needed. Relationships with patients whom the physician was treating for a mental health disorder are particularly problematic and may result in civil liability or professional disciplinary action in some jurisdictions, regardless of patient consent or the time elapsed since terminating the physician-patient relationship. In general, a physician considering a sexual relationship with a former patient is advised to solicit the opinions of legal counsel or an ethicist before proceeding with the relationship.

The Impaired Physician and Colleague Responsibility

Members of the medical profession have an obligation to protect the welfare of patients, which includes taking action when a colleague puts patients at risk. Many states have mandatory reporting statutes that require a physician to report to appropriate authorities when a colleague continues to practice despite his or her inability to do so safely because of impairment from substance use or illness.

In a 2009 survey, the majority of respondents endorsed a duty to report, but of the 17% who had direct knowledge of an impaired colleague, only two-thirds actually reported him or her to the relevant authority. Beliefs that someone else was taking care of the problem or that nothing would happen were the most common reasons for failure to report. Common signs of physician impairment at work are shown in **Table 14**.

All U.S. states now have physician health programs (PHPs) that allow for anonymous reporting of impaired

TABLE 14. Signs of Physician Impairment in the Work Setting

Late to appointments; increased absences; unknown whereabouts

Unusual rounding times, either very early or very late

Increase in patient complaints

Increased secrecy

Decrease in quality of care; careless medical decisions

Incorrect charting or writing of prescriptions

Decrease in productivity or efficiency

Increased conflicts with colleagues

Increased irritability and aggression

Smell of alcohol; overt intoxication; needle marks

Erratic job history

Adapted with permission from Ross S. Identifying an Impaired Physician. Virtual Mentor. December 2003, Volume 5, Number 12. Accessed at http://virtualmentor.ama-assn.org/2003/12/cprl1-0312.html. 22 December 2011. The viewpoints expressed in Virtual Mentor are those of the authors and do not necessarily reflect the views and policies of the AMA. Copyright 2003, American Medical Association.

physicians, and many states stipulate those licensed to practice by the state must report impaired colleagues. Once the PHP is notified of a possibly impaired physician, assessment, treatment, and monitoring can be arranged. If a physician voluntarily participates in the PHP's treatment and monitoring program, the PHP will often advocate for him or her with the state medical board, resulting in mitigation or even avoidance of formal disciplinary action as long as the physician remains in compliance.

Palliative Care

Introduction

The primary focus of palliative care is to relieve patient suffering and to improve the quality of patients' lives and those of their caregivers. Palliative care involves a multifaceted approach that includes clarifying goals of treatment, managing symptoms, mobilizing resources to optimize care and social support, and integrating care across settings—whether home, nursing home, or hospital. Despite its widespread availability, palliative care continues to be underutilized. Much of the resistance to initiating palliative care stems from the traditional care dichotomy between "doing everything" versus providing comfort care—a dichotomy that often fails to focus on relieving suffering and improving quality of care.

Palliative care is often thought of as end-of-life care only, but palliative care addresses pain, suffering, and quality of life across all stages of treatment and does not exclude life-prolonging treatment and rehabilitation. *Nonhospice* palliative care may be offered along with curative or life-prolonging therapies for patients with complex, life-threatening disorders. *Hospice* palliative care is offered when patients reach their final weeks or months of life, when the likely harm of life-prolonging or curative therapies exceeds benefit, and these therapies are discontinued. Hospice services can be provided in a patient's home, in specialized hospice units in hospitals, or in community-based facilities, depending on patients' and their family's individual needs and preferences.

Emerging data for concurrent palliative care intervention in the treatment of cancer strongly suggest that patients using palliative care services have higher scores for quality of life and mood than those undergoing cancer treatment alone. In a study of 151 patients with newly diagnosed metastatic non–small cell lung cancer randomly assigned to standard oncologic therapy alone versus early palliative care with standard oncologic therapy, patients in the palliative care group had a mean survival of 11.6 months as compared with 8.9 months in the group not provided early palliative care. The intervention group also experienced less depression and better quality of life.

Palliative care consultation programs are also associated with significant hospital cost savings, with an adjusted net savings of $1696 in direct costs for patients discharged alive from the hospital and $4908 net savings for patients dying in the hospital as compared with patients who receive usual care.

KEY POINT

- Palliative care addresses pain, suffering, and quality of life across all stages of treatment and does not exclude life-prolonging treatment and rehabilitation.

Deciding When Hospice Palliative Care Is Indicated

Approximately 30% of Medicare's expenditures occur in patients' last year of life. Evidence suggests that more aggressive care at the end of life—whether prolonged hospitalization, intensive care unit admission, or performance of procedures—does not improve either quality or duration of life. The problem with estimating when the last year of life has arrived is that patients do not progress in identical patterns.

Prognostication can be even more difficult when a patient does not have cancer (**Figure 3**). In patients with cancer, the clinical course frequently ends with an obvious decline in the final weeks or months of disease. Patients with organ failure often have gradual decline with serious exacerbations followed by improvement; it can be very challenging to predict timing of death in these patients. A third group of patients are those with frailty, sometimes with concomitant dementia. These patients have long, slow declines but without discrete exacerbations of disease.

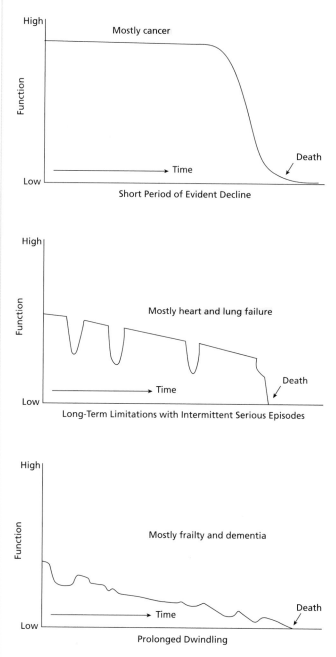

FIGURE 3. Trajectories of late-life illness.

Reprinted with permission from Lorenz KA, Lynn J, Dy SM, et al. Evidence for improving palliative care at the end of life: a systematic review. Ann Intern Med. 2008;148(2):147-159. [PMID: 18195339] Copyright 2008, American College of Physicians.

Recent evidence suggests that minority patients receive more intensive care at the end of life than they would if they were more adequately communicated with regarding advance care planning, prognosis, and treatment alternatives, such as nonhospice or hospice palliative care. The National Comprehensive Cancer Network has recommended that patients be screened for palliative care needs at initial presentation with cancer as well as at subsequent visits, and that palliative care services be available to all patients with cancer.

KEY POINT

- More aggressive care at the end of life does not improve either quality or duration of life.

Assessment and Communication

The cornerstone of both hospice and nonhospice palliative care is communication with patients, families, and caregivers. The first step in this communication is to establish goals of care in a patient-centered, open-ended format. Adequate time needs to be allotted to ensure that these discussions provide the opportunity for actively listening to the patient and key care providers (rather than being physician-centered—oriented toward efficiency and completing the task). The initial meeting or meetings should emphasize discovery of what the patient knows and understands regarding the diagnosis and prognosis. This discussion should allow opportunity to clarify how much the patient actually wants to know and should respect the diverse ways in which patients and their families process information about life-altering or life-threatening medical conditions. Medical jargon should be avoided and medical information conveyed succinctly and empathetically. Several meetings may be necessary to allow further processing of information and preparation of more questions by the patient or family members. As issues are addressed and worked through, a plan should be presented in a clear and succinct manner. Next steps should be outlined and, when necessary, carefully reiterated.

KEY POINT

- The first step in communication with patients, families, and caregivers regarding palliative care is to establish goals of care in a patient-centered, open-ended format.

Symptom Management

Symptoms common in patients with cancer and other life-threatening illnesses are myriad. Numerous symptom assessment instruments have been validated in the medical literature. The Edmonton Symptom Assessment Scale is a brief survey that asks patients to rate several symptoms on a scale (pain, dyspnea, fatigue, nausea, depression, anxiety, drowsiness, appetite, sense of well being) and also allows them to add one additional symptom and rate it. These symptoms may occur because of the underlying disease or secondary to treatments for symptoms of the disease.

Pain

Undertreated patient pain is a major problem in both the inpatient and outpatient settings. Assessment of pain can be difficult, particularly in patients with dementia, delirium, or somnolence caused by medications being used to treat pain.

Strong evidence from randomized trials supports treating cancer-related pain with NSAIDs, opioids, and radiation therapy; evidence regarding the use of bisphosphonates for cancer pain is less convincing. There is a lack of studies providing strong evidence on effective ways to treat pain in advanced heart failure or dementia. Opioid use in the treatment of noncancer pain continues to be controversial.

The World Health Organization analgesic ladder provides a stepwise approach to the management of pain (**Figure 4**). Pain management in palliative care, as with other conditions, should begin with nonopioid analgesia, including acetaminophen and NSAIDs (see Common Symptoms, Chronic Noncancer Pain). Adjuvant pain medications are used to treat pain symptoms that respond poorly to analgesic agents, such as neuropathic or bony

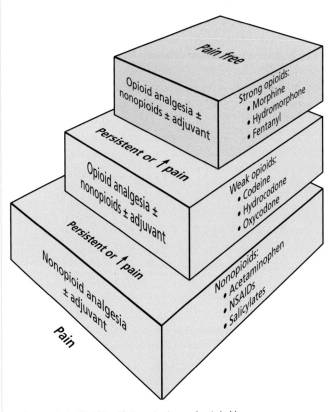

FIGURE 4. World Health Organization analgesic ladder.

H
CONT.

metastatic pain. Examples of these medications include anticonvulsants, corticosteroids, and antidepressants. Corticosteroids are useful for treating spinal cord compression or brain metastases, but data are lacking in support of their use in other cancer-related pain. Benzodiazepines should generally be avoided as they may actually worsen pain and also cause confusion and agitation in patients who are elderly or have dementia.

Various opioid analgesics are listed in **Table 15**. A weaker opioid analgesic (such as oxycodone) can be added at any point along the World Health Organization ladder. If pain persists or worsens, stronger opioid analgesia should be started. The usual starting dose of short-acting morphine is 5 to 15 mg orally in opiate-naïve patients and the elderly or 1 to 5 mg intravenously. Shorter-acting morphine can be used for breakthrough pain but should be changed to long-acting morphine if a patient develops persistent pain throughout the day or beyond 24 hours of treatment with shorter-acting opioids. A starting dosage of long-acting morphine is usually 30% to 50% of a patient's total average 24-hour usage. This dosage is increased every 3 to 4 days. Analgesia dosage for breakthrough pain should be 10% to 20% of the total daily opioid dose or 25% to 30% of the single standing dose. Analgesia should be gradually increased, with the firm goal of controlling pain. Beliefs about "maximum" dosages do not usually apply.

Although many health care providers worry about respiratory depression as a side effect of morphine, respiratory depression occurs rarely in patients who are actively in pain. In the elderly, however, it is generally best to start at the lower range. Hydromorphone is a semisynthetic opioid agonist that is similar to morphine but has a more favorable pharmacokinetic profile. Fentanyl is more expensive but can be administered as a lollipop, transdermally, or intravenously. Methadone, a long-acting opioid, has an unpredictable half-life and has been reported to cause QT interval prolongation and arrhythmias. It should be used with caution, with monitoring of the QT interval. Meperidine should be avoided because it can cause seizures, especially in the setting of kidney failure, as well as confusion and mood alterations. A fentanyl transdermal patch is an excellent alternative to decrease frequency of dosing but is substantially more expensive than long-acting morphine and takes up to 24 hours to take effect, making dose adjustment slightly more complicated.

When using opioids, it is important to be sensitive to patient concerns about addiction, as these concerns may present an obstacle to attaining adequate pain control. It is extremely rare for patients to become addicted to opioids in the acute hospital setting and rare to become addicted when being treated in the setting of cancer-related pain. Occasionally, opioid use may result in opioid-induced hyperalgesia. This is a poorly understood phenomenon whereby increased dosages of opioids exacerbate pain rather than

relieve it. Other important side effects of morphine include xerostomia, constipation, sedation, myoclonus, urinary hesitancy, nausea, and itching.

Constipation

Constipation is common in cancer patients, particularly in the elderly. It is defined as fewer than three bowel movements per week, the subjective sensation of incomplete bowel movements, or difficult passage of stool. It is important to obtain a history about a patient's premorbid bowel habits in order to establish a baseline. Forty percent to 95% of cancer patients suffer from constipation, and 95% of patients on opioids report constipation. Opioids cause constipation by binding to the μ receptor in the bowel, diminishing intestinal activity and reducing intestinal secretions. Constipation is also exacerbated by decreased activity and, toward the end of life, by reduced mobility and access to the toilet. Other contributing factors in cancer patients include hypercalcemia and bowel obstruction (from primary or metastatic disease or treatment-related adhesions).

A bowel regimen should be prescribed for any patient starting opioid analgesic agents and should include both a stool softener and a laxative. "Rescue laxatives," such as lactulose, magnesium citrate, or enemas, may be needed if the patient fails to have at least three bowel movements weekly or reports symptoms of constipation on a standard bowel regimen. **H**

Some data indicate that opioid rotation can improve constipation. Three studies have showed reduced reliance on laxatives when oral morphine was switched to a fentanyl transdermal patch.

Fatigue

Fatigue, the subjective feeling of physical, emotional, or mental exhaustion, is one of the most common and distressing symptoms related to cancer and cancer treatment. In contrast to fatigue in a healthy person, fatigue in a cancer patient is not relieved by rest. It affects 60% to 90% of patients with cancer and up to 96% of patients undergoing radiation or chemotherapy. Notably, as cancer progresses, fatigue worsens. Fatigue can also be an early harbinger of recurrent cancer.

Treatment of fatigue in cancer and other end-stage illnesses, such as heart failure and COPD, begins with education of the patient and family members about modes of energy conservation and distraction. Various modalities have been evaluated in reducing cancer-related fatigue, including biofeedback and exercise programs, but the small patient populations in these studies make it difficult to establish firm evidence-based recommendations about interventions. However, given the low morbidity of such treatments, it is reasonable to try an exercise or rehabilitation program.

TABLE 15.	Common Noninjected Narcotics Used in Palliative Care for Chronic Pain					
Agent	**Drug:Morphine Potency Ratio[a]**	**Form**	**Starting Dose**	**Onset**	**Duration**	**Comments**
Morphine	—	Immediate release	10 mg q 3-4 h	30 min	4 h	Tablet, solution, and rectal suppository
		Controlled/ sustained release[b]	15-30 mg q 12 h	2-4 h	12 h	Tablets, ranging from 15-200 mg
Oxycodone	2:1	Immediate release	2.5-5 mg q 6 h	10-15 min	3-6 h	Tablet and solution form
		Extended release[b]	10 mg q 12 h	1 h	12 h	Tablets 60 mg or higher for use only in opioid-tolerant patients.
Fentanyl	4:1[c]	Immediate release	200-µg lozenge: may repeat once in 15 min, then q 6 h 100-µg buccal tablet: may repeat once in 30 min, then q 4 h	5-15 min	4-8 h	Not recommended for opioid-naïve patients. Transmucosal lozenge or buccal tablet should be used only in patients who are already receiving narcotics and are opioid tolerant. Limit to 4 or fewer daily—additional doses mark need for adjustment of basal pain medication.
		Extended release	25-µg patch q 72 h	12-24 h	72 h	Not recommended for opioid-naive patients. Patients should be on at least 60 mg oral morphine equivalents/d before starting. Dose should not be adjusted upward based on supplemental opiate need for 3 days after initial placement or 6 days after subsequent dose changes. 17 hours are required for 50% decrease in fentanyl levels after removal.
Codeine	1:3-8 (variable)	Immediate release	30-60 mg q 4-6 h	30-60 min	4-6 h	Tablet and liquid, usually taken with adjunct analgesics due to weak strength. Variable efficacy due to differences in metabolism to morphine with CYP2D6 enzyme.
Hydromorphone	4:1	Immediate release	2-4 mg q 3-6 h	15-30 min	4-5 h	Also available as liquid, rectal suppository. Dose adjustment required with kidney failure.
		Extended release	8-64 mg q 24 h	1-2 h	24 h	For use in opioid-tolerant patients only. Dose adjustment required with kidney failure.
Hydrocodone	1:1	Immediate release	5-15 mg q 3-8 h	30-60 min	4-8 h	Available as combination product with adjunct analgesics.

q = every; µg = microgram.

[a]A ratio of 2:1 indicates that the medication is twice as powerful as an equivalent mg strength of morphine. No fixed conversion ratio is likely to be satisfactory in all patients, especially patients receiving large opioid doses.

[b]Divide cumulative daily dose of short-acting narcotic into two divided doses of the longer-acting narcotic.

[c]The fentanyl comparison is a µg-to-mg conversion.

⊞ Dyspnea

Dyspnea is a common and troubling symptom for patients with cancer as well as advanced COPD and heart failure. Up to 70% of cancer patients suffer from dyspnea in the last 6 weeks of life, and for 30%, it is rated as moderate to severe in intensity. Strong evidence supports the use of β-agonists, morphine, pulmonary rehabilitation, and oxygen for symptom relief in COPD. Although opioids are frequently used in cancer-related dyspnea, evidence is weak for their use in this situation. However, options are limited in treating cancer-related dyspnea, and opioid use is standard of care. Morphine use in cancer-related dyspnea is prescribed the same way it is used in cancer pain. Benzodiazepines are also sometimes used to treat cancer-related dyspnea but have not been well studied. Oxygen may also be used in treating cancer-related dyspnea, but evidence for functional improvement is lacking.

Nausea

Chronic nausea, defined as nausea lasting longer than 1 week, affects up to 60% of cancer patients in the last 6 months of life regardless of whether they receive chemotherapy. Metoclopramide is a dopamine agonist with prokinetic activity through the cholinergic system. It has a short half-life but can be given intravenously, subcutaneously, or orally and results in symptomatic improvement in 50% of patients. Serotonin antagonists (ondansetron) are effective for chemotherapy-related nausea but are expensive and unproven in the chronic palliative care setting. Dronabinol is a cannabinoid that is effective in chemotherapy-related nausea and AIDS-related wasting, but it has not been well studied for chronic palliative care patients. It may cause somnolence, confusion or euphoria. Dexamethasone has been increasingly used for palliative care as an antiemetic. A trial of 2 to 4 mg intravenously can be tried for patients not responding to other antiemetic agents.

Anorexia and Nutrition

Loss of appetite can be one of the most disturbing symptoms for patients and their providers. Reassurance often needs to be provided, and advance directives regarding feeding tubes should ideally be clarified in advance of the anorexia that occurs at the end of life. Feeding tubes are controversial and probably do not confer a survival advantage to cancer patients unless used as a temporizing measure in the treatment of head and neck or gastrointestinal cancers. Feeding tubes are not recommended for terminal cancer. Two classes of drugs have been shown to improve appetite in patients with cancer but do not provide a survival advantage. Progestational agents, such as megestrol, improve appetite and weight gain. Side effects include thromboembolism, impotence, edema, and vaginal bleeding. Corticosteroids have also been found to improve appetite in patients with cancer, but the proper dosing regimen has not been established. ⊞

Depression

Depression is a common symptom in patients approaching the end of life. Tricyclic antidepressants and selective serotonin reuptake inhibitors have been found to be equally effective, provided treatment duration is 6 weeks or longer. Randomized controlled trials have also found consistent efficacy in nonpharmacologic interventions, such as psychotherapy, education, and individual and group support.

Delirium ⊞

Delirium is common at the end of life and can be caused by advanced medical conditions, the medications being used to palliate symptoms, or a combination of both. Family members frequently need to be reassured that delirium is common. Opioid analgesia can be reduced provided pain remains controlled. If opioid dosage cannot be reduced owing to pain or dyspnea, haloperidol can be given at a dose of 0.5 to 1 mg intramuscularly. Additional sedative agents (such as benzodiazepines) may be required but can further exacerbate delirium in patients who are elderly or have dementia. ⊞

KEY POINTS

- Respiratory depression as a side effect of morphine occurs rarely in patients who are actively in pain.
- A bowel regimen should be prescribed for any patient starting opioid analgesic agents.

Bereavement and Grief

Although providing psychosocial, spiritual, and bereavement support for patients and their families is considered an essential part of hospice palliative care, effective ways to do this are not well demonstrated in the medical literature. Approximately 15% of bereaved survivors in the U.S. experience complicated grief, defined as grief persisting more than 6 months after a death. Its chief symptom is a yearning for a loved one so intense that it incapacitates all other desires. Many interventions have been studied, but thus far, none have shown results adequate to provide evidence-based guidance in this area. It is important, however, for physicians to be sensitive to the needs of bereaved survivors given the depth of despair for which they are at risk.

Common Symptoms

Overview

Common symptoms generally fall into a few major categories, including pain, upper respiratory, neurologic, dermatologic, musculoskeletal, and psychological. Common symptoms account for more than half of visits to the general internist. Most symptoms improve within 2 weeks, but up to 25% of these common symptoms become recurrent or chronic. Patients may present with symptoms as the primary reason for a visit or as a secondary concern during an appointment for follow-up of chronic medical conditions. Symptoms for which no demonstrable pathology is found are designated as somatic. Up to one third of symptoms presented in primary care visits have no demonstrable cause. Some patients may feel uncomfortable discussing sensitive or difficult issues, and talking about a common symptom may feel more acceptable to them. Examples of these hidden agendas include concerns about sexual dysfunction, sexually transmitted infection, incontinence, and depression or other psychological issues. Asking patients if they have other concerns during the visit can often uncover these issues. Depression, anxiety, or somatization should be considered in patients presenting with multiple symptoms in different parts of the body.

Clinical decision rules (CDRs) aid in the diagnosis and management of many common symptoms. Examples of CDRs include the Centor score to diagnose group A streptococcal pharyngitis and the Ottawa ankle rule to determine which patients with ankle injuries require imaging. There is a growing literature regarding the evidence-based approach to evaluating and managing many common symptoms; for example, the Rational Clinical Examination series published by the Journal of the American Medical Association.

Chronic Noncancer Pain

Chronic pain is defined as persistent pain of sufficient duration and intensity to have a significant impact on a patient's quality of life, functional status, and well-being. Pain may be considered chronic if it persists for longer than the anticipated healing time, although various time frames have been proposed (persistence of pain for more than 6 weeks, 3 months, or 6 months). Chronic noncancer pain (CNCP) affects as many as 50 million Americans and is associated with many conditions encountered in primary care, including fibromyalgia, postherpetic neuralgia, diabetic neuropathy, and osteoarthritis. CNCP exacts a significant personal and economic burden, with costs estimated at $85 billion annually as a result of job loss, missed work days, and medical visits. (Cancer pain is discussed in Palliative Care).

Assessment

CNCP may affect many aspects of a patient's life, and guidelines from the Institute for Clinical Systems Improvement emphasize that an initial assessment should evaluate each patient's pain within the context of his or her psychological state and beliefs, family supports, and social and work environments. Physicians should first obtain information about pain location, character, intensity, duration, relieving and exacerbating factors, and previous treatments. Patients should be questioned regarding the impact of pain on their activity level, ability to work, mood, sleep, and relationships with others. The patient's symptoms and goals for treatment need to be explored in a thorough, patient-centered manner. The Brief Pain Inventory (BPI), a patient-completed questionnaire, is a standardized tool for obtaining information about a patient's pain symptoms efficiently. Screening for depression and anxiety, as well as substance abuse, is essential, since these diagnoses may significantly affect treatment options. A history of physical, verbal, or sexual abuse has been associated with chronic pain syndromes, and providers should carefully assess for current or previous threats to a patient's well-being and safety. **Table 16** lists the key elements of the CNCP assessment, as well as suggested strategies for obtaining this information.

All patients with CNCP should receive a complete physical examination, with special attention to the musculoskeletal and nervous systems. Muscle strength and tone should be assessed, joints inspected for signs of effusion or erythema, and trigger points identified. Testing of sensation is essential for diagnosing absent or abnormal sensory states, such as allodynia (pain with stimuli that are usually not painful) or hyperalgesia (increased sensitivity to pain).

There is no specific role for diagnostic testing in the assessment and management of CNCP, as abnormalities that are identified may not be the source of the patient's pain. Tests for certain conditions may be considered, such as an MRI for evaluating back pain if conditions such as spinal stenosis or herniated disk disease are suspected. Similarly, nerve conduction studies may be helpful in select patients if the diagnosis or etiology of neuropathy is uncertain.

Based on findings from the history and physical examination, a patient's pain should be classified into one of five types: neuropathic pain, muscle pain, inflammatory pain, mechanical/compressive pain, and mixed (**Table 17**). This classification is helpful for choosing mechanism-specific treatment options that are most likely to alleviate the pain. Before initiating treatment, providers should assess for common behavioral, social, or systems barriers that may prevent a patient from experiencing functional improvement, irrespective of the treatment plan. Behavioral barriers include low motivation, unrealistic expectations, poor adherence, chemical dependency, and passivity. Social barriers include time constraints, lack of social support, cultural and language barriers, and financial issues. Systems barriers include formulary and coverage restrictions and difficulty accessing behavioral health care. Identifying these barriers can help providers develop a realistic expectation of what can be accomplished in management of a patient's pain. Patients involved in litigation may display limited response to treatment.

TABLE 16. Key Elements in the Assessment of the Patient with Chronic Noncancer Pain

Key Element	Notes[a]
General Assessment	
Pain location, intensity, quality, onset, relieving and exacerbating factors	The Brief Pain Inventory, Chronic Pain Grade, and Neuropathic Pain Scale are all helpful for assessing multiple aspects of a patient's pain.
Functional status	The Physical Functional Ability Questionnaire (FAQ 5) is brief and easy to complete.
Mental health disorders (depression, anxiety, substance abuse)	The Patient Health Questionnaire (PHQ-9) screens for major depressive disorder. The CAGE Questionnaire is a brief screen for alcohol use disorders (see Routine Care of the Healthy Patient).
Verbal, physical, or sexual abuse	Sensitivity and empathy are essential when eliciting this information.
Assessment for Opioid Therapy	
Risk stratification for initiating therapy	The Screener and Opioid Assessment for Patients with Pain (SOAPP) and Opioid Risk Tool (ORT) are patient-completed. The Diagnosis, Intractability, Risk, and Efficacy (DIRE) tool is provider-completed.
Follow-up	The 6 A's are a useful framework for follow-up visits: Analgesia, Activities of daily living, Adverse events, Aberrant behavior, Assessment, Action plan.

[a]Several tools are available for assessments; listed scales are examples.

TABLE 17. Classification of Chronic Pain Mechanisms and Recommended Pharmacologic Therapies

Mechanism of Pain	Description	Examples	Medications
Neuropathic	Burning, shooting, stabbing	Diabetic peripheral neuropathy, postherpetic neuralgia, fibromyalgia[a], multiple sclerosis, trigeminal neuralgia	*Systemic:* gabapentin, pregabalin, TCAs, duloxetine, venlafaxine, tramadol, opioids, carbamazepine *Local:* topical lidocaine 5% patch, capsaicin
Muscle	Tender trigger points Pain often involves the neck, shoulders, arms, low back, hips, lower extremities	Myofascial pain syndrome, fibromyalgia[a]	TCAs, milnacipran (for fibromyalgia)
Inflammatory	Involved joints are warm, erythematous, and swollen	Rheumatoid arthritis and other inflammatory arthropathies	DMARDs, NSAIDs, TCAs
Mechanical/compressive	Aggravated by activity, relieved by rest	Back pain, neck pain, musculoskeletal pain	NSAIDs, acetaminophen, TCAs, duloxetine

DMARD = disease-modifying antirheumatic drug; TCA = tricyclic antidepressant.

[a]Fibromyalgia pain may be both neuropathic and muscular in origin.

Management

General Principles

The goal of CNCP treatment is to improve function and quality of life in the context of pain that may be ongoing. A comprehensive treatment plan may include physical rehabilitation, cognitive-behavioral therapy (CBT), management of comorbid psychiatric conditions, complementary and alternative therapy, and pharmacologic therapies. A graded exercise program will help to improve functional status, and machine muscle strengthening, aerobic low-impact exercises, and flexion/extension exercises are equally beneficial. "Passive" modalities (transcutaneous electrical nerve stimulation [TENS], massage, and ultrasound) should only be used in the context of an active exercise program; massage therapy may be particularly beneficial for patients with low back pain, fibromyalgia, and knee osteoarthritis. All patients should be taught self-management strategies that can improve pain, such as ice and heat therapy.

CBT techniques include biofeedback, mindfulness-based stress reduction, imagery, and hypnosis, and have been shown to have small but positive effects on pain, disability, and mood. Depression and CNCP are frequently coexistent, and simultaneous treatment should be initiated if the depression is mild to moderate in severity. In contrast, psychiatric therapy is the initial focus of treatment in the setting of severe major depressive disorder and CNCP, as untreated patients will not be able to actively work toward achieving rehabilitation and treatment goals.

Acupuncture has been studied for various CNCP syndromes. The limited evidence for effectiveness for neck pain does not appear to be clinically significant. The improvement with acupuncture in chronic back pain, osteoarthritic knee pain, and fibromyalgia has not been demonstrated to be superior to sham acupuncture. Recent studies have shown that manipulative therapy, when included as part of an interdisciplinary treatment program, can reduce chronic pain. Herbal medications should be used cautiously because of the risk for drug interactions and adverse effects. Feverfew and willow bark appear to be effective for treating headaches and back pain, respectively, but little evidence supports the use of glucosamine, chondroitin, dimethylsulfoxide, or devil's claw.

Nonopioid Medical Therapies

Although medication is not the sole focus of the treatment plan, it is a useful adjunct to care for many patients with CNCP. The World Health Organization analgesic ladder (see Palliative Care), although developed for the palliative care setting, is widely used in the management of CNCP. Pharmacologic pain management should begin with nonopioid agents, such as acetaminophen, NSAIDs, and the selective cyclooxygenase-2 (COX-2) inhibitor celecoxib. Adjuvant therapies include antidepressants, anticonvulsants, muscle relaxants, and topical medications. Tramadol is a unique analgesic that activates μ-opioid receptors and also inhibits serotonin reuptake. It is effective for the treatment of moderate to severe chronic pain, but may increase the risk for suicide in certain patients; moreover, tramadol may be abused or subject to criminal diversion. Caution is necessary when initiating tramadol in patients who are taking serotonin reuptake inhibitors, as cotreatment can increase the risk for serotonin syndrome.

Factors to consider when selecting a medication include the type of pain being treated, side effects, drug interactions, and patient comorbidities. Medications that are appropriate for each type of pain are listed in Table 17.

Acetaminophen is generally safe but should not exceed 4 g/d and should be avoided or used cautiously in patients with liver disease. NSAIDs are reasonable alternatives or supplements to acetaminophen, especially if pain is associated with inflammation. NSAIDs and COX-2 inhibitors should be used cautiously, as they can increase the risk of gastritis, kidney dysfunction, and adverse cardiovascular outcomes. In older patients, the risk for adverse reactions is increased, and the American Geriatrics Society recommends acetaminophen, rather than NSAIDs, as first-line therapy. Older patients who are treated with an NSAID should also be prescribed a proton pump inhibitor to reduce gastric toxicity; this should be considered in any patient on long-term NSAIDs. Contraindications to NSAID therapy include current peptic ulcer disease, chronic kidney disease, and heart failure. For patients with high cardiovascular risk, naproxen may be a safer choice than diclofenac or ibuprofen. Diclofenac has been associated with increased cardiovascular risk as compared with other NSAIDs, and ibuprofen interferes with the antiplatelet effects of aspirin.

Adjuvant therapies such as gabapentin and pregabalin are efficacious for the treatment of neuropathic pain and have few drug interactions. According to a Cochrane systematic review, pregabalin dosed at 600 mg/d provided substantial pain relief for postherpetic neuralgia, diabetic neuropathy, and fibromyalgia (number needed to treat = 3.9, 5.0, and 11.0, respectively), but treatment-associated dizziness and somnolence were common. Tricyclic antidepressants (TCAs) can be effective for fibromyalgia and other central sensitization pain syndromes, but may produce significant adverse reactions, including constipation, dry mouth, conduction abnormalities, and urinary retention; their use should be avoided in the elderly. Duloxetine, a norepinephrine transporter (NET) inhibitor that has been approved for the treatment of fibromyalgia and diabetic neuropathy, and tramadol both also inhibit serotonin uptake, making them effective for neuropathic pain. In patients with postherpetic neuralgia and diabetic neuropathy, combination therapy with gabapentin and nortriptyline, as compared with monotherapy with each agent, produces better pain relief with fewer adverse reactions.

Opioid Therapy

Opioid therapy should be reserved for patients with moderate to severe neuropathic pain that has been unresponsive to other pharmacologic therapy. It is typically not beneficial in patients with inflammatory or mechanical/compressive pain. The significant side effects associated with opioid therapy (constipation, fatigue, nausea), as well as the attendant risks for abuse and addiction, make appropriate patient selection essential. The most important risk factors for aberrant drug-taking behaviors are a personal or family history of drug or alcohol abuse, age younger than 45 years, and a history of psychiatric disease. Other risk factors include female sex, cigarette smoking, preadolescent sexual abuse (in women), previous legal problems, history of motor vehicle accidents, and poor family support. The DIRE score (Diagnosis, Intractability, Risk, and Efficacy) is a physician-completed risk-stratification tool that can be helpful for determining which patients are most suitable for opioid therapy; higher scores (that is, a more severe diagnosis, clearly intractable pain, lower psychosocial risk, no chemical dependence history, and higher efficacy of opioids already used) predict greater success with treatment. The DIRE score can be accessed at www .icsi.org/pain__chronic__assessment_and_management_of _14399/pain__chronic__assessment_and_management_of __guideline_.html (Appendix E). Table 16 lists additional tools that may be helpful for assessing risk.

Patients who are selected for opioid therapy should have a thorough understanding of its risks and benefits. The patient and the physician should work together to develop an opioid management plan, or pain contract, that outlines agreed-upon goals and rules of treatment. (An example is available in the chronic pain guideline linked to above, Appendix F.) Typically, pain contracts include stipulations that pain medications will not be sought elsewhere, that the patient will abstain from illicit drugs, will keep clinic appointments as scheduled, and will obtain randomly scheduled urine toxicology screens. A copy of this signed document can be given to the patient and reviewed periodically at follow-up visits to ensure that treatment expectations are being met.

Medication selection should be influenced by the severity and frequency of pain; long-acting opioids, which maintain more consistent drug levels, are preferred for the treatment of CNCP. Physicians should be cautious when initiating methadone, which can cause QT-interval prolongation, hypotension, and cardiac arrhythmias. An electrocardiogram should be obtained at baseline, after 30 days of treatment, and annually thereafter. Methadone should be started at low doses and gradually increased to effective doses. Although methadone requires regular monitoring of QT intervals, it can be effective when other opioids are not. In addition, methadone lacks the euphoric effects of morphine and other opioids that can contribute to dose escalation and potential abuse.

Careful monitoring of patients treated with opioid therapy is essential, and clinicians can use the "6 A's" as a framework for assessment during follow-up visits. Patients should be queried about the effectiveness of *Analgesia*, the benefit of therapy on their *Activities of daily living*, *Adverse events* associated with treatment, and *Aberrant behaviors* suggesting drug abuse; providers should also *Assess mood* and review the *Action (treatment) plan*. Clues to aberrant drug-taking behaviors include multiple episodes of prescription loss, repeated requests for dose increases or early refills, drug requests by name, missed appointments, repeatedly seeking prescriptions from other clinicians, not following through with other components of the treatment plan, and aggressive complaining about needing more of the drug. Random urine drug testing, which is recommended for all patients on opioid therapy, may be conducted more frequently if patients exhibit any of these behaviors. When interpreting the results of urine drug testing, providers should consider the possibility of false-positive and false-negative tests, and correlate results clinically (that is, a specific type of urine testing is required for hydrocodone).

Patients should be seen monthly for the first 3 months after opioid therapy is initiated; once a stable regimen is achieved, visits may occur every 3 to 6 months. More frequent visits, with possible therapy restructuring or discontinuation of opioid therapy, should occur if there is evidence of drug abuse or misuse, significant side effects, or lack of functional improvement. Patients on high doses of opioid therapy should also be seen more frequently, as a recent retrospective cohort study suggests that such patients are at higher risk for medically serious or fatal overdose. That study found that patients prescribed 100 mg/d of opioid medication were nine times more likely to have an overdose than patients prescribed 20 mg/d or less. Patients prescribed 50 mg/d to 99 mg/d were at four times the risk of those on lower doses.

KEY POINTS

- Before initiating treatment for chronic noncancer pain, providers should assess for common behavioral, social, or systems barriers that may prevent a patient from experiencing functional improvement.

- All patients with chronic noncancer pain should be taught self-management strategies that can improve pain.

- Pharmacologic management of chronic pain should start with acetaminophen, NSAIDs, and adjuvant pain therapies.

- Opioid therapy should be reserved for patients with chronic moderate to severe neuropathic pain that has been unresponsive to other treatments.

Cough

Cough is one of the most common symptoms for which patients seek medical attention from either a primary care physician or a pulmonologist. In addition, it has significant impact on health care expenditures. According to the American College of Chest Physicians, up to 30,000,000 physician visits annually are for cough-related symptoms, and billions of dollars are spent on medication for symptomatic relief.

A cough is triggered by chemical or mechanical stimulation of cough receptors. These receptors are located in the upper and lower respiratory tracts as well as in the stomach, gastroesophageal junction, diaphragm, esophagus, pericardium, and ears. The knowledge of the location of cough receptors and the chemical and mechanical triggers of the cough reflex contributes to understanding the differential diagnosis. Recent guidelines suggest an empiric and integrative approach to the management of cough based on duration of cough.

Acute Cough

Acute cough is a cough that is present for less than 3 weeks. Upper respiratory tract infections (rhinosinusitis, pharyngitis) and acute bronchitis are the most common causes. Other considerations include exacerbations of COPD, pneumonia, allergic rhinitis, left ventricular failure, asthma, medications, and aspiration.

Rhinosinusitis (the common cold) and acute bronchitis are most commonly caused by viruses (influenza A and B, parainfluenza, coronavirus, rhinovirus, and respiratory syncytial virus). Nonviral causes include *Mycoplasma pneumoniae*, *Chlamydophila pneumoniae*, and *Bordetella pertussis* (whooping cough). Fever may or, more likely, may not be present. Cough with purulent sputum is not a reliable indicator of a bacterial infection. In acute bronchitis, the cough generally lasts more than 5 days and, although most resolve in 3 weeks, bronchial hyperreactivity can lead to persistence of cough for up to 8 weeks.

The incidence of pertussis has increased over the past two decades. If suspected, culture via nasopharyngeal aspirate or swab and macrolide antibiotic treatment are indicated.

Routine antibiotic treatment of uncomplicated upper respiratory tract infections and acute bronchitis in nonelderly immunocompetent patients is not recommended. Despite recommendations to avoid antibiotics in most patients, antibiotic overuse is common. Up to 60% of patients who present with upper respiratory tract infection symptoms or acute bronchitis are given antibiotics. Patient satisfaction with care for acute bronchitis depends primarily on physician-patient communication rather than on antibiotic prescription.

Lower respiratory tract infection or pneumonia can present with cough, but these infections generally are accompanied by fever, constitutional symptoms, pleuritic chest pain, and abnormalities on pulmonary examination. In patients with such findings and moderate to severe symptoms, a chest radiograph should be obtained. Influenza should be considered in any patient during the appropriate season who presents with cough, fever, myalgia, and headache.

Approximately 15% of patients on an ACE inhibitor develop cough. The cough usually begins within 1 week of starting therapy, although in some patients it may be delayed. The medication should be discontinued. Cough generally abates within 1 to 4 weeks. Since this is a class-specific effect, rechallenge with a different ACE inhibitor is not recommended. An angiotensin receptor blocker can be substituted for an ACE inhibitor as these medications generally do not cause cough.

Treatment of the patient with acute cough is based on primary diagnosis and is mainly supportive. For patients with the common cold, first-generation antihistamines, decongestants, inhaled ipratropium bromide, cromolyn sodium, and naproxen are helpful in decreasing sneezing and rhinorrhea. Newer-generation nonsedating antihistamines are ineffective. A review of 17 trials in adults concluded that centrally acting (codeine, dextromethorphan) or peripherally acting (moguisteine, benzonatate) antitussive therapy results in little, if any, improvement in cough associated with upper respiratory tract infection. The American College of Chest Physicians does not recommend their use. β_2-agonists should not be used unless cough is accompanied by wheezing.

Subacute and Chronic Cough

Subacute cough, a cough of 3 to 8 weeks' duration, is most commonly postinfectious. If an infectious origin is unlikely, upper airway cough syndrome (UACS, previously called postnasal drip syndrome), asthma, pertussis, acid reflux, or acute exacerbation of primary lung disease should be considered. Chronic cough is defined as the persistence of cough for longer than 8 weeks. The most common causes are UACS, asthma, nonasthmatic eosinophilic bronchitis (NAEB), and gastroesophageal reflux disease (GERD). In several case series, UACS, asthma, and GERD accounted for 90% of patients with chronic cough (excluding those with cough related to smoking or ACE inhibitors). Other, less common, causes are chronic bronchitis, bronchiectasis, lung cancer, aspiration, irritation of the external auditory canal, and psychogenic. There are often multiple causes for a case of chronic cough.

The medical history and physical examination may suggest a potential cause or causes, but neither is reliable for definitively ruling in or ruling out specific disease. Patients with chronic cough, especially smokers, should undergo chest radiography. If the chest radiograph is normal, the physician should consider UACS, asthma, NAEB, and GERD and begin a stepwise, sequential approach for evaluation and treatment (**Figure 5**). The definitive diagnosis may be known only after successful individual or joint empiric treatment.

The use of a systematic algorithmic approach in the immunocompetent patient with chronic cough can lead to successful outcomes in more than 90% of patients. In general, unless symptoms point to a specific diagnosis or there is a definitive finding on chest radiograph, empiric therapy for UACS for 2 to 3 weeks is started first. If there is no response, evaluation and treatment for asthma, NAEB, and GERD should ensue. All patients with chronic cough who smoke should receive smoking cessation counseling.

Specific therapy for each diagnosis should be optimized. For patients with UACS, first-generation antihistamines and decongestants remain first-line therapy. Patients with cough-variant asthma may demonstrate reversible airflow obstruction or airway hyperreactivity with bronchoprovocation testing.

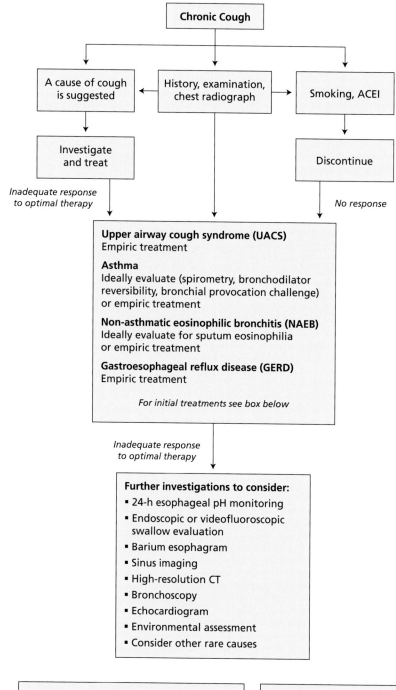

FIGURE 5. Evaluation of chronic cough. ACEI = angiotensin-converting enzyme inhibitor; LTRA = leukotriene receptor antagonist.

However, as bronchoprovocation testing may yield false-positive results, asthma should be diagnosed as a cause of chronic cough only if symptoms abate after 2 to 4 weeks of standard antiasthmatic therapy with an inhaled bronchodilator and inhaled corticosteroids. NAEB is diagnosed in patients who have sputum eosinophilia but are without airway hyperreactivity. These patients are treated with inhaled corticosteroids. GERD may be diagnosed in patients with typical symptoms or in those who fit a typical clinical profile and in whom near-complete or complete resolution of symptoms occurs with antireflux treatment. Typical heartburn symptoms may be present in only 60% patients with chronic cough caused by GERD. Although 24-hour pH monitoring may be helpful in the evaluation of patients with suspected GERD, empiric treatment can be initiated before testing. Effective treatment modalities include dietary and lifestyle modification and acid suppressive therapy with proton pump inhibitors for 1 to 3 months (see MKSAP 16 Gastroenterology and Hepatology).

When disease-based specific therapy fails, cough suppressants may be helpful. Unlike in treatment of acute cough, some clinical trials suggest that centrally acting narcotic (morphine or codeine) or nonnarcotic (dextromethorphan) medications may be effective in the treatment of chronic cough. Peripherally acting antitussives may also be beneficial. As with any long-term medication, risks and benefits need to be considered.

Cough in the Immunocompromised Patient

In addition to being at risk for the common community-acquired infections seen in the immunocompetent host, the immunocompromised patient is at risk for various opportunistic infections that may present with cough, such as tuberculosis, *Pneumocystis jirovecii* pneumonia, and aspergillosis. The degree and duration of immunosuppression, along with whether the primary impairment is in humoral or cell-mediated immunity, can assist in determining the more likely causes. Definitive work-up is indicated in immunocompromised patients with cough. Empiric antibiotic therapy should be initiated while diagnostic testing is used. Treatment can be modified based on subsequent microbiologic test results.

Hemoptysis

Hemoptysis is defined as coughing up any amount of blood from the lower respiratory tract. Hemoptysis must be distinguished from hematemesis or nasopharyngeal bleeding. Massive hemoptysis (>200 mL/d) can be life-threatening. The most common causes of hemoptysis are infection (airway inflammation) and malignancy. Other sources include the tracheobronchial tree (bronchitis, bronchiectasis, tumor), pulmonary parenchyma (abscess; pneumonia, including tuberculosis; Goodpasture syndrome, granulomatosis with polyangiitis [also known as Wegener granulomatosis]), and pulmonary vasculature (arteriovenous malformation, pulmonary

embolism, mitral stenosis, left-sided heart failure). All patients with hemoptysis should undergo chest radiography and, if indicated, chest CT or bronchoscopy.

KEY POINTS

- Routine antibiotic treatment of uncomplicated upper respiratory tract infections and acute bronchitis in nonelderly immunocompetent patients is not recommended.
- Neither centrally acting nor peripherally acting antitussive agents have demonstrated improvement in acute cough associated with upper respiratory tract infection.

Chronic Fatigue and Chronic Fatigue Syndrome

Fatigue is a common symptom in primary care, occurring in a fifth to a quarter of patients. Fatigue is difficult to define and quantify and is often viewed as a minor problem. Chronic fatigue is variably defined as lasting longer than 30 days or longer than 3 months, with a resulting inability to perform desired activities. Chronic fatigue may be secondary to various diseases, including malignancy; autoimmune and endocrine disorders; neurologic diseases (multiple sclerosis, Parkinson disease); chronic kidney, lung, heart, or liver disease; HIV infection; substance abuse; medication side effects; and heavy metal poisoning.

Chronic fatigue syndrome (CFS) is a distinct entity of fatigue that persists for 6 months or more. Diagnostic criteria developed for research purposes have been applied widely in the clinical setting. The International CFS Study Group definition includes medically unexplained fatigue of longer than 6 months' duration after clinical evaluation, with four or more of the following symptoms: subjective memory impairment, sore throat, tender lymph nodes, muscle or joint pain, headache, unrefreshing sleep, and postexertional malaise lasting longer than 24 hours; exclusion criteria include the presence of substance abuse, an eating disorder, an underlying psychiatric disorder, dementia, or severe obesity (BMI ≥ 45). Chronic fatigue of longer than 6 months' duration that does not meet criteria for CFS is designated idiopathic chronic fatigue.

Diagnosis and Evaluation of Chronic Fatigue

There are no specific recommendations regarding diagnostic evaluation for chronic fatigue. Patients with fatigue greater than 1 month rarely have abnormalities on either physical or laboratory evaluation; testing should thus be judicious and performed only when clearly indicated. The degree of functional limitation of patients with fatigue is often underestimated by health care providers, resulting in inadequate or incomplete attention and treatment.

Historical elements associated with CFS include unrefreshing sleep, subjective memory impairment, and substantial curtailment in previous level of functioning. CFS has been associated with various conditions, including post–viral infection (parvovirus B19), childhood trauma, and preexisting psychiatric disorders; many associations have not been reproduced in other studies, or are only seen in small numbers of patients, and thus cannot be clearly attributed as causes of CFS.

Physical examination in patients with chronic fatigue is usually normal and performed with the intent to exclude other possible organic causes. Findings of fever, lymphadenopathy, and muscle wasting warrant further evaluation for organic causes and should not be attributed to CFS. Selected laboratory or other diagnostic studies may help identify the cause of chronic fatigue or rule out treatable causes.

Management of Chronic Fatigue and Chronic Fatigue Syndrome

Management of CFS is challenging and requires a comprehensive strategy tailored to the patient's individual goals and needs. Providers must consider the risks of over-investigation, including reinforcement of the patient's belief that a treatable organic cause may be found, the potential hazards of testing itself, and false-positive findings, as well as time and cost issues. Treatment is directed at the underlying illness, if identified; nonspecific therapies include counseling, exercise, and possibly medications. Nonpharmacologic therapy includes lifestyle modification, sleep hygiene, and graded activity; selected patients may benefit from referral for CBT, physical rehabilitation, or psychiatric management. One goal should be to prevent further deterioration in functional ability, which may be accomplished with supportive management and by limiting largely ineffective treatments, such as corticosteroids and immunotherapy. Patients with comorbid depression should be offered antidepressant therapy, but no specific class of medications is recommended specifically for CFS. The limited number of small randomized controlled trials (RCTs) do not provide conclusive evidence for the effectiveness of dietary supplements and herbal remedies for CFS.

Patients with CFS should have regular follow-up to monitor their symptoms, for support and validation, and to avoid unnecessary diagnostic and treatment interventions. Prognosis is variable and related primarily to severity and degree of impairment. In studies, patients with less impairment or fatigue of shorter duration were more likely to recover, although functional outcome is often not reported or standardized, thus limiting the definition of recovery. Other predictors of poor outcome include self-reported poor health and coexisting somatic or mental health disorders.

KEY POINTS

- Fever, lymphadenopathy, or muscle wasting in a patient with chronic fatigue warrants further evaluation for organic causes and should not be attributed to chronic fatigue syndrome.

- Treatment of chronic fatigue syndrome is largely nonpharmacologic and includes lifestyle modification, sleep hygiene, graded activity, and cognitive-behavioral therapy.

- Patients with chronic fatigue syndrome should have regular follow-up to monitor their symptoms, for support and validation, and to avoid unnecessary diagnostic and treatment interventions.

Dizziness

Dizziness is a frustrating and acutely debilitating symptom for many patients. It is more common in women, and prevalence in the elderly may be as high as 37%. Patients with dizziness are at increased risk for falls and nursing home placement. Although most causes of dizziness have a benign course, they may be associated with life-threatening consequences, including stroke and death.

The evaluation of dizziness is challenging and without universally accepted guidelines. The history and physical examination are the most effective diagnostic tools and are used to classify dizziness into four categories: (1) vertigo, (2) presyncope, (3) dysequilibrium, and (4) other causes. The history and physical examination can also help to distinguish peripheral or otologic disease from central disease. Although categorization is attractive, it is not always possible, especially in the elderly. Up to one half of geriatric patients with dizziness have multiple causes in more than one category. Nonetheless, this schema forms the current best framework for diagnosis, evaluation, and management.

In general, key elements of the history include timing of symptoms, duration, provocative or palliative measures, and risk factors for atherosclerotic disease. All patients should have orthostatic vital signs taken and undergo thorough cardiac and neurologic examinations. Routine laboratory testing is not helpful.

Vertigo

Vertigo is the illusion of movement, either personal or environmental, caused by unilateral or asymmetric disruption of peripheral or central vestibular structures. It is typically, but not always, rotational. In studies that examined dizziness in primary care, specialty, or emergency settings, vertigo was the most common type, present in approximately half of patients. It may be accompanied by severe nausea, vomiting, nystagmus, and postural instability. Central causes of vertigo include vascular disease and stroke, mass lesions of the brainstem and cerebellum, multiple sclerosis, migraine, and seizures.

Peripheral causes of vertigo include benign paroxysmal positional vertigo (BPPV), vestibular neuronitis, and Meniere disease. Less common peripheral causes include aminoglycoside toxicity, herpes zoster, otitis media, and perilymph fistulas.

Diagnosing the cause of vertigo is critical because targeted, disease-specific treatment can improve symptoms and prognosis. The duration of symptoms can guide the differential diagnosis (**Table 18**), and results from the Dix-Hallpike maneuver can distinguish central from peripheral disease (**Table 19**). In the Dix-Hallpike maneuver, the patient is instructed to sit upright, turn the head 45 degrees, and keep both eyes open during the entire maneuver. The examiner supports the head and, while instructing the patient to lie down, rapidly places the head below the level of the examining table. The examiner notes nystagmus and subjective symptoms. The test is repeated with the head turned to the opposite side.

Peripheral Vertigo

Clinical Presentation
The most common cause of vertigo is BPPV. Patients with BPPV classically report recurrent, intense, and brief episodes of vertigo (1 minute or less) with a rapid change in head position, such as turning the head while driving or turning over in bed. Auditory or associated neurologic symptoms are absent. BPPV is caused by movement of otoliths or other debris in the semicircular canals (most commonly the posterior semicircular canal) induced by head movement. This leads to perturbation of sensory receptors in the vestibular labyrinth. Recurrences are common, reported to be 18% at 1 year and 30% at 3 years.

Vestibular neuronitis is acute in onset (hours) and is frequently associated with a viral infection that affects the vestibular portion of the eighth cranial nerve. Nausea and vomiting are common; no brainstem symptoms are present (distinguishing it from central vertigo). Hearing usually is not affected, but if it is, the term labyrinthitis is used. Symptoms can be very severe, and although symptoms usually peak during the first 24 hours and resolve within 7 days, full recovery may take longer. Residual dizziness can last for months.

Meniere disease, also known as idiopathic endolymphatic hydrops, is characterized by the classic triad of vertigo, unilateral low frequency hearing loss, and tinnitus, occasionally associated with aural fullness. Endolymphatic hydrops refers to a condition of increased hydraulic pressure in the inner ear endolymphatic system leading to these symptoms. In Meniere disease, the cause of the increased pressure is not known. Vertigo may be the first presenting sign. The diagnosis may be secured only after repeated attacks of vertigo with associated hearing loss.

Treatment
BPPV can be treated by the Epley maneuver (**Figure 6**), which can be curative. This maneuver attempts to move the debris floating in the semicircular canal to a position where it can exit into the utricular cavity. An evidence-based review of all major studies analyzing repositioning procedures concluded that this therapy is beneficial. In one study, 61% of the treated group had complete resolution of symptoms at 4 weeks compared with 20% in the control (sham-treated) group. The number needed to treat was 2.4. Medications generally are ineffective in BPPV.

For other causes of vertigo, particularly vestibular neuronitis, treatment options are generally limited to symptom relief. Vestibular suppressants and antiemetic drugs (antihistamines, benzodiazepines, and phenothiazines) are the three major drug

TABLE 18.	Duration of Vertigo and Suggested Causes
Duration of Vertigo	**Underlying Cause**
Seconds	Benign paroxysmal positional vertigo
Minutes to hours	Transient ischemic attack
	Meniere disease
	Perilymph fistula
	Migraine
Days	Acute vestibular neuronitis/labyrinthitis
	Ischemia/stroke
	Migraine
	Multiple sclerosis
Weeks	Psychogenic

TABLE 19.	Interpretation of Dix-Hallpike Maneuver Findings in Evaluation of Vertigo	
Characteristic	**Peripheral Disease**	**Central Disease**
Latency of nystagmus	2- 40 s	No latency
Duration of nystagmus	<1 min	>1 min
Severity of symptoms	Severe	Less severe
Habituation	Yes	No
Fatigability	Yes	No
Direction of nystagmus	Horizontal, with rotational component; never vertical	Can be vertical, horizontal, or torsional; may change with position

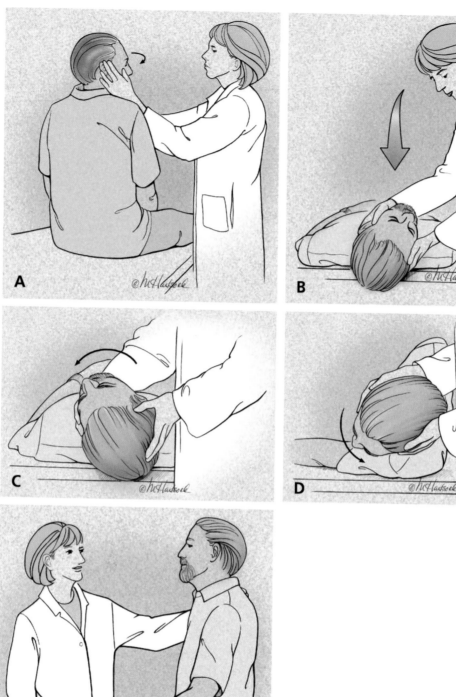

FIGURE 6. Epley maneuver for relieving benign paroxysmal positional vertigo. The patient sits on the examination table, with eyes open and head turned 45 degrees to the right (*A*). The physician supports the patient's head as the patient lies back quickly from a sitting to supine position, ending with the head hanging 20 degrees off the end of the examination table and still turned to the right (*B*). The physician turns the patient's head 90 degrees to the left side. The patient remains in this position for 30 seconds (*C*). The physician turns the patient's head an additional 90 degrees to the left while the patient rotates his or her body 90 degrees in the same direction. The patient remains in this position for 30 seconds (*D*). The patient sits up on the left side of the examination table (*E*). The procedure may be repeated on either side until the patient experiences relief of symptoms.

© Maria Hartsock, CMI. Reprinted from Swartz R, Longwell P. Treatment of Vertigo. Am Fam Physician. 2005;71(6):1115-1122, 1129-1130. [PMID: 15791890]

classes that may modify the intensity of symptoms. The most common drugs are centrally active antihistamine anticholinergic medications. These medications have been shown to reduce symptom severity. Benzodiazepines act centrally to suppress vestibular responses. Phenothiazine antiemetics are useful when nausea and vomiting accompany vertigo. Side effects of all of these medications include sedation. Some experts advocate corticosteroid therapy, but robust outcome data are lacking. Data for calcium channel blockers, betahistine, corticosteroids and ginger root are either weak or conflicting. Medications are recommended only for short periods (24-48 hours). More prolonged use may suppress vestibular feedback and central compensation mechanisms, leading to prolongation of symptoms.

Referral to a trained therapist for vestibular rehabilitation (VR) is helpful for peripheral vertigo, especially if initiated early. In a review of 27 moderate- to high-quality trials enrolling community-dwelling adults, VR proved to be effective. Compared with control groups, VR led to improvement in symptoms, walking, balance, vision, and activities of daily living. Exercises include learning to bring on symptoms to desensitize the vestibular system, learning to coordinate head and eye movements, and improving balance and walking skills.

Although caffeine restriction, salt restriction, and diuretic therapy have been advocated for Meniere disease, a recent review concluded that there is insufficient high-quality evidence to recommend these interventions. Similarly, there are no strong data for corticosteroids or immunosuppressive therapy.

Central Vertigo

Ischemia, infarction, and hemorrhage of the brainstem or cerebellum are life-threatening causes of vertigo. Patients at risk are those with hypertension, tobacco use, hyperlipidemia, diabetes mellitus, atrial fibrillation, and preexisting atherosclerotic vascular disease. Up to one quarter of patients with risk factors for stroke who present with severe vertigo or nystagmus or who are unable to stand without support have infarction of the inferior cerebellum.

The distinction between vertigo due to vascular disease and vertigo due to vestibular neuronitis is critical. Neurologic symptoms are absent in patients with vestibular neuronitis. However, patients with vertigo due to brainstem ischemia, infarction, or hemorrhage may demonstrate diplopia, dysarthria, dysphagia, and focal numbness or weakness. Those with cerebellar disease may present with gait abnormalities and headache. MRI of the brain with angiography is the preferred diagnostic test. Patients with brainstem or cerebellar disease require immediate medical or neurosurgical intervention.

Presyncope

Presyncope is the sensation of near loss of consciousness. The main cause is a global and temporary decrease in cerebral perfusion owing to cardiovascular disease (ischemia, arrhythmia, valvular heart disease), hypotension, carbon monoxide poisoning, anemia, or vasovagal reaction (see Syncope, below).

Dysequilibrium

Dysequilibrium is defined as imbalance or unsteadiness while standing or walking, without the sensation originating in the head. It is relieved with sitting or recumbency. Dysequilibrium is caused by defective sensory input (vision, vestibular), impaired proprioception or motor function, generalized weakness, Parkinson disease, joint pain, or anxiety or other psychiatric disorders. Medications can be contributing factors. A multidisciplinary approach to treatment is frequently indicated. The plan may include physical therapy, assistance devices for ambulation, audiometry testing, vision testing, and medication reconciliation.

Nonspecific Dizziness

Vague signs of dizziness, lightheadedness, or "wooziness" comprise the last and typically most frustrating category of dizziness. Although frequently attributed to psychiatric disorders, especially anxiety and depression, there may be overlap with other categories. Other specific causes include hypoglycemia, hyperglycemia, electrolyte abnormalities, thyroid disorders, anemia, and multiple classes of medications.

KEY POINTS

- All patients being evaluated for dizziness should have orthostatic vital signs taken and undergo thorough cardiac and neurologic examinations; routine laboratory testing is not helpful.

- Benign paroxysmal positional vertigo (BPPV) can be treated by the Epley maneuver, which attempts to move the debris floating in the semicircular canal to a position where it can exit into the utricular cavity; medications generally are ineffective for BPPV.

- Patients with vertigo accompanied by diplopia, dysarthria, dysphagia, focal numbness, gait abnormalities, or headache may have brainstem or cerebellar disease requiring immediate medical or neurosurgical intervention.

Insomnia

Insomnia is defined as any difficulty with sleep initiation, duration, consolidation, or quality that occurs despite adequate opportunity for sleep (in contradistinction to sleep deprivation) and results in daytime sleepiness or other adverse effects on daytime activities. It can be primary or secondary, the latter being more common. Causes include underlying medical problems such as chronic pain, depression, GERD, and obstructive sleep apnea. Insomnia also may be secondary to a poor sleep environment, medications, or other substances. It can be acute (transient) or chronic (occurring at least three times weekly for at least 1 month). Insomnia is sometimes defined as initial (difficulty falling asleep), middle (awakenings during the night), and terminal (early morning awakening).

Insomnia is more common in women, the elderly, patients with comorbid medical problems, shift workers, and persons of lower socioeconomic status. Patients with chronic insomnia are more likely to use health resources, be absent or late to work, and be involved in motor vehicle collisions, and they have an increased risk of suicide, depression, anxiety, and substance abuse. As many as 50% of patients identify some aspect of sleep disorder; clinicians should consider screening for insomnia by asking every patient about their sleep.

Evaluation of Insomnia

Several sleep questionnaires exist for use in patients in whom a sleep problem has been identified. Alternatively, physicians can ask about key components of the problem, including characterization of the sleep disturbance (duration, frequency, severity, progression), precipitating factors, past problems, and previous treatments and response. A thorough sleep history includes patterns of sleep and wakefulness (time to bed, time to sleep, number of awakenings), nocturnal symptoms, pre-sleep and sleep environment, and daytime activities. Interviewing a bed partner may provide additional information. A formal sleep diary may also be used. Important questions include information about medication and other substance use, especially over-the-counter (OTC) medications, caffeine, and alcohol.

Physical examination should assess for obesity, body habitus consistent with obstructive sleep apnea (enlarged tongue or tonsils, increased neck circumference), thyroid dysfunction, heart failure, and neurologic disease. Mental status examination should focus on mood and level of alertness. Laboratory and other diagnostic evaluations should be performed judiciously. An overnight polysomnography may be indicated if obstructive sleep apnea or other primary sleep disturbance (for example, restless legs syndrome or periodic limb movements of sleep) is strongly suspected, or in patients refractory to initial therapy.

Management of Insomnia

Therapy for insomnia is directed at treating any underlying cause or associated comorbid conditions. Pain, esophageal reflux, heart failure, and obstructive sleep apnea should be treated as appropriate. Nonpharmacologic interventions are preferred, especially in the elderly and in those with chronic insomnia.

Sleep hygiene refers to behavioral and environmental factors that affect sleep. Improving sleep hygiene is an important component of insomnia management; alone, however, this is often insufficient to treat chronic insomnia. Components of sleep hygiene include maintenance of a stable bedtime and awakening time, appropriate exposure to light during daytime and darkness during nighttime, avoidance of stimulants and exercise after 6 PM, use of the bed for sleeping and sex only, a maximum of 8 hours in bed, adjusting the bed and room comfort level, and relaxation strategies before bedtime.

CBT has been to shown to be more effective for both primary and secondary insomnia than drug therapy. Several sessions weekly are required over a several-week period. Adjunct medications may be used with CBT initially, but long-term studies indicate that CBT alone is best for maintenance therapy. Other, less common, treatments include sleep restriction, biofeedback, and relaxation techniques.

The decision to initiate pharmacologic treatment should take into account the patient's response to other therapies, patient preferences, treatment goals, comorbid conditions, medication interactions, adverse effects, and cost. Initial recommendations are for short- and intermediate-acting benzodiazepine γ-aminobutyric acid (GABA)-receptor agonists, nonbenzodiazepine GABA-receptor agonists, and type A melatonin-receptor agonists (**Table 20**). Nonbenzodiazepine GABA-receptor agonists are preferred over other sedating agents, including sedating antidepressants, owing to their lack of effect on sleep architecture and their superior safety profile. With benzodiazepines, caution is warranted regarding dependence and tolerance, as well as side effects of daytime sedation and psychomotor impairment. They should not be used in patients with a history of drug or alcohol abuse. Nonbenzodiazepine GABA-receptor agonists, such as zolpidem and zaleplon, have fewer adverse effects, mostly owing to their shorter half-life. Adverse effects of these agents include nausea, vertigo, nightmares, disorientation, and agitation. Zolpidem is associated with cases of somnambulism, such as nocturnal eating, driving, and walking. Data are limited regarding hypnotic agents for long-term therapy. The FDA recommends that treatment be limited to 1 month, and sleep specialists do not recommend long-term therapy. Small studies have show effectiveness for zolpidem for up to 8 weeks and for eszopiclone for up to 6 months.

Other sedative-hypnotic agents (chloral hydrate, barbiturates), gabapentin, and antipsychotic medications are not recommended for use for primary insomnia. Antidepressant medications are recommended for use only when insomnia is one of the manifestations of an underlying depressive disorder. Use of tricyclic antidepressants is discouraged owing to their significant side effect profile; antidepressants that are most efficacious for use in insomnia are low-dose trazodone or mirtazapine. Antihistamines are often used to treat insomnia, especially diphenhydramine, owing to its OTC availability and inclusion in OTC products marketed specifically for sleep. Because these drugs antagonize central H_1 receptors, their side-effect profile is significant and is predominantly anticholinergic with carry-over sedation and should be avoided for chronic insomnia. Diphenhydramine has a long half-life and is an inhibitor of CYP2D6 drug metabolism. Thus, with its anticholinergic profile, it is a particularly bad choice for elderly patients, especially those with mild cognitive impairment or Alzheimer disease or who are exposed to polypharmacy. OTC melatonin is available, and in this form is a nonspecific agonist of melatonin receptors. It may be helpful for short-term use for jet lag and other circadian rhythm disorders; however, its effectiveness compared with specific melatonin receptor agonists available

TABLE 20. Drug Treatment of Primary Insomnia

Agent, Dosage	Half-Life (hour)	Side Effects
Benzodiazepines		Daytime sedation, dizziness, anterograde amnesia, falls, rebound insomnia
Estazolam, 1-2 mg	10-24	
Flurazepam, 15-30 mg	2-3	
Quazepam, 7.5-30 mg	40	
Temazepam, 7.5-30 mg	8-15	
Triazolam, 0.125-0.5 mg	2-5	
Nonbenzodiazepine sedative – hypnotic agents		Daytime sedation, dizziness, anterograde amnesia, falls, rebound insomnia
Zolpidem, 5-10 mg	3	
Zaleplon, 5-10 mg	1	
Eszopiclone, 2-3 mg	5-7	Unpleasant taste, dry mouth, drowsiness, dizziness
Melatonin-receptor agonist		
Ramelteon, 8 mg	2-5	Drowsiness, dizziness, increased serum prolactin levels

Adapted with permission from Wilson JF. In the clinic. Insomnia. Ann Intern Med. 2008;148(1):ITC13-1-ITC13-16. [PMID: 18166757] Copyright 2008, American College of Physicians.

by prescription for acute and chronic insomnia is not known. Many patients drink alcohol to help with sleep; although alcohol may help in falling asleep, it interferes with sleep architecture and often causes sleep disruption in the latter half of the night. Dopaminergic agents may be helpful for patients with insomnia associated with restless legs syndrome (see MKSAP 16 Neurology).

Referral to a sleep specialist is indicated if the etiology of insomnia remains unclear, if daytime functioning is impaired, if the insomnia is refractory to therapy, or if the patient requests it. Consultation may also be helpful for patients with restless legs syndrome or other primary sleep disorders, such as narcolepsy. Pulmonary, otolaryngology, or dental referral may be helpful for patients with obstructive sleep apnea or if specific upper airway anatomic abnormalities are suspected. Psychiatric referral is helpful for patients with concurrent psychiatric disorders, patients requiring high doses of medications for treatment, patients with insomnia refractory to treatment, or patients requiring tapering or titration of medications or combinations of medications.

KEY POINTS

- The first-line treatment of insomnia is improving sleep hygiene; additional options include cognitive-behavioral therapy and medications.
- Short- and intermediate-acting benzodiazepine γ-aminobutyric acid (GABA)-receptor agonists, nonbenzodiazepine GABA-receptor agonists, and melatonin-receptor agonists are all effective in the treatment of insomnia, but have different risks of long-term dependence and tolerance as well as side effects.

- Antihistamines such as diphenhydramine have a long half-life, have significant anticholinergic side effects, and often have carry-over sedation; they are a poor choice for treating insomnia in the elderly.

Syncope

Syncope is defined as the transient loss of consciousness with loss of postural tone and spontaneous recovery, resulting from global cerebral hypoperfusion. Loss of consciousness distinguishes syncope from pseudosyncopal events, such as drop attacks and simple falls, and global cerebral hypoperfusion distinguishes syncope from other causes of loss of consciousness, such as seizure and stroke. The loss of consciousness of syncope is usually less than 1 minute, with complete restoration of orientation and function at the time of recovery.

Neurocardiogenic Syncope

Neurocardiogenic syncope, the most common type, is predominantly a clinical diagnosis. Vasovagal neurocardiogenic syncope (the common "faint") results from a reflex withdrawal of sympathetic tone accompanied by an increase in vagal tone, precipitating a drop in blood pressure and heart rate. Without the surge in vagal tone, bradycardia is absent; this variant is called vasodepressor syncope. Patients with neurocardiogenic syncope often experience a prodromal phase, usually longer than 10 seconds, characterized by palpitations, nausea, blurred vision, warmth, diaphoresis, or lightheadedness, although these symptoms are less common in the elderly. Provoking factors include prolonged standing, postural change, hot environments, emotional distress, and preload-reducing situations (dehydration, use of diuretics or vasodilators). The first episode usually occurs at a young age, and recurrences are common. Variants of neurocardiogenic syncope that are specifically situational include cough, sneeze, defecation, swallow, micturition, laughter, post-exercise, and post-prandial syncope. Carotid sinus syncope occurs after mechanical manipulation of the carotid sinuses, altering sympathetic and parasympathetic tone; it may be reproduced by carotid sinus massage and is more common in the elderly, in men, and in those with underlying structural heart disease.

Orthostatic Hypotension

Orthostatic hypotension is characterized by an abnormal drop in blood pressure with standing (greater than 20 mm Hg systolic or 10 mm Hg diastolic). Since orthostatic changes may be "initial" (immediate), "classic" (within 3 minutes), or delayed, syncope may occur immediately (0-3 minutes) or be delayed (up to 30 minutes). Orthostatic syncope is more common in the elderly; in those taking vasoactive drugs, diuretics, or alcohol; and in the setting of volume depletion or autonomic failure, such as primary or idiopathic autonomic neuropathy. It may occur in association with Parkinson disease, diabetes, amyloidosis, Shy-Drager syndrome, and lower motor neuron injuries. Patients commonly have symptoms of dizziness, weakness, and fatigue, both before and after the event.

A unique variant of orthostatic intolerance is postural orthostatic tachycardia syndrome, usually seen in young women and related to inadequate venous return with significant tachycardia; patients may experience symptoms of light-headedness and palpitations, but not syncope.

Cardiac Causes of Syncope

Cardiac diseases account for the remaining causes of true syncope and predominate in the elderly. Arrhythmias are the most common and the most worrisome causes of syncope and include bradycardias (sinus and atrioventricular node dysfunction) as well as tachyarrhythmias (supraventricular and ventricular; atrial tachyarrhythmias rarely cause syncope). Patients with an arrhythmogenic cause of syncope usually have had only one or two episodes, with less than 5 seconds of warning symptoms before each episode. Patients often have underlying structural heart disease as a contributing cause. A prolonged QT interval may result in arrhythmia causing syncope and can be drug-related (see MKSAP 16 Cardiovascular Medicine). Clues to arrhythmia include brief or absent prodrome, palpitations immediately preceding the episode, and syncope occurring in the supine position. (An exception is ventricular tachycardia, which usually has a warning prodrome of more than 5 seconds and associated diaphoresis).

Other cardiac causes resulting in inadequate cardiac output and subsequent cerebral hypoperfusion include valvular heart disease, cardiac tumors, pericardial disease, and cardiomyopathy. Clues to structural heart disease include relationship to exercise or exertion, sensitivity to volume status, and association with medications. Cardiac ischemia, pulmonary embolism, and aortic dissection are unusual causes of syncope and rarely occur without other symptoms.

Diagnostic Evaluation of Syncope

The diagnostic evaluation of syncope begins with a thorough history and physical examination. The history and physical examination reveal an etiology in one-third to two-thirds of patients. In addition, the history often helps with risk stratification as well as with diagnosis. Any witnesses should be interviewed, as patients may not remember important aspects of the event. Important aspects of the history include age, position, prodrome, triggers, associated symptoms, duration of symptoms, previous episodes and duration between episodes, medications, family history (especially in young patients), and underlying medical conditions. Vital signs, including orthostatic vital signs, often contribute to the diagnosis. Elderly patients may have asymptomatic orthostasis. Thus, it is important to document symptom reproduction with elicitation of orthostatic change; otherwise, an alternative cause for syncope should be sought. Carotid artery palpation and auscultation and detailed cardiopulmonary, abdominal, and neurologic examinations should be performed. Carotid sinus massage should be performed in patients suspected of having carotid sinus hypersensitivity but is contraindicated in patients with recent myocardial infarction or cerebral ischemia.

Despite its low diagnostic yield, a 12-lead electrocardiogram (ECG) remains the first and most widely recommended test to perform in patients being evaluated for syncope, partly owing to its noninvasive nature, availability, and low cost. Although this test is relatively insensitive for finding a specific cause of syncope, its specificity is high, and an abnormal ECG is used to identify and stratify patients for additional testing.

The remainder of the evaluation should be directed by the unique circumstances of the patient's event. Guidelines for syncope generally do not dictate the degree of detail considered necessary for further testing. Echocardiography is recommended in patients suspected of having structural heart disease. If an arrhythmia is suspected, documentation of the arrhythmia is indicated either by inpatient telemetry or ambulatory monitoring (see MKSAP 16 Cardiovascular Medicine). No specific routine laboratory studies are recommended, although women of reproductive age warrant a pregnancy test. Tests with the lowest likelihood of affecting diagnosis or management include head CT scan, carotid Doppler ultrasonography, electroencephalography, and measurement of cardiac enzyme levels; these studies may be indicated if symptoms point to specific etiologies but otherwise should be omitted from the work-up. Recommendations to not routinely perform cardiac enzyme testing are supported by evidence that patients with cardiac ischemia almost always present with chest pain or ECG changes. Neurologic studies have only been shown to be useful in patients with new neurologic findings on initial evaluation. Tilt-table testing should be reserved for patients with suspected neurocardiogenic syncope not confirmed by history and physical examination, for those with recurrent syncopal episodes, and for patients suspected of having arrhythmogenic syncope or who have a high risk profile for cardiovascular events in whom previous testing has not been revealing.

Risk Stratification and Management of Syncope

Several risk scores have been developed and validated in order to identify patients with syncope at high risk of adverse events. Causes of syncope vary according to the clinical setting in which the evaluation was conducted (office versus emergency department), and a significant number of patients (40%-50%) never present for evaluation; this number is higher in younger persons. Risk stratification thus is subject to patient population and setting. None of the current risk assessment tools is widely accepted in emergency practice.

Neurocardiogenic and orthostatic syncope both are generally benign in nature and do not require hospitalization. An exception is an elderly patient in whom a secondary cause of orthostasis is suspected or in whom recurrent episodes carry risk for harm from trauma. For neurocardiogenic causes, management may consist of patient education with specific instructions on abortive and preventive strategies. These isometric counter-pressure maneuvers include leg crossing, hand-grip, squatting, and muscle tensing. β-Blockers are no longer indicated in vasovagal syncope.

Orthostatic hypotension is associated with a two-fold increase in mortality from underlying causes; these should be treated appropriately. For benign orthostatic causes, treatment consists of the maneuvers listed above, as well as positional changes, maintenance of adequate fluid intake, compression stockings, and possibly midodrine or fludrocortisone if indicated (frequent episodes with subsequent risk of trauma; syncope during high-risk or competitive activities, such as in pilots or athletes). These patients have an excellent prognosis and no increase in mortality. Patients with carotid sinus hypersensitivity benefit from insertion of a dual-chamber permanent pacemaker.

Cardiac causes of syncope carry a high mortality in all age groups; 6-month mortality is greater than 10% and is related to the underlying cause, not the syncope itself. Although younger patients are more likely to have benign causes of syncope, patients with suspected cardiac causes warrant further inpatient evaluation regardless of age. High-risk patients requiring immediate in-hospital telemetry are those with exertional or supine syncope, palpitations before the event, a family history of sudden death, nonsustained ventricular tachycardia, and abnormal ECG findings (conduction abnormalities, bradycardia). Other indications for hospitalization include chest pain, heart failure, syncope without warning signs, hemorrhage, suspected or known heart disease, and frequent recurrent episodes. **H**

KEY POINTS

- Tests in the evaluation of syncope with the lowest likelihood of affecting diagnosis or management include head CT scan, carotid Doppler ultrasonography, electroencephalography, and measurement of cardiac enzyme levels; these studies should not be performed in the absence of symptoms pointing to specific etiologies.

- Indications for hospitalization in patients with syncope include chest pain, heart failure, syncope without warning signs, hemorrhage, suspected or known heart disease, and frequent recurrent episodes.

- High-risk patients with syncope requiring immediate in-hospital telemetry are those with exertional or supine syncope, palpitations before the event, a family history of sudden death, nonsustained ventricular tachycardia, or abnormal electrocardiographic findings.

Chest Pain

Chest pain accounts for 2% of all outpatient visits to primary care physicians and 5.5 million visits to emergency departments in the United States annually. It is the most common symptom in persons 50 to 64 years of age presenting for emergency care. Approximately 3 million patients are hospitalized each year for further evaluation and treatment. Although a few patients presenting with chest pain have true medical emergencies or require inpatient care, prompt and accurate diagnosis is nonetheless essential. The physician must not only distinguish ischemic from nonischemic chest pain but also distinguish emergent causes of chest pain from nonemergent ones. Misdiagnosis can be catastrophic for the patient and a source of a malpractice claim against the physician.

The most likely cause of chest pain varies according to patient characteristics and the presentation setting. In the outpatient setting, musculoskeletal causes are the most common, accounting for approximately 40% of cases, followed by gastrointestinal disease (19%). In the emergency department, acute coronary syndromes are more common, accounting for up to 13% of patient visits.

Differential Diagnosis

The differential diagnosis of chest pain largely consists of cardiac, pulmonary, gastrointestinal, and musculoskeletal disease. Dermatologic disease (herpes zoster affecting thoracic dermatomes) and psychiatric conditions (anxiety, panic attack) also can result in chest pain. Whereas most causes of chest pain can be evaluated and treated in a nonurgent fashion, others, such as acute coronary syndromes,

CONT.

aortic dissection, tension pneumothorax, and pulmonary embolism, require rapid triage for definitive diagnosis and intervention.

Cardiac Causes of Chest Pain

Cardiac causes of chest pain include ischemia (acute coronary syndromes, stable angina), aortic dissection, myocarditis, pericarditis, and aortic stenosis. A standard diagnostic approach is to distinguish ischemic chest pain from nonischemic causes as the first step. Characterization of the chest pain is helpful, as pain descriptors provided by the patient can increase or decrease the likelihood of ischemia. (Assessment of pretest probability of ischemic heart disease based on age, sex, and description of the pain is discussed in MKSAP 16 Cardiovascular Medicine.) In a meta-analysis describing the value and limitations of the chest pain history in the evaluation of patients with suspected acute myocardial infarction, radiation to the right arm or shoulder and radiation to both arms or shoulders had the highest positive likelihood ratios (LR+) of 4.7 and 4.1, respectively. Other pain descriptors that increase the likelihood of acute myocardial infarction are pain associated with exertion (LR+ 2.4), radiation to the left arm (LR+ 2.3), diaphoresis (LR+ 2.0), nausea or vomiting (LR+ 1.9), and pain that is pressure-like (LR+ 1.3). Descriptors that decrease the likelihood of acute myocardial infarction include pleuritic pain (LR+ 0.2); pain described as either positional, sharp, or reproducible with palpation (LR+ 0.3); and pain that is either inframammary in location or not associated with exertion (LR+ 0.8). In one study of 48 patients, no patient with sharp or stabbing pain that was positional, pleuritic, or reproducible with palpation and who had no history of angina or myocardial infarction was diagnosed with acute myocardial infarction at discharge. There is no predictable association between acute myocardial infarction and relief of chest pain with nitroglycerin. A high index of suspicion is necessary in women, the elderly, and patients with diabetes, as they may not present with classic symptoms.

Patients presenting with acute chest pain can be stratified into high, intermediate, or low risk of having an acute coronary syndrome based on information easily available in the office setting, including pain descriptors, history of heart disease, cardiac risk factors, and 12-lead ECG (**Table 21**). The ECG can be diagnostic (new ST-segment elevation or depression, T-wave inversion in multiple leads). In some patients, however, the ECG is normal or near-normal even in the presence of acute ischemia, and serial evaluations may be necessary.

Several more detailed prediction tools and algorithms have been published in an attempt to guide further evaluation and therapy and minimize unnecessary testing. These tools,

TABLE 21. Likelihood that Signs and Symptoms Represent an Acute Coronary Syndrome Secondary to CAD			
	High Likelihood	**Intermediate Likelihood**	**Low Likelihood**
Feature	**Any of the following:**	**Absence of high-likelihood features and presence of any of the following:**	**Absence of high- or intermediate-likelihood features but may have:**
History	Chest or left arm pain or discomfort as chief symptom reproducing prior documented angina Known history of CAD, including MI	Chest or left arm pain or discomfort as chief symptom Age >70 y Male sex Diabetes mellitus	Probable ischemic symptoms in absence of any of the intermediate-likelihood characteristics Recent cocaine use
Physical examination	Transient MR murmur, hypotension, diaphoresis, pulmonary edema, or crackles	Extracardiac vascular disease	Chest discomfort reproduced by palpation
ECG	New, or presumably new, transient ST-segment deviation (1 mm or greater) or T-wave inversion in multiple precordial leads	Fixed Q waves ST-segment depression 0.5 to 1 mm or T-wave inversion greater than 1 mm	T-wave flattening or inversion less than 1 mm in leads with dominant R waves Normal ECG
Cardiac markers	Elevated serum cardiac troponin I, troponin T, or creatine kinase MB	Normal	Normal

CAD = coronary artery disease; ECG = electrocardiogram; MI = myocardial infarction; MR = mitral regurgitation.

Common Symptoms

utilizing history, physical examination, ECG, and cardiac bio-markers (creatine kinase MB, troponin), are predominantly used in emergency departments.

Aortic dissection is characterized by sudden and severe pain at onset, often with a tearing, splitting, or ripping quality that radiates to the back. Asymmetric intensity of peripheral pulses (pulse deficit) is a strong predictor (LR+ 5.7), and the chest radiograph may demonstrate a widened mediastinum. These classic features are often absent, however, and an acute aortic condition must be considered in any patient with severe thoracic pain. Pericarditis and myocarditis usually present with pleuritic chest pain. The pain in pericarditis is unaffected by exercise, worsens with recumbency, and is relieved with sitting forward. A pericardial rub may be present. Classic ECG findings are diffuse ST-segment elevation and PR-segment depression. Aortic stenosis may cause exertional chest pain, which may be accompanied by syncope, dyspnea, and other signs of heart failure.

Pulmonary Causes of Chest Pain

Pulmonary causes of chest pain include pulmonary embolism, pneumothorax, pleuritis, pneumonia, pulmonary hypertension, and other parenchymal lesions. In general, the pain with pulmonary embolism, pneumothorax, pleuritis, and pneumonia is pleuritic in nature and accompanied by dyspnea.

With pulmonary embolism, pain may be accompanied by cough, wheezing, hemoptysis, tachypnea, and tachycardia. Risk factors include immobilization, recent surgery, paresis, history of deep venous thrombosis, malignancy, obesity, tobacco use, and estrogen therapy. The diagnosis is made by ventilation-perfusion scan, chest CT angiography, or pulmonary artery angiography (see MKSAP 16 Pulmonary and Critical Care Medicine). In low-probability scenarios, a negative D-dimer test can be helpful in ruling out thromboembolism.

Pneumothorax can be primary (spontaneous) or secondary. Rupture of a subpleural bleb underlies a spontaneous pneumothorax, and lifetime recurrence rates are up to 50%. Secondary pneumothorax occurs in patients with underlying pulmonary disease such as COPD, cystic fibrosis, or tuberculosis. Physical examination demonstrates decreased chest expansion, decreased breath sounds, and hyperresonance to percussion, all on the affected side. Diagnosis is made by chest radiograph. Tension pneumothorax, heralded by hypotension and tracheal deviation to the unaffected side, is a medical emergency.

Pulmonary hypertension includes pulmonary arterial hypertension and pulmonary hypertension secondary to other conditions, including heart, lung, and thromboembolic disease. The chest pain associated with pulmonary hypertension is not pleuritic but usually is accompanied by exertional dyspnea and fatigue. In most patients, the pain is due to ischemia from either subendocardial hypoperfusion or compression of coronary arteries by enlarged pulmonary arteries. On physical examination, jugular venous pressure is often elevated, there may be a parasternal heave, the S_2 heart sound is widely split, and the P_2 (pulmonic valve) component of S_2 is loud.

Gastrointestinal Causes of Chest Pain

The most common gastrointestinal cause of chest pain is GERD. Although often described as burning, it can mimic angina and be relieved by nitroglycerin. It generally is worsened with bending over or recumbency and relieved with antacids, H_2 blockers, or proton pump inhibitors. Other, less common, gastrointestinal causes of chest pain include cholecystitis, cholangitis, esophageal spasm, peptic ulcer disease, and pancreatitis.

Musculoskeletal Causes of Chest Pain

Musculoskeletal chest pain is common, especially in women. Etiologies include costochondritis, osteoarthritis, and muscle strain. The pain is sharp, occasionally pleuritic, worsened or reproduced with movement or palpation, and relieved with NSAIDs. It may last for weeks. Pain that worsens with movement can raise concern for ischemia, and a careful history is essential. Imaging is usually not indicated or helpful.

Chest Pain and Decision to Hospitalize

The decision to hospitalize a patient with chest pain is challenging. The goal is to identify patients with life-threatening disease who require immediate attention while minimizing unnecessary work-up and treatment in others. A rapid clinical determination of the likelihood of an acute coronary syndrome (see Table 21) is the essential first task for the physician and should guide the decision. In addition, the physician should consider the likelihood of short-term adverse outcomes (death, nonfatal myocardial infarction) in patients with an acute coronary syndrome. Patients suspected of having an acute coronary syndrome should be admitted. Low-risk patients can be further stratified with stress testing.

The use of formal risk scores (TIMI, GRACE, PURSUIT) can be useful in further risk stratification and management. While some centers utilize chest pain evaluation units (CPEUs) to streamline evaluation and limit unnecessary coronary care unit admissions, the true cost-effectiveness of these units is unknown.

Despite a comprehensive history, physical examination, and ECG, approximately 2% of patients with an acute coronary syndrome are missed in the emergency department. Women younger than 55 years old and those who are nonwhite, those who report dyspnea as a chief symptom, or those who have normal ECGs are more likely to be discharged. In one study, the risk-adjusted mortality ratio for those not hospitalized compared with those who were was 1.9 (95% CI, 0.7-5.2).

Patients with pneumothorax, pulmonary embolism, and pericarditis are generally hospitalized for further care.

49

CONT.

Aortic dissection and tension pneumothorax always require admission. **H**

Edema

Excess fluid accumulation in the interstitial space leads to edema. Such fluid accumulation results from increased capillary hydrostatic pressure, increased capillary permeability, or decreased plasma oncotic pressure, as well as from retention of sodium and water by the kidneys. Lymphedema, a type of nonpitting edema due to extravasation of high–protein content lymphatic fluid, is caused by congenital lymphatic disease or damage to the lymphatic vessels from surgery, radiation, obstruction, or recurrent cellulitis.

The differential diagnosis of the patient with edema is broad but can be narrowed by history and physical examination. Causes of bilateral edema include heart failure, nephrotic syndrome, cirrhosis, hypoproteinemia, constrictive pericarditis, chronic venous insufficiency, lymphedema, and medications (including minoxidil, nifedipine, amlodipine, thiazolidinediones, NSAIDs, and fludrocortisone). If central venous pressure is elevated, cardiac disease or pulmonary hypertension is likely; if normal, other causes should be considered. The most common causes of unilateral leg edema are deep venous thrombosis, cellulitis, and malignant lymphedema.

The management of edema involves identifying and reversing the underlying disorder. Diuretics should be used carefully, especially in patients whose sodium retention is secondary to a reduction in cardiac output. In these patients, diuretics may further reduce intravascular volume. In patients with chronic venous insufficiency (stasis edema) or lymphedema, diuretic therapy should be avoided because fluid mobilization from the interstitial to the vascular space does not predictably occur. Sodium restriction, leg elevation, and compressive stockings can be helpful.

Musculoskeletal Pain

Acute Low Back Pain

Diagnosis and Evaluation

The prognosis for acute musculoskeletal low back pain is excellent. More than 70% of patients presenting to primary care clinics recover completely, and fewer than 10% seek ongoing care after 3 months. Because of this, initial diagnostic evaluation of acute low back pain should focus on identifying patients at risk for nonmusculoskeletal causes, such as malignancy, infection, or underlying systemic illness. Particular attention should be paid to diagnosis of conditions that require urgent evaluations (tumor, infection, rapidly progressive neurologic symptoms, cauda equina syndrome) and those for which specific treatments may be more effective than symptomatic therapy (rheumatologic diseases, compression fractures).

Psychosocial factors are more useful than the physical examination in predicting the course of recovery in acute back pain. Presence of depression, passive coping strategies, job dissatisfaction, higher disability levels, disputed compensation claims, and somatization all may predict poorer outcomes. In patients with risk factors for ongoing pain, quantitative assessment of the patient's pain and function can be valuable.

History

Age is the most useful screening factor in low back pain. Cancer, compression fractures, and spinal stenosis are all significantly more likely in older patients. Age older than 50 years has a 75% to 90% sensitivity and 60% to 70% specificity for these three diagnoses. Spondyloarthropathies almost always present before the age of 40 years, but this finding is very nonspecific (sensitivity 100%, specificity 7%). Other important factors in the history are shown in **Table 22**.

Neurologic history and physical examination should focus on differentiating disk herniation and accompanying sciatica (unilateral sharp or burning pain radiating down the back or side of the leg, usually to the foot or ankle) from lesions that compress the central spinal cord (cauda equina syndrome). Key findings associated with central spinal cord compression include bowel and bladder dysfunction (particularly urinary retention or incontinence), diminished sensation over the perineum, bilateral or multilevel neurologic deficits, and rapidly progressive neurologic deficits.

TABLE 22. History Features and Suggested Diagnoses in Low Back Pain

Suggested Diagnosis	History Feature
Cancer	Unexplained weight loss
	Failure to improve after 1 month
	No relief with bed rest
Infection	Fever
	Injection drug abuse
	Urinary tract infection
	Skin infection
Inflammatory/rheumatologic condition	Presence of morning stiffness
	Pain not relieved when supine
	Pain persisting for >3 months
	Gradual onset
	Involvement of other joints
Nerve root irritation (radiculopathy)	Sciatica
	Increased pain with cough, sneeze, or Valsalva maneuver
Spinal stenosis	Severe leg pain
	No pain when seated
	Pseudoclaudication
Compression fracture	Trauma
	Corticosteroid use
	Osteoporosis
Cauda equina syndrome	Bowel or bladder dysfunction
	Saddle sensory loss
	Rapidly progressive neurologic deficits

Physical Examination

Clinicians should inspect for scoliosis and kyphosis, noting any erythema or edema that suggests underlying infection or inflammation. Skin findings (for example, psoriasis) that may suggest an underlying inflammatory arthritis should also be noted. Palpation and percussion of the back can help differentiate vertebral tenderness from pain originating in the paraspinous soft tissues. The presence of vertebral tenderness should increase suspicion of compression fracture or infection. The straight-leg raise test (reproduction of pain extending below the knee with 10 degrees to 60 degrees of leg elevation), weakness and diminished reflexes at the ankles, and sensory loss in the feet are all associated with disk herniation. The crossed straight-leg raise test (lifting the unaffected side causing pain in the opposite leg) is less sensitive but more specific than performing the straight-leg raise test on the affected side. The quality of pain is not important

in the straight-leg raise tests; what matters is that the pain radiates below the knee.

Lumbar spinal stenosis is more common in patients older than 65 years and is anecdotally associated with increased pain when walking and relief when sitting, often called neurogenic claudication or pseudoclaudication. Evidence regarding the diagnostic value of neurogenic claudication is limited, however, and the available data suggest a poor positive likelihood ratio. An abnormal Romberg test or a wide-based gait in the presence of pain suggesting spinal stenosis are specific but not sensitive findings.

Further Diagnostic Testing

Patients with nonspecific low back pain and no symptoms or signs to suggest systemic illness should not routinely receive additional diagnostic testing. The American College of Physicians recommends that diagnostic imaging for low back pain be obtained in patients acutely only if they have evidence of a severe progressive neurologic deficit or signs or symptoms suggestive of a serious or specific underlying condition. There is no evidence to suggest an optimal imaging strategy for such patients if pain persists beyond 1 to 2 months, although plain radiography may be reasonable in this circumstance. For patients with a history that suggests malignancy or fracture, plain radiography is recommended for initial imaging. Complete blood count and erythrocyte sedimentation rate can also be helpful in evaluating patients for infection or evidence of systemic illness. In patients with rapidly progressive neurologic symptoms (but not stable mild neurologic symptoms), cauda equina syndrome, or suspicion for epidural abscess or osteomyelitis, MRI is the preferred modality because of better visualization of soft tissues and the spinal canal. If MRI is not feasible, CT myelography is a viable alternative. Noncontrast CT is useful for detecting sacroiliitis and is a reasonable diagnostic study in patients in whom an inflammatory spondyloarthropathy is suspected.

Patients whose symptoms specifically suggest radiculopathy or spinal stenosis should not receive additional imaging unless they have an inadequate response to noninvasive management and are considering surgery or epidural corticosteroid injection. For patients who are considering an invasive intervention, MRI is usually the initial study of choice. Asymptomatic herniated disks are common findings on MRI, so disk herniations that do not cause nerve root impingement or correlate anatomically with the patient's symptoms should be approached with suspicion.

Treatment

Because the overall prognosis for acute musculoskeletal low back pain is excellent, therapeutic interventions should focus on mitigating symptoms and maintaining function while the patient recovers. Most patients without sciatica show substantial improvement within 2 weeks. Patients with sciatica may be slower to improve, but three quarters of patients are substantially better after 3 months. Pain from spinal stenosis is less likely to improve, although even with this condition, some fluctuation is common.

Nonpharmacologic Treatment

Patients should be encouraged to maintain their daily activities as best they can. Bed rest has been shown in several trials to decrease functional recovery and increase pain in patients both with and without sciatica. Spinal manipulation therapy has been shown to be associated with modest benefits in treatment of acute low back pain, comparable to conventional therapy. Most randomized trials of manipulation involved 2 to 3 weeks of therapy; there is no evidence to suggest that long-term manipulation is any more helpful. Massage and yoga have been shown to be helpful in small studies. The improvement seen with acupuncture in chronic back pain is not superior to sham acupuncture. Supervised exercise therapy and physical therapy have not been shown to be effective early in the course of low back pain, but are helpful in patients whose pain persists for more than 4 weeks and to prevent recurrences.

Pharmacologic Treatment

First-line pharmacotherapy for most patients with acute low back pain includes acetaminophen and NSAIDs. NSAIDs should be used with caution in patients at increased risk for nephrotoxicity (older patients and patients with diabetes mellitus, heart failure, or preexisting kidney disease) or gastrointestinal ulcer. Concurrent treatment with a proton pump inhibitor or misoprostol or use of a cyclooxegenase-2 (COX-2) selective NSAID reduces risk of ulcers in patients at high risk and is specifically recommended for patients older than 75 years. Some patients may also be at increased risk of hypertension and cardiovascular events when using NSAIDs, although different drugs have shown these effects to varying degrees in observational studies. When NSAIDs are used, the lowest effective dose should be used for the shortest possible period, especially in older patients and those with comorbidities that put them at risk for complications. Acetaminophen has fewer adverse effects, but doses should be limited to a maximum of 4 g/d to reduce the risk of hepatotoxicity, although even this dose may be linked to hepatotoxicity in patients with moderate to high alcohol use.

Opioid analgesics or tramadol may be helpful in patients with acute low back pain for whom NSAIDs or acetaminophen do not provide adequate relief. Although reasonably safe for short-term use in modest doses, opioids should be used with caution in elderly patients and patients with chronic mechanical low back pain and used only with extreme caution or avoided altogether in patients with a history of addiction or substance abuse.

There are several drugs with diverse mechanisms of action that are collectively referred to as skeletal muscle relaxants. Evidence suggests these drugs may have some modest benefit in pain relief in acute low back pain. All can cause dizziness and sedation, however, and should be used with caution in older patients.

Interventional and Surgical Treatment

Many injection therapies have been tried in the management of low back pain. Epidural corticosteroid injections may provide short-term relief in patients with disk herniations causing radiculopathy, but evidence is mixed and long-term outcomes are unchanged. Facet joint injections, trigger point injections, and prolotherapy lack compelling supportive evidence; American Pain Society guidelines recommend against their use.

Surgery has clearly shown benefit only in patients with disk herniation causing persistent radiculopathy, patients with painful spinal stenosis, and patients with cauda equina syndrome. For patients with radiculopathy, diskectomy and microdiskectomy show improved outcomes at 6 to 12 weeks compared with nonsurgical therapy, although both surgical and nonsurgical groups tend to continue to improve with time, and differences in outcomes diminish over 1 to 2 years. In spinal stenosis, decompressive laminectomy shows moderate benefits compared with nonsurgical therapy for the first 1 to 2 years, again with diminishing effects in long-term follow-up.

Cauda equina syndrome is considered an emergency **H** because of the risk of rapid, irreversible loss of neurologic function and because of its association with urgent underlying conditions, such as neoplasia or infection. Management typically involves prompt surgical decompression of the affected area of the spinal cord. **H**

For patients with neither radiculopathy nor spinal stenosis, the value of surgery is questionable. Available evidence is of moderate quality and suggests that outcomes from surgery are similar to those of nonsurgical therapy. When benefit has been shown in clinical trials, it is limited to a narrow group of patients with more than 1 year of moderately severe pain and disability and without serious medical or psychiatric comorbidities.

KEY POINTS

- Patients with nonspecific low back pain and no symptoms or signs to suggest systemic illness should not routinely receive additional diagnostic testing.
- Most patients with acute low back pain improve within 3 months with conservative therapy.

Neck Pain

Diagnosis and Evaluation

Neck pain typically arises from three broad categories of conditions: mechanical neck pain arising from muscles, joints, and associated tissues; neurogenic neck pain arising from a cervical nerve root to the spinal cord; and neck pain associated with systemic disease. Initial approach to the history and physical examination should aim to differentiate these categories.

Mechanical neck pain is typically an aching pain localized to the neck, although it may be referred up toward the head or down toward the shoulder girdle. The history may include injury (for example, whiplash or acute strain) or unaccustomed activity, suggesting an overuse syndrome. Physical examination often reveals decreased range of motion, tenderness over soft tissues, and pain caused or exacerbated by flexion or extension of the neck.

Neurogenic pain is typically burning and often radiates to the shoulder or down the arm. Patients may have dermatomal numbness or muscle weakness in the distribution of a cervical nerve root. Involvement of multiple spinal levels, spasticity, hyperreflexia, gait abnormality, or leg weakness all suggest central spinal cord compression.

Patients with underlying systemic illnesses frequently have symptoms suggesting the underlying problem. These may include fever, weight loss, joint pain or arthritis elsewhere, symptoms of polymyalgia rheumatica (headache, visual changes, shoulder and hip girdle pain), or history of immunosuppression, cancer, or injection drug use. Anterior neck pain is an unusual presentation of cervical spine disease and should lead the clinician to suspect other anatomic structures as possible sources of pain. Physical examination should be directed toward identifying underlying systemic illness based on symptoms and risk factors.

Imaging studies should be directed based on suspicions raised during history and physical examination. Mechanical neck pain outside of the setting of acute trauma rarely requires imaging, although plain films can be helpful in patients older than 50 years to exclude malignancy and to assess for osteoarthritic changes. Patients with weakness, hyporeflexia, or symptoms or signs of spinal cord involvement should be evaluated with MRI or CT myelography. Patients with symptoms or signs of systemic illness and a suspected anatomic abnormality in the neck (tumor, abscess, pathologic fracture, or disease of anterior neck structures) should have imaging directed at the suspected underlying cause.

Blood tests are not routinely needed for evaluation of patients with neck pain, but should be ordered as appropriate to exclude or confirm underlying systemic illness. Erythrocyte sedimentation rate, C-reactive protein, and complete blood count can be useful in evaluating for infection or inflammatory conditions.

Treatment

Most patients with neck pain recover with conservative therapy. For patients with mechanical neck pain, mobilization and a gentle home exercise program have been shown to be beneficial. For patients with cervical radiculopathy, the role of either hard or soft cervical collars is unclear, and acupuncture does not appear to offer clinically significant benefit. As in low back pain, acetaminophen and NSAIDs are first-line pharmacotherapy for most patients with acute neck pain. Opioids and skeletal muscle relaxants should be reserved for patients with a poor response to acetaminophen and NSAIDs or who are having difficulty sleeping (in which case sedation is a desirable effect). Patients with neurogenic neck pain may find additional benefit from medications targeting neuropathic pain (see Common Symptoms, Chronic Noncancer Pain, Management).

Interventional therapy is not beneficial for patients with mechanical neck pain. Epidural corticosteroid injection may be beneficial in patients with stable radiculopathy that fails to respond to conservative therapy. Surgery is clearly indicated in patients with progressive neurologic symptoms that stem from a defined anatomic abnormality. The role of surgery in patients with chronic neck pain without progressive neurologic deficits is controversial; limited data suggest faster short-term pain relief but no long-term difference compared with conservative management.

KEY POINTS

- Mechanical neck pain outside of the setting of acute trauma rarely requires imaging, although plain films can be helpful in patients older than 50 years to exclude malignancy and to assess for osteoarthritic changes.

- Most patients with neck pain recover with conservative therapy.

Shoulder Pain

Diagnosis and Evaluation

Important historical features to elicit in the evaluation of shoulder pain include location, severity, chronicity, circumstances of onset, history of trauma, and associated symptoms. Shoulder pain may arise from structures of the shoulder (intrinsic disorders) or may be referred from other sites (extrinsic disorders). Pain with movement of the shoulder along with stiffness, locking, catching, and instability all suggest an intrinsic disorder, whereas a normal shoulder examination or the presence of constitutional symptoms and respiratory or gastrointestinal symptoms suggests an extrinsic or systemic etiology. Neck pain, decreased range of motion of the neck, paresthesias, and pain that radiates down the arm past the elbow suggest cervical spine disease. Pain that worsens with intake of food raises the possibility of pain referred from a gallbladder disorder. Discomfort with physical (nonshoulder) exertion should raise concern for cardiac ischemia. Other extrinsic causes of shoulder pain include pneumonia, apical lung masses, and diaphragmatic irritation due to a variety of causes.

Examination of the shoulder should include inspection, palpation, range-of-motion testing (both passive and active), and provocative maneuvers. It is important to begin by fully exposing both shoulders and examining for any asymmetry or muscle wasting. Palpation should include the acromioclavicular (AC) joint, bicipital groove, all bony structures, and the cervical spine. Pain that is only present with active but not passive range-of-motion testing suggests an extraarticular condition; pain with both active and passive range-of-motion testing suggests an intraarticular condition. Pain that occurs between 60 and 120 degrees of abduction suggests a rotator cuff impingement syndrome, whereas pain with more than 120 degrees of abduction favors AC joint pathology.

Many provocative tests are commonly performed in the assessment of shoulder pain (**Table 23**). The Apley scratch test can be used to assess range of motion. The Neer (**Figure 7**) and Hawkins (**Figure 8**) tests are both useful for diagnosing rotator cuff impingement. The Yergason test (**Figure 9**) is used to assess inflammation of the long head of the biceps and lesions of the glenoid labrum. The apprehension test (**Figure 10**) assesses anterior glenohumeral instability.

Rotator Cuff Disorders

Rotator cuff tendinitis (inflammation of the rotator cuff tendons) can result from repetitive overhead motions, shoulder instability, or trauma. The supraspinatus tendon is most commonly affected and is sometimes accompanied by tendinitis of the long head of the biceps muscle.

Impingement syndrome results from compression of the rotator cuff between the inferior surface of the acromion and the superior surface of the humeral head. Impingement

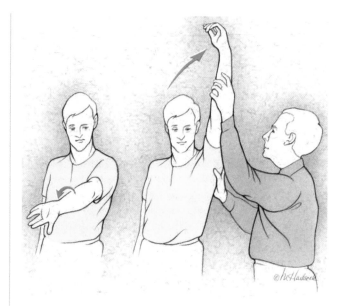

FIGURE 7. Neer test. The examiner applies forced flexion to the affected arm while the arm is fully pronated. This test is considered positive if pain is elicited and suggests either rotator cuff tendinitis or subacromial impingement.

© Maria Hartsock, CMI. Reprinted from Woodward TW, Best TW. The painful shoulder: part I. Clinical evaluation. Am Fam Physician. 2000;61(10):3079-3088. [PMID: 10839557]

symptoms are worse with abduction of the arm, as the space between the acromion and humeral head is smallest with this movement. Impingement can be caused by spurs on the

TABLE 23. Tests Used in Shoulder Evaluation and Significance of Positive Finding		
Test	**Maneuver**	**Diagnosis Suggested by Positive Result**
Apley scratch test	Patient touches superior and inferior aspects of opposite scapula	Loss of range of motion: rotator cuff problem
Neer test	Forced flexion of pronated arm	Subacromial impingement (89% sensitivity; 31% specificity)
Hawkins test	Forward flexion of the shoulder to 90 degrees and internal rotation	Supraspinatus tendon impingement (92% sensitivity; 25% specificity)
Drop-arm test	Attempted slow lowering of arm to waist	Rotator cuff tear
Cross-arm test	Forward elevation to 90 degrees and active adduction	Acromioclavicular joint arthritis
Spurling test	Spine extended with head rotated to affected shoulder while axially loaded	Cervical nerve root disorder
Apprehension test	Anterior pressure on the humerus with external rotation	Anterior glenohumeral instability
Relocation test	Posterior force on humerus while externally rotating the arm	Anterior glenohumeral instability
Sulcus sign	Pulling downward on elbow or wrist	Inferior glenohumeral instability
Yergason test	Elbow flexed to 90 degrees with forearm pronated	Biceps tendon instability or tendinitis
Speed maneuver	Elbow flexed 20 to 30 degrees and forearm supinated	Biceps tendon instability or tendinitis
"Clunk" sign	Rotation of loaded shoulder from extension to forward flexion	Labral disorder

Reprinted with permission from The Painful Shoulder: Part I. Clinical Evaluation., May 15, 2000, Vol 61, No 10, American Family Physician Copyright © 2000 American Academy of Family Physicians. All Rights Reserved.

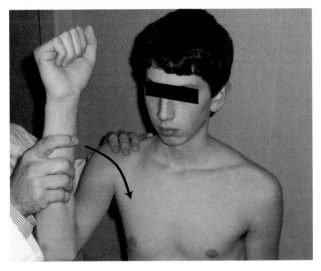

FIGURE 8. Hawkins test for shoulder impingement. The patient holds the arm extended anteriorly at 90 degrees with the forearm bent to 90 degrees (at 12 o'clock), as if holding a shield. The scapula should be stabilized by the examiner. The arm is then internally rotated to cross in front of the body. A positive test elicits pain in the shoulder.

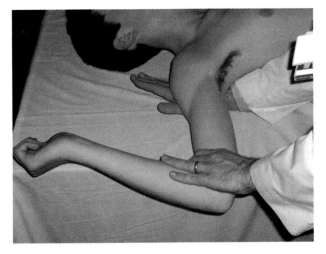

FIGURE 10. Apprehension test. The patient is placed supine on a table. With the arm abducted at 90 degrees and the forearm flexed, the examiner stands at the bedside facing the patient and places one hand under the affected shoulder. With the other hand, gentle pressure is placed on the forearm. Pain or apprehension constitutes a positive test.

acromion, calcification of the coracoacromial ligament, or superior migration of the humeral head during abduction. If left untreated, impingement may lead to a full-thickness rotator cuff tear.

Patients with either rotator cuff tendinitis or impingement have pain located over the lateral deltoid that is present with abduction and internal rotation of the arm. Nighttime symptoms are common. Examination reveals pain with

abduction between 60 degrees and 120 degrees. Pain may be elicited with deep palpation of the lateral deltoid inferior to the acromion process. Both the Neer and Hawkins tests are sensitive but less specific for diagnosing impingement syndrome.

Weakness and loss of function should raise concern for a rotator cuff tear. Examination findings include supraspinatus weakness, weakness with external rotation, evidence of impingement, and a positive drop-arm test. When the diagnosis is not clear or if concern exists for a rotator cuff tear, imaging of the shoulder should be obtained. MRI is the preferred imaging modality (>90% sensitivity), although ultrasonography, in experienced hands, is also an option.

Management of rotator cuff disease is multifaceted. Initially, management includes rest, modification of activities, and NSAIDs to help reduce inflammation and provide pain relief. Subacromial corticosteroid injection has been shown to improve pain for up to 9 months. Physical therapy focused on strengthening the rotator cuff muscles using low-resistance exercises may be beneficial in stabilizing the head of the humerus and reducing impingement. Partial-thickness tears can be managed similar to tendinitis. Full-thickness tears may require surgical intervention depending on other patient characteristics (such as age, type of daily activities, or profession).

Adhesive Capsulitis

Adhesive capsulitis (frozen shoulder) is caused by thickening of the capsule surrounding the glenohumeral joint. It is associated with diabetes, Parkinson disease, stroke, previous trauma, and hypothyroidism but may be idiopathic, particularly in the elderly. It can also occur in the setting of a shoulder or arm injury with concomitant restriction in movement

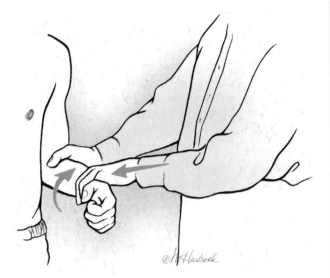

FIGURE 9. The Yergason test consists of resisted supination with the arm at the patient's side and the elbow at 90 degrees of flexion. The test is positive if shoulder pain is elicited.

of the shoulder by the patient. Pain is characteristically slow in onset and is located near the insertion of the deltoid muscle. Patients often avoid lying on the affected side. On examination, there is loss of both active and passive range of motion. Radiographic findings are usually absent.

Initial treatment consists of physical therapy and medication with NSAIDs. Subacromial corticosteroid injection (and intra-articular corticosteroids for refractory cases) is most useful in patients with concurrent rotator cuff pathology. Recovery is typically prolonged (up to 2 years). Consideration for surgical intervention is reserved for those in whom conservative therapy has failed.

Acromioclavicular Joint Degeneration

AC joint degeneration typically results from trauma (in younger patients) or osteoarthritis (in older patients). Bilateral involvement should raise concern for rheumatoid arthritis. On examination, there is pain on palpation of the AC joint. Palpable osteophytes may be present. Pain characteristically occurs with shoulder adduction and abduction above 120 degrees. Plain radiography, if obtained, reveals degenerative changes. Therapy consists of NSAIDs and possibly intra-articular corticosteroid injections. Exercises focused on improving scapular retraction may be beneficial. If these therapies fail, surgical referral is warranted.

KEY POINTS

- Management of rotator cuff disease includes rest, activity modification, and anti-inflammatory therapy; after resolution of symptoms, an exercise program to strengthen the rotator cuff muscles should be initiated.
- Management of adhesive capsulitis consists of physical therapy and oral anti-inflammatory agents; recovery is typically prolonged.

Elbow Pain

Diagnosis and Evaluation

One should begin by obtaining a complete description of the patient's pain. Examination of the elbow includes inspection, palpation, range-of-motion testing, and special tests (see individual conditions below). The neck, shoulder, and wrist should also be examined, as pain can be referred to the elbow from each of these sites.

Epicondylitis

Lateral epicondylitis (tennis elbow) is caused by overuse of the wrist extensor muscles and is most commonly observed in nonathletes, such as computer users who use a mouse. The pain is located laterally, characteristically radiates down the forearm to the dorsal hand, and worsens with activity and at night. On examination, there is tenderness to palpation where the extensor muscles attach to the lateral epicondyle. Pain increases with forced extension of the wrist.

Medial epicondylitis (golfer's elbow) is characterized by pain in the medial elbow and proximal forearm that occurs with activities that require wrist flexion. On examination, there is tenderness to palpation from the medial epicondyle to the pronator teres and flexor carpi radialis muscles. Pain increases with wrist flexion and resisted forearm supination.

Rest, avoidance of activities that worsen pain, stretching, and resistance exercises constitute initial therapy. Corticosteroid injection and oral NSAIDs may provide short-term (but not long-term) relief of symptoms when other measures fail. Surgery may be required for refractory cases.

Olecranon Bursitis

Olecranon bursitis, characterized by painful swelling of the posterior elbow, can result from repetitive trauma, inflammation (gout, rheumatoid arthritis), or infection. On examination, there is localized swelling posterior to the olecranon process without limitation of range of motion of the elbow. When pain, inflammation, or fever is present, fluid should be aspirated for Gram stain, culture, and crystal analysis to rule out septic bursitis and to evaluate for gout. Treatment options include NSAIDs and corticosteroid injection (once infection has been ruled out). Chronic effusions may require surgical intervention.

Ulnar Nerve Entrapment

Entrapment of the ulnar nerve at the elbow (cubital tunnel syndrome) commonly manifests with pain in the elbow with flexion that radiates to the hand accompanied by paresthesias and sensory loss involving the fourth and fifth fingers (**Figure 11**). Weakness is a late finding. Treatment consists of splinting, NSAIDs, and surgical decompression when severe.

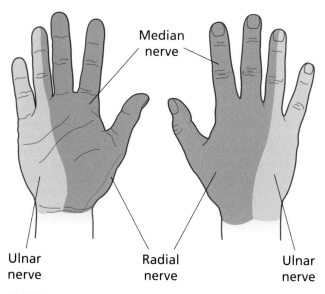

FIGURE 11. Innervation of the hand.

Wrist and Hand Pain

Indications for Imaging

Radiographs (posteroanterior, posteroanterior oblique, and lateral views) should be obtained in all patients with wrist or hand pain with both a history of trauma and localized tenderness to palpation to exclude fracture. Radiographs are also helpful in patients with suspected osteoarthritis.

Carpal Tunnel Syndrome

Carpel tunnel syndrome is caused by compression of the median nerve at the level of the wrist. Risk factors include female sex, obesity, pregnancy, diabetes, hypothyroidism, connective tissue disorders, and rheumatoid arthritis.

The most common clinical presentation is of pain and paresthesias in the distribution of the median nerve (see Figure 11). Patients may also report paresthesias involving all five fingers. Pain is usually worse at night and may radiate into the proximal arm. If left untreated, thenar muscle atrophy may occur. Symptoms may be unilateral or bilateral, with bilateral symptoms occurring in up to 65% of patients at the time of presentation.

The most useful history and examination findings in diagnosing carpal tunnel syndrome are use of a hand symptom diagram, thumb abduction and opposition weakness, and hypalgesia in the territory of the median nerve. The Phalen maneuver and Tinel sign are frequently used but have poor test characteristics. Nerve conduction studies are widely considered to be the diagnostic standard for carpal tunnel syndrome (sensitivity >85%, specificity >95%) and are helpful to obtain when the diagnosis is uncertain.

First-line therapies include avoidance of repetitive motions involving the wrist and hand and nocturnal splinting of the wrist at a neutral angle. Corticosteroid injection of the carpal tunnel appears to provide short-term benefit in patients with mild to moderate disease. A 2-week course of oral corticosteroids appears to be effective on at least a short-term basis. NSAIDs, diuretics, and pyridoxine have all been used, but evidence of their efficacy is lacking.

Surgery is indicated in patients with at least moderately severe disease with persistent symptoms (6 or more months), severe motor impairment, and nerve conduction studies that confirm the diagnosis.

Other Causes of Wrist and Hand Pain

Fracture should be suspected when there is a history of direct trauma and localized tenderness to palpation on examination. Distal radius and scaphoid fractures most commonly result from a fall on an outstretched hand. If clinical suspicion for a scaphoid fracture is high, treatment should not be delayed even if radiographs are normal, as lack of treatment can lead to avascular necrosis. Hamate fractures can result from direct trauma or from repetitive trauma, such as from swinging a golf club or baseball bat.

De Quervain tenosynovitis is caused by inflammation of the abductor pollicis longus and extensor pollicis brevis tendons in the thumb. It is usually associated with repetitive use of the thumb but can also be associated with other conditions, including pregnancy, rheumatoid arthritis, and calcium apatite deposition disease. The typical presentation is of pain on the radial aspect of the wrist that occurs when the thumb is used to pinch or grasp. Examination findings include localized tenderness over the distal portion of the radial styloid process and pain with resisted thumb abduction and extension. Patients also report pain with the Finkelstein test, in which the patient is asked to make a fist over the fully flexed thumb and then to ulnar deviate the hand. This test is positive when pain is present on the radial side of the thumb. Acute therapy consists of applying ice and taping or splinting the thumb to prevent movement. Persistence of symptoms may require injection with a corticosteroid and local anesthetic or use of a short-arm cast with thumb spica. Surgery should be considered in patients with persistent symptoms after a repeat injection.

Ganglion cysts, swellings that overlie either joints or tendons typically on the dorsal surface, arise as a result of chronic irritation of the wrist. If the cyst is not painful, no intervention is required. Treatment options for painful cysts include surgical resection or injection with either a crystalline corticosteroid (preceded by aspiration of the contents) or with hyaluronic acid (followed by aspiration).

Osteoarthritis of the hand is common, often involving the first carpometacarpal joint and the proximal and distal interphalangeal joints. Osteoarthritis of the wrist (radiocarpal arthritis) is uncommon and is almost always post-traumatic. Clinical manifestations of osteoarthritis of the hands and wrists include decreased range of motion, pain that worsens with activity and improves with rest, and swelling. Onset is usually insidious. On examination, one may note bony enlargement of the involved joints. A combination of pharmacologic and nonpharmacologic treatments, individualized to the patient, is recommended. It is important to educate patients about joint protection and refer to physical therapy or provide instructions on hand exercises. Application of heat and ultrasound have been found to be helpful. For mild to moderate pain and when only a few joints are affected, local or topical treatments (topical NSAIDs, capsaicin) are often more effective than systemic treatments.

KEY POINTS

- Radiographs should be obtained in all patients with wrist or hand pain with both a history of trauma and localized tenderness to palpation.

- First-line therapies for carpal tunnel syndrome include avoidance of repetitive motions involving the wrist and hand and nocturnal splinting of the wrist at a neutral angle.

- If clinical suspicion for a scaphoid fracture is high, treatment should not be delayed even if radiographs are normal.

Hip Pain

Diagnosis and Evaluation

Because hip pain can have nonmusculoskeletal causes, it is essential to inquire about symptoms related to the gastrointestinal, gynecologic, and genitourinary systems. On examination, one should observe gait, inspect both the affected and unaffected hips, palpate the sacroiliac joints and bony structures of the hip, including the greater trochanter, and assess range of motion. The FABER test (**Figure 12**) is used to assess Flexion, ABduction, and External Rotation of the hip. It is essential to also perform abdominal, genital, back, and knee examinations, as pain can be referred to the hip from each of these sites. Neurologic and vascular examination of the lower extremities also may help to reveal a cause.

Radiography should be obtained in all patients presenting with acute hip pain to evaluate for fracture. MRI is helpful to evaluate for fracture when radiography is negative but clinical suspicion is high and also to evaluate for avascular necrosis, infection, and tumor, if concern exists.

Specific Causes of Hip Pain

The location of the pain helps to focus the broad differential diagnosis. Anterior (groin) pain is most often caused by osteoarthritis of the hip. The pain is usually chronic, insidious in onset, and worsens with activity. Early morning stiffness may also be present but usually improves with activity. Examination is usually remarkable for decreased and painful internal rotation. Pain may also be produced by logrolling (rocking thigh back and forth with both hands while the patient is supine). When anterior hip pain is acute in onset, the differential diagnosis includes osteonecrosis (most

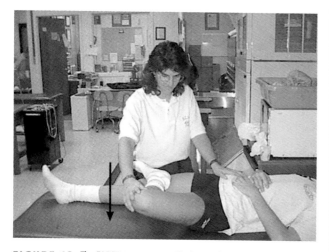

FIGURE 12. The FABER test assesses Flexion, ABduction, and External Rotation of the hip. With the leg in a figure-four position, the normal leg should attain a parallel plane with the table. Gentle downward pressure on the knee in this position simultaneously places stress on the ipsilateral sacroiliac joint.

Reproduced with permission from Davis MF, Davis PF, Ross DS. ACP Expert Guide to Sports Medicine. Philadelphia, PA: American College of Physicians, 2005:360. Copyright 2005, American College of Physicians.

common in the setting of corticosteroid or excessive alcohol use), fracture (suspect when trauma is present), septic arthritis, and acute synovitis. The examination findings for each of these conditions are similar to those seen with osteoarthritis. An extra-articular cause of anterior hip pain should be suspected when hip range of motion is normal and when pain is not elicited by movement of the hip. Extra-articular causes include inguinal hernia, lower abdominal pathology, and lumbar disk disease at the L1 level.

Lateral hip pain is most often caused by trochanteric bursitis, usually resulting from gait abnormalities. Patients with trochanteric bursitis report pain when lying on the affected side in the area of greater trochanter. On examination, there is point tenderness to palpation approximately 2.5 cm (1 in) posterior and superior to the greater trochanter. Treatment consists of correction of the underlying etiology, heat, stretching, and corticosteroid injection. Another cause of lateral hip pain is entrapment of the lateral femoral cutaneous nerve (meralgia paresthetica), frequently presenting as an oval-shaped area of burning, numbness, or tingling on the distal lateral thigh. Lumbar disk disease at the L4-L5 level may also present with pain in the region of the lateral hip and thigh.

Posterior hip pain can result from sacroiliitis, lumbosacral disk disease, and, rarely, pathology affecting the hip joint. Sacroiliac pathology can lead to pain referred to the gluteal region and is characterized by tenderness to palpation of the sacroiliac joint. Spinal disease often causes pain accompanied by paresthesias and back pain. Piriformis syndrome is caused by compression of the sciatic nerve by the piriformis muscle, leading to pain in the buttocks and the distribution of the sciatic nerve. Piriformis syndrome should be considered when sciatica is present without clear evidence of lumbosacral disk disease.

KEY POINT

- In the evaluation of hip pain, it is essential to perform abdominal, genital, back, and knee examinations, as pain can be referred to the hip from each of these sites.

Knee Pain

Diagnosis and Evaluation

Determining the chronicity of pain helps to focus the broad differential diagnosis. The most common cause of chronic knee pain is osteoarthritis. The presence of multijoint involvement along with systemic symptoms raises concern for an inflammatory condition, such as rheumatoid arthritis. The differential diagnosis for acute knee pain includes trauma, overuse, spontaneous meniscal tear, infection, crystalline disease, and inflammatory arthritis. Septic arthritis must be treated without delay.

On examination, both knees should be fully exposed, and the affected knee compared with the unaffected knee. Any asymmetry or swelling should be noted, as should any erythema, ecchymoses, or muscle atrophy. The presence of swelling, especially if the pain is acute and the overlying skin is erythematous, should be considered an indication to perform arthrocentesis to evaluate for both septic arthritis and a crystalline disorder.

All knee structures should be palpated, and range of motion should be evaluated. The integrity of the anterior cruciate ligament can be assessed by performing the anterior drawer and Lachman tests (**Figure 13**). The posterior drawer test is used to assess the posterior cruciate ligament; with the knee at 90 degrees of flexion and the hip at 45 degrees of flexion, posterior force is applied to the proximal tibia and both the extent of movement and the firmness of the endpoint are assessed. A varus stress test assesses the integrity of the lateral collateral ligament, and a valgus stress test assesses the integrity

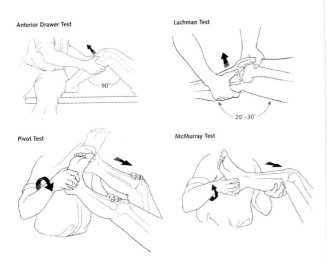

FIGURE 13. Tests for assessing integrity of knee ligaments and injury to knee menisci. (*Top left*) Anterior drawer test (anterior cruciate ligament): Place patient supine, flex the hip to 45 degrees and the knee to 90 degrees. Sit on the dorsum of the foot, wrap your hands around the hamstrings (ensuring that these muscles are relaxed), then pull and push the proximal part of the leg, testing the movement of the tibia on the femur. Do these maneuvers in three positions of tibial rotation: neutral, 30 degrees externally, and 30 degrees internally rotated. A normal test result is no more than 6 to 8 mm of laxity. (*Top right*) Lachman test (anterior cruciate ligament): Place patient supine on examining table, leg at the examiner's side, slightly externally rotated and flexed (20-30 degrees). Stabilize the femur with one hand and apply pressure to the back of the knee with the other hand with the thumb of the hand exerting pressure placed on the joint line. A positive test result is movement of the knee with a soft or mushy end point. (*Bottom left*) Pivot test (anterior cruciate ligament): Fully extend the knee, rotate the foot internally. Apply a valgus stress while progressively flexing the knee, watching and feeling for translation of the tibia on the femur. (*Bottom right*) McMurray test (meniscus): Flex the hip and knee maximally. Apply a valgus (abduction) force to the knee while externally rotating the foot and passively extending the knee. An audible or palpable snap during extension suggests a tear of the medial meniscus. For the lateral meniscus, apply a varus (adduction) stress during internal rotation of the foot and passive extension of the knee.

of the medial collateral ligament (**Figure 14**). The McMurray test (see Figure 13) can be used to detect medial and lateral meniscal injuries, but its low sensitivity increases the likelihood of false-negative results. The medial-lateral grind test is considered the most sensitive (69%) and specific (86%) test for assessing the intactness of the menisci. It is performed with the patient in the supine position. The examiner places the patient's calf in one hand and places the thumb and index finger of the opposite hand over the joint line and then applies varus and valgus stresses to the tibia during both extension and flexion. The test is considered to be positive when the examiner detects a grinding sensation over the joint line with these maneuvers.

Radiographs should be obtained if there is a history of trauma. MRI is useful if concern exists for ligamentous or meniscal injury.

Degenerative Joint Disease

Osteoarthritis most commonly involves the medial compartment of the knee. Pain typically worsens with use and improves with rest. Although morning stiffness may be present, it usually resolves with activity and there are no systemic symptoms. Examination may reveal joint line tenderness, decreased range of motion, crepitus, effusion, and palpable bony changes. Radiographs may aid in determining severity (see MKSAP 16 Rheumatology).

Trauma

Ligamentous injuries of the knee are common. Injury to the anterior cruciate ligament frequently occurs when the patient plants one foot and quickly turns in the opposite direction. Often, a "pop" is heard, swelling quickly develops, and the patient is not able to complete the activity that was being performed when the injury occurred. Medial collateral ligament injuries occur when the knee experiences a valgus force, and lateral collateral ligament injuries occur when the knee experiences a varus force. Medial collateral ligament injuries are much more common than lateral collateral ligament injuries. Meniscal injuries occur with sudden twisting motions of the knee, although "spontaneous" meniscal tears without evidence of significant trauma may occur, primarily in older patients owing to chronic degeneration of the meniscus. Although painful, the patient is able to immediately bear weight. Swelling may occur.

Appropriate treatment of knee trauma is highly dependent on the nature and extent of injury, the degree of dysfunction, and the overall medical status of the patient. Many traumatic knee injuries may be managed without surgical intervention; orthopedic input may be helpful in establishing an optimal therapeutic approach.

Patellofemoral Pain Syndrome

Patellofemoral pain syndrome, an overuse syndrome, typically manifests as anterior knee pain that is worse with prolonged sitting and with walking up and down stairs. It is commonly

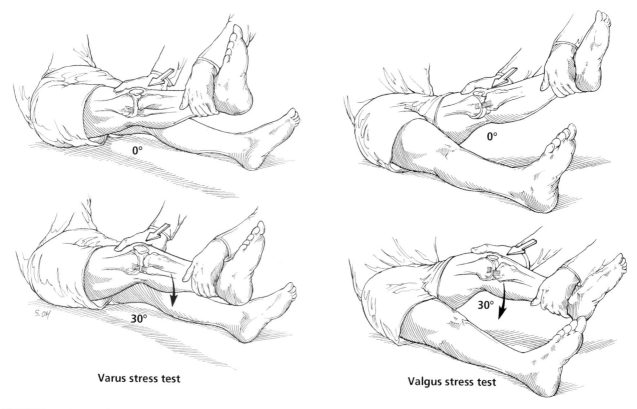

Varus stress test

Valgus stress test

FIGURE 14. Varus and valgus forces applied to knee.

seen in runners but also occurs in nonrunners, and it affects women more than men. On examination, the pain may be reproduced by applying pressure to the surface of the patella (patellofemoral compression test) with the knee in extension and moving the patella laterally or medially. Radiographs are unnecessary as the diagnosis is clinical.

Treatment can be divided into acute (first week) and recovery phases. Treatment during the acute phase focuses on pain control and consists of activity modification, short-term use of NSAIDs, and other conservative measures, such as icing. Treatment during the recovery phase should consist of a rehabilitation program that focuses on strengthening the hip abductor and quadriceps muscles and stretching, although there is no single accepted program.

Bursitis

Pes anserine bursitis manifests as pain located near the antero-medial aspect of the proximal tibia and is most commonly caused by overuse or direct trauma. On examination, tenderness is elicited at the level of the tibial tuberosity (approximately 4 cm [1.5 in] below the level of the medial joint line). Swelling may be present at the insertion of the medial hamstring muscles. Treatment consists of avoiding squatting and limiting repetitive bending and direct pressure on the bursa. Placing a pillow between the legs at night and avoiding

crossing the legs may be helpful, as may the application of ice. Oral NSAIDs have limited usefulness owing to the lack of penetration to the bursal space.

Prepatellar bursitis, inflammation of the bursa lying between the patella and the overlying skin, frequently results from repeated trauma ("housemaid's knee") but can also be caused by infection or gout. Patients with prepatellar bursitis present with pain in the anterior aspect of the knee. Erythema, swelling, and tenderness to palpation may be observed near the lower pole of the patella. Treatment consists of rest and avoidance of kneeling.

Iliotibial Band Syndrome

Iliotibial band syndrome presents as lateral knee pain that is worse with walking up or down steps. It is caused by friction between the iliotibial band and the lateral femoral condyle and is frequently seen in runners and cyclists. Tenderness is present at the lateral femoral epicondyle (approximately 3 cm [1.2 in] proximal to the joint line). A Noble test is performed by having the patient, in the supine position, repeatedly flex and extend the knee with the clinician's thumb placed over the lateral femoral epicondyle. A positive Noble test reproduces the patient's pain.

Treatment is conservative and typically consists of rest, stretching, NSAIDs, and addressing contributing factors (such as running).

Baker Cyst

Patients with a popliteal (Baker) cyst report the insidious onset of posterior knee pain and may also note a sense of posterior fullness. It can represent either a true cyst or may be an extension of an intra-articular knee effusion. Examination reveals palpable fullness in the posteromedial knee. Treatment is usually aimed at the underlying condition but may require aspiration and, in a small number of patients, surgical resection.

KEY POINT

- The medial-lateral grind test is the most sensitive and specific test for assessing the intactness of the menisci.

Ankle and Foot Pain

Ankle Sprains

Ankle sprains usually involve a combination of plantar flexion and inversion leading to damage to the lateral ligaments. The anterior talofibular ligament is the most commonly injured. Patients with ankle sprains initially present with pain, swelling, and diminished proprioception. Although typically a self-limited condition, residual symptoms, including pain, instability, and stiffness, are common and may persist for years. Ankle sprains can be graded by severity: ligamentous stretching with no instability and mild pain (grade I); partial ligamentous tear with moderate tenderness to palpation and pain with ambulation (grade II); and complete ligamentous tear with instability, severe pain, and inability to ambulate (grade III).

Evaluation should begin with a determination of the circumstances under which the ankle was injured and whether the ankle was inverted or everted. The inability to bear weight immediately after injury suggests a possible fracture or a more serious sprain. A popping sound when the injury occurred suggests ligament rupture.

Examination should include inspection, palpation, range-of-motion testing, assessment of weightbearing status, and focused testing of the ankle. Palpation should include the bony structures of the ankle and the entire length of the tibia and fibula. The Achilles tendon should also be palpated along its entire course. Specific tests allow for assessment of the integrity of the structures of the ankle. Compression of the fibula and tibia at the midcalf ("squeeze test") should be performed, as pain with this maneuver in the area of the distal tibia and fibular syndesmosis indicates a syndesmosis sprain ("high ankle sprain"). The talar tilt test, used to assess the calcaneofibular ligament, is performed by holding the distal end of the tibia and fibula in one hand while using the other hand to invert the ankle. It is considered positive if the tilt is 5% to 10% greater on the affected side as compared with the unaffected side. The Ottawa ankle and foot rules are a highly sensitive tool to help the clinician determine when it is appropriate to obtain radiographic studies in patients presenting with a history of trauma (**Figure 15**).

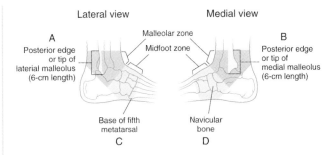

FIGURE 15. Ottawa ankle and foot rules. An ankle radiographic series is indicated if a patient has pain in the malleolar zone and any of these findings: bone tenderness at *A*, bone tenderness at *B*, or inability to bear weight immediately and in the emergency department (or physician's office). A foot radiographic series is indicated if a patient has pain in the midfoot zone and any of these findings: bone tenderness at *C*, bone tenderness at *D*, or inability to bear weight immediately and in the emergency department (or physician's office).

Reproduced with permission from Davis MF, Davis PF, Ross DS. ACP Expert Guide to Sports Medicine. Philadelphia, PA: American College of Physicians, 2005:404. Copyright 2005, American College of Physicians.

Early management of uncomplicated ankle sprains (grade I) includes controlling swelling with ice, compression, and elevation. NSAIDs can be used to help with pain control and to reduce inflammation. Range-of-motion exercises should be started promptly. Further rehabilitation, including proprioceptive training, is essential to prevent chronic instability. Management of grade II sprains is similar but may require limiting weightbearing in addition to stabilization during recovery. Grade III sprains may require surgical intervention given the presence of complete tearing and loss of ankle stability, particularly with failure to respond to more conservative therapies.

Hind Foot Pain

Plantar fasciitis, the most common cause of heel pain, is characterized by intense, sharp pain in the heel with the first steps after long periods of inactivity (such as in the morning or after resting) and initially improves with walking but subsequently worsens. Risk factors include pes planus, running, occupations requiring prolonged standing, and obesity. Examination is notable for tenderness to palpation at the anteromedial aspect of the heel. Radiographs have limited utility but frequently reveal heel spurs and can help to rule out stress fractures of the calcaneus. Cornerstones of therapy include weight loss when appropriate, exercises that stretch the plantar fascia and calf, appropriate footwear, activity modification, and analgesics. Orthotics or night splints may be helpful for some patients. Corticosteroid injections appear to provide short-term improvement in symptoms, although long-term efficacy has not been established. Most cases (>80%) resolve within a year of onset of symptoms, regardless of therapy.

Achilles tendinopathy is caused by recurrent microtrauma and can be either acute or chronic. Acute Achilles tendon pain most commonly results from an abrupt increase in activity level whereas chronic pain (lasting >3 months) results from poor mechanics (pes planus, pes cavus, limb length discrepancy) and improper footwear. Risk factors include male sex, increasing age, history of fluoroquinolone or corticosteroid use, and obesity. Treatment includes avoidance of potentially aggravating activities, using a heel lift, and a 7- to 10-day course of NSAIDs.

Rupture of the Achilles tendon commonly occurs when the patient is pushing off with the foot. Patients may hear a popping sound and usually experience severe pain at the time of injury, although up to one-third of patients do not experience pain. On examination, clinicians can perform the Thompson test (sensitivity, 96%; specificity, 93%) by squeezing the patient's calf while the patient kneels with the feet hanging over the edge of the examining table. Absence of resultant plantar flexion supports the presence of an Achilles tendon rupture. Diagnostic ultrasound can be obtained when the diagnosis is in question. Partial Achilles tendon rupture can be managed similarly to chronic Achilles tendinopathy; surgical intervention is required for complete tendon rupture.

Midfoot Pain

Tarsal tunnel syndrome is due to compression of the tibial nerve at the level of the ankle and is typically manifested as pain and paresthesias in the midfoot. The most common cause of tarsal tunnel syndrome is from scar tissue or loose bony or cartilaginous fragments from fracture of the calcaneus, medial malleolus, or talus. Symptoms also commonly occur in the heel and toes and are worse at night and with prolonged standing. Examination findings can include the presence of a Tinel sign posterior to the medial malleolus (an electric shot sensation upon percussion of the posterior tibial nerve) and sensory loss on the plantar surface of the foot. If severe, atrophy of the intrinsic muscles of the foot may result. Treatment options include NSAIDS, orthotics, and modifications to footwear.

Although uncommon, stress fractures involving the bones of the midfoot can affect runners.

Forefoot Pain

In hallux valgus deformity (bunion), the first toe deviates laterally, and a bony deformity develops on the medial aspect of the first metatarsophalangeal (MTP) joint. This is typically accompanied by the inflammation of a bursa on the medial aspect of the first MTP joint, especially with tight-fitting shoes. Treatment is usually conservative and includes NSAIDs and accommodating footwear. When these interventions fail, orthotics, bracing, and surgical intervention may be required.

Morton neuroma, a common cause of metatarsalgia, results in burning pain in the space between the third and fourth toes or, less commonly, between the second and third toes. It results from entrapment of one of the common digital nerves. Pain is usually worse with standing and is most common in women who wear high heels. On examination,

there is tenderness to palpation of the affected interdigital space. Treatment consists of avoiding high heels and wearing cushioning under the forefoot. NSAIDs are not usually helpful, but corticosteroid injection is helpful in select patients.

KEY POINT

- The Ottawa ankle and foot rules are highly sensitive for ruling out fracture.

Dyslipidemia

Screening

The U.S. Preventive Services Task Force (USPSTF) strongly recommends initiating screening in men at age 35 years, and in women who are at increased risk of cardiovascular disease at age 45 years; screening may also be considered in both men and women beginning at age 20 years who have increased cardiovascular risk. A repeat screening interval of 5 years is considered appropriate in low-risk individuals, with a shorter interval in those with borderline results, and a longer interval in patients with consistently normal testing. The National Cholesterol Education Program Adult Treatment Panel III (ATP III) guidelines recommend initiating screening for lipid disorders at the age of 20 years for all adults, with screening at 5-year intervals for low-risk individuals. More frequent measurements are required for persons with multiple risk factors or in those with zero or one cardiovascular risk factors and an LDL cholesterol level only slightly lower than the goal level. The preferred screening test is a fasting lipoprotein profile including measurements of total cholesterol, HDL cholesterol, and triglycerides in order to calculate the LDL cholesterol level. (LDL cholesterol = total cholesterol − HDL cholesterol − [triglycerides ÷ 5]) The ATP III classification of lipid levels is shown in **Table 24**.

KEY POINTS

- The U.S. Preventive Services Task Force strongly recommends initiating lipid screening in men at age 35 years and in women who are at increased cardiovascular risk at age 45 years, and possibly earlier in both men and women at increased risk for cardiovascular disease.
- The National Cholesterol Education Program Adult Treatment Panel III recommends initiating lipid screening in all adults at age 20 years.

Evaluation of Lipid Levels

LDL Cholesterol

LDL cholesterol comprises 60% to 70% of serum cholesterol and is the most atherogenic of the lipoproteins. Cholesterol treatment guidelines focus on reducing LDL cholesterol as

TABLE 24. Adult Treatment Panel III Classification of Lipid Levels (mg/dL)

LDL Cholesterol—Primary Target of Therapy	
<100 mg/dL (2.59 mmol/L)	Optimal
100-129 mg/dL (2.59-3.34 mmol/L)	Near optimal/above optimal
130-159 mg/dL (3.36-4.11 mmol/L)	Borderline high
160-189 mg/dL (4.14-4.89 mmol/L)	High
≥190 mg/dL (4.92 mmol/L)	Very high
Total Cholesterol	
<200 mg/dL (5.18 mmol/L)	Desirable
200-239 mg/dL (5.18-6.19 mmol/L)	Borderline high
≥240 mg/dL (6.21 mmol/L)	High
HDL Cholesterol	
<40 mg/dL (1.03 mmol/L)	Low
≥60 mg/dL (1.55 mmol/L)	High

Reprinted from ATP III Guidelines At-A-Glance Quick Desk Reference. National Heart, Lung, and Blood Institute. NIH Publication 01-3305. May 2001. Accessed August 8, 2011, at www.nhlbi.nih.gov/guidelines/cholesterol/atglance.pdf.

the primary target of therapy. LDL cholesterol levels have been linked to new and recurrent coronary heart disease (CHD) in numerous trials; higher levels of LDL cholesterol are associated with a greater cardiovascular risk, and a 1% reduction in LDL cholesterol reduces risk by 1%. As outlined in the ATP III guidelines, a patient's goal LDL cholesterol level is determined by counting the number of cardiac risk factors and assessing the short-term risk for an acute coronary syndrome (**Table 25**). For patients without diabetes or

CHD, the risk for a cardiovascular event over the next 10 years may be estimated using the Framingham risk calculator (http://hp2010.nhlbihin.net/atpiii/calculator.asp?user type=prof). Patients are thus stratified into three different cardiac risk categories (<10%, 10%-20%, >20% risk over 10 years) and treatment goals vary accordingly. Certain medications and medical conditions can cause abnormal LDL cholesterol levels, including diabetes, hypothyroidism, and kidney disease. Suggestive history and physical examination findings should prompt evaluation for these disorders before initiating LDL cholesterol–lowering therapy.

Triglycerides

Elevated triglyceride levels reflect the presence of atherogenic VLDL remnants and are a marker for low HDL cholesterol levels, increased insulin resistance, and other components of the metabolic syndrome. It is controversial whether serum triglyceride levels themselves are an independent predictor of cardiac risk. However, as triglyceride-rich VLDL remnants have been associated with cardiovascular disease, the ATP III guidelines designate non-HDL cholesterol, which comprises LDL cholesterol together with VLDL cholesterol, as a secondary target for lipid-lowering therapy when triglyceride levels are greater than 200 mg/dL (2.26 mmol/L). The goal for non-HDL cholesterol (total cholesterol – HDL cholesterol) is 30 mg/dL (0.34 mmol/L) higher than the goal for LDL cholesterol.

The American Heart Association (AHA) suggests that the "optimal" triglyceride level is less than 100 mg/dL (1.13 mmol/L), but studies have not shown benefit for using medication to reach this target. Because lifestyle factors, including physical inactivity and a high-carbohydrate diet, have been

TABLE 25. Adult Treatment Panel III Recommendations for LDL Cholesterol Level Management

Risk Category	LDL Cholesterol Goal	Initiate TLC	Consider Drug Therapy[a]
High risk: CHD or CHD equivalents[b] (10-year risk >20%)	<100 mg/dL (2.59 mmol/L) (optional goal: <70 mg/dL [1.81 mmol/L])[c]	≥100 mg/dL (2.59 mmol/L)	≥130 mg/dL (3.37 mmol/L) 100 to 129 mg/dL (2.59 to 3.34 mmol/L): drug optional[d]
Moderately high risk: ≥2 risk factors (10-year risk 10% to 20%)	<130 mg/dL (3.37 mmol/L)	≥130 mg/dL (3.37 mmol/L)	≥130 mg/dL (3.37 mmol/L)
Moderate risk: ≥2 risk factors (10-year risk <10%)	<130 mg/dL (3.37 mmol/L)	≥130 mg/dL (3.37 mmol/L)	≥160 mg/dL (4.14 mmol/L)
Lower risk: 0 to 1 risk factor	<160 mg/dL (4.14 mmol/L)	≥160 mg/dL (4.14 mmol/L)	≥190 mg/dL (4.92 mmol/L); 160 to 189 mg/dL (4.14 to 4.90 mmol/L): drug optional

CHD = coronary heart disease; TLC = therapeutic lifestyle changes.

[a]When LDL cholesterol–lowering drug therapy is employed, intensity of therapy should be sufficient to achieve at least a 30% to 40% reduction in LDL cholesterol levels.

[b]CHD risk equivalents include peripheral arterial disease, abdominal aortic aneurysm, carotid artery disease, transient ischemic attacks or stroke of carotid origin or 50% obstruction of a carotid artery, diabetes, and 10-year risk for CHD ≥20%.

[c]ATP III Update 2004: Implications of recent clinical trials for the ATP III Guidelines. Available at www.nhlbi.nih.gov/guidelines/cholesterol/atp3upd04.htm.

[d]If a high-risk person has high triglyceride or low HDL cholesterol levels, combining a fibrate or nicotinic acid with an LDL cholesterol–lowering drug can be considered.

Data from the National Heart Lung and Blood Institute. National Cholesterol Education Program. Third Report of the Expert Panel on Detection, Evaluation, and Treatment of High Blood Cholesterol in Adults (Adult Treatment Panel III): Executive Summary. www.nhlbi.nih.gov/guidelines/cholesterol/atp_iii.htm. Published May 2001. Accessed July 14, 2009.

linked to elevated triglyceride levels, weight loss, exercise, and decreased consumption of carbohydrates and fructose are recommended for patients with borderline (150-199 mg/dL [1.69-2.24 mmol/L]) and high (200-499 mg/dL [2.26-5.63 mmol/L]) triglyceride levels. In accordance with ATP III guidelines, pharmacotherapy is recommended if the non-HDL cholesterol level is above goal, or if triglyceride levels are greater than 500 mg/dL (5.65 mmol/L), because of the increased risk for pancreatitis. Additionally, treating chronic diseases (diabetes, obesity, kidney disease) or eliminating medications that are associated with high triglyceride levels (corticosteroids, protease inhibitors, β-blockers, estrogens) may be beneficial.

HDL Cholesterol

HDL cholesterol makes up about 20% to 30% of serum cholesterol, and low levels have been linked to increased mortality from cardiovascular disease; a 1% decrease in serum HDL cholesterol level is associated with a 2% to 3% increase in cardiovascular risk. Reflecting this inverse relationship, the presence of a high HDL cholesterol level, defined as greater than 60 mg/dL (1.55 mmol/L), subtracts one risk factor when counting risk factors for LDL cholesterol treatment goals. Although HDL cholesterol level is the lipid risk factor most tightly correlated with cardiovascular risk, this may be related in part to the close association among low HDL cholesterol, small, dense LDL particles, and high triglyceride levels. Thus, the updated ATP III guidelines do not designate HDL cholesterol level as a specific target for lipid-lowering therapy. Causes of low HDL cholesterol level include elevated triglyceride levels, obesity, physical inactivity, smoking, high carbohydrate diets, type 2 diabetes, β-blockers, anabolic steroid use, progestational medications, and genetic factors.

Nonstandard Lipid Risk Factors

Several nontraditional risk factors may be related to cardiovascular outcomes, including levels of Lp(a) lipoprotein, small LDL particles, HDL subspecies, apolipoproteins B and A-1, and the total cholesterol/HDL cholesterol ratio. However, the USPSTF and updated ATP III guidelines do not recommend measuring or treating any of these risk factors when managing lipid levels.

Management of Dyslipidemias

Therapeutic Lifestyle Changes

Therapeutic lifestyle changes are the cornerstone of lipid-lowering therapy, and the ATP III guidelines recommend them for all patients with abnormal lipid levels. Saturated fat intake should be reduced to less than 7% of total calories (about 19 g of saturated fat for a 2500-calorie diet) and dietary cholesterol consumption decreased to less than 200 mg/d. Incorporating these changes alone into a standard Western diet can reduce LDL cholesterol levels by 9% to 12%;

combining these changes with exercise can result in an LDL cholesterol reduction of up to 15%. Referral to a nutrition professional is also helpful. If goal LDL cholesterol levels are not reached after 6 weeks, the addition of 2 g/d of dietary plant sterols and stanols, found in certain fortified margarines and spreads, can enhance LDL cholesterol lowering by approximately 10%. Similarly, intake of viscous fiber, found in oatmeal, fruits, legumes, and certain vegetables, results in a modest LDL cholesterol reduction.

Drug Therapy

Providers should consider initiating drug therapy in patients who have not achieved LDL cholesterol goals after 3 months of therapeutic lifestyle changes, and simultaneously with lifestyle changes in patients with CHD or CHD risk equivalents who are unlikely to achieve LDL cholesterol goals with dietary therapy alone. The ATP III guidelines for LDL cholesterol goals and treatment strategies are listed in Table 25. Several medications are effective for reducing LDL cholesterol (**Table 26**).

Statins are considered first-line therapy, as they are the most effective for LDL cholesterol lowering and also reduce the risk for CHD outcomes in both primary and secondary prevention. Additionally, statins have been shown to reduce markers of inflammation, including high-sensitivity C-reactive protein levels, and this effect may contribute to their clinical benefits. Several studies have shown that statins reduce total mortality by 20% to 30% in patients with established CHD disease, but a recent meta-analysis of statin treatment for primary prevention in high-risk patients (which included data from the JUPITER trial) failed to show a mortality benefit. The updated ATP III guidelines recommend a goal LDL cholesterol level of less than 100 mg/dL (2.59 mmol/L) in high-risk patients and an optional goal of less than 70 mg/dL (1.81 mmol/L) in very high-risk patients, such as those with established cardiovascular disease plus diabetes.

Physicians should consider potencies, drug interactions, and metabolism when choosing among the currently available statins. The benefits of statin therapy are generally class specific, and there is no compelling evidence that newer agents are more effective than established statin medications, which may be more cost effective. The ATP III guidelines recommend titrating the statin dose to reduce LDL cholesterol levels by 30% to 40%; each doubling of the statin dose reduces LDL cholesterol level by a mean of approximately 6%. However, higher doses of statins are associated with an increased risk for myopathy. The FDA has recently recommended that an 80-mg dosage of simvastatin be prescribed only to those who have been tolerating it well for 12 months or more. Other risk factors for statin-induced myopathy include increased age, multiple medical problems, female sex, and cotreatment with certain medications. Inhibitors of the cytochrome P-450 3A4 (CYP3A4) isoenzyme, including cyclosporine, amiodarone, fibrates, and protease inhibitors,

TABLE 26. Medications for Treating Abnormal Lipid Levels

Agent	Changes in Lipid Values	Evidence	Notes
Statins	LDL cholesterol ↓ 18%-55% HDL cholesterol ↑ 5%-15% TGs ↓ 7%-30%	Reduced CHD in 1° and 2° prevention. Mortality benefit in 2° prevention.	Most effective agents for reducing LDL cholesterol. See Table 27 for adverse effects. Higher doses increase risk for adverse events. Contraindicated in pregnancy.
Bile acid sequestrants	LDL cholesterol ↓ 15%-30% HDL cholesterol ↑ 3%-5% No effect or possible ↑ in TGs	Reduced CHD in 1° prevention.	Avoid in patients with high TGs (>200 mg/dL [2.26 mmol/L]). Constipation, abdominal pain, and nausea are common side effects, but are seen less frequently with colesevelam.
Fibrates	LDL cholesterol ↓ 5%-20% (↑ in patients with elevated TGs) HDL cholesterol ↑ 10%-35% TGs ↓ 20%-50%	Reduced CHD in 1° and 2° prevention.	Most effective agents for reducing TGs, but may raise LDL cholesterol. Combination therapy with statins reduces overall cholesterol profile but may increase risk for myopathy. Avoid in patients with gallstones or kidney disease.
Nicotinic acid	LDL cholesterol ↓ 5%-25% HDL cholesterol ↑ 15%-35% TGs ↓ 20%-50%	Reduced CHD and atherosclerotic progression in 2° prevention.	Most effective agent for increasing HDL cholesterol. Flushing is common, but may be less frequent with sustained-release formulations or with prior administration of aspirin. Other adverse events include hepatotoxicity, gout, and hyperglycemia.
Ezetimibe	LDL cholesterol ↓ 18%	No evidence for cardiovascular benefit in 1° or 2° prevention.	Can reduce LDL cholesterol by an additional 19% when added to statin therapy. May be associated with myopathy.
Omega-3 fatty acids	TGs ↓ 30%-50%	Mixed evidence for reduction of CHD in 2° prevention.	Used as an alternative to fibrates or nicotinic acid for lowering TGs. Therapeutic doses range from 3-12 g/d.

1° = primary; 2° = secondary; CHD = coronary heart disease; TG = triglycerides.

should be used cautiously or not at all in patients taking CYP3A substrates, such as simvastatin, lovastatin, and atorvastatin. In contrast, pravastatin is metabolized renally, and fluvastatin and rosuvastatin are metabolized by CYP2C9, potentially making these better choices in patients treated with multiple medications. Additional adverse events associated with statin use and potential management strategies are listed in **Table 27**. Patients should be monitored for adverse events by obtaining serum creatine kinase and aminotransferase levels before initiating statin therapy. Because the risk of significant liver or muscle damage is very low, routine follow-up testing is not indicated and should be performed based on the development of symptoms or other clinical findings while on therapy.

Critics of the ATP III "treat to target" approach, outlined above, note that many patients do not achieve target LDL cholesterol levels, possibly because of the complexity of the treatment guidelines and the potential adverse effects associated with high-dose statins. A recent decision analysis compared the "treat to target" approach with a "tailored" approach, which eliminates the process of adjusting statin dosing according to achieved LDL cholesterol levels, and instead uses a fixed dose of statin based on the calculated 5-year cardiovascular risk. In this analysis, both approaches

would treat similar numbers of patients with statins, but the tailored treatment approach prevented more cardiac morbidity and mortality.

Bile acid sequestrants are most effective when used in combination with statins, but may be used as monotherapy in patients who are considering pregnancy or need only modest LDL cholesterol reduction. Ezetimibe monotherapy can reduce LDL cholesterol by 18%, but evidence of improvement in cardiovascular outcomes with this medication is lacking; it may be considered in patients who are intolerant of statin therapy.

Combination Drug Therapy

Combination drug therapy may be required to achieve LDL cholesterol goals in select patients. Bile acid sequestrants are particularly effective at lowering LDL cholesterol when combined with statins and can produce an additional 12% to 16% LDL cholesterol reduction. This combination is efficacious with low to moderate doses of statins, and should be considered early in therapy for patients with very high LDL cholesterol levels and in patients who may not tolerate high doses of statins. If combined statin-sequestrant therapy is unsuccessful at achieving the target LDL cholesterol level, nicotinic acid may be added as a third agent.

TABLE 27. Major Adverse Events Associated with Statin Use

Adverse Event	Definition	Incidence	Management strategy
Myalgia	Muscle ache or weakness *without* an increase in CK	5%-10%	Investigate for other causes of muscle pain, including vitamin D deficiency, thyroid disease, fibromyalgia, medications, exercise, and strenuous work.
			Follow symptoms and CK levels weekly; discontinue statin or decrease dose if symptoms worsen or CK levels increase.
			Once symptoms resolve and CK levels return to baseline, consider use of a statin or alternative LDL cholesterol–lowering medications associated with less risk for myopathy: fluvastatin, rosuvastatin, pravastatin, ezetimibe, bile acid sequestrants.
			Consider supplementation with coenzyme Q10.
Myositis	Muscle ache or weakness *with* an increase in CK less than 10× ULN	NA	Same as for myalgia.
Rhabdomyolysis	Muscle ache or weakness *with* an increase in CK > 10× ULN and creatinine elevation, accompanied by myoglobinuria	0.09%	Discontinue statin therapy immediately. Monitor symptoms and CK levels. Statin may be restarted, preferably at a lower dose, once symptoms resolve completely and CK levels normalize.
Elevated aminotransferases	Incidental asymptomatic elevation of serum aminotransferase levels to less than 3× ULN with no associated histopathologic changes	3%	Continue statin therapy. Elevation is typically transient and occurs during the first 12 weeks of therapy. Recheck liver chemistry tests only if clinically indicated.
Hepatotoxicity	Alanine aminotransferase > 3× ULN with total bilirubin levels > 2× ULN	1%	Discontinue statin therapy and recheck liver chemistry test results.
			If liver chemistry test results normalize, consider rechallenge with the same statin at a lower dose or a different statin.
			If liver chemistry test results remain elevated, continue to withhold statin, screen for underlying liver disease, and consider drug interactions.

CK = creatine kinase; NA = not available; ULN = upper limit of normal.

Statins and fibrates can be used together cautiously to target both LDL and non-HDL cholesterol goals. Gemfibrozil raises the serum concentrations of statins by twofold or more, thereby increasing the risk for myopathy; fenofibrate is thus preferred for combination therapy.

The ARBITER 6-HALTS study compared the effectiveness of niacin or ezetimibe, when added to statin therapy, for reducing carotid intima-media thickness and altering lipid levels. HDL cholesterol levels in the niacin group increased by 18%, and LDL cholesterol levels in the ezetimibe group decreased by 19%; an improvement in carotid intima-media thickness was noted only for the niacin group. In two recent trials, combination treatment with simvastatin and fenofibrate (the ACCORD-Lipid trial) and simvastatin and niacin (the AIM-High trial) as compared with simvastatin monotherapy did not reduce cardiovascular risk.

Management of Hypertriglyceridemia

Lifestyle changes are the primary therapy for treatment of hypertriglyceridemia, and patients should be encouraged to lose weight, exercise regularly, and restrict alcohol use and excessive carbohydrate intake. In patients with above-goal LDL cholesterol and triglyceride levels, treatment with a statin, which reduces triglycerides by 20% to 40%, is first-line therapy. Patients with hypertriglyceridemia and elevated non-HDL cholesterol (≥30 mg/dL [0.77 mmol/L] above LDL cholesterol goal) and normal LDL cholesterol levels may be treated with nicotinic acid or a fibrate initially according to ATP III guidelines. Nicotinic acid reduces triglyceride levels by 30% to 50% and increases HDL cholesterol levels by 20% to 30% and may be the most efficacious monotherapy in patients with elevated non-HDL cholesterol levels. Fibrates are also effective for reducing triglycerides and increasing HDL cholesterol levels (changes of 40%-60% and 15%-25%, respectively), but they can raise LDL cholesterol levels by up to 30%. Thus, fibrate monotherapy may be ineffective for achieving non-HDL cholesterol goals. Therapeutic doses of eicosapentaenoic acid (3 to 9 g/d), which is found in fish oil supplements, can lower triglyceride levels by up to 50%, and may be an alternative to nicotinic acid or fibrate therapy. Evidence is lacking, however, that treatment with fish oil supplementation reduces mortality or cardiovascular events. In a recent randomized controlled trial among patients with established cardiovascular disease, investigators failed to show a reduction in cardiovascular events with low-dose daily supplementation of marine fatty acids, including eicosapentaenoic acid and docosahexaenoic acid.

Management of Low HDL Cholesterol

Low levels of HDL cholesterol are associated with increased cardiac risk, and treatment with medications that increase HDL cholesterol levels, such as nicotinic acid and fibrates, have been shown to reduce cardiovascular outcomes in several large studies. However, this effect may be mediated by treatment modification of the lipoprotein derangements that are associated with low HDL cholesterol levels, including small, dense LDL particles and elevated triglycerides. Thus, evidence of a direct relationship between raising HDL cholesterol levels and decreased cardiac risk is lacking.

In patients with CHD or CHD risk equivalents, treatment of abnormal LDL cholesterol levels should be the primary target of therapy. Once the goal LDL cholesterol level has been achieved, the addition of nicotinic acid or a fibrate may raise HDL cholesterol levels. In the VA-HIT trial, patients with established cardiovascular disease, low LDL cholesterol levels, and low HDL cholesterol levels were treated with gemfibrozil for 5 years. Gemfibrozil increased HDL cholesterol and decreased triglyceride levels, and this was associated with a 22% reduction in cardiovascular events.

Therapeutic lifestyle changes are the primary therapy for patients with low cardiac risk and abnormal HDL cholesterol levels. Weight reduction and increased physical activity can increase HDL cholesterol levels by up to 30%; smoking cessation can also increase HDL cholesterol slightly. There is no clear evidence, however, that initiating drug therapy to raise HDL cholesterol levels in low-risk patients is beneficial. Moreover, a trial attempting to raise HDL cholesterol levels using the cholesteryl-ester transfer protein inhibitor torcetrapib was terminated early because of excess deaths in the torcetrapib group.

KEY POINTS

- Therapeutic lifestyle changes are the cornerstone of lipid-lowering therapy and are recommended for all patients with abnormal lipid levels.
- Lipid-lowering drug therapy should be considered in patients who have not achieved LDL cholesterol goals after 3 months of therapeutic lifestyle changes, and simultaneously with lifestyle changes in patients with coronary heart disease or risk equivalents who are unlikely to achieve LDL cholesterol goals with dietary therapy alone.
- Baseline serum creatine kinase and aminotransferase levels should be obtained before initiating statin therapy; routine follow-up testing is not indicated.

Metabolic Syndrome

Epidemiology and Pathophysiology

The metabolic syndrome consists of a group of risk factors for cardiovascular disease and type 2 diabetes. Various criteria exist for making this diagnosis; the ATP III criteria are presented in **Table 28**. The designation of metabolic syndrome as a "syndrome" remains controversial. Some experts in the fields of diabetes, dyslipidemia, and obesity feel that focusing on interventions aimed at improving the individual constituents of the metabolic syndrome are more important than lumping those metabolic abnormalities into a syndrome. Others, however, feel that grouping the risk factors into a syndrome creates a lower threshold for education and intervention and that attaching a name may also help motivate patients to exercise, consume healthier diets, and lose weight.

The epidemic of obesity and insulin resistance in the United States has led to a sharply rising prevalence of metabolic syndrome, from an estimated 50 million cases in 1990 to 64 million by the year 2000. Metabolic syndrome is associated with a 7-fold increased risk for the future development of type 2 diabetes. It is also associated with a 2-fold increase in cardiovascular events and a 1.5-fold increase in all-cause mortality. The cardiovascular risk is present before the development of diabetes.

The clinical features and cardiovascular risks associated with this syndrome appear to be related to the dysregulation of adipose tissue. Cytokines secreted by adipose cells lead to a proinflammatory state believed to accelerate atherosclerosis, plaque rupture, and atherothrombosis. Insulin-like growth factor is also believed to play a role in metabolic syndrome and increased cardiovascular risk.

Management of Metabolic Syndrome

The "ABCDE" approach has been advocated as a reasonable approach to management of metabolic syndrome (**Table 29**).

TABLE 28. Criteria for Metabolic Syndrome

Any Three of the Following:

Risk Factor	Defining Level
Abdominal obesity (waist circumference)	>40 in (>102 cm) in men; >35 in (>88 cm) in women
Triglyceride level[a]	≥150 mg/dL (1.70 mmol/L)
HDL cholesterol	<40 mg/dL (1.04 mmol/L) in men; <50 mg/dL (1.30 mmol/L) in women
Blood pressure	≥130/≥85 mm Hg
Fasting glucose	≥110 mg/dL (6.11 mmol/L)

[a]Triglyceride level ≥150 mg/dL (1.70 mmol/L) as a single factor correlates highly with presence of metabolic syndrome.

Data from the National Heart Lung and Blood Institute. National Cholesterol Education Program. Third Report of the Expert Panel on Detection, Evaluation, and Treatment of High Blood Cholesterol in Adults (Adult Treatment Panel III): Executive Summary. www.nhlbi.nih.gov/guidelines/cholesterol/atp_iii.htm. Published May 2001. Accessed July 14, 2009.

TABLE 29. "ABCDE" Approach to Management of Metabolic Syndrome

A	Assessment, aspirin	Diagnose metabolic syndrome, calculate Framingham risk score
		Begin aspirin if ≥6% 10-year Framingham risk
B	Blood pressure control	Goal <130/80 mm Hg if intermediate Framingham risk (≥ 6% 10-year risk)
C	Cholesterol management	LDL cholesterol: Statin therapy preferred; LDL cholesterol goal <100 mg/dL (2.59 mmol/L) for high-risk patients, <130 mg/dL (3.36 mmol/L) for intermediate-risk patients (per ATP III guidelines; see Table 25)
		Non-HDL cholesterol: Statin intensification and fenofibrate therapy; non-HDL cholesterol goal <130 mg/dL (3.36 mmol/L) for high-risk patients, <160 mg/dL (4.14 mmol/L) for intermediate-risk patients (per ATP III guidelines)
		Niacin for increasing HDL cholesterol controversial
D	Diabetes prevention, diet	Intensive lifestyle modification
		Metformin when indicated
		Weight loss
		Low glycemic diet
		Consider Mediterranean diet
E	Exercise	Daily vigorous activity
		Recommend use of pedometer; goal >10,000 steps/d

ATP III = National Cholesterol Education Program Adult Treatment Panel III.

Adapted with permission from Blaha MJ, Bansal S, Rouf R, Golden SH, Blumenthal RS, Defilippis AP. A practical "ABCDE" approach to the metabolic syndrome. Mayo Clin Proc. 2008;83(8):932-941. [PMID: 18674478] Copyright 2008, Elsevier.

The first step is assessment and diagnosis of metabolic syndrome. The Framingham risk calculator can then be used to calculate the patient's 10-year risk of myocardial infarction or death due to cardiovascular disease. As patients with metabolic syndrome are at increased risk of thrombosis owing to increased platelet aggregation, aspirin (81 mg/d) should be started in patients with intermediate or high Framingham risk (without contraindications to aspirin) to decrease platelet aggregation. The use of aspirin in low-risk patients is controversial owing to conflicting results in various studies.

Data are not clear about target blood pressures in metabolic syndrome, but some authors suggest a goal blood pressure of below 130/80 mm Hg in patients with intermediate or high Framingham 10-year risk. Owing to mounting evidence that β-blockers and thiazide diuretics worsen glucose tolerance, the American Heart Association and others have removed these drugs as recommended first-line agents to treat blood pressure that is above goal in patients with metabolic syndrome. ACE inhibitors and angiotensin receptor blockers to treat high blood pressure may be better choices in these patients because they have consistently been shown to improve glycemic control.

Although LDL cholesterol is not considered in diagnosing the metabolic syndrome, it is considered to be the principal lipoprotein determinant of atherosclerosis. It is generally recommended that in intermediate- and high-risk patients, statins be used. Fibrate therapy should be instituted in intermediate- and high-risk patients with metabolic syndrome and elevated triglyceride levels.

Lifestyle modification, increased physical activity, weight loss, and diet should be emphasized in all metabolic syndrome interventions. Weight loss reduces oxidative stress and improves all of the components of metabolic syndrome. A diet with a high glycemic load leads to more insulin resistance; therefore, a low-glycemic diet should be emphasized. Cardiac and respiratory fitness is associated with increased insulin sensitivity, decreased incidence of metabolic syndrome and decreased cardiovascular mortality.

KEY POINT

- Aspirin should be started in patients with metabolic syndrome without contraindications who have an intermediate or high Framingham cardiovascular risk.

Dyslipidemia Management in Older Patients

Older patients (ages 65-80 years) with established cardiovascular disease derive similar benefit as younger patients from statin therapy and tolerate these medications well. Primary prevention with statins in this age group, however, is controversial. Cardiovascular risk factor assessment may be less reliable in older patients, and older age confers an increased risk for statin-associated myopathy. Thus, risks and benefits of primary prevention with statin therapy must be weighed carefully in this age group.

- Risks and benefits of primary prevention with statin therapy must be weighed carefully in older patients, as cardiovascular risk factor assessment is less reliable and adverse effects are more frequent in this age group.

Dyslipidemia Management and Stroke Prevention

The American Heart Association (AHA) guidelines on stroke prevention highlight the importance of lipid-lowering therapy. For prevention of recurrent transient ischemic attack or stroke in patients with a history of CHD or elevated cholesterol levels, treatment should be aimed at lipid lowering according to ATP III guidelines. Lipid lowering for secondary stroke prevention in patients *without* a history of cardiac disease should aim for an LDL cholesterol level below 70 mg/dL (1.81 mmol/L) or an LDL cholesterol reduction of at least 50%. Secondary stroke prevention may also include treatment with niacin or gemfibrozil to increase low HDL cholesterol levels.

Aspirin as an Adjunct to Dyslipidemia Management

Aspirin reduces cardiovascular risk by irreversibly inhibiting platelets by inactivating cyclooxygenase-1, thus blocking the formation of thromboxane A_2. Although well established for the secondary prevention of cardiovascular disease, the USPSTF recommends against the routine use of aspirin in primary prevention in men aged 44 years and younger as well as in women aged 54 years and younger. Because the risk of first myocardial infarction is reduced by aspirin use in men ages 45 to 79 years, they recommend its use if the harm of gastrointestinal bleeding does not outweigh the benefit. Calculating Framingham risk scores can be used to help determine CHD risk in this patient population. Similarly, in women ages 55 to 79 years treated with aspirin, there is a statistically significant decreased risk of ischemic stroke but not a decrease in cardiovascular death or myocardial infarction. Again, the USPSTF recommends weighing the potential harm (gastrointestinal bleeding) against the benefit. The data are unclear regarding harm versus benefit of aspirin in men and women older than 80 years. Table 30 shows the 10-year CHD risk levels for men and stroke risk for women at which the benefit of aspirin exceeds harms. The USPSTF emphasizes an individualized approach based on shared decision-making between physicians and patients.

The optimal dose of aspirin for primary prevention is unclear, as dosages used in studies have varied from 50 mg/d to 1500 mg/d. Given no evidence of improved outcomes and the increased risk of bleeding with higher doses, the USPSTF recommends the use of 75 mg/d aspirin when indicated for this purpose.

The risk of gastrointestinal bleeding increases with age. A history of peptic ulcer disease increases the risk of serious bleeding 2 to 3 fold. Other risk factors for serious gastrointestinal bleeding include male sex (twice the risk of women) and NSAID therapy (4 times the risk compared with aspirin alone).

- The U.S. Preventive Services Task Force recommends aspirin in men ages 45-79 years for primary prevention of cardiovascular disease and in women ages 55-79 years for primary prevention of stroke if the bleeding risks do not outweigh benefit.

Obesity

Definition and Epidemiology

Nearly 34% of adults and 17% of children in the United States are obese, defined as a BMI of 30 or greater. These are double and triple the rates, respectively, of a quarter century ago, and these numbers continue to rise. The highest rates are in black women (50%) and Hispanic women (43%). The Institute of Medicine identifies obesity as an "emerging priority area" for national action.

TABLE 30. CHD Risk Levels at Which Cardiovascular Disease Events Prevented is Closely Balanced to Serious Bleeding Events in Patients Taking Aspirin for Primary Prevention

Men		Women	
Age	10-Year CHD Risk, %	Age	10-Year Stroke Risk, %
45–59 y	≥4	55–59 y	≥3
60–69 y	≥9	60–69 y	≥8
70–79 y	≥12	70–79 y	≥11

CHD = coronary heart disease.

Reprinted from US Preventive Services Task Force. Aspirin for the prevention of cardiovascular disease: U.S. Preventive Services Task Force recommendation statement. Ann Intern Med. 2009;150(6):396-404. [PMID: 19293072]

In adults, obesity is defined by BMI (body mass divided by the square of the height), and online BMI calculators are widely available (www.nhlbisupport.com/bmi/). Categories of obesity and overweight based on BMI proposed by the World Health Organization and National Institutes of Health (NIH) are listed in **Table 31**, along with the most recent prevalence estimates for U.S. men and women.

Obese and overweight persons are at increased risk for heart disease, hypertension, dyslipidemia, type 2 diabetes mellitus, stroke, osteoarthritis, sleep apnea, gallbladder disease, certain cancers (endometrial, breast, colon), and overall mortality. These risks increase progressively with rising BMI. Obesity also is associated with reduced quality of life, societal discrimination, and increased health care costs. It is estimated that obesity added $147 billion to health care costs in 2008. In persons aged 65 years and older, obesity is associated with impaired physical functioning, including difficulty with activities of daily living.

Screening and Evaluation

The NIH and the U.S. Preventive Services Task Force (USPSTF) recommend screening all adults for obesity. The USPSTF recommends screening by calculating the BMI. The NIH recommends screening both with BMI and waist circumference measurement. Waist circumference is measured with a measuring tape placed around the abdomen at the level of the iliac crest. Central adiposity (waist circumference in men >102 cm [40 in]; in women >88 cm [35 in]) is associated with an increased risk for type 2 diabetes, dyslipidemia, hypertension, and heart disease, not only in obese persons, but also in those who are overweight.

The assessment of the obese patient begins with the history and physical examination. The history should specifically elicit chronology of weight gain, family history of obesity, medications that can promote weight gain (**Table 32**), exercise, eating patterns, and symptoms and risk factors for cardiovascular disease. The general physical examination of the obese patient can

TABLE 32. Medications That Cause Weight Gain

Drug Category	Medications
Atypical antipsychotic agents	Clozapine, olanzapine, quetiapine, risperidone
Antidiabetic drugs	Sulfonylureas, thiazolidinediones, insulin
Corticosteroids	Glucocorticoids (e.g., prednisone)
Tricyclic antidepressants	Amitriptyline, imipramine, doxepin
Selective serotonin reuptake inhibitors	Paroxetine
Anticonvulsant agents	Valproic acid, carbamazepine
β-Blockers	Propranolol, atenolol, metoprolol

be challenging owing to excessive intervening adipose tissue, and formal instruction in specific maneuvers in the physical examination receives limited attention in standard textbooks. However, practical suggestions to augment accuracy of the examination have been published (http://jama.jamanetwork.com/article.aspx?doi=10.1001/jama.2010.1950).

Assessment for comorbidities associated with obesity should be considered. The USPSTF does not recommend specific laboratory tests based on the presence of obesity alone, but the American Diabetes Association (ADA) recommends screening for diabetes in patients with a BMI of 25 or greater who have other risk factors for diabetes. Although the major cause of obesity is imbalance between caloric intake and energy expenditure, physicians should consider less common causes, including hypothyroidism and Cushing syndrome.

KEY POINTS

- All adults should be screened for obesity using BMI calculation.
- Central adiposity is associated with an increased risk for type 2 diabetes, dyslipidemia, hypertension, and heart disease in both overweight and obese persons.

TABLE 31. Classification of Obesity

Category	Adult BMI	2007-2008 U.S. Prevalence of Obesity[a]	
		Men ≥20 y (%)	Women ≥20 y (%)
Underweight	<18.5		
Normal weight	18.5-24.9		
Overweight	25.0-29.9	30	29
Obese	≥30.0	32	36
Obesity class I	30.0-34.9	21	18
Obesity class II	35.0-39.9	7	11
Obesity class III	≥40.0	4	7
Summary (obese plus overweight)	≥25.0	62	65

[a]Data from U.S. Health and Human Services Centers for Disease Control and Prevention. Health United States, 2010. Available at www.cdc.gov/nchs/data/hus/hus10.pdf. Accessed January 4, 2012.

Treatment

After the initial assessment of the obese patient, the physician should determine the patient's level of motivation for weight loss, and an individualized treatment plan should follow. Success can be enhanced by a combined team of health professionals, including a dietitian, a behavioral therapist, and an exercise therapist. Adherence to strategies that decrease caloric input and increase energy expenditure will result in weight loss. A combined approach of diet and physical activity is likely to be more successful than an individual one, but strategies that focus on decreasing caloric input are more successful than those that only focus on energy expenditure. The goal is to achieve a reduction in body weight of 10% at a rate of 0.5 to 1 kg (1-2 lb) per week during a 6-month period. This degree of weight loss will reduce the risk of many medical complications of obesity. In addition to lifestyle modification (behavioral changes, exercise, and diet), medication and surgery have become increasingly popular options. The overall management of the obese patient is presented in **Figure 16**.

KEY POINT

- A recommended weight loss goal is a reduction in body weight of 10% at a rate of 0.5 to 1 kg (1-2 lb) per week during a 6-month period.

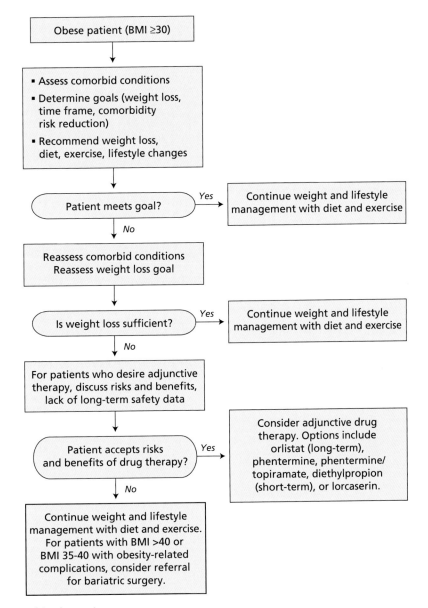

FIGURE 16. Management of the obese patient.

Adapted with permission from Snow V, Barry P, Fitterman N, Qaseem A, Weiss K; Clinical Efficacy Assessment Subcommittee of the American College of Physicians. Pharmacologic and surgical management of obesity in primary care: a clinical practice guideline from the American College of Physicians. Ann Intern Med. 2005;142(7):526. [PMID: 15809464] Copyright 2005, American College of Physicians.

Lifestyle Modification

The USPSTF recommends that clinicians offer all obese patients intensive counseling and behavioral interventions. This includes counseling in diet and exercise. Lifestyle modification has been shown to be the most effective intervention to prevent type 2 diabetes, and the ADA recommends lifestyle modification for diabetes prevention.

Behavioral Therapy

Behavioral therapy focuses the patient's attention on his or her personal maladaptive eating patterns and assists the patient to control or modify food intake, increase exercise, and avoid stimuli that trigger eating. Behavioral therapy is best when accomplished by a therapist trained in this technique and in combination with other modalities but can be initiated by the primary care physician. Principles of behavioral therapy using motivational interviewing are discussed in Routine Care of the Healthy Patient. In a systematic evidence review for the USPSTF on the effectiveness of primary care–relevant treatment for obesity in adults, 21 studies that used behavioral interventions resulted in a weight loss of 1.5 to 5.0 kg (3.3-11 lb) at 12 to 18 months, compared with little or no weight loss in the control groups. Behavioral therapy is time intensive, and regain of weight is common. However, in a recent randomized controlled trial of patients who successfully completed an initial behavioral weight loss program, monthly brief personal contact follow-up was associated with sustained weight loss. The use of technology-based interventions (Web-based interactive interventions) provided early but transient benefit.

Exercise

Exercise as monotherapy is likely not adequate for significant weight loss. In a 12-month study of moderate to vigorous exercise for 1 hour daily, 6 days per week, women lost only 1.4 kg (3.1 lb) and men lost 1.8 kg (4 lb). However, exercise at a level of walking 60 to 90 minutes per day is effective in maintaining weight that is lost and, therefore, is a useful adjunct to any weight loss program. Exercise has other health benefits, including improving cardiovascular health and decreasing waist circumference.

Consistent Dietary Caloric Restriction

Consistent dietary caloric restriction leads to successful weight loss. Obese patients can lose approximately 0.45 kg (1 lb) weekly by decreasing their intake by 500 to 1000 kcal/d below what is needed to maintain current weight. Total calories should not be restricted to less than 800 kcal/d as "very-low-calorie" diets are no more effective than low-calorie diets for successful long-term weight loss and have higher adverse consequences. No one diet has consistently been shown to be superior to others when long-term outcomes are measured. A meta-analysis comparing low-fat to low-carbohydrate diets found that whereas weight loss was better in the short term for the low-carbohydrate diet, there was no difference at 1 year. A randomized trial comparing outcomes of an intensive behavioral intervention combined with either a low-fat or a low-protein diet resulted in an 11% weight loss at 1 year and a 7% weight loss in 2 years in both groups. The low-carbohydrate diet group demonstrated a 23% increase in HDL cholesterol levels at 2 years. Exercise can enhance weight loss, especially when begun during the early phases, but caloric restriction is the key aspect to continued loss of weight. Recent evidence suggests that inadequate sleep (<7-9 hours) also compromises the success rates of typical dietary interventions.

KEY POINTS

- All obese patients should be offered intensive counseling and behavioral interventions to encourage weight loss, including counseling in diet and exercise.
- No one diet has been demonstrated superior to others in achieving long-term weight loss.

Pharmacologic Therapy

With the rising prevalence of obesity, drug therapy has emerged as an attractive option for weight loss in obese patients, especially when lifestyle modification is ineffective. However, both short-term and long-term safety and efficacy may limit use in many patients. Current FDA-approved options for drug therapy in the United States include sympathomimetic drugs that suppress appetite (phentermine, diethylpropion) and drugs that alter fat absorption (orlistat). Several appetite suppressant medications, including sibutramine, have been removed from the market over the years owing to safety concerns.

Sympathomimetic drugs are approved only for short-term use as an adjunct to other weight loss programs. Although studies have documented weight loss with continuous and intermittent use (net loss, 3.6 kg [7.9 lb]), most users regain weight upon discontinuation. Significant increases in blood pressure and arrhythmias can occur with phentermine; caution is indicated in patients with hypertension and cardiovascular disease. However, in a recent study of low-dose, controlled-release phentermine plus topiramate combined with office-based lifestyle intervention, modest weight loss was achieved (8.1 kg [17.8 lb] at 56 weeks compared with 1.4 kg [3.1 lb] in the placebo group). Significant improvement was noted in waist circumference, blood pressure, and lipid levels in the treatment group. Combination phentermine/topiramate has been FDA-approved for the treatment of obesity.

Orlistat, now available over-the-counter, is a lipase inhibitor that leads to fat malabsorption. In a recent meta-analysis on the pharmacologic treatment of obesity, the mean weight loss in patients treated with orlistat was 2.9 kg (6.4 lb) at 12 months. Secondary benefits included reductions in LDL cholesterol level and blood pressure and, in patients with diabetes, improvement in glycemic control. Approximately 15%

to 30% of patients experience gastrointestinal side effects (flatus, abdominal cramps, fecal incontinence, oily spottage), especially while consuming high-fat diets. Orlistat has not been associated with serious cardiovascular side effects. However, a recently completed review by the FDA noted rare reports of severe liver injury with orlistat. Malabsorption of fat-soluble vitamins A, D, and E has been reported, and vitamin supplementation is advisable while taking the medication.

In 2012, lorcaserin, a brain serotonin 2C receptor agonist, was FDA approved for adults with BMI greater than 30 or greater than 27 with obesity-related complications. In conjunction with a reduced-calorie diet and exercise counseling, lorcaserin was associated with an average weight loss of 3% at 1 year. Lorcaserin should be used with caution in patients who are on medications that increase serotonin levels. It has not been studied in patients with significant valvular heart disease.

KEY POINT

- Pharmacologic options for weight loss include orlistat for long-term use, the appetite suppressants phentermine and diethylpropion for short-term use, and lorcaserin.

Surgery

For class II or III obese patients (BMI ≥35) in whom diet, exercise, and/or medication have failed, especially those with significant obesity-related comorbidities, weight loss surgery should be considered. The NIH Consensus Development Conference Statement suggested the following criteria for considering a patient for bariatric surgery:

1. Patients should be well-informed, motivated, able to participate in treatment and long-term follow-up, and have acceptable operative risks.

2. Patients should have a BMI that exceeds 40.

3. Patients with a BMI between 35 and 40 with obesity-related comorbidities, such as severe sleep apnea, diabetes, or severe joint disease, should be considered.

4. Patients should be evaluated by a multidisciplinary team with medical, surgical, psychiatric, and nutritional expertise.

Surgical therapies involve restriction of stomach size and malabsorption of ingested calories as their mechanisms of action. According to worldwide survey data, the most common procedures are Roux-en-Y gastric bypass (65.1%), laparoscopic adjustable band procedures (24%), vertical banded gastroplasties (5.4%), and biliopancreatic diversion (4.8%) (**Figure 17**). The laparoscopic adjustable band procedure is increasing in popularity among patients and physicians, although the weight loss with this procedure, and restrictive surgeries in general, is less robust compared with gastric bypass. The two most common procedures are compared in **Table 33**.

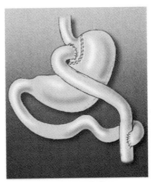
Roux-en-Y gastric bypass

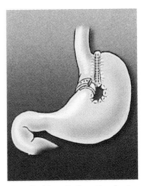
Vertical banded gastroplasty

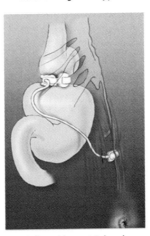
Adjustable gastric band

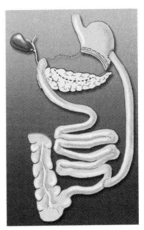
Biliopancreatic diversion with duodenal switch

FIGURE 17. Surgical procedures for obesity.

Reprinted with permission from Maggard MA, Shugarman LR, Suttorp M, et al. Meta-analysis: surgical treatment of obesity. Ann Intern Med. 2005;142(7):547-559. [PMID: 15809466] Copyright 2005, American College of Physicians.

Randomized controlled and cohort studies comparing bariatric surgery with nonsurgical interventions have found that surgery results in more dramatic and sustained weight loss and leads to improvement in obesity-related comorbidities. In a meta-analysis comprising 16,944 patients with a mean BMI of 47 (range 32-69) who underwent some type of bariatric procedure, the average weight loss at 12 months was 43.46 kg (95.6 lb) for Roux-en-Y gastric bypass, 32.16 kg (70.8 lb) for vertical band gastroplasty, 30.19 kg (66.4 lb) for adjustable gastric banding, and 51.93 kg (114.2 lb) for biliopancreatic diversion. Diabetes resolved in 76.8% of patients, hypertension resolved in 61.7%, obstructive sleep apnea resolved in 85.7%, and hyperlipidemia improved in 70%. Another meta-analysis reached similar conclusions. In a large retrospective cohort study, all-cause mortality decreased by 40% in the surgery group compared with the control group at a mean follow-up of 7.1 years. However, in a recent subset of obese, high-risk, primarily male patients, bariatric surgery was not significantly associated with survival during a mean of

TABLE 33. Comparison of Commonly Used Bariatric Procedures

Characteristic	Laparoscopic Adjustable Gastric Banding	Roux-en-Y Gastric Bypass
Mechanism of weight loss	Restrictive	Restrictive and malabsorptive
Technique	Adjustable silicone ring is placed around the top part of the stomach, creating a 15-30 mL pouch.	7-10 mL gastric pouch is separated from the rest of the stomach and connected to the small intestine, bypassing the rest of the stomach and duodenum.
Dietary program	<800 kcal/d for 18-36 months; 1000-1200 kcal/d thereafter. Certain foods can get "stuck" (rice, bread, meats, nuts), causing pain and vomiting.	<800 kcal/d for 12-18 months; 1000-1200 kcal/d thereafter in three small, high-protein meals per day. Avoid sugar and fats to prevent "dumping syndrome."
Hospital length of stay	<1 day	3-4 days
Weight loss at 12 months	30.19 kg (66.4 lb)	43.46 kg (95.6 lb)
30-day mortality	0.1%	0.5%
Incidence of postoperative complications	10%	15%
Nonoperative complications	Nausea, vomiting, reflux	Cholelithiasis, nutritional deficiencies (vitamin B_{12}, other B vitamins, iron, calcium, folic acid, vitamin D; rare: magnesium, copper, zinc, vitamin A, vitamin C)

6.7 years of follow-up. Some studies document short-term improvements in quality of life.

Bariatric surgery carries procedure-specific short-term and long-term risks. Surgical mortality rates are low (<1%) and appear to be reduced with the laparoscopic approach and with surgeons who perform a high volume of the procedures. Complications of bariatric surgery are discussed in MKSAP 16 Gastroenterology and Hepatology. Long-term multidisciplinary follow-up of the patient after bariatric surgery is essential. An average of 20% to 25% of lost weight is regained in 10 years. Dietary counseling, increased physical activity (at least 150 minutes weekly), and behavioral modification are recommended. For patients who have undergone a Roux-en-Y procedure, recent guidelines suggest twice yearly monitoring of vitamin D, calcium, phosphorus, parathyroid hormone, and alkaline phosphatase levels. To assess nutritional deficiencies after a malabsorptive procedure, ferritin, vitamin B_{12}, folate, vitamin D, and calcium levels should be assessed every 6 months for the first 2 years and annually thereafter. Bone mineral density testing is recommended yearly until stable.

KEY POINT

- Bariatric surgery may be considered for patients with a BMI above 40 or with a BMI above 35 with obesity-related complications.

Men's Health

Male Sexual Dysfunction

Male sexual dysfunction is common and causes significant distress. Many men, however, hesitate to bring such symptoms to the attention of their health care providers. Sexual dysfunction can be categorized as either erectile dysfunction (ED), ejaculatory dysfunction, or decreased libido.

Erectile Dysfunction

ED, the most common form of sexual dysfunction in men, is the inability to maintain an erection sufficient for satisfactory sexual performance. Up to one in three men experience ED at some point in their lives.

Risk Factors

The prevalence of ED increases with age, with up to 30% of men older than 70 years being affected. Obese men have close to a two-fold greater risk of developing ED than men of normal weight. Risk is similarly increased in men who smoke cigarettes compared with nonsmokers. Other modifiable risk factors include sedentary lifestyle and use of a variety of substances, including alcohol, barbiturates, cocaine, heroin, marijuana, and methamphetamines. Not only do ED and cardiovascular disease share many risk factors (diabetes mellitus, hyperlipidemia, and hypertension), ED is itself a cardiac risk factor that independently predicts mortality and confers a risk similar to that of moderate smoking. Hormonal disorders associated with ED include hypogonadism, hypothyroidism, and hyperprolactinemia. The risk of ED increases with a history of previous pelvic irradiation, surgery (including, but not limited to, prostate surgeries), or trauma. Neurologic conditions associated with an increased risk of ED include dementia, multiple sclerosis, prior cerebrovascular accident, and quadri- or paraplegia.

ED is a common side effect of medications. Up to one-quarter of all cases of ED are thought to be due to medications. **Table 34** provides a list of medications commonly associated

TABLE 34. Medications Commonly Associated with Erectile Dysfunction

Antidepressants
  Monoamine oxidase inhibitors
  Selective serotonin reuptake inhibitors
  Tricyclic antidepressants

Benzodiazepines

Opioids

Anticonvulsants
  Phenytoin
  Phenobarbital

Antihypertensives
  α-Blockers
  β-Blockers
  Calcium channel blockers
  Clonidine
  Spironolactone
  Thiazide diuretics

5α-Reductase inhibitors
  Dutasteride
  Finasteride

with ED. Various psychiatric conditions are associated with ED, including anxiety, depression, and prior sexual abuse. Relationship discord and stress can also lead to ED.

Diagnosis and Evaluation

The initial evaluation of a man reporting ED consists of obtaining medical, psychosocial, and sexual histories in addition to performing a focused physical examination and a limited laboratory investigation. During the medical history, it is important to first obtain an accurate description of what the patient is experiencing, as some patients confuse premature ejaculation with ED. Clinicians should seek to determine the presence or absence of medical conditions, medications, and other risk factors associated with ED. A psychosocial history should be performed with the purpose of identifying any underlying psychological conditions that may be contributory. Sexual history includes libido (loss is seen with androgen deficiency, depression, and as a side effect of medication use); ability to achieve and maintain erections, including circumstances (the sudden onset of the loss of ability to achieve an erection suggests a psychogenic origin but can also occur following radical prostatectomy and after trauma); ability to achieve orgasm, including quality and timing (if situational, suggests psychogenic origin); and penile curvature (its presence, along with penile pain, suggests Peyronie disease); and presence of early morning erections (presence suggests intact corpus cavernosae blood flow and intact neurogenic reflexes). The severity of ED symptoms can be assessed using the International Index of Erectile Function–5 (IIEF-5), a validated, five-item questionnaire (available at www.hiv.va.gov/ provider/manual-primary-care/urology-tool2.asp). It is also important to inquire about lifestyle factors and the sexual function of the patient's partners.

During the physical examination, the patient's BMI, blood pressure, and heart rate should be determined. A genital, digital rectal, and screening neurologic examination in addition to an assessment of lower extremity pulses and secondary sexual characteristics should also be performed. Because many episodes of ED are transient, an extensive laboratory evaluation is not mandatory at presentation without symptoms or findings suggestive of an underlying systemic disorder or before implementing lifestyle modification or counseling therapy. If indicated for suspected abnormalities or persistent symptoms, a reasonable initial laboratory investigation consists of obtaining a fasting serum glucose level, lipid panel, thyroid-stimulating hormone level, and early morning total testosterone level. Additional laboratory tests should only be obtained on the basis of findings in the history and physical examination.

Treatment

The first step in successfully treating ED is to attempt to identify an underlying etiology. If possible, treatment should be directed toward the underlying condition. Regardless of etiology, first-line therapies for ED consist of both lifestyle modifications and pharmacotherapy with phosphodiesterase type 5 (PDE-5) inhibitors. In one study, nearly one third of obese men had improved ED symptoms simply by exercising regularly and losing weight. Attempts should therefore be made to lower the patient's BMI below 30. Patients should be counseled to stop smoking and consideration should be given to stopping (if possible) any medications that are associated with ED. Psychosexual therapy performed by a sex therapist has been found to improve ED in 40% to 80% of patients.

PDE-5 inhibitors function by increasing cyclic guanosine monophosphate (cGMP) levels, which leads to smooth muscle relaxation and engorgement. Improvement in ED appears to be dose related for both sildenafil (up to 50 mg) and vardenafil (all doses) but not tadalafil. All PDE-5 inhibitors improve erections and sexual intercourse success compared with placebo and possess approximately equivalent efficacy. The efficacy of PDE-5 inhibitors is further improved when combined with other ED therapies such as psychotherapy and attempts at weight loss. Because ED shares many risk factors with atherosclerotic disease and itself is an independent risk factor, an assessment of the patient's cardiovascular risk should be made before prescribing a PDE-5 inhibitor. This can be accomplished using guidelines established by the Second Princeton Consensus Conference (**Table 35**).

PDE-5 inhibitors are generally well tolerated. Headache, the most common side effect, occurs in approximately 10% of patients. Dizziness, dyspepsia, flushing, rhinitis, syncope, and visual disturbances occur less commonly. Nonarteritic anterior optic neuropathy, although

TABLE 35. Second Princeton Consensus Conference Guidelines for Treatment of Erectile Dysfunction in Patients with Cardiovascular Disease or Cardiac Risk Factors

Risk Level	Treatment Recommendation
Low risk	
Asymptomatic and <3 major cardiac risk factors[a]	Can initiate or resume sexual activity or treat for ED with PDE-5 inhibitor (if not using nitrates)
Controlled hypertension	
Mild stable angina	
Post successful coronary revascularization	
MI (>6-8 weeks before)	
Mild valvular disease	
Left ventricular dysfunction (NYHA functional class I)	
Intermediate/indeterminate risk	
Asymptomatic and ≥3 major cardiac risk factors[a]	Further cardiac evaluation (stress test or cardiology consultation) and restratification before resumption of sexual activity or treatment for ED
Moderate stable angina	
Recent MI (2-6 weeks)	
Left ventricular dysfunction (ejection fraction <40%) or heart failure (NYHA class II)	
Noncardiac atherosclerotic disease (clinically evident PAD, history of stroke/TIA)	
High risk	
Unstable or refractory angina	Defer sexual activity or ED treatment until cardiac condition is stabilized and reassessed
Uncontrolled hypertension	
Moderate to severe heart failure (NYHA class III-IV)	
Recent MI (<2 weeks)	
High-risk arrhythmia	
Obstructive hypertrophic cardiomyopathy	
Moderate to severe valvular disease (particularly aortic stenosis)	

ED = erectile dysfunction; MI = myocardial infarction; NYHA = New York Heart Association; PAD = peripheral arterial disease; PDE = phosphodiesterase; TIA = transient ischemic attack.

[a]Major cardiac risk factors are: age, hypertension, diabetes mellitus, smoking, dyslipidemia, sedentary lifestyle, family history of premature coronary artery disease. (Male sex is excluded.)

Recommendations from Kostis JB, Jackson G, Rosen R, et al. Sexual dysfunction and cardiac risk (the Second Princeton Consensus Conference). Am J Cardiol. 2005;96(2):313-321. [PMID: 16018863]

extremely rare, has been documented and is caused by crossover inhibition of PDE-6 receptors. The use of PDE-5 inhibitors is contraindicated in patients taking nitrates owing to the potential for profound hypotension. Caution should be exercised when using PDE-5 inhibitors in patients concomitantly taking drugs that inhibit the cytochrome P-450 3A4 pathway, such as protease inhibitors, erythromycin, and ketoconazole. A comprehensive list of interacting medications can be accessed at http://medicine.iupui.edu/clinpharm/ddis/ClinicalTable.aspx.

Second-line therapies for ED include prostaglandin E_1 (alprostadil) administered either via intracavernosal or intraurethral routes, with the former being more effective and better tolerated. Additional therapies include use of penile pumps and placement of penile prostheses. Testosterone therapy appears to be effective in men with ED and androgen deficiency (see below).

Premature Ejaculation

Premature ejaculation, ejaculation that occurs sooner than desired, is diagnosed by obtaining a thorough sexual history. Treatment should be individualized and include a discussion with the patient of risks and benefits of each option. Pharmacologic therapies can be either oral or topical. Oral therapies function by causing anorgasmia and include several selective serotonin reuptake inhibitors (fluoxetine, paroxetine, and sertraline) and clomipramine, a tricyclic antidepressant. Topical anesthetic agents, such as lidocaine or prilocaine cream, function by reducing stimulation and can be used with or without a condom.

Decreased Libido

Decreased libido, a decreased desire for sexual activity, is less common in men than in women but often is more disabling. When decreased libido is associated with marked distress and interferes with relationships, the term hypoactive sexual desire disorder is used. Causes include hypogonadism, hyperprolactinemia, medications, relationship difficulties, and psychiatric disorders (most commonly depression). Decreased libido also is more common as men age. Treatment is frequently directed toward the underlying cause, if one is identifiable. It is also important to explore the quality of the relationship with the patient's sexual partner, as relationship difficulties may be the underlying issue rather than decreased libido.

KEY POINTS

- First-line therapy for erectile dysfunction consists of lifestyle modifications, psychosexual counseling, and pharmacotherapy with a phosphodiesterase type 5 inhibitor.
- Men with erectile dysfunction (ED) and three or more cardiac risk factors require cardiac evaluation before initiating treatment for ED or resuming sexual activity.
- The use of phosphodiesterase type 5 inhibitors is contraindicated in patients taking nitrates owing to the potential for profound hypotension.

Androgen Deficiency

Androgen deficiency in the setting of male hypogonadism is suggested by the signs and symptoms listed in **Table 36**. Men with specific signs and symptoms of androgen deficiency should be evaluated by measuring morning total testosterone level as the initial diagnostic test. However, because the less specific symptoms of potential androgen deficiency overlap considerably with many other common symptoms, testing in men with these symptoms should be approached judiciously, particularly those without more definitive findings on history or examination that suggest the diagnosis. The assessment of men for androgen deficiency should include a general health evaluation to exclude systemic illness and a review of medications (including opioids and high-dose corticosteroid therapy) and recreational drugs (such as marijuana) that affect testosterone production or metabolism. Eating disorders and excessive exercise can transiently lower testosterone levels. Clinical guidelines published by the Endocrine Society recommend against screening of asymptomatic men in the general population for androgen deficiency, regardless of age.

Men with low-normal testosterone levels should have confirmatory testing before initiating testosterone therapy, and further evaluation of the cause of hypogonadism should be pursued before treatment is started, if indicated (see

TABLE 36. Symptoms and Signs Suggestive of Androgen Deficiency in Men
More specific symptoms and signs
Incomplete or delayed sexual development, eunuchoidism
Reduced sexual desire (libido) and activity
Decreased spontaneous erections
Breast discomfort, gynecomastia
Loss of body (axillary and pubic) hair, reduced shaving
Very small (especially <5 mL) or shrinking testes
Inability to father children, low or zero sperm count
Height loss, low-trauma fracture, low bone mineral density
Hot flushes, sweats
Less specific symptoms and signs
Decreased energy, motivation, initiative, and self-confidence
Feeling sad or blue, depressed mood, dysthymia
Poor concentration and memory
Sleep disturbance, increased sleepiness
Mild anemia (normochromic, normocytic, in the female range)
Reduced muscle bulk and strength
Increased body fat, BMI
Diminished physical or work performance

Adapted with permission from Bhasin S, Cunningham GR, Hayes FJ, et al; Task Force, Endocrine Society. Testosterone therapy in men with androgen deficiency syndromes: an Endocrine Society clinical practice guideline. J Clin Endocrinol Metab. 2010;95(6):2537. [PMID: 20525905] Copyright 2010, The Endocrine Society.

MKSAP 16 Endocrinology and Metabolism). Testosterone therapy for men is recommended with symptomatic androgen deficiency to induce and maintain secondary sex characteristics and to improve sexual function, sense of well-being, muscle mass and strength, and bone mineral density. Because of potential adverse effects of testosterone therapy, the Endocrine Society recommends against its use in patients with breast or prostate cancer, a palpable prostate nodule or induration, a prostate-specific antigen (PSA) level greater than 4 ng/mL (or >3 ng/mL in men at high risk for prostate cancer), a hematocrit greater than 50%, untreated severe obstructive sleep apnea, severe lower urinary tract symptoms, or uncontrolled or poorly controlled heart failure. Management of patients on testosterone replacement therapy is addressed in more detail in MKSAP 16 Endocrinology and Metabolism.

KEY POINTS

- Men with symptoms of androgen deficiency and low-normal testosterone levels should have confirmatory testing before initiating testosterone therapy.
- Guidelines recommend against screening of asymptomatic men in the general population for androgen deficiency, regardless of age.

Benign Prostatic Hyperplasia

Benign prostatic hyperplasia (BPH) is a common cause of lower urinary tract symptoms (LUTS) in men. LUTS can be classified as related to overactive bladder symptoms versus bladder outlet obstruction (BOO). Overactive bladder symptoms, caused by BPH and detrusor muscle hyperactivity, include nocturia and urinary frequency and urgency. BOO symptoms, caused by physical obstruction, include decreased urinary stream, urinary retention, incomplete bladder emptying, and incontinence. The differential diagnosis of BPH includes neurologic conditions (stroke, multiple sclerosis, spinal cord conditions) as well as effects of certain medications, such as diuretics. Guidelines from the American Urological Association (AUA) recommend performing a digital rectal examination and obtaining a baseline AUA symptom index score (questionnaire available at http://www2.niddk.nih.gov/NR/rdonlyres/8E99FCF4-8A92-43EE-8E47-5B70D634938A/0/AUABPH.pdf) to track progression and effectiveness of treatment. A urinalysis should be obtained when evaluating BPH symptoms to rule out underlying infection.

Treatment modalities include watchful waiting and conservative measures for mild symptoms, drug therapy (**Table 37**), and surgical interventions for severe or refractory symptoms. Conservative measures include reduced fluid intake, timed voiding, limiting caffeine and alcohol, discontinuing exacerbating medications, and improving mobility.

TABLE 37. Medical Therapies for Patients with Moderate to Severe Symptoms of Benign Prostatic Hyperplasia

α-Blockers
Alfuzosin
Doxazosin
Tamsulosin
Terazosin
Silodosin
5α-Reductase inhibitors
Dutasteride
Finasteride
Anticholinergic agents
Oxybutynin
Tolterodine
Combination therapy
α-Blocker and 5α-reductase inhibitor
α-Blocker and anticholinergic agents
Phosphodiesterase type 5 inhibitor
Tadalafil

Information adapted from AUA Guidelines: www.auanet.org/content/guidelines-and-quality-care/clinical-guidelines.cfm?sub=bph. Accessed August 3, 2012.

Peripheral α-blockers and 5α-reductase inhibitors (5-ARIs) are the two most common drugs used for BPH, either alone or in combination. α-Blockers, effective in 70% of patients, have more immediate clinical effect, whereas 5-ARIs may lead to clinical shrinkage of the enlarged prostate gland. Coexisting overactive bladder symptoms can be treated with combination α-blocker and anticholinergic therapy (tolterodine, oxybutynin). Anticholinergic drugs should be avoided in those with post-void residual volumes greater than 250 mL.

When BPH coexists with BOO symptoms, combination α-blocker and 5-ARI therapy has shown the highest efficacy compared with other treatments when the prostate is enlarged. Data from two trials indicate that combination therapy may be better in the short term than treatment with either drug individually, although 5-year outcomes remain similar. Although commonly used by patients, complementary or alternative medications, such as saw palmetto, have not been found to have benefit in recent clinical trials.

The PDE-5 inhibitor tadalafil has been FDA-approved for treatment of lower urinary tract symptoms in BPH. No long-term studies have compared outcomes with tadalafil to those with α-blockers or 5-ARIs.

Indications for surgical interventions in patients with BPH include refractory lower urinary tract symptoms, recurrent urinary retention with or without urinary tract infection, bladder stones, and kidney failure with hydronephrosis. Open prostatectomy is indicated for a severely enlarged prostate; however, those with less severe enlargement may benefit from less invasive techniques. Transurethral resection of the prostate (TURP) has been the usual surgery of choice, with studies showing symptom improvement in 70% of men and average time to recurrent treatment of 3 years. Although long-term results from trials of minimally invasive surgical interventions, such as transurethral needle ablation (TUNA) and transurethral microwave thermotherapy (TUMT) show good initial results, the time to recurrent intervention is shorter, and the choice of procedure should balance the risk of recurrence with the decreased invasiveness and fewer side effects associated with these procedures. Studies are not sufficient to recommend any particular intervention.

KEY POINT

- Overactive bladder symptoms related to benign prostatic hyperplasia include nocturia and urinary frequency and urgency; bladder outlet obstruction symptoms include decreased urinary stream, urinary retention, incomplete bladder emptying, and incontinence.

Acute Testicular and Scrotal Pain

Diagnosis of acute scrotal pain can often be made on the basis of history and physical examination. The main sources of such symptoms are testicular torsion and epididymitis. Orchitis is painful inflammation of the testicle itself and can be virally induced (mumps) or an extension of bacterial infections of the urinary tract or epididymis. Other causes of scrotal pain may include referred pain from abdominal aneurysm, inguinal hernia with strangulation of bowel or omentum, nephrolithiasis, lumbosacral nerve impingement, and retroperitoneal inflammation.

The patient should be asked about the onset (sudden or gradual), quality and severity of pain, history of trauma, and recent sexual activity, as well as lower urinary tract symptoms such as urinary frequency, urgency, and dysuria. Physical examination should include inspection and palpation and transillumination of the testes. The cremasteric reflex (obtained by stroking the upper inner thigh and observing a rise in the ipsilateral testicle) is absent in most patients with testicular torsion. Urinalysis is indicated in the evaluation of acute scrotal pain to assess for infection. Doppler ultrasonography to assess blood flow can be a useful adjunct aiding in diagnosis and in one study was 82% sensitive and 100% specific for torsion.

Testicular Torsion

Testicular torsion constitutes an emergency and occurs when the testes twist on the spermatic cord, leading to decreased blood flow and ischemia. It is more common in children and in men younger than 30 years. Pain is usually sudden in onset and often accompanied by nausea and vomiting. Physical examination often reveals an elevated, high-riding testis with longitudinal access abnormally oriented transversely. Considerable edema may be present. Elevation of the testis hurts more in torsion, whereas epididymal pain may be relieved by this maneuver. Treatment of torsion includes rapid surgical decompression to resume blood flow. In the absence of rapid access to surgery, manual decompression may be attempted.

Epididymitis

Infection or inflammation of the epididymis often causes pain localized to the superior and posterior aspect of the testicle. The onset may be acute, subacute, or chronic, and pain may occur more gradually compared with torsion. Pain may be accompanied by lower urinary tract symptoms of dysuria, urgency, or frequency. Epididymitis may be infectious or noninfectious, with infectious epididymitis more likely to be acute. Patients with acute infectious epididymitis may be quite sick, with high fevers and leukocytosis. There may be concomitant prostatitis. Subacute presentations are more common and may not be accompanied by lower urinary tract symptoms.

Risk factors for epididymitis include recent sexual activity, heavy exertion, and bicycle riding. Distribution is bimodal, with occurrences highest in those younger than 35 years and older than 55 years. In younger patients, sexually transmitted diseases such as chlamydial infection and gonorrhea are the most likely causes (see MKSAP 16 Infectious

Disease). Older men and men who practice anal intercourse are more susceptible to *Escherichia coli*, Enterobacteriaceae, and pseudomonal infection and should be treated with ceftriaxone and a fluoroquinolone. A 21-day course of a fluoroquinolone antibiotic is appropriate for most other causes of infectious epididymitis.

Noninfectious epididymitis is caused by reflux of urine into the epididymis, which causes inflammation. Treatment is conservative, with scrotal support, application of ice, and NSAIDs. **H**

KEY POINTS

- Urinalysis is indicated in the evaluation of acute scrotal pain to assess for infection.
- Testicular torsion, characterized by sudden pain and an elevated, high-riding, abnormally oriented testis, is a surgical emergency.

Hydrocele and Varicocele

One percent of adult males have a hydrocele, which is a fluid collection between the layers of the tunica vaginalis. A communicating hydrocele occurs when a patent processus vaginalis allows fluid to pass from the peritoneal space into the scrotum, whereas a simple hydrocele has no such connection. Hydroceles vary in size and often develop gradually. Although most are asymptomatic, larger hydroceles can become painful. Physical examination usually reveals a tense, smooth, scrotal mass that is easily transilluminated. Transillumination can help distinguish a hydrocele from a hernia, varicocele, or solid mass. If a question remains, ultrasonography is the preferred modality for evaluation.

In adults, hydroceles that are small and do not bother the patient do not require intervention. Large or painful hydroceles can be treated either surgically or with aspiration and sclerotherapy. Communicating hydroceles usually require correction.

Epididymal Cyst

Epididymal cysts are often palpated at the head of the epididymis. Cysts larger than 2 cm are considered spermatoceles. Cysts can be palpated separately from the testis and usually are not painful. Ultrasonography is the study of choice for definitive diagnosis. Surgical repair is recommended only in rare cases of chronic pain related to the cyst.

Varicocele

A varicocele is a dilation of the testicular vein and pampiniform plexus within the scrotum; 90% occur on the left side. Varicoceles are one of the most commonly identified scrotal abnormalities, found in 15% of adult men and in 40% of men with infertility. The classic description is a scrotal mass on the left side with a "bag of worms" consistency that increases in size with standing and decreases while supine. Varicoceles are often painless and discovered during adolescence by self-examination. Ultrasonography is the test of choice if the diagnosis is in question.

Varicoceles are a leading cause of infertility. Repair may be warranted in men with abnormal sperm counts who desire children, although a Cochrane review did not confirm increased fertility with repair. Conservative care is adequate for men who do not desire children and are otherwise asymptomatic.

Surgical repair techniques include open inguinal varicocelectomy, laparoscopic varicocelectomy, and subinguinal microscopic varicocelectomy. All of these techniques are effective at reversing abnormal sperm parameters but not necessarily fertility. Sclerotherapy is a less invasive option that is associated with fewer complications but may be less effective in reducing symptoms.

KEY POINT

- In adult men, asymptomatic hydroceles and varicoceles can usually be diagnosed clinically and generally do not require advanced imaging or treatment.

Acute and Chronic Prostatitis and Pelvic Pain

Acute and chronic prostatitis and pelvic pain are common, with up to 2 million physician visits annually attributed to these syndromes. Symptoms fall into two categories: pain symptoms, which may include the perineum, testes, penis, or suprapubic area; and urinary symptoms, including dysuria, urinary frequency, and incomplete bladder emptying. The NIH's Chronic Prostatitis Symptom Index can aid in diagnosis and can be used to follow symptoms objectively over time (www.prostate.net/wp-content/uploads/pdf/chronic-prostatitis-symptom-test.pdf).

The diagnosis of chronic prostatitis and pelvic pain is one of clinical exclusion. Examination should rule out active urethritis, urethral stricture, testicular sources of pain, rectal masses, hemorrhoids, and neurologic diseases of the bladder. Urinalysis and urine culture should be performed, although the results are usually negative. Leukocytes may be found in post–prostatic massage urine, expressed prostatic secretions, or semen, but the presence of leukocytes is not correlated with treatment response.

A four-stage classification system was developed by the NIH to describe prostate syndromes (**Table 38**). Patients with acute bacterial prostatitis (class I) present with fever and urinary symptoms and often have an exquisitely tender prostate gland upon digital rectal examination. These infections generally respond well to standard antibiotic treatment (fluoroquinolones, trimethoprim-sulfamethoxazole). Chronic bacterial prostatitis (class II) presents with pain and urinary symptoms with recurrent bacterial infection; an extended course (1 month) of a fluoroquinolone is typically the first-line treatment.

Treatment of class III syndromes, which present with pain or LUTS, is difficult and often refractory to intervention. α-Blockers may help control urinary symptoms but have less of an effect on pain. Antibiotics are often used in the treatment of inflammatory chronic pelvic pain syndrome (CPPS) despite studies that fail to show long-term efficacy. For inflammatory CPPS, AUA guidelines recommend one course of antibiotics but not recurrent courses if the first is ineffective. NSAIDs have also been recommended based on a trial of rofecoxib, which provided some reduction in symptoms.

Other agents that have been studied for the treatment of CPPS include muscle relaxants and finasteride. Agents used in the treatment of neuropathic pain, such as gabapentin, have been recommended when primary therapies are ineffective. Complementary therapies that may be helpful in some patients include cernilton, a pollen extract; quercetin, a natural bioflavonoid; and saw palmetto extract, but the efficacy of these agents has not been determined. Surgical interventions for CPPS should be avoided unless there is a structural cause for symptoms, such as urethral stricture or BOO.

TABLE 38. Classification of Prostatitis	
Category	**Definition**
I. Acute bacterial prostatitis	Acute infection of the prostate
II. Chronic bacterial prostatitis	Recurrent infection of the prostate
III. Chronic abacterial prostatitis/chronic pelvic pain syndrome (CPPS)	No demonstrable infection
IIIA. Inflammatory CPPS	Leukocytes in semen, expressed prostatic secretions, or post-prostatic massage urine
IIIB. Noninflammatory CPPS	No leukocytes in semen, expressed prostatic secretions, or post-prostatic massage urine
IV. Asymptomatic inflammatory prostatitis	No symptoms; detected either by prostate biopsy, or the presence of leukocytes in semen samples during evaluation for other disorders

Adapted from Litwin MS, McNaughton-Collins M, Fowler FJ Jr., et al. The National Institutes of Health chronic prostatitis symptom index: development and validation of a new outcome measure. Chronic Prostatitis Collaborative Research Network. J Urol. 1999;162(2)369–375. [PMID: 10411041] with permission from American Urological Association. Copyright 1999, American Urological Association.

- Acute (class I) and chronic bacterial (class II) prostatitis are treated with antibiotic therapy.
- Chronic prostatitis/pelvic pain syndromes (class III) are often refractory to intervention; treatment options include α-blockers, a single course of antibiotics, and NSAIDs.

Hernia

A hernia occurs when an organ bulges through an area of weakness in muscle or connective tissue. They most commonly occur in the groin, and the incidence is higher in men than women. Hernias also may occur in the abdomen (ventral and umbilical) and at incision sites. Hernias may be caused by acquired or congenital weakness of connective or muscle tissue and by increased intra-abdominal pressure owing to straining, heavy lifting, or cough.

There are two types of inguinal hernia, direct and indirect. Direct inguinal hernias occur when intra-abdominal contents herniate through a weak spot in the fascia between the rectus abdominis and the inguinal ligament. Indirect inguinal hernias occur when intra-abdominal contents protrude through the internal inguinal ring. The less common femoral hernia occurs when intra-abdominal contents protrude through the femoral canal. The vast majority of inguinal hernias are indirect.

Clinical presentations of inguinal hernias can vary from an asymptomatic bulge, to a feeling of groin or abdominal pressure, to severe pain owing to movement of abdominal contents into the inguinal canal and occasionally into the scrotum. Hernias may be complicated by incarceration or strangulation, which can also lead to bowel obstruction. Direct hernias tend to present with a low abdominal bulge and cause less pain and less frequently develop incarceration, whereas femoral hernias more commonly develop these complications.

Diagnosis is made by physical observation and digital examination of the inguinal canal, with a bulge that is often visible or palpable and is usually more prominent upon standing.

Asymptomatic inguinal hernias may be monitored, whereas symptomatic hernias may require surgical repair. There is evidence that watchful waiting in asymptomatic patients may be acceptable, but patients should be warned of potential complications, such as incarceration and strangulation. The optimal type of surgery (laparoscopic versus open surgical repair) remains controversial, although reviews indicate lower recurrence rates when polypropylene mesh is used. Potential complications of repair include early recurrence, infection, seroma, hematoma, chronic neuropathic pain, and late recurrence.

- Asymptomatic inguinal hernias may be monitored; symptomatic hernias require surgical repair.

Women's Health

Female Sexual Dysfunction

Approach to the Patient

Female sexual dysfunction, defined as sexual difficulties that are persistent and personally distressing to the patient, affects up to 35% of sexually active women, peaking in middle-age. Because women are often uncomfortable initiating discussions about sexual problems, it is incumbent upon the practitioner to routinely ask about sexual function, even during brief office visits. Asking if a patient is sexually active and if there are any related problems, including pain with intercourse, is appropriate. For individuals with potential issues, a complete sexual history should be obtained, including a thorough review of medical problems, psychiatric disorders, and reproductive surgeries that can contribute to sexual dysfunction. Patients should be queried about the use of medications that may interfere with sexual function. **Table 39** lists additional questions that aid in identifying problems with desire, arousal, orgasm, or pain, which may help in determining cause and potential treatment strategies. A pelvic examination is important and may be helpful in identifying specific areas of pain, vaginal atrophy, inadequate lubrication, and vaginismus. Laboratory testing is recommended only if there is suspicion for a particular diagnosis, such as a prolactinoma, thyroid abnormalities, or adrenal disease.

Classification of Female Sexual Disorders

The DSM-IV identifies six disorders that correspond to abnormalities in the female sexual response cycle: hypoactive

TABLE 39. Essential Questions to Include in an Assessment for Female Sexual Dysfunction
How does the patient describe the problem?
How long has the problem been present?
Was the onset sudden or gradual?
Is the problem specific to a situation/partner or is it generalized?
Were there likely precipitating events (biologic or situational)?
Are there any problems in the woman's primary sexual relationship (or any relationship in which the sexual problem is occurring)?
Are there current life stressors that might be contributing to sexual problems?
Is there guilt, depression, or anger that is not being directly acknowledged?
Are there physical problems such as pain?
Are there problems in desire, arousal, or orgasm?
Is there a history of physical, emotional, or sexual abuse?
Does the partner have any sexual problems?

With kind permission from Springer Science+Business Media: Int Urogynecol J Pelvic Floor Dysfunct, Evaluation and treatment of female sexual disorders, 2009;20 Suppl 1:S33-S43, Kingsberg S, Althof SE. [PMID: 19440781] Copyright 2009, Springer Science+Business Media.

sexual desire disorder and sexual aversion disorder (sexual desire disorders), sexual arousal disorder, orgasmic disorder, and dyspareunia and vaginismus (sexual pain disorders).

The Female Sexual Function Index (www.fsfi-question-naire.com) is a validated 19-item, patient-completed questionnaire that assesses each of these areas of sexual functioning and can be used as an adjunct in the clinical assessment. Women who score less than 26 are considered to be at risk for sexual dysfunction.

Sexual Desire Disorders

Hypoactive sexual desire disorder (HSDD) is diagnosed if a woman reports a persistent lack of sexual thoughts or desire for or receptiveness to sexual activity. HSDD is the most common female sexual disorder, affecting 12% to 19% of U.S. women. Desire encompasses three separate components—drive, cognition, and motivation. Drive, perceived as spontaneous sexual interest, is biological and is based on neuroendocrine functions. Cognition refers to the belief and value framework that a patient has regarding sex. Motivation is the willingness to engage in sexual activity and may be influenced by the quality of the relationship and several psychosocial factors.

Testosterone is essential for normal sex drive and may also play a role in sexual motivation. Levels of testosterone decline progressively with age in women; however, measured testosterone levels have not been shown to correlate meaningfully with sexual functioning. Despite this, treatment with testosterone has been shown to increase sexual function scores and the number of satisfying sexual episodes but is associated with adverse effects, including excess hair growth and acne, and altered lipoprotein levels with oral therapy. In 2006, the Endocrine Society acknowledged the short-term efficacy of testosterone therapy for the treatment of sexual dysfunction in women but recommended against generalized use because of the lack of long-term safety data. The low estradiol levels that characterize surgical and natural menopause may also be linked to lack of desire and sexual responsiveness. Although study results are inconsistent, systemic estrogen or estrogen-progesterone therapy (EPT) may increase sexual desire, enjoyment, and orgasmic frequency.

To date, the FDA has not approved any medication for the treatment of female HSDD. Individual and couples sex therapy or psychotherapy may be beneficial.

Sexual aversion disorder is defined as a persistent or recurrent aversion to any genital contact with a sexual partner. Women with sexual aversion usually experience feelings of abhorrence and revulsion; panic may accompany specific sexual situations. Avoidance of sexual behavior typically reinforces the aversion, so treatment often involves graduated reintroduction of sexual behavior and relaxation exercises, which may be augmented by therapy with a selective serotonin reuptake inhibitor.

Orgasmic Disorder

Female orgasmic disorder is the persistent or recurrent delay or absence of orgasm following a normal excitement phase. Cognitive-behavioral therapy is most effective for teaching a woman to be comfortable, minimizing negative attitudes, and decreasing anxiety.

Sexual Arousal Disorder

Female sexual arousal disorder is the inability to complete sexual activity with adequate lubrication and absent or impaired genital responsiveness to sexual stimulation. Cognitive-behavioral therapy with sensate focus and training to improve partner communication are effective strategies. Systemic or local estrogen therapy can increase lubrication in postmenopausal women; in premenopausal women, vaginal moisturizers can be helpful.

Sexual Pain Disorders

Dyspareunia is persistent urogenital pain that occurs around intercourse and is not related exclusively to inadequate lubrication or vaginismus. Therapy is aimed at identifying and treating the underlying cause, which may include vulvodynia, interstitial cystitis, pelvic adhesions, infections, endometriosis, and pelvic venous congestion. Coexisting vaginal atrophy and inadequate lubrication may worsen the pain syndrome and usually can be diagnosed on physical examination. Vaginal estrogen frequently improves atrophy, whereas systemic estrogen or estrogen-progesterone therapy can increase vaginal blood flow and lubrication. Successful treatment strategies must address the complex psychological and behavioral changes that accompany this syndrome, as well as the desire and arousal disorders that often develop as a result of the painful sexual experience.

Vaginismus is the involuntary, recurrent, and persistent spasm of the outer third of the vagina, preventing desired vaginal penetration. Episodes may be situation-specific, for example, pelvic examinations or intercourse. The anticipation of pain with vaginal entry underpins this diagnosis and may result in sexual avoidance. Treatment involves cognitive-behavioral therapy to help the patient feel safe, calm, and in control of the encounter, thereby reducing her anticipatory response. Systematic desensitization teaches deep muscle relaxation and uses objects of increasing diameter, such as dilators, to achieve gradual vaginal tolerance.

KEY POINT

- Laboratory testing is recommended in the evaluation of female sexual dysfunction only if there is suspicion for a particular diagnosis.

Evaluation of a Breast Mass

Breast symptoms in women are common. In a retrospective study of 2400 primary care patients followed for 10 years, 16% of women ages 40 to 79 years presented with a "breast lump" or "lumpiness." Whether discovered by the patient or detected by a physician, a palpable breast mass requires a systematic and logical evaluation. The performance of a careful history and physical examination may lead to a likely diagnosis. However, in most cases, further testing (imaging, tissue sampling) is necessary.

Clinical Presentation

A breast mass or lump is a discrete, firm, three-dimensional abnormality that is different from the surrounding breast tissue. The differential diagnosis of a palpable breast mass is outlined in **Table 40**. The critical challenge in evaluating a breast mass is distinguishing benign from malignant disease. Risk factors for breast cancer should be determined (see MKSAP 16 Hematology and Oncology). History and physical examination features that favor a benign lesion include younger age, absence of breast cancer risk factors, normal overlying skin, a milky (vs. bloody) nipple discharge, change in size during menstrual cycles, and a mass that is round, mobile, and soft. Whereas pain is more likely to be associated with a benign lesion, the presence of pain does not rule out malignancy.

Although most breast masses (up to 90%) are benign cysts or fibroadenomas, neither the history nor the physical examination can definitively rule in or rule out underlying malignancy with sufficient accuracy. In a study of 201 referral patients with palpable solid breast masses, the sensitivity of the physical examination for the detection of breast cancer was 88%. The positive and negative predictive values for breast cancer were 73% and 87%, respectively. Therefore, a palpable breast mass requires further evaluation, including imaging and/or tissue sampling, for definitive diagnosis. Physicians should pursue all breast findings until resolution.

Evaluation

Mammography and ultrasonography are the best imaging modalities for evaluating a palpable breast mass. The choice of ultrasonography versus diagnostic mammography in evaluating a breast mass depends in part on the patient's age. The increased density of breast tissue in women younger than 30 to 35 years may limit the utility of mammography, making ultrasound a better first choice. Ultrasonography may also be a better choice in the pregnant patient as ultrasonography avoids potentially harmful radiation exposure. The main utility of ultrasonography is its ability to differentiate cystic from solid lesions. A simple cyst with symmetric round borders and no internal echoes that, with aspiration, drains nonbloody fluid and disappears completely, is likely to be benign. If bloody fluid is obtained from cyst aspiration, it should be sent for cytology. A solid lesion with uniform borders and uniformly sized internal echoes is most likely a benign fibroadenoma. Fibroadenomas should be followed to assure that they spontaneously regress or decrease in size. Alternatively, depending on the preference of the patient, they can be surgically removed.

TABLE 40.	Differential Diagnosis of Breast Mass
Cysts	
Simple	
Complex	
Infection	
Abscess	
Mastitis	
Tuberculosis	
Trauma	
Fat necrosis	
Hematoma	
Benign tumors	
Fibroadenoma	
Hamartoma	
Papilloma	
Phyllodes tumor (benign variant)	
Lipoma	
Adenoma (tubular or lactating)	
Granular cell tumor	
Neurofibroma	
Hemangioma	
Malignant tumors	
Ductal carcinoma in situ	
Invasive ductal or lobular carcinoma	
Phyllodes tumor (malignant variant)	
Squamous cell carcinoma	
Sarcoma	
Angiosarcoma	
Leukemia	
Lymphoma	
Other	
Diabetic mastopathy	
Sarcoidosis	
Granulomatosis with polyangiitis (also known as Wegener granulomatosis)	
Idiopathic granulomatous mastitis	
Gynecomastia (in men)	

Reproduced with permission from Ganschow PS, et al. Breast Health and Common Breast Problems. American College of Physicians. Philadelphia, PA. 2004:159. Copyright 2004, American College of Physicians.

In women older than 30 to 35 years, the test of choice is diagnostic mammography. An irregular mass with microcalcifications and spiculations is suspicious for malignant disease, and biopsy is mandatory in these cases (see below).

Approximately 10% to 20% of palpable breast cancers are undetected by ultrasonography or mammography. Therefore, the evaluation of a palpable breast mass suspicious for malignancy should continue with biopsy even if the mammogram or ultrasound is unrevealing.

After palpation and imaging, definitive diagnosis is obtained through tissue sampling. Tissue sampling procedures include fine needle aspiration, core needle biopsy with or without stereotactic or ultrasound guidance, or excisional biopsy. Fine needle aspiration, generally reserved for cystic lesions, is operator-dependent and requires an experienced cytopathologist for interpretation. Core needle biopsy, although more costly and with a greater risk for postprocedure hematoma, provides better tissue sampling for pathologic examination and hormone receptor status (if positive for cancer) and can distinguish in situ versus invasive cancer. Core needle biopsy is the test of choice for most solid lesions. Excisional biopsy is used when core needle biopsy is nondiagnostic or when biopsy and imaging studies are not in agreement. Further management of abnormal pathology requires consultation with a breast surgeon and oncologist.

KEY POINT

- When imaging a palpable breast mass, ultrasonography is preferred for pregnant women or women younger than 30 to 35 years; mammography is preferred for women older than 30 to 35 years.

Breast Pain

Clinical Presentation

Breast pain may be characterized as cyclical, noncyclical, or extramammary. Although most women experience mild breast discomfort with the onset of menses, cyclical mastalgia typically lasts for several days and is moderate to severe in intensity. Noncyclical mastalgia has no relationship to the menstrual cycle and may be caused by pregnancy, medications (nicotine, hormone therapy), stretching of Cooper ligaments (secondary to large breasts), or cancer. Extramammary breast pain may be caused by musculoskeletal, cardiac, gastrointestinal, or spinal disorders. Chest wall inflammation, a common cause of extramammary pain, typically presents with unilateral, localized, burning discomfort.

Evaluation

Breast cancer may be associated with mastalgia; therefore, a thorough physical examination is essential in all women presenting with breast pain. Women with a palpable breast mass should be referred for diagnostic imaging. Chest wall pain is typically reproduced by palpation or by examination maneuvers that place stress on the inflamed musculoskeletal structures. All women who are evaluated for mastalgia should be up to date on routine mammographic screening, according to age and personal risk factors for breast cancer.

Treatment

Women with cyclical mastalgia benefit from education and reassurance, as most will experience spontaneous resolution of their symptoms. Medical treatment may be considered for women with severe and persistent pain that interferes with quality of life. Danazol (100 mg twice daily) is the only therapy that has been FDA-approved for the treatment of cyclical mastalgia, but side effects, including menorrhagia and weight gain, often limit its use. Patients with cyclical mastalgia experience benefit with tamoxifen (10 mg/d), and treatment-associated hot flushes and menstrual irregularities are relatively infrequent.

Contraception

Nearly half of pregnancies in the United States are unintended. Adherence to contraception may be improved by counseling patients at risk for unintended pregnancy regarding appropriate contraceptive options, especially patients with serious medical conditions in whom the risk of adverse events of unintended pregnancy is high. Contraceptive options are compared in **Table 41**.

Oral Contraceptive Pills

Oral contraceptive pills (OCPs) include combination estrogen-progesterone products and progesterone-only pills. Differences in combination preparations lie in the type and strength of estrogen and in the androgenicity of their progesterone component. Combinations with lower estrogen dose are as effective with fewer side effects. The mechanisms of action of combination pills include inhibition of ovulation, alteration of the cervical mucus to an environment less conducive to sperm migration, and inhibition of endometrial proliferation. Most hormonal methods are highly effective; annual failure rates are 0.3% with "perfect" use, 8% with typical use. Combined products are also available as a patch and a vaginal ring. Contraindications to combination products include history of thrombosis, liver disease, breast cancer, migraine with aura, and uncontrolled hypertension. Women older than 35 years who smoke more than 15 cigarettes a day should not be prescribed estrogen-containing preparations. Progesterone-only pills, also called the "mini-pill," may be used by women with contraindications to estrogen.

Medications that induce the CYP3A class of liver enzymes may reduce the effectiveness of hormonal contraceptives. Common drugs with this effect include barbiturates, carbamazepine, many antiseizure medications, rifampin, and certain antiretroviral agents. In addition, some antibiotics and some other neurologic medications may alter efficacy of combination preparations via other mechanisms. Additional contraception or barrier methods should be used concurrently and for 4 weeks after discontinuing such drugs.

TABLE 41. Comparison of Contraceptive Options

Agent	Failure Rate[a] (perfect use/ typical use[b])	Advantages	Disadvantages
Combination estrogen-progesterone preparations		Decreased incidence of endometrial, ovarian cancers	Increased risk of myocardial infarction, ischemic stroke, VTE, hypertension
		Decreased dysmenorrhea, menorrhagia, symptomatic ovarian cysts	Increased risk of cancers of the cervix, liver, breast
			Breakthrough bleeding.
		Less iron-deficiency anemia	
Oral	0.3/8		May worsen acne, exacerbate migraine
Patch	0.3/8	Easier compliance	Local skin reaction
			Increased estrogen dose, thus higher VTE risk
Vaginal ring	0.3/8	Easier compliance	Requires self-insertion
		Lowest level of systemic estrogen	
Progesterone-only preparations		Use when estrogen is contraindicated	May worsen acne
Mini-pill			Must maintain precise daily dosing schedule
Long-acting preparations			Irregular bleeding, amenorrhea, decreased bone mineral density (especially in adolescents)
Depot medroxyprogesterone acetate (IM or SQ)	0.3/8	Administered every 3 months	Delayed return to ovulation (10 months)
		Decreased risk of endometrial cancer, PID	
		Improves endometriosis	
Progesterone implants	0.8-1/—	Effective up to 3 years	Delayed return to ovulation (6 months)
Intrauterine devices		Least dependence on user	Bleeding, pain, expulsion (rare); no protection from STIs
Copper	0.6/0.8	Nonhormonal	
		Effective up to 10 years	
Levonorgestrel	0.1/0.1	Decreased blood loss, decreased anemia	
		Effective up to 5 years	
Barrier methods		Only use when needed	Most user-dependent
Cervical cap	9-26/16-32		Requires spermicide
Diaphragm	6/16		Requires spermicide
Male condom	2/15	Protection from STIs	
Female condom	5/21	Protection from STIs	
Vaginal sponge	6-9/16-32		
Sterilization			
Female (tubal ligation)	2% in 10 years	May reduce ovarian cancer risk	Surgical complications
			Regret
			Increased risk of ectopic if pregnancy occurs
Male (vasectomy)	<1% in 10 years	Lower costs, fewer complications, and more effective than tubal ligation	Surgical complications

PID = pelvic inflammatory disease; SQ = subcutaneous; STI = sexually transmitted infection; VTE = venous thromboembolism.

[a]Per 100 women/year.

[b]Perfect use implies correct and consistent use exactly as directed/intended. Typical use reflects rates in actual practice with patients.

Long-Acting Contraceptives

Long-acting progesterone compounds include depot medroxyprogesterone acetate (DMPA) injections, subcutaneous progesterone implants, and progesterone-containing intrauterine devices (IUDs). DMPA may be administered either intramuscularly or subcutaneously following a negative pregnancy test. Etonogestrel implants are small rods inserted subdermally in the upper inner arm and are effective for 3 years. These long-acting progesterone methods are less reliant on user compliance, and therefore may be particularly effective in patients who may have difficulty with daily treatment or barrier methods. They are not recommended for women desiring pregnancy in the subsequent 2 years after cessation of treatment because of potential contraceptive-associated delayed fertility.

Intrauterine Devices

IUDs are the most commonly used form of reversible contraception worldwide. The copper IUD and the levonorgestrel-containing IUD may be placed at any time (except during pregnancy) in an office setting without need for anesthesia. IUDs combine the highest efficacy (typical failure rate <1%) with the lowest cost. The copper IUD may be implanted within 7 days of unprotected intercourse for use as emergency contraception.

Barrier Methods

Barrier methods (see Table 41) allow for "as-needed" contraception but are much less reliable than hormonal methods. All barrier methods are more effective when used with spermicides; spermicides alone are not considered reliable. All barrier methods reduce risk of sexually transmitted infection (STI); evidence is strongest for prevention of HIV infection with male condoms. Limited evidence suggests barrier methods protect future fertility, perhaps by reducing STIs. Combining a barrier method with a hormonal method is recommended when pregnancy must be avoided (for example, during use of teratogenic agents) and in adolescents, in whom risk of both unintended pregnancy and STI is very high.

Emergency Contraception

Emergency contraception refers to contraception administered after intercourse but before implantation. Efficacy for all products increases the earlier they are used. Four methods are available in the United States: levonorgestrel tablets, combined contraceptive tablets, the copper IUD, and progesterone modulators.

The levonorgestrel-only, single-dose (1.5 mg) regimen is the most widely used and most effective option, and is available over-the-counter (by prescription for adolescents younger than 17 years). Other options include two-dose levonorgestrel (0.75 mg taken 12 hours apart), or two tablets of a high-dose combination OCP (100 micrograms ethinyl estradiol, taken twice, 12 hours apart). Levonorgestrel has greater efficacy and fewer side effects (nausea, vomiting, dizziness, headache). If vomiting occurs within 2 hours of taking emergency contraception, the dose should be repeated, given vaginally, or given after an antiemetic has been used. These methods work by delaying or preventing ovulation, and are not abortifacients. They may be taken up to 5 days (120 hours) post-intercourse. The copper IUD is inserted up to 5 days after intercourse. It functions primarily by stopping fertilization and interfering with implantation. It may remain in place as long-term contraception.

Mifepristone, a progesterone-receptor modulator, is approved by the FDA as an abortifacient, but has been used outside the United States as emergency contraception. Ulipristal, another progesterone-receptor modulator with agonist and antagonist effects, has been approved for use as emergency contraception in the United States.

Sterilization

Sterilization is highly effective, with an annual failure rate of 1 in 1000. Female sterilization (tubal ligation) incurs more risk and cost than vasectomy and is less effective. Incidence of regret and requests for reversal of tubal ligation are significantly higher in women younger than 30 years and in those who are postpartum or postabortion at the time of the procedure.

KEY POINTS

- Women older than 35 years who smoke more than 15 cigarettes a day should not be prescribed estrogen-containing contraceptives.
- Intrauterine devices are highly effective at preventing pregnancy and are low cost.

Preconception Counseling

Adequate preconception care can significantly reduce the risk for preterm birth and birth anomalies. Each health care visit with a reproductive-age woman represents an opportunity for preconception counseling; providers should routinely ask if a patient is either considering pregnancy or could possibly become pregnant. For patients considering pregnancy, preconception risk should be assessed (**Table 42**) and brief interventions undertaken to optimize reproductive health, including encouraging a healthy lifestyle; stressing the importance of tobacco, alcohol, and drug cessation; and referring underweight or overweight patients for formal nutritional evaluation. Prescription medications should be changed, if possible, to minimize exposure to potential teratogens (**Table 43**). Consultation with specialists for co-management of specific diseases in pregnancy, such as diabetes mellitus and epilepsy, may be indicated.

A physical examination and focused laboratory testing can provide additional information regarding a patient's reproductive health and preconception risk. Measurements of

TABLE 42. Preconception Risk Assessment

Risk Category	Specific Items to Assess
Reproductive awareness	Desire for pregnancy, number and timing of desired pregnancies, age-related changes in fertility, sexuality, contraception
Environmental hazards and toxins	Exposure to radiation, lead, mercury
Nutrition and folic acid consumption	Healthy diet, daily consumption of folic acid, restricting consumption of shark, swordfish, king mackerel, and tilefish to fewer than 2 servings weekly (owing to high mercury content)
Genetics	Family history of inherited genetic disorders
Substance abuse	Use of tobacco, alcohol, illicit drugs
Medical conditions	Seizure disorder, diabetes mellitus, hypertension, thyroid disease, asthma, HIV infection, systemic lupus erythematosus
Medications	Over-the-counter and prescription medications, potential teratogens
Infectious diseases and vaccinations	Immunity to varicella, rubella, pertussis, tetanus; risk for hepatitis B
Psychosocial concerns	Depression, interpersonal/family relationships, risk for abuse (physical, sexual, emotional)

Based on Johnson K, Posner SF, Biermann J, et al.; CDC/ATSDR Preconception Care Work Group; Select Panel on Preconception Care. Recommendations to improve preconception health and health care—United States. A report of the CDC/ATSDR Preconception Care Work Group and the Select Panel on Preconception Care. MMWR Recomm Rep. 2006;55(RR-6):1-23. [PMID: 16617292]

TABLE 43. Teratogenic Medications Commonly Prescribed by Internists

ACE inhibitors
Androgens, testosterone derivatives
Carbamazepine
Fluoxetine, paroxetine
Folic acid antagonists
Lithium
Phenytoin
Primidone
Statins
Tetracycline
Valproic acid
Vitamin A derivatives: isotretinoin, retinoids, etretinate
Warfarin

Adapted from Berghella V, Buchanan E, Pereira L, Baxter JK. Preconception Care. Obstet Gynecol Surv. 2010;65(2):119-131. [PMID: 20100361]

BMI and blood pressure are essential, and the pelvic examination may include collecting specimens for cervical cytology and chlamydial testing (if indicated per screening recommendations for these tests). All women who are considering pregnancy should be routinely assessed for immunity to varicella and rubella, and screening for HIV may be considered.

Certain interventions optimize pregnancy outcomes in all reproductive-age women, including appropriate vaccinations, daily folic acid, and proper diet and exercise. Vaccination for rubella and varicella to nonimmune women should be administered at least 4 weeks before conception to minimize risks to the fetus. Influenza vaccination is appropriate for those who will be pregnant during flu season, and pertussis vaccination, in combination with tetanus and diphtheria, is recommended for all persons who have not been immunized as adults. Supplementation with folic acid (400 micrograms/d) reduces the risk of neural tube defects. Because these defects occur very early in gestation, when a woman might not even know she is pregnant, folic acid supplementation is generally recommended for all women who are of reproductive age. Higher doses of folic acid may be appropriate in women who have prior children with a neural tube defect, take antiseizure medications, or who are obese.

KEY POINT

- Preconception counseling should include risk assessment in the following areas: reproductive awareness, environmental hazards and toxins, nutrition and folic acid supplementation, genetics, substance abuse, medical conditions, medications, infectious diseases and vaccinations, and psychosocial concerns.

Menopause

Overview

Menopause is defined as the permanent cessation of menses and is diagnosed retrospectively, after a woman has experienced amenorrhea for 12 months. Menopause occurs through a series of stages characterized according to variations in the menstrual cycle and alterations in follicle-stimulating hormone (FSH) levels. Women typically begin to experience irregular menses in early perimenopause, with cycles of variable length, and then progress into late perimenopause, with intervals of amenorrhea lasting more than 60 days and two or more skipped cycles. FSH levels begin to rise in this perimenopausal transition but may fluctuate significantly depending on the frequency of anovulation. After 1 year of amenorrhea (menopause), a woman is considered to be early postmenopausal, and FSH levels become very elevated (FSH >40 units/L, estradiol <20 ng/mL). Late postmenopause starts 5 years after the last menstrual period. On average, women in the United States experience menopause at the age of 51 years.

The hallmark symptoms of the menopausal transition are hot flushes and night sweats (vasomotor symptoms) and vaginal dryness and dyspareunia (urogenital symptoms). A hot flush is characterized by the sudden onset of intense warmth that starts in the face or chest and then spreads throughout the body; it is usually associated with sweating and palpitations. Night sweats are hot flushes that occur during sleep and often result in nocturnal awakenings. Up to 50% of women experience hot flushes during the menopausal transition, but symptoms typically resolve spontaneously within a few years of onset. Conversely, vaginal dryness and dyspareunia, which result from progressive estrogen depletion and subsequent urogenital atrophy, become much more prevalent in late postmenopause. Mood changes, cognitive difficulties, and primary sleep disorders may be more common in menopausal women, but these symptoms have not been definitely linked to changes in hormone levels. The differential diagnosis of menopausal symptoms includes thyroid disease, elevated prolactin levels, and pregnancy, and testing for these conditions may be considered in selected patients.

Management of Vasomotor Symptoms

Women should be reassured that hot flushes and night sweats are common in the menopausal transition and that spontaneous resolution typically occurs within a few years. As smoking, obesity, and sedentary lifestyle are all risk factors associated with hot flushes, behavioral changes may result in symptom improvement.

Systemic Hormone Therapy

Systemic hormone therapy is the most effective treatment for moderate to severe vasomotor symptoms, and has FDA approval for this indication. It may be considered as a treatment option for women who have a thorough understanding of the risks and benefits associated with therapy. Several formulations of estrogen are currently available and include conjugated equine estrogen, micronized 17 β-estradiol, and transdermal 17 β-estradiol. Most experts recommend starting with the lowest dose of estrogen that effectively relieves symptoms and titrating up as necessary to achieve maximal relief. Although supporting data are limited, transdermal estrogen, as compared with oral estrogen, may be associated with less thromboembolic risk as it avoids the hepatic first-pass effect. Moreover, transdermal and oral estrogen seem to be equally effective for treating vasomotor symptoms. Common adverse effects of systemic estrogen therapy are breast tenderness and uterine bleeding.

All women with an intact uterus who are treated with hormone therapy must receive progesterone to avoid estrogen-induced endometrial hyperplasia and cancer. Several preparations are available and may be given continuously or cyclically. Women treated with cyclic progesterone may have occasional withdrawal bleeding and should be counseled regarding this effect. Absolute contraindications to hormone therapy include pregnancy; unexplained vaginal bleeding; a history of coronary artery disease, stroke, thromboembolic disease, or breast or endometrial cancer; hypertriglyceridemia; recent vascular thrombosis or cardiovascular event; and immobilization.

Table 44 lists a stepwise approach for initiating hormone therapy in women aged 50-59 years who have experienced menopause at the median age (51 years). In general, women should be treated with the lowest possible dose of estrogen for the shortest amount of time necessary; treatment for longer than 5 years is not advised. Systemic hormone therapy can be discontinued abruptly or tapered gradually; there is no difference in the rates of vasomotor symptom recurrence. The North American Menopause Society (NAMS) suggests that bone density be measured if hormone therapy is discontinued after several years of treatment.

Benefits and Risks of Systemic Hormone Therapy

The Women's Health Initiative (WHI) demonstrated that combination estrogen and progesterone therapy (EPT) decreased the risk of osteoporotic fractures and colorectal cancer but increased the risk of coronary heart disease (CHD), venous thromboembolism, invasive breast cancer, and stroke. In contrast, estrogen-only therapy increased the risk for stroke, but no other outcomes. Notably, the absolute benefits and risks associated with treatment were quite small; among 10,000 women treated with EPT, there were five fewer hip fractures and eight additional strokes.

Additional analyses of data from the WHI suggest that while the overall risk of CHD in postmenopausal women on hormone therapy is increased, the greatest risk is in older women (ages 70-79 years) and is minimal in younger women (ages 50-59 years) treated earlier in menopause. This has led NAMS to recommend that hormone therapy not be used as primary prophylaxis for CHD among women at any age. Hormone therapy may be used to treat menopausal symptoms in women ages 50 to 59 years or those within 10 years of menopause as there is minimal CHD risk; hormone therapy should not be initiated in women older than 60 years.

In contrast to CHD risk, the increased risk of stroke observed with hormone therapy does not vary according to length of time since menopause onset. Notably, the risk of stroke with hormone therapy use among women aged 50 to 59 years did not differ significantly from that among women older than 60 years.

In a follow-up study of more than 12,000 women who participated in the WHI, investigators found that EPT, as

TABLE 44. Initiating Systemic Hormone Therapy in Women Ages 50-59 Years[a]

Step 1: Confirm that hot flushes/night sweats are moderate-severe in intensity and/or vaginal symptoms are moderate-severe in intensity and have been refractory to local therapies.

Step 2: Assess for absolute contraindications to systemic hormone therapy.

Step 3: Assess the patient's baseline risk for stroke, cardiovascular disease, and breast cancer (consider using the Framingham stroke risk score, Framingham CHD risk score, and Gail risk score to quantify this risk). If the Framingham stroke or CHD risk score is >10% or Gail risk score is elevated, consider avoiding systemic hormone therapy.[b,c]

Step 4: Use the lowest dose of estrogen that relieves menopausal symptoms.

Step 5: Add systemic progesterone therapy to estrogen therapy in women who have an intact uterus.

Step 6: Assess symptoms and side effects within 4-6 weeks of initiating therapy. Increase the dose of estrogen if symptoms are persistent.

Step 7: Reassess symptoms and risk factors for cardiovascular disease, stroke, and breast cancer regularly. Ideally, treatment with systemic hormone therapy should continue for no more than 5 years.

Step 8: Discontinue systemic hormone therapy if the risks of treatment outweigh the benefits, if symptoms resolve spontaneously, or according to patient preference. Therapy does not need to be tapered.

CHD = coronary heart disease.

[a]According to North American Menopause Society, systemic hormone therapy should be avoided in women older than 60 years who have experienced menopause at the median age (51 years). If a woman has experienced menopause later than the median age, these guidelines apply within the first 10 years of menopause.

[b]Some authors indicate that systemic hormone therapy is safe in women who have experienced menopause within the last 5 years and have a Framingham CHD risk score of 10%-20%.

[c]The majority of participants in the Women's Health Initiative had a Gail risk score of less than 2%.

compared with placebo, increases the risk of node-positive invasive breast cancer and breast cancer mortality. The timing of hormone therapy initiation may be influential: exposure to EPT during the early postmenopause is associated with an increased incidence of breast cancer, whereas exposure during late postmenopause is not. The increased breast cancer risk associated with therapy (8 excess cases per 10,000 person years) becomes apparent after 3 to 5 years of exposure to hormone therapy. Moreover, EPT increases breast density and may impede the interpretation of mammograms. Post-hoc analysis of the WHI data suggests that EPT may promote lung cancer among older smokers, but these results need further validation.

The low absolute risk of adverse events supports the option to prescribe hormone therapy for women with moderate to severe vasomotor or urogenital symptoms who are at low risk for CHD, stroke, and invasive breast cancer.

Nonhormonal Therapy

Several nonhormonal therapies are available for women who have contraindications to hormone therapy or want to avoid its attendant risks. Certain antidepressants (selective serotonin reuptake inhibitors and serotonin-norepinephrine reuptake inhibitors), gabapentin, and clonidine may reduce hot flush frequency by one or two per day as compared with placebo. Red clover extract and black cohosh are ineffective for treating hot flushes, and study results suggest mixed benefits with soy isoflavone extracts.

Management of Urogenital Symptoms

Progressive estrogen depletion during the menopausal transition leads to thinning of the vaginal epithelium and vaginal atrophy. Clinically, women may report vaginal dryness, itching, dyspareunia, dysuria, and frequent urinary tract infections. Mild to moderate symptoms can be effectively treated with vaginal moisturizers, and lubrication may ease pain with intercourse. The FDA has approved the use of vaginal estrogen therapy for women who do not respond to these measures or who have moderate to severe urogenital symptoms. Several preparations are currently available and include conjugated estrogen vaginal cream, estradiol vaginal cream, vaginal estradiol tablets, and an estradiol vaginal ring. Although each of these treatments is equally effective in relieving symptoms, low-dose vaginal estradiol tablets (10-25 micrograms) and the estradiol vaginal ring (8-9 micrograms) are preferred over vaginal estrogen creams, as they result in minimal systemic estrogen absorption. According to the NAMS guidelines, progesterone therapy is typically not indicated when low-dose local estrogen therapy is used to treat vaginal atrophy.

KEY POINTS

- Women with vasomotor menopausal symptoms that warrant hormone therapy should be treated with the lowest possible dose of estrogen for the shortest amount of time necessary.

- To minimize cardiovascular risk, hormone therapy should not be initiated in women older than 60 years who have not previously received hormone therapy and who experienced menopause at the median age.

- Hormone therapy does not increase the risk for coronary heart disease among women aged 50-59 years who have experienced menopause at the median age.

Abnormal Uterine Bleeding

Clinical Presentation and Evaluation

Abnormal uterine bleeding refers to bleeding that is excessive in frequency, duration, or amount, and is often described by the pattern of occurrence and degree of flow. *Polymenorrhagia* is bleeding occurring more than once every 24 days, the lower limit of the average menstrual cycle. *Oligomenorrhea* is bleeding less frequently than every 35 days, although women are more likely to complain of too frequent than infrequent menses. *Metrorrhagia* is irregular or intermenstrual bleeding. *Menorrhagia* refers to regular cycles with excessive bleeding, defined as monthly menstrual loss of more than 80 mL or bleeding for more than 7 days. *Menometrorrhagia* is bleeding at irregular intervals with excessive flow.

Abnormal bleeding is usually characterized as ovulatory or anovulatory. Ovulatory bleeding is cyclical and may be caused by anatomic abnormalities (polyps, leiomyomas), bleeding disorders, medications that interfere with hemostasis, or uterine cancer. Anovulatory bleeding is usually unpredictable and of variable flow and duration owing to loss of cyclical hormonal influences on the endometrium; if no anatomic or medical cause is identified for bleeding, anovulatory bleeding may be referred to as dysfunctional uterine bleeding (DUB). Anovulatory cycles are characterized by estrogen-mediated endometrial proliferation without the stabilizing effects of progesterone, resulting in endometrial desquamation and erratic bleeding. Anovulation has many potential causes, but also commonly occurs in women without underlying medical or anatomic issues.

These terms apply only to women of reproductive age; in postmenopausal women (absence of menses for 1 year), any uterine bleeding is abnormal and warrants further evaluation, especially for endometrial cancer. Perimenarchal and perimenopausal stages are often characterized by abnormal bleeding patterns and are usually not cause for concern.

Initial evaluation includes history with attention to stressors, diet, exercise, weight changes, trauma, medications, and substance abuse. Important historical factors for estimating changes in blood loss include change in pattern with flow excessive for the patient, increase in number of pads or tampons used, leaking despite use of pads or tampons, and presence of clots. Additional history may give clues to an underlying endocrine or bleeding disorder, chronic liver or kidney disease, or STI. Physical examination should include a complete pelvic examination with attention to pelvic pathology; screening for cervical malignancy should be up-to-date. Pregnancy testing should be performed in all women with abnormal uterine bleeding as pregnancy is the most common cause of a divergence from a normal bleeding pattern. An assessment for chronic diseases, including liver, kidney, thyroid, autoimmune, and bleeding diathesis, should be performed as indicated. In adolescents and young adults, coagulation disorders are most common. Pelvic ultrasonography should be performed in women with structural abnormalities noted on examination, abnormal bleeding despite evidence of ovulatory cycles, or new-onset intermenstrual bleeding.

In women with prolonged anovulation, exposure to unopposed estrogen increases risk for endometrial carcinoma. Therefore, pelvic ultrasonography is indicated in women older than 35 years to assess endometrial stripe thickness; an endometrial stripe 5 mm or thicker warrants endometrial biopsy before initiation of medical therapy. Ultrasonography is also indicated in younger women in whom empiric medical therapy has failed to control bleeding.

Management

Management of abnormal uterine bleeding should be directed toward the underlying cause. Anatomic or structural abnormalities causing ovulatory bleeding generally require directed therapy.

Management of anovulatory bleeding is directed toward restoring the hormonal balance and stabilizing the endometrium. Treatment depends on the contraceptive plans of the patient. For women desiring fertility, a progestin such as medroxyprogesterone acetate may be used for the last 2 weeks of each cycle to promote withdrawal bleeding. For women not desiring pregnancy, OCPs may be used, as well as other contraceptive methods, including depot medroxyprogesterone, the vaginal contraceptive ring, and levonorgestrel IUD. For severe bleeding, short courses of gonadotropin-releasing hormone (GnRH) agonists or intravenous high-dose estrogens may be used. For patients who do not respond to medical treatment, evaluation for alternative causes or surgical treatment is appropriate.

For patients with chronic diseases not otherwise amenable to therapy (for example, chronic kidney disease), treatment is symptomatic. NSAIDs can decrease uterine bleeding by up to 40% owing to the high concentrations of prostaglandins in the endometrium. Danazol (200-400 mg/d) is approved for the treatment of heavy or irregular bleeding.

KEY POINT

- In postmenopausal women, any uterine bleeding is abnormal and warrants further evaluation, especially for endometrial cancer.

Dysmenorrhea

Dysmenorrhea is complicated or painful menstruation. It is usually seen in adolescents and young adults and is the most common gynecologic symptom in this age group. In 90% of cases, dysmenorrhea is associated with normal ovulatory cycles and no pelvic pathology (primary dysmenorrhea). In the remaining 10% of cases, a secondary cause, such as endometriosis, fibroids, or uterine pathology may be found. Symptoms of dysmenorrhea include abdominal cramps, headache, nausea, and vomiting. Symptoms coincide with onset of menses and last 1 to 2 days. Severity typically correlates with the amount and duration of menstrual blood flow.

Initial evaluation includes a thorough history, with particular attention to sexual activity and risks for abuse or infection. Unless pelvic pathology is suspected (previous radiation, trauma, infection, foreign body), treatment may begin without further evaluation. Effective treatments include NSAIDs and cyclooxygenase-2 inhibitors. These agents block prostaglandins in the endometrial lining, inhibiting the inflammation, vasoconstriction, and uterine ischemia thought to be the etiology. For patients with incomplete relief of symptoms, use of combined contraceptive therapy is effective; pills, patches, or the vaginal ring may be used. Extended-cycle combined OCPs may be particularly useful for this indication. Other treatment options include long-acting progesterones; these options should be used with caution in adolescents owing to the risk for osteoporosis from estrogen deficiency.

Women not responding to therapy should be suspected of having a secondary cause. The most common of these is endometriosis, which causes both cyclic and noncyclic pain. Treatment options are similar; additionally, GnRH agonists and aromatase inhibitors have been used but require calcium and vitamin D supplementation. If pelvic pathology is suspected or if symptoms are refractory, gynecologic referral may be appropriate.

Chronic Pelvic Pain

Chronic pelvic pain (CPP) in women is defined as noncyclic pain of at least 6 months' duration that localizes to the anatomic pelvis, anterior abdominal wall at or below the umbilicus, the lumbosacral back, or the buttocks, and is of sufficient severity to cause functional disability or necessitate medical care. Approximately 15% to 20% of reproductive-age women have experienced CPP for more than 1 year. The most common causes of CPP are endometriosis, pelvic adhesions, pelvic varices, interstitial cystitis, and irritable bowel syndrome (IBS); many women have more than one diagnosis. Fifty percent to 80% of women with CPP have symptoms consistent with IBS. Risk factors for CPP include physical and sexual abuse, pelvic inflammatory disease, a difficult obstetric delivery, a history of abdominopelvic surgery, and other chronic pain syndromes, such as fibromyalgia. Endometriosis, interstitial cystitis, and IBS all tend to worsen during the menstrual cycle; additional historical clues and tests that aid in diagnosis are listed in **Table 45**. Laboratory studies should include a complete blood count, serum chemistries, erythrocyte sedimentation rate, urinalysis and urine culture, and vaginal/endocervical swabs for culture. Transvaginal ultrasonography is helpful for identifying anatomic pelvic pathology, and a normal study aids in providing reassurance. Laparoscopy may be indicated for evaluation of severe symptoms of unclear etiology or identified pathology on examination or ultrasonography.

NSAIDs can be used as first-line short-term therapy for most women with moderate CPP. Although evidence to support the use of antidepressants is limited, psychotherapy and writing about the stress of pelvic pain may be helpful.

TABLE 45.	Diagnosis and Treatment Strategies for the Most Common Causes of Chronic Pelvic Pain[a]			
Etiology	**Characteristic History**	**Diagnostic Strategies**	**Treatment Strategies**	**Prevalence**
Endometriosis	Pain that may worsen with menstruation, dyspareunia, dysmenorrhea	Empiric treatment with GnRH agonist therapy; diagnostic laparoscopy	GnRH agonist therapy; combination OCPs for women with significant dysmenorrhea; laparoscopic surgical destruction of endometriosis lesions (stages I-III endometriosis)	Up to two-thirds of women with CPP have endometriosis
Pelvic adhesions	History of PID, endometriosis, abdominal or pelvic surgery	Diagnostic laparoscopy	Surgical adhesiolysis for severe adhesions	25%-50% of women with CPP have adhesions, although causality is usually not clear
Pelvic varices	Dull, chronic pain worsened with prolonged standing, improved by lying down and elevating legs	Combined transabdominal and transvaginal ultrasound	Medroxyprogesterone acetate	May cause pain in up to 42% of women with CPP
Interstitial cystitis	Dysuria, urgency, frequency, repeatedly negative urine cultures	Interstitial cystitis symptom index; cystoscopy	Pentosan polysulfate sodium; tricyclic antidepressants; GnRH agonist therapy may be helpful	38%-85% of women presenting to gynecologists with CPP may have this diagnosis

CPP = chronic pelvic pain; GnRH = gonadotropin-releasing hormone; OCP = oral contraceptive pill; PID = pelvic inflammatory disease.

[a]Irritable bowel syndrome, a common cause of CPP, is discussed in MKSAP 16 Gastroenterology and Hepatology.

Condition-specific treatment strategies are listed in Table 45. GnRH agonists are effective in treating women with CPP associated with endometriosis or IBS and may improve pain control in women with interstitial cystitis. The American College of Obstetricians and Gynecologists (ACOG) guidelines recommend empiric treatment with GnRH agonists in women with undiagnosed CPP; benefit may obviate the need for diagnostic laparoscopy. Add-back therapy with estrogen or progesterone can mitigate the detrimental effects that GnRH agonist therapy has on bone density without affecting treatment efficacy.

Surgical options for treatment include laparoscopic excision of endometriotic implants, adhesiolysis, sacral nerve stimulation, presacral neurectomy, and uterine nerve ablation. Hysterectomy is an effective treatment for CPP, although a substantial proportion of young women with normal pelvic anatomy at surgery will continue to experience pain. Except for pathology-directed interventions (such as for endometriosis), surgical treatment is generally pursued only after failure of medical therapy.

Vaginitis

Clinical Presentation and Evaluation

Vaginitis comprises a spectrum of infectious and noninfectious conditions that produce characteristic vulvovaginal symptoms, including vaginal discharge, vulvar itching, burning, and irritation. The most common causes of vaginitis are bacterial vaginosis, trichomoniasis, and vulvovaginal candidiasis. Less frequently, vaginal irritation can result from atrophy, allergic reactions, or certain dermatologic conditions.

All patients should be queried about the duration of symptoms; relationship to the menstrual cycle, douching, and sexual activity; discharge odor; and associated vulvar itching, irritation, burning, and swelling. The vulva and vagina should be inspected carefully for erythema, excoriations, and tenderness, and vaginal wall secretions should be collected for pH, amine testing, and saline and 10% potassium hydroxide microscopy. Additional point-of-care testing may aid in the diagnosis.

Bacterial Vaginosis

Bacterial vaginosis (BV) is a polymicrobial infection characterized by an overgrowth of multiple anaerobic bacteria (*Gardnerella vaginalis*, *Ureaplasma*, *Mycoplasma*, and *Bacteroides* species, among others), resulting in a reduction of the normal vaginal hydrogen peroxide–producing *Lactobacillus* species. Risk factors include douching, lack of condom use, and multiple or new sexual partners (although BV may also be diagnosed in women who have never been sexually active). BV infection increases the risk of complications in pregnancy and obstetric surgery, and affected women are more likely to acquire HIV, gonorrhea, chlamydial

infection, and genital herpes. Symptomatic patients may report a thin, white or gray homogeneous discharge that has a "fishy" smell.

BV can be diagnosed if at least three of the four Amsel criteria are present: homogenous, thin, white discharge; vaginal pH greater than 4.5; fishy odor before or after the addition of 10% potassium hydroxide to vaginal secretions ("whiff" test); and the presence of clue cells on saline microscopy. Clue cells are squamous vaginal epithelial cells with a large number of coccobacillary organisms densely attached to their surface, giving them a granular appearance (**Figure 18**). The Amsel criteria have a sensitivity of 92% and a specificity of 77% for diagnosis of BV. Other diagnostic options include a point-of-care test card that detects proline aminopeptidase and has a sensitivity of 90% and a specificity of 97%. Culture for *G. vaginalis* is not recommended owing to low specificity.

Treatment is with either oral (7 days) or topical (5-7 days) metronidazole or clindamycin (oral or topical). Metronidazole is safe in pregnancy, but topical clindamycin should be avoided as it may increase the risk of adverse outcomes. Approximately 30% of women will experience a recurrence of BV within 3 months.

Trichomoniasis

Women who have multiple sexual partners, exchange sex for payment, or use injected drugs are at particularly high risk for trichomoniasis, an STI caused by infection with the protozoan *Trichomonas vaginalis*. Although some infected women are asymptomatic, many experience a profuse malodorous yellow-green discharge with vulvar itching, burning, and postcoital bleeding. Trichomoniasis is associated with a vaginal pH greater than 4.5 and the presence of motile trichomonads on saline microscopy, but the specificity of an abnormal vaginal pH and the sensitivity of saline microscopy for identifying motile trichomonads are both low. If point-of-care tests are unavailable, vaginal secretions may be sent for culture.

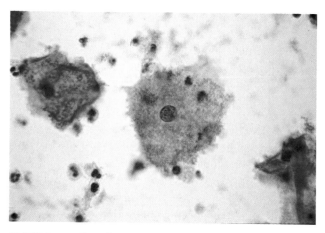

FIGURE 18. Clue cells.

Oral single-dose metronidazole therapy is associated with a high rate of cure and should be provided to all symptomatic women; in addition, treatment of the sexual partner is essential for preventing reinfection. Metronidazole may be safely given at any stage in pregnancy. Inadequate response to treatment may be caused by reinfection (up to 17% of treated women are reinfected within 3 months) or diminished responsiveness to metronidazole. If the latter is suspected, a 7-day course of metronidazole (500 mg twice daily) often results in clinical resolution. Subsequent diagnostic testing to confirm treatment success should be considered for women who are HIV-positive as they may be less responsive to single-dose metronidazole. Persistent coinfection with *T. vaginalis* can increase HIV shedding and viral transmission.

Vulvovaginal Candidiasis

Most women experience at least one episode of vulvovaginal candidiasis (VVC) in their lifetime, and more than one third will have two or more infections. Pregnancy, diabetes, and treatment with antibiotics or corticosteroids increase the risk for VVC. Although VVC produces classic symptoms, such as vulvar pruritus, external dysuria, and a thick, "cottage-cheese" discharge, studies have shown that the history alone is insufficient for reliably establishing the diagnosis. On examination, vulvar edema, erythema, and excoriations are suggestive of disease, but VVC is confirmed only if symptoms are accompanied by the presence of yeasts, hyphae, or pseudohyphae on microscopy or Gram stain, or if a vaginal culture is positive for yeast. Vaginal pH is normal in VVC. As the sensitivity of microscopy may be as low as 65%, empiric treatment for VVC can be considered if vaginal culture is unavailable and symptoms are accompanied by characteristic physical examination findings. Culture for *Candida* in the absence of symptoms is not recommended, as 10% to 20% of women are colonized.

Once the diagnosis of VVC is made, infection is characterized as uncomplicated or complicated and treatment is prescribed accordingly. Uncomplicated VVC responds well to therapy with over-the-counter topical imidazoles or a single dose of oral fluconazole. Complicated VVC, which is diagnosed in women who are severely symptomatic, pregnant, immunosuppressed, or diabetic, necessitates more aggressive treatment, including topical imidazole treatment for up to 14 days or two doses of oral fluconazole given 3 days apart. In pregnant women, VVC is treated with a 7-day course of topical imidazole. Recurrent VVC is defined as more than four symptomatic episodes per year. Recurrence is treated initially with a 7- to 14-day course of topical imidazole therapy or oral fluconazole every third day for a total of three doses, followed by oral fluconazole weekly for 6 months. Twenty percent of cases of recurrent VVC are caused by *Candida* species other than *C. albicans*, and these may be treated with a 2-week course of intravaginal boric acid.

Eye Disorders

Red Eye

Clinical Evaluation

Red eye is the most common eye condition seen in primary care. Most cases of red eye can be safely managed by the primary care physician, but it is important to know when to refer to an ophthalmologist. During the initial evaluation, the history should focus on the acuity of onset of symptoms, whether one or both eyes are involved, history of trauma or risk factors for foreign bodies or abrasion, other accompanying symptoms (nausea, vomiting, photophobia, headache), presence of systemic disease, and whether the vision is intact. The physical examination should begin with assessment of visual acuity, location and distribution of redness, presence or absence of discharge, and pupillary shape. Funduscopy has little diagnostic yield in evaluating the red eye.

Conjunctivitis

Conjunctivitis, inflammation of the thin, usually transparent outermost lining of the eye, is the most common cause of red eye. When inflamed, the conjunctiva appears pink or red and the conjunctival blood vessels may be seen. Conjunctivitis is caused by viruses, bacteria, allergies, or contact lens wear. The history is usually helpful in distinguishing these etiologies. Viral conjunctivitis (**Figure 19**) is usually caused by an adenovirus; a history of a preceding upper respiratory tract infection and recent exposure to a person with conjunctivitis are clues to this diagnosis. Onset is usually acute, with unilateral redness and watery discharge. Other symptoms include itching, mild photophobia, a diffuse foreign body sensation, and crusting of the eyelids after sleep. Persons with viral conjunctivitis are contagious for up to 2 weeks after the second eye becomes involved and, therefore, should perform frequent hand washing and avoid sharing personal items. Food handlers and health care providers should not return to work until eye discharge ceases. The treatment for viral conjunctivitis is largely supportive, including cold compresses and artificial tears. There is no role for antibiotic eye drops in the treatment of viral conjunctivitis.

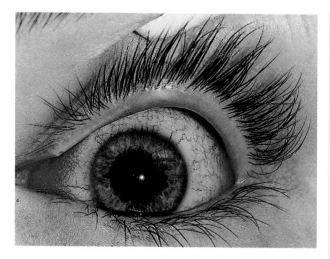

FIGURE 19. Viral conjunctivitis.

Eye with Viral Conjunctivitis. Digital image. Wikimedia Commons. 1 Feb. 2010. Web. 16 May 2012. <http://commons.wikimedia.org/wiki/File:An_eye_with_viral_conjunctivitis.jpg>.

Bacterial conjunctivitis (**Figure 20**) is also highly contagious and is categorized as hyperacute, acute, and chronic. Acute bacterial conjunctivitis, the most common form of bacterial conjunctivitis seen in the outpatient setting, is usually caused by *Staphylococcus aureus*; but *Streptococcus pneumoniae* and *Haemophilus influenzae* can also be culprit organisms. Bacterial conjunctivitis is usually distinguished from viral conjunctivitis by the presence of mucopurulent discharge that is worse when waking in the morning and when dried may form a significant crust, whereas viral conjunctivitis has clearer discharge and may be preceded by an upper respiratory tract infection. Hyperacute bacterial conjunctivitis is associated with a copious purulent discharge, pain, and diminished vision. In sexually active adults, hyperacute bacterial conjunctivitis may be caused by *Neisseria gonorrhoeae*. Gonococcal conjunctivitis is sudden in onset and can rapidly progress to corneal perforation. Patients with gonococcal conjunctivitis

should be treated systemically for *N. gonorrhoeae* as well as *Chlamydia trachomatis* infection, as one-third of patients with gonorrhea are coinfected with *C. trachomatis*.

Bacterial cultures and Gram staining are not generally performed in the evaluation of bacterial conjunctivitis. Exceptions include when gonococcal infection is suspected, the patient is immunocompromised, wears contact lenses, has hyperacute bacterial conjunctivitis, or has failed to improve after 1 week of therapy. Broad-spectrum antibiotic eyedrops should be prescribed for use for 5 to 7 days. Bacterial conjunctivitis that persists for at least 4 weeks is considered chronic; these patients should be evaluated by an ophthalmologist.

Allergic conjunctivitis is a clinical diagnosis. It may resemble viral conjunctivitis in terms of clear discharge; however, it tends to be associated with seasonal allergies, with itching in one or both eyes as the predominant symptom. Treatment includes oral antihistamines, topical antihistamines, and artificial tears; antibiotic treatment is not indicated.

Subconjunctival Hematoma

Subconjunctival hematoma (**Figure 21**) occurs when subconjunctival vessels bleed into the subconjunctival space. This can occur spontaneously or result from trauma, a Valsalva maneuver, cough, or antiplatelet or antithrombotic agents. Subconjunctival hematomas are painless and do not affect vision but are sometimes frightening for the patient. Patients should be reassured and informed that resolution occurs gradually over several weeks. Although most subconjunctival hemorrhages are benign, other causes of this finding include endocarditis, bleeding disorders, and medications (such as imatinib mesylate); these causes should be considered if appropriate.

Corneal Conditions

Corneal abrasions cause a foreign body sensation, photophobia, tearing, and pain. They often result from trauma caused by foreign bodies or fingernails. To examine the cornea, fluorescein dye should be instilled into the eye and the eye

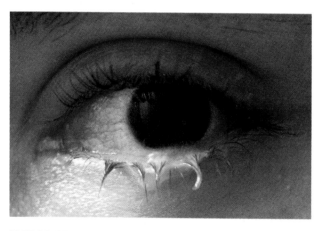

FIGURE 20. Bacterial conjunctivitis.

Swollen Eye with Conjunctivitis. Digital image. Wikimedia Commons. 8 Feb. 2008. Web. 16 May 2012. <http://commons.wikimedia.org/wiki/File:Swollen_eye_with_conjunctivitis.jpg>.

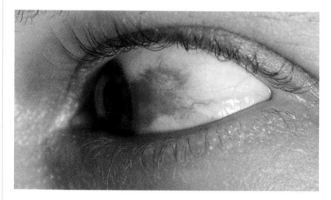

FIGURE 21. Subconjunctival hematoma. A well-localized superficial collection of extravasated blood is visible; the sclera and conjunctiva are not involved.

Subconjunctival Hemorrhage. Digital image. Wikimedia Commons. 28 Jun. 2011. Web. 16 May 2012. <http://commons.wikimedia.org/wiki/File:Subconjunctival_hemorrhage_eye.jpg>.

examined under a Wood lamp or with a slit lamp. The area underneath the upper lid should be examined to rule out a foreign body, which should be removed if present. Although there is little supporting evidence that topical antibiotics improve outcomes, many practitioners still prescribe a short course (48-72 hours). Eye patches have not been shown to speed healing or improve patient symptoms. Most abrasions improve markedly within 24 to 48 hours owing to rapid epithelial cell proliferation.

Corneal ulcers can result from bacterial infection, herpes simplex virus infection, contact lens wear, or trauma. The ulcer can be detected with fluorescein dye; herpes infection classically causes a dendritic-appearing ulcer. Corneal ulcers can erode and cause corneal perforation and permanent visual loss. Patients should be seen by an ophthalmologist early for antimicrobial therapy and consideration of corneal scraping.

Episcleritis and Scleritis

Episcleritis (**Figure 22**) is inflammation of the superficial vessels of the episclera, the vascular membrane that underlies the conjunctiva. The inflammation tends to be more localized than with conjunctivitis, which tends to be diffuse. Its etiology is unclear. It typically is not associated with pain, visual changes, or tearing, and it usually resolves without specific treatment.

Scleritis is inflammation of the fibrous layer of the eye underlying the conjunctiva and episclera. Anterior scleritis, involving the superficial sclera and the deep vessels within the episclera, is the most common form. Posterior scleritis involves the deeper structures of the eye. Patients presenting with this disorder usually have severe, dull pain that may have awoken them from sleep. There may be visual loss, particularly

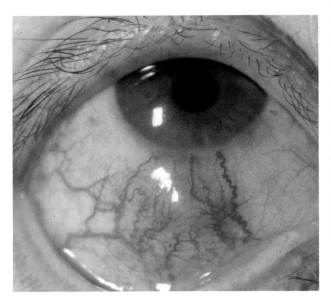

FIGURE 22. Episcleritis. Superficial dilated blood vessels are seen, with white sclera visible between the blood vessels.

Image courtesy of Linda Lippa, MD, University of California, Irvine.

with posterior scleritis. Patients with scleritis should be referred emergently to an ophthalmologist as this can be a sight-threatening condition.

The history is important for differentiating scleritis (pain, vision impairment) from episcleritis (less pain, vision unaffected); however, it is challenging to differentiate the two entities by physical examination. If there is uncertainty whether the patient has scleritis or episcleritis, an urgent referral should be made to an ophthalmologist for clarification.

Approximately 50% of patients with scleritis have an underlying systemic disease, such as rheumatoid arthritis, or an infectious disease, such as tuberculosis or syphilis. Treatment depends upon the underlying cause but may include NSAIDs for mild scleritis and systemic corticosteroids or tumor necrosis factor inhibitors for severe disease.

Uveitis

Uveitis, inflammation of the uvea, commonly presents as a red eye with pain, photophobia, and blurred vision. Anterior uveitis, or iridocyclitis, is inflammation of the iris and ciliary body and is more common than posterior uveitis. It is characterized by circumferential redness (ciliary flush) at the corneal limbus (junction of the cornea and sclera). Vision is usually normal in anterior uveitis. The classic finding upon slit lamp examination is the presence of inflammatory "flare cells" in the anterior chamber. The differential diagnosis for causes of uveitis includes infection (syphilis, tuberculosis), autoimmune disorders, sarcoidosis, and malignancy, although no cause is identified in more than 50% of patients. Anterior uveitis is usually idiopathic but can be associated with herpes simplex virus infection, trauma, or the presence of HLA-B27 antigen. Patients with uveitis should be urgently referred to an ophthalmologist for treatment.

Blepharitis

Blepharitis is inflammation of the eyelid margins. It is usually caused by *S. aureus* infection or seborrheic dermatitis, and occasionally by rosacea. It is treated with warm compresses and cleansing of the eyelid margins with diluted nontearing shampoo using a cotton tip applicator. Topical antibiotic ointment may also be used for staphylococcal blepharitis. Oral tetracyclines may be prescribed when blepharitis is associated with rosacea.

KEY POINTS

- Conjunctivitis, most often caused by a viral infection, is the most common cause of red eye; antibiotic therapy is not indicated for viral conjunctivitis.

- Both viral and bacterial conjunctivitis are highly contagious, and hand hygiene and other measures should be emphasized to minimize transmission.

- Corneal ulceration, scleritis, and uveitis should be evaluated by an ophthalmologist if diagnosed or if there is diagnostic uncertainty.

Macular Degeneration

Pathophysiology and Clinical Presentation

Age-related macular degeneration (AMD) is a leading cause of visual loss, particularly in the elderly. Progression of disease can lead to difficulty driving, reading, and performing activities of daily living, and may increase the risk of falling.

There are two types of AMD, dry (atrophic) and wet (neovascular) (**Figure 23**). In dry AMD (approximately 85% of cases), soft drusen (deposits of extracellular material) form in the area of the macula. Dry AMD may present in one or both eyes. It may be asymptomatic in the early stages and subsequently progress, with the gradual loss of central vision. Wet AMD is usually more aggressive and sight-threatening than dry AMD. It is caused by neovascularization of the macula with subsequent bleeding or scar formation. Visual loss may be more sudden (over a period of weeks) and is often more severe. It most frequently presents in one eye.

The strongest risk factors for AMD are age, smoking, family history, and cardiovascular disease. Quitting smoking reduces the risk of developing AMD. No antioxidant or other supplement has been proved conclusively to prevent AMD; however, some studies report that diets high in antioxidants may be protective.

The diagnosis of either wet or dry AMD is made with dilated funduscopic examination and fluorescein angiography performed by an ophthalmologist.

Treatment

There are no proven treatments for dry AMD. Patients with advanced dry AMD may benefit from antioxidant agents (vitamin C, vitamin E, β-carotene) and zinc; smokers should avoid β-carotene owing to risk of increased lung cancer. Laser phototherapy for dry AMD and drusen is not recommended as it may increase the incidence of neovascularization.

Several inhibitors of vascular endothelial growth factor (VEGF) have been used to slow the neovascularization of wet AMD. Laser photocoagulation therapy is no longer routinely recommended for wet AMD owing to potential complications outweighing possible benefits, except in patients with extrafoveal lesions.

> **KEY POINT**
>
> - Quitting smoking reduces the risk of developing age-related macular degeneration.

Glaucoma

Primary Open Angle Glaucoma

Primary open angle glaucoma (POAG) is a progressive optic neuropathy associated with increased intraocular pressure (IOP) without an identifiable blockage of the normal drainage pathways of the aqueous humor. It is the most common form of glaucoma and is the leading cause of irreversible blindness in the world. POAG is characterized by painless, gradual loss of peripheral vision in both eyes, which may be unnoticed by the patient. It is often asymmetric. In later stages, it may progress to involve central visual acuity. Clinical findings include an increased optic cup:disc ratio (>0.5), disc hemorrhages, and vertical extension of the central cup. Risk factors include age older than 40 years, race (incidence in blacks is four times higher than in whites), and positive family history.

Lowering IOP has been shown to delay or prevent the progression of POAG symptoms over time. Pharmacologic agents are the mainstay of glaucoma treatment, but adverse effects can be significant (**Table 46**). Laser therapy to increase

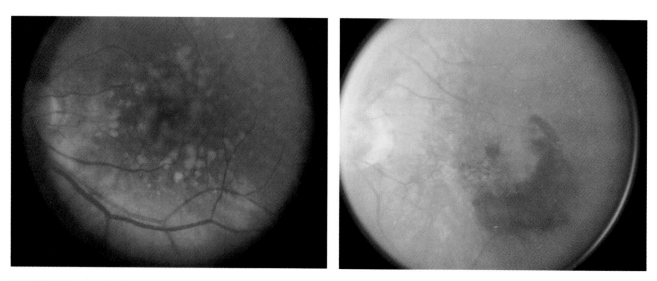

FIGURE 23. Age-related macular degeneration. The dry form (*left*), is characterized by distinct yellow-white lesions (drusen) surrounding the macular region and areas of pigment mottling. The wet form (*right*), is characterized by clumps of hyperpigmentation, hypopigmentation, and evidence of subretinal hemorrhage.

Images courtesy of Edward A. Jaeger, MD, Jefferson Medical College, Wills Eye Institute, Philadelphia, PA.

TABLE 46. Drug Treatment for Primary Open Angle Glaucoma

Agent	Mechanism of Action	Systemic Side Effects
β-Blockers (timolol)	Decreases inflow	Bradycardia, heart block, bronchospasm, decreased libido, central nervous system depression, mood swings
Nonselective adrenergic agonists (epinephrine)	Decreases inflow and increases outflow	Hypertension, headaches, extrasystole
Selective α_2-adrenergic agonists (brimonidine)	Decreases inflow and increases outflow	Hypotension, vasovagal attack, dry mouth, fatigue, insomnia, depression, syncope, dizziness, anxiety
Parasympathomimetic agents (pilocarpine, echothiophate iodide)	Increases outflow	Increased salivation, increased gastric secretion, abdominal cramps, urinary frequency, shock
Oral carbonic anhydrase inhibitors (acetazolamide)	Decreases inflow	Acidosis, depression, malaise, hirsutism, paresthesias, numbness, blood dyscrasias, diarrhea, weight loss, kidney stones, loss of libido, bone marrow suppression, hypokalemia, bad taste, increased serum urate level
Topical carbonic anhydrase inhibitors (dorzolamide)	Decreases inflow	Lower incidence of systemic effects compared with oral carbonic anhydrase inhibitors
Prostaglandin analogues (latanoprost)	Increases outflow	Flu-like symptoms, joint and muscle pain
Hyperosmotic agents (mannitol)	Reduces vitreous and aqueous volume	Headache, heart failure, expansion of blood volume, nausea, vomiting, diarrhea, electrolyte disturbance, kidney failure

Adapted from Smith OU, Seligsohn AL, Khan SJ, Spaeth GL. Primary open angle glaucoma. http://pier.acponline.org/physicians/diseases/d602/tables/d602-tables.html (login required). In PIER (online database). Philadelphia: American College of Physicians, 2009. Accessed July 7, 2009.

aqueous outflow, although able to lower the IOP, may lose efficacy over time. Surgical options, such as trabeculectomy or iridectomy, have attendant risks of complications, including blindness.

Acute Angle Closure Glaucoma

Acute angle closure glaucoma results from blocked drainage of the aqueous humor. Patients present with red eye with severe pain and headache and occasionally nausea and vomiting and visual halos. Visual acuity is usually reduced. It is caused by increased IOP owing to blocked drainage of the aqueous humor. Physical examination reveals a semidilated, nonreactive pupil with an IOP greater than 50 mm Hg. Acute angle closure glaucoma is an immediate threat to vision, and urgent referral to an ophthalmologist is important to avert optic nerve atrophy.

KEY POINT

- Pharmacologic agents are the mainstay of primary open angle glaucoma treatment, but adverse effects can be significant.

Cataract

A cataract is an opacity of the lens. Cataracts are the leading cause of blindness and low vision globally, and the prevalence in the United States approaches 20% in those older than 40 years. Risk factors include older age, ultraviolet B radiation exposure, smoking, diabetes mellitus, a family history of cataracts, and systemic corticosteroid use. Symptoms include painless decreased visual acuity, decreased night vision, glare, and diplopia. On ophthalmoscopic examination, there is a decrease or absence of the red reflex, and opacification of the lens can be visualized.

Treatment is surgical removal of the cataract. Surgery is indicated if symptoms from the cataract interfere with the patient's ability to meet his or her needs of daily living; there are no criteria based upon the level of visual acuity. The posterior capsule is left intact, and a corrective replacement intraocular lens may be inserted to restore normal vision. Perioperative consultation is not required for those undergoing a procedure under local anesthesia and sedation as the surgery is considered low risk; aspirin and warfarin can be continued.

Complications from surgery are rare but include inflammation, corneal edema, and macular edema. Rarely, infective endophthalmitis develops (see Eye Emergencies). A common late-stage complication is opacification of the posterior capsule, leading to decreased visual acuity; this may be managed surgically.

Dry Eye

Dry eye (keratoconjunctivitis sicca) causes symptoms of gritty irritation, dryness, and burning of the eyes. Symptoms usually occur gradually and may worsen over the course of the day. Symptoms can be caused by any process that disrupts the tear film, either by decreasing tear production and secretion or by increasing tear evaporation. Symptoms may be aggravated by environmental irritants (smoke, allergens, low humidity) and relieved with eye closing and increased humidity.

Decreased tear secretion is usually caused by inflammation of the lacrimal gland, which may be a localized process or associated with a systemic disease, such as Sjögren syndrome or rheumatoid arthritis. Additionally, decreased corneal sensation, which may occur with diabetes, hard contact lens wearing, herpes zoster infection, or laser-assisted in situ keratomileusis (LASIK) eye surgery, causes reduced tear secretion. Increased tear evaporation may be caused by increased size of the palpebral fissure (as seen in Graves ophthalmopathy) or by meibomian gland dysfunction, which reduces the protective lipid layer of the tear film. Other risk factors for dry eyes include increasing age, female sex, decreased androgen levels, and certain medications, including anticholinergic agents, antihistamines, selective serotonin reuptake inhibitors, nicotinic acid, and isotretinoin. Patients with persistent or severe dry eye, as with Sjögren syndrome, Graves disease, or Bell palsy, may suffer corneal damage.

Treatment of dry eye is directed at decreasing inflammation and addressing any lid pathology disrupting the tear film. Artificial tears are helpful for lubrication. Warm compresses may also be helpful. Lid inflammation may be treated with oral tetracyclines. Meibomianitis may respond to gentle scrubs with mild nontearing shampoo. Punctal or canalicular plugs may lower tear film osmolality and thus decrease evaporation. Topical corticosteroid drops (short-term use only) and topical cyclosporine have also been used in patients with dry eye caused by systemic illness.

Excessive Tearing

Excessive tearing results from either overproduction of tears (lacrimation) or impaired drainage through the lacrimal duct system (epiphora). Lacrimation is often bilateral and painless, whereas epiphora may be unilateral and can be painful, particularly if infection of the ductal system is involved (dacryocystitis). The eyes should be examined for evidence of foreign body or acute conjunctivitis. The lids should be examined for ectropion and adequate lid closure and the punctum examined for blockage, inflammation, or purulence.

Treatment is focused on the underlying cause, with ophthalmologic referral for mechanical intervention for patients with lacrimal drainage problems.

Retinal Detachment

Retinal detachment occurs when the neurosensory layer of the retina separates from the retinal pigment epithelial layer and choroid. This can result from either fluid accumulation behind or vitreous traction on the retina. Separation can cause ischemia in the retina or a tear that may lead to visual loss. Retinal detachment occurs predominantly in myopic patients. Patients may report floaters, squiggly lines, flashes of light, and then a sudden visual defect that is peripheral, appearing as a black curtain, which then progresses across the visual field. Funduscopic examination usually visualizes the detachment (**Figure 24**). The treatment is surgical. Prognosis depends upon the extent of the detachment or tear and time to surgery, so early recognition and emergent referral is crucial.

Posterior vitreous detachment (PVD), in which contraction of the vitreous places traction on the retina, is the most common type of retinal detachment and typically occurs in persons aged 50 to 75 years. Patients with PVD can be asymptomatic but most often present with floaters or flashes of light (photopsias). Most photopsias are benign and idiopathic, becoming more common as age progresses.

Symptoms of PVD usually progress over a period of 1 week to 3 months and can progress to visual loss. Patients with uncomplicated PVD have less than a 5% chance of developing a full retinal tear within 6 weeks, and symptomatic patients should simply be reassured and educated about potential symptoms of visual loss. Symptoms in patients without full tears usually resolve over 3 to 12 months. No specific limits on activity are necessary. For those patients with PVD who develop retinal tears, one half go on to full retinal detachment. A full retinal detachment may present with cobweb-like floaters with acute visual loss or with a monocular decreased visual field; these patients should be evaluated acutely. Those with full detachments will require ophthalmologic intervention.

KEY POINT

- Patients with cobweb-like floaters with acute visual loss or who are found to have a monocular decreased visual field may have a full retinal detachment and should be seen urgently by an ophthalmologist.

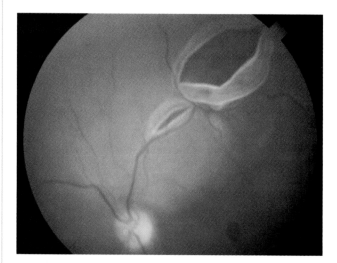

FIGURE 24. Retinal detachment, with characteristic folding and tearing of the retina.

Image courtesy of Edward A. Jaeger, MD, Jefferson Medical College, Wills Eye Institute, Philadelphia, PA.

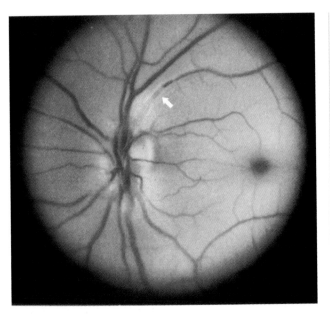

FIGURE 25. Occlusion of the central retinal artery (*arrow*) characterized by the appearance of an opalescent retina, retinal pallor, and "cherry-red spot" defining the fovea.

Image courtesy of Edward A. Jaeger, MD, Jefferson Medical College, Wills Eye Institute, Philadelphia, PA.

Retinal Vascular Occlusion

Central Retinal Vein Occlusion

Patients with central retinal vein occlusion (CRVO) typically report a sudden, unilateral loss of vision. This differs from occlusion of a branch retinal vein, which is often asymptomatic. The etiology of CRVO is usually a thrombus occluding the central retinal vein. Risk factors include age, hypertension, diabetes, hyperlipidemia, smoking, obesity, hypercoagulable states, glaucoma, and retinal arteriolar abnormalities. Diagnosis is based on the history of abrupt onset of monocular blindness coupled with classic funduscopic examination findings of congested, tortuous retinal veins; scattered intraretinal hemorrhages; and cotton wool spots in the area of the vein occlusion. An afferent pupillary defect may be seen.

Suspicion of CRVO warrants rapid ophthalmologic consultation. Clinical outcomes usually correlate well with visual acuity level at presentation, and those with severe visual loss are less likely to regain normal function.

Central Retinal Artery Occlusion

Arterial occlusions are usually seen in the elderly and may be caused by embolic or thrombotic events or vasospasm. Patients present with sudden, painless visual loss in one eye, an afferent pupillary defect, and a pale retina with a cherry red fovea that appears accentuated in color owing to the pale retinal background (**Figure 25**). Visual acuity at the time of presentation predicts final visual acuity, and irreversible vision loss tends to occur after 4 hours of ischemia. Attempts can be made to lower IOP while awaiting emergent ophthalmology consultation.

- Abrupt onset of painless monocular blindness may indicate a retinal vascular occlusion and warrants emergent ophthalmologic consultation.

Eye Emergencies

Indications for urgent or emergent ophthalmology consultation are listed in **Table 47**. Any patient with acute vision loss should be seen emergently by an ophthalmologist. Important causes of acute visual loss include retinal artery occlusion, retinal vein occlusion, temporal arteritis, retinal detachment, and optic neuritis.

Nearly all patients with globe trauma should be seen emergently by an ophthalmologist. Orbital fractures do not need to be seen emergently unless there is globe penetration, visual loss, or impairment of extraocular muscles. Direct trauma or laceration to the eyelid, nasolacrimal system, lid margin, or tarsal plate should be seen by either an ophthalmologist or plastic surgeon.

Chemical injuries to the eye are an ocular emergency. The eye should be irrigated for at least 30 minutes using normal saline solution or lactated Ringer solution while an ophthalmology consultation is occurring.

Endophthalmitis is inflammation of the aqueous and vitreous humors and usually results from infection, most often as a postoperative complication of eye surgery. It may also be associated with endocarditis. Treatment may include intravitreal antibiotics. Orbital cellulitis involves the periocular tissues and eyelids and usually results from contiguous sinus or dental infection. Patients present with marked ocular and eyelid erythema, swelling, pain, and fever. To differentiate preseptal cellulitis from orbital cellulitis, extraocular muscles and pupillary reflexes should be carefully evaluated. A CT scan is usually performed to evaluate for deeper infection. Any patient presenting

TABLE 47. Indications for Urgent or Emergent Ophthalmology Consultation

Condition
Acute angle closure glaucoma
Acute vision loss
Central retinal vascular occlusion
Corneal ulceration
Endophthalmitis
Herpes zoster ophthalmicus
Optic neuritis
Orbital cellulitis
Retinal detachment
Scleritis
Trauma to globe or lid
Uveitis

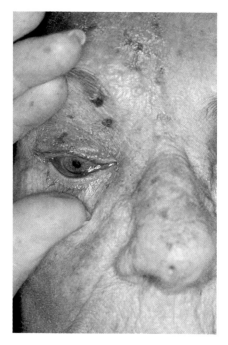

FIGURE 26. Herpes zoster ophthalmicus.

with herpes zoster involving the tip of the nose (Hutchinson sign) should be seen by an ophthalmologist to rule out herpes zoster ophthalmicus (**Figure 26**). The Hutchinson sign has a fairly high correlation with the presence of corneal involvement, which can cause permanent visual loss.

Optic neuritis occurs predominantly in middle-aged, white persons, and affects women more than men. Patients present with pain with eye movement, blurred vision, visual field deficits, and change in color perception. The optic disc usually appears normal. Optic neuritis is usually self-limited, but an ophthalmology consultation and a brain MRI should be obtained. Optic neuritis can be an early harbinger of multiple sclerosis. Intravenous corticosteroids may help speed recovery. **H**

KEY POINTS

- Any patient with acute vision loss should be seen emergently by an ophthalmologist.

- Globe trauma, chemical injury, orbital cellulitis, endophthalmitis, and optic neuritis are ocular emergencies, and urgent ophthalmologic evaluation should be obtained.

Ear, Nose, Mouth, and Throat Disorders

Evaluation of Hearing Loss

Causes of hearing loss are generally categorized as conductive or sensorineural (**Table 48**). Conductive hearing loss is caused by a mechanical problem preventing the transmission

of acoustic vibrations from external sources to the cochlea and may originate in the ear canal, tympanic membrane, or the ossicles of the middle ear. Sensorineural hearing loss involves the perception and transmission of acoustic vibrations and may reflect a cochlear problem or an issue with the acoustic nerve.

If hearing loss is unilateral, the Weber and Rinne tests can help to differentiate between conductive and sensorineural hearing loss. A 256 Hz tuning fork is commonly used for the Weber test and a 512 Hz fork for the Rinne test, although a 512 Hz fork may be used for both. In the Weber test, the vibrating tuning fork is placed in contact with the forehead or scalp in the midline equidistant from both ears. In conductive hearing loss, the fork will be heard more loudly in the affected ear, and in sensorineural hearing loss, it will be louder in the unaffected ear. In the Rinne test, the vibrating tuning fork is held against the mastoid process of the affected ear until it can no longer be heard; it is then removed and held outside the ear. If the tuning fork can be heard after removal, the conductive system is likely intact, favoring a sensorineural cause of hearing loss. If the tuning fork is better heard in contact with the mastoid bone, conductive hearing loss is more likely.

In practice, patients who report hearing loss and lack an obvious cause on physical examination (such as cerumen impaction or middle ear effusion) should be referred for formal audiometry, which is better able to discriminate between conductive and sensorineural hearing loss, and help determine which patients will likely benefit from amplification.

Imaging of the central nervous system is not considered part of a routine evaluation for hearing loss. A clinical setting in which imaging should be considered is the progressive onset of unilateral sensorineural hearing loss; a small but significant number of these patients have retrocochlear pathology as a cause of their hearing loss, such as an acoustic neuroma. If imaging is pursued, MRI is the study of choice to evaluate the posterior fossa and internal auditory canal.

Sudden sensorineural hearing loss, defined as a 30 dB loss over a period of 3 days or less, is a discrete and poorly understood clinical syndrome. Viral infection, bacterial meningitis, Lyme disease, migraine, Meniere disease, acoustic neuroma, head injury, drug reactions, and neurosarcoidosis can all cause sudden hearing loss; however, a cause is identified in only approximately 10% of these patients. Most cases are idiopathic and unilateral and otoscopy is normal; acute otorhinolaryngologic evaluation is appropriate. Limited data suggest that corticosteroid therapy may improve the likelihood of hearing recovery. Fortunately, more than half of patients recover completely within 2 weeks.

KEY POINT

- Patients who report hearing loss and lack an obvious cause on physical examination should be referred for formal audiometry.

TABLE 48. Common Causes of Hearing Loss

Disease	Notes
Conductive	
Cerumen impaction	Cerumen may completely obstruct ear canal, causing conductive hearing loss. Impacted cerumen can be removed with gentle irrigation or an ear curette. No removal needed if asymptomatic.
Otosclerosis	Bony overgrowth of the stapes footplate with eventual fixation. Family history of otosclerosis is common. Treatment is stapedectomy or stapedotomy. Hearing aid may be helpful.
Tympanic membrane perforation	Often heals without intervention. Ear should be kept dry. Refer for possible repair if associated with significant hearing loss or possible middle ear pathology.
Cholesteatoma	An expanding mass composed of keratinizing squamous epithelial cells that may contain cholesterol crystals. Although histologically benign, it may erode extensively into local structures, including the cochlea, ossicles, tympanic membrane, and facial nerve. Treatment is surgical removal.
Sensorineural	
Presbycusis	Age-related hearing loss; typically symmetric high-frequency hearing loss. Hearing aids are mainstay of treatment.
Sudden sensorineural hearing loss	Unclear etiology; presents as a sudden loss of hearing that is sensorineural in nature. Rapid treatment with corticosteroids may improve outcome, although one study showed little difference whether treatment was initiated within 24 hours or 7 days.
Meniere disease	Classically presents as a triad of sensorineural hearing loss, tinnitus, and vertigo, although all three are not necessarily present in each patient. Symptoms may fluctuate, and attacks are often precipitated by high salt intake.
Vestibular schwannoma (acoustic neuroma)	Benign neoplasm, usually causing sensorineural hearing loss, tinnitus, and sometimes vertigo. A family or personal history of neurofibromatosis 2 puts patients at high risk for these tumors, often bilaterally.
Noise-induced	History of chronic noise exposure or sudden, short exposure to noise blast. Prevention is mainstay of treatment; hearing aids if condition is already advanced.
Drug-induced	History of ototoxic medication use (aminoglycosides, chemotherapeutic agents [irreversible], aspirin and NSAIDs [partially reversible], antimalarials [reversible], loop diuretics [sometimes irreversible]).
Both conductive and sensorineural	
Infection	Middle ear infection may impair movement of the tympanic membrane or ossicles, producing reversible conductive hearing loss. Viral cochleitis may cause reversible sensorineural hearing loss. Chronic ear infection may lead to conductive hearing loss.
Head trauma	May produce a conductive hearing loss from ossicular disruption and hemotympanum or a sensorineural hearing loss from cochlear fracture or auditory nerve injury.

Tinnitus

Tinnitus is the perception of sound that is not audible. Patients frequently characterize it as "ringing," "buzzing," or "whistling," although it may manifest as other sounds. It may be unilateral or bilateral, depending on the nature of the underlying disorder. Although tinnitus is part of the defining triad for Meniere disease, it is not specific to Meniere disease and can occur with virtually any cause of sensorineural hearing loss, such as presbycusis, noise exposure, or acoustic neuroma. It can also occur with conductive hearing loss, such as from eustachian tube dysfunction or cerumen impaction, although this is less common.

Pulsatile tinnitus (tinnitus synchronized with the patient's pulse) and objective tinnitus (tinnitus that can be heard by an external observer, for example with a stethoscope) may be indicators of an underlying vascular etiology such as arteriovenous malformation, atherosclerosis, carotid artery disease, or a paraganglioma (glomus tumor). Physical examination for pulsatile tinnitus includes auscultation for bruits over the ear and eye as well as the neck. Pulsatile tinnitus of indeterminate etiology should be evaluated by an otorhinolaryngologist.

Absent a treatment for the underlying cause, treatment for tinnitus is challenging. Medications are largely ineffective, and the mainstay of therapy is neurocognitive interventions to help patients cope with the problem and diminish dysfunctional cognitive processes associated with the experience of tinnitus. External noise generators are sometimes used to mask the sound of tinnitus, but evidence supporting their efficacy is sparse.

KEY POINTS

- Tinnitus can occur with virtually any cause of sensorineural hearing loss, including Meniere disease, presbycusis, noise exposure, or acoustic neuroma.
- Pulsatile tinnitus and objective tinnitus may be indicators of an underlying vascular etiology.

101

- Medications are largely ineffective in the treatment of tinnitus; the mainstay of therapy is neurocognitive interventions to help patients cope with the problem.

Otitis Media

Acute otitis media is inflammation of the middle ear. It occurs predominantly in children. Despite the fact that it is diagnosed more than 5 million times each year in the United States, there is a paucity of quality studies of the disorder in children and remarkably little substantive literature about acute otitis media in adults. In some countries, such as the Netherlands, management is frequently observation only, in contrast to the United States, where this diagnosis is the leading cause of antibiotic prescriptions for children.

Otitis media usually follows an upper respiratory tract infection and is frequently accompanied by ear pain for 24 to 48 hours. Fever, although less common than ear pain, increases the likelihood of otitis media. In the pediatric literature, tympanic membrane bulging has the highest likelihood ratio for acute otitis media, followed by tympanic membrane cloudiness and immobility. Other signs include erythema of the tympanic membrane, with the likelihood ratio increasing for greater degrees of redness. Complications of acute otitis media include hearing loss, tympanic membrane perforation, mastoiditis, and meningitis. However, suppurative complications may occur in as few as 0.12% of untreated children.

There are no adequate trials of treatment in adults, but in children, the American Academy of Pediatrics and the American Academy of Family Practice currently recommend observation along with analgesic therapy in cases in which there is diagnostic uncertainty or in milder cases of otitis media. In patients in whom a decision is made to treat, amoxicillin should be used in patients who are not allergic to penicillin-containing antibiotics, with escalation to amoxicillin-clavulanate in 48 to 72 hours if the patient fails to improve or worsens. A macrolide antibiotic should be used as initial therapy in penicillin-allergic patients. An anti-inflammatory agent should be recommended for pain relief.

KEY POINT

- Complications of otitis media include hearing loss, tympanic membrane perforation, mastoiditis, and meningitis.

Otitis Externa

Otitis externa, a diffuse inflammation of the outer ear canal, may be acute or chronic. The acute form, which accounts for approximately 90% of cases of otitis externa, is usually caused by bacteria. The chronic form, which lasts 3 or more months, is usually caused by fungal infection, allergy, or a systemic dermatitis. Manifestations of otitis externa include pain, itching, and erythema early in the course but may progress to include edema, otorrhea and conductive hearing loss. Risk factors for the development of otitis externa include increased moisture, use of cotton-tipped swabs or bobby pins to clean the ear canal, use of hearing aids, and decreased production of cerumen, which contains an antimicrobial lysozyme and has a pH of 6.9, helping to inhibit bacterial growth.

Acute otitis externa can range from mild inflammation of the external canal to a severe and life-threatening infection if the temporal bone becomes involved. Onset is usually over a few days to a week and is initially manifested by pruritus, erythema, and discomfort, which progresses to edema of the canal, serous or purulent secretions, and pain with tugging on the pinna or moving the tragus. Approximately 50% of bacterial cases are caused by *Pseudomonas aeruginosa* and the remainder by *Staphylococcus aureus* and other aerobic and anaerobic bacteria. Fungi cause 10% or fewer cases of acute otitis externa; other etiologies, such as herpes zoster, cause fewer than 5% of cases. Hospital admission is usually not required, but is indicated if disease progresses to necrosis of the ear canal and osteomyelitis of the underlying bone (malignant otitis externa) or to involve the temporal or mastoid bones. These patients usually have disproportionate pain along with fever higher than 39.0 °C (102.2 °F); skin necrosis, facial paralysis, vertigo, and meningeal signs also may be present.

Chronic otitis externa is frequently caused by allergic contact dermatitis from earrings, cosmetics, soaps, shampoos, or the plastic components in hearing aids. Ironically, some patients initially treated for acute otitis externa develop a type IV delayed hypersensitivity reaction to the otic solutions used to treat the acute infection. Fungal infections causing otitis externa usually can be identified by the presence of white, cotton-like strands (*Candida*) with or without white or black fungal balls (*Aspergillus*).

Management of acute otitis externa involves clearing the canal of as much debris as possible to optimize penetration of ototopical agents as well as to visualize the tympanic membrane to ensure it is intact before initiating an ototopical agent. Most forms of otitis externa may be effectively treated with topical therapy. Mild otitis externa can be treated with a dilute acetic acid solution, although many practitioners still choose to prescribe a 7- to 10-day course of an ototopical agent containing neomycin, polymyxin B, and hydrocortisone for both mild and more severe forms. However, ototoxicity can occur from topical aminoglycosides when use is prolonged or the tympanic membrane is not intact; in addition, these agents can cause contact dermatitis in 5% to 18% of patients. Topical fluoroquinolones are more expensive but are approved for use when the tympanic membrane is not intact. Oral antibiotics should be considered for extra-canal involvement, for older patients, for those who have not responded to topical treatment, and for immunocompromised or diabetic patients. Patients with malignant otitis externa or disease involving the temporal or mastoid bones should be hospitalized and given intravenous antibiotics.

Fungal infections are usually treated with 2% acetic acid or isopropyl alcohol. Severe fungal infections may require treatment with topical antifungal agents, such as 1% clotrimazole.

KEY POINTS

- Management of otitis externa involves clearing the canal of as much debris as possible before initiating an ototopical agent.

- Patients with malignant otitis externa or involvement of the temporal or mastoid bones usually have disproportionate pain and fever higher than 39.0 °C (102.2 °F); hospital admission and intravenous antibiotics are indicated.

Cerumen Impaction

Cerumen cleans, protects, and lubricates the external auditory canal. Cerumen is normally eliminated by a mechanism involving jaw motion, causing it to migrate out of the ear canal. Accumulation of cerumen occurs when this self-cleaning mechanism is inadequate. Excess cerumen is present in 1 in 20 adults and one third of geriatric patients and is a common cause of visits to physicians for ear symptoms. Cerumen impaction refers to a collection of cerumen sufficiently large that it is either symptomatic or blocks visualization of the ear canal or tympanic membrane. Cerumen-related symptoms include pain, itching, tinnitus, odor, drainage, vertigo, and hearing loss. Hearing loss can range from 5 to 40 dB, depending on the degree of impaction.

Treatment options for cerumen impaction include observation without specific treatment, use of ceruminolytic agents, manual removal of cerumen, and irrigation. Evidence-based guidelines indicate that it is not necessary to remove the cerumen unless the patient is symptomatic or the canal or tympanic membrane needs to be evaluated. Patients should be reassured that cerumen is naturally occurring and has beneficial effects, and that specific efforts to cleanse the ear canals are not needed. Complications of treatment, which occur in approximately 1 in 1000 treated patients, include tympanic membrane perforation, ear canal laceration, infection, and hearing loss.

KEY POINT

- It is not necessary to remove cerumen from the ear canal unless the patient is symptomatic or the canal or tympanic membrane needs to be evaluated.

Upper Respiratory Tract Infections

Sinusitis

Acute sinusitis is a challenging clinical domain because the correlation between symptoms, pathophysiology, and treatment is tenuous. Evidence about diagnosis of sinusitis is limited. A history of cigarette smoking, allergic rhinitis, or previous episodes of sinusitis may indicate patients at increased risk. Common symptoms associated with sinusitis such as headache, facial pain and pressure that increases when bending forward, fever, and toothache have not been well assessed in comparison with gold standard tests such as sinus aspiration or radiography. Physical examination findings that have been shown to add diagnostic value include purulent rhinorrhea with unilateral predominance, local pain with unilateral predominance, bilateral purulent rhinorrhea, and pus in the nasal cavity. The presence of three or more of these symptoms has a positive likelihood ratio of 6.75. Imaging is rarely necessary in an average-risk patient, but should be considered in immunocompromised patients at risk for unusual organisms, such as fungal or pseudomonal sinusitis.

Initial treatment of patients with symptoms suggestive of acute sinusitis is largely symptomatic. Systemic antihistamines, intranasal corticosteroids, and topical decongestants have all been shown to be helpful. Topical decongestants should be limited to a few days of use to avoid rebound rhinitis (rhinitis medicamentosa). Evidence in acute sinusitis suggests a small increase in the number of patients whose symptoms resolve if antibiotics are used in patients with symptoms that have been present for at least 7 days. However, the cure rate is high in placebo-treated patients (80%); therefore, the number needed to treat is also high: between 8 and 15 patients would need to be treated with antibiotics to produce one additional cure. Because of this, some guidelines and clinicians recommend initial symptomatic treatment with initiation of antibiotics only in patients with 3 to 4 days of severe symptoms (such as fever ≥39.0 °C [102.2 °F], purulent drainage, and facial pain), worsening of symptoms that were initially improving following a typical upper respiratory tract infection, or failure to improve after 10 days. If antibiotics are used, there is no evidence of superiority for any particular antibiotic in patients without risk for infection with resistant organisms. Amoxicillin-clavulanate and doxycycline are both appropriate first-line agents.

Allergic Rhinitis

Allergic rhinitis should be strongly considered in a patient with rhinitis symptoms (sneezing, congestion, rhinorrhea) associated with a particular season, environment (for example, home or work), or exposure (such as pets). A detailed history of when and where symptoms occur can often point to a probable allergen. Although not a part of routine evaluation, either in vitro specific IgE antibody testing or skin testing can confirm an allergy to specific antigens if needed. Such testing is most valuable when considering allergen immunotherapy but should also be considered if the patient is considering expensive or difficult lifestyle changes to reduce allergen exposure.

Initial therapy should include an assessment of the options to reduce exposure to allergens; for example, closing windows and doors and using an air filter at home to mitigate pollen exposure. These measures can be cumbersome, however, and patients, especially those with mild or transient symptoms, may prefer pharmacotherapy. Treatment options include intranasal corticosteroids, oral antihistamines, intranasal antihistamines, oral leukotriene inhibitors, and intranasal cromolyn. Intranasal corticosteroids are considered first line therapy because of superior effectiveness in controlled trials. Cost and frequency of dosing are also important to consider in developing a treatment plan. Combining intranasal corticosteroids and oral antihistamines may be helpful in patients who have persistent symptoms with a single agent. Patients with specific allergies confirmed by testing may be candidates for allergen immunotherapy. Immunotherapy reduces symptoms and medication use but is expensive, requires multiple injections or sublingual administrations over a long period of time, and carries a small risk of systemic reactions with each injection.

Nonallergic Rhinitis

Patients with chronic rhinitis symptoms without an associated exposure may have nonallergic or vasomotor rhinitis. Nonallergic rhinitis may also have specific triggers, such as odors, spicy foods, and changes in temperature. The diagnosis is often evident by clinical history but may be confirmed by allergy testing, which reveals either no specific allergies or allergies that correlate poorly with the patient's symptoms. Treatments for nonallergic rhinitis include intranasal corticosteroids, antihistamines, and anticholinergic agents; oral medications are less effective for nonallergic rhinitis. Nasal saline irrigation may also be helpful.

Rhinitis medicamentosa is the syndrome of chronic rhinitis resulting from long-term use of topical nasal decongestants. Withdrawal of the offending medication is the only effective therapy, but management of the resulting rebound rhinitis is notoriously difficult. Intranasal corticosteroids may be helpful.

Many anatomic conditions and systemic illnesses should be considered in the differential diagnosis of chronic rhinitis. Anatomic conditions include deviated septum, nasal polyps, hypertrophic turbinates, and cerebrospinal fluid leak; systemic illnesses include sarcoidosis, granulomatosis with polyangiitis (also known as Wegener granulomatosis), cystic fibrosis, and hypothyroidism. Pregnancy also may be associated with chronic rhinorrhea and congestion.

Pharyngitis

Most cases of acute pharyngitis are viral and require no specific intervention other than symptomatic therapy. Because of the association between group A streptococcal (GAS) pharyngitis and rheumatic fever, however, GAS pharyngitis should be identified and treated to prevent rheumatic heart disease. However, empiric antimicrobial treatment not based on a clinical decision tool incorporating specific clinical information is discouraged as this has been shown to lead to significant inappropriate antibiotic use. The four-point Centor criteria are widely used to identify patients at risk of GAS pharyngitis: (1) fever (subjective or measured >38.1 °C [100.5 °F]); (2) absence of cough; (3) tonsillar exudates; and (4) tender anterior cervical lymphadenopathy. Patients with zero or one Centor criterion are low-risk and do not need additional testing. Patients with two or three criteria should have a confirmatory test (either a rapid GAS antigen test or throat culture; both studies are not necessary) and be treated based on the result. Patients meeting all four criteria should also have a confirmatory test but may be treated empirically while awaiting results.

Penicillin is the treatment of choice for GAS pharyngitis: options include a 10-day course of oral penicillin or a single intramuscular injection of penicillin G. The latter is a particularly good option in high-risk situations (for example, secondary prevention of rheumatic fever) or if there is concern about the patient completing a full course of oral therapy. A 10-day course of erythromycin or a 5-day course of azithromycin are alternatives in patients who are allergic to penicillin.

Group C and group G streptococci can cause a clinical syndrome similar to GAS pharyngitis, although often less severe. Although they have been associated with glomerulonephritis and reactive arthritis, group C and G streptococci are not known to cause acute rheumatic fever. Treatment with antibiotics may shorten the duration of symptoms, but controlled trials are lacking.

Lemierre Syndrome

Acute pharyngitis is rarely complicated by septic thrombosis of the internal jugular vein (Lemierre syndrome). This is most often caused by *Fusobacterium necrophorum*, an anaerobic gram-negative rod that is part of the normal oropharyngeal flora. Infection is thought to occur by contiguous spread through the tissues of the pharynx. The diagnosis should be suspected in anyone with antecedent pharyngitis and persistent fever despite antimicrobial therapy. Anterior neck pain and tenderness are frequently but not universally present. Soft tissue CT of the neck with contrast typically shows a jugular vein thrombus with surrounding tissue enhancement. Empiric therapy should be directed at both streptococci and anaerobes and should be active against β-lactamase–producing organisms. Therapy typically lasts at least 4 weeks.

- Initial treatment of patients with symptoms suggestive of acute sinusitis is largely symptomatic, including systemic antihistamines, intranasal corticosteroids, and topical decongestants.
- First-line therapy for the treatment of allergic rhinitis is an intranasal corticosteroid.
- Patients with pharyngitis with zero or one of the Centor criteria (fever, absence of cough, tonsillar exudates, tender anterior cervical lymphadenopathy) have a low risk of group A streptococcal infection, and do not need additional testing or antibiotic therapy.

Epistaxis

Epistaxis is a common occurrence, affecting 60% of the population some time in their lifetime; approximately 6% seek medical treatment. More than 90% of nosebleeds occur along the anterior portion of the nasal septum (the Kiesselbach area). This area receives its blood supply from branches of both the internal and external carotid arteries. Most episodes of anterior epistaxis can be controlled with patient-exerted direct pressure. The other 10% of epistaxis episodes occur posteriorly, along the nasal septum and lateral wall. This area's blood supply is from the external carotid artery via the sphenopalatine branch of the maxillary artery. Posterior epistaxis is more common in older patients.

The most common cause of epistaxis in children is nose picking; other causes in adults include the administration of intranasal medications such as corticosteroids or decongestants, dry nasal mucosa during winter months, viral or bacterial rhinosinusitis, and neoplasms. Systemic diseases associated with epistaxis include hematologic malignancies, hemophilia, and acquired bleeding disorders from liver or kidney disease. Iatrogenic causes associated with epistaxis include anticoagulant and antiplatelet medications and possibly *Ginkgo biloba* and ginseng supplements. Patients with epistaxis frequently have hypertension upon presenting to a health care provider; however, it is unclear whether chronic hypertension is associated with epistaxis or whether the hypertension is simply the result of anxiety owing to the epistaxis. Nosebleeds are rarely life threatening.

Evaluation of epistaxis begins with a history focused on frequency, location, whether the nosebleed is unilateral or bilateral, and evaluation of risk factors that may be associated with the bleeding. Ideally, the site of the bleed should be visualized in order to localize the epistaxis as anterior or posterior. Anesthetic or vasoconstrictor topical sprays (lidocaine with oxymetazoline, for example) may be needed both to control bleeding and allow visual localization of the bleeding site.

Unless the patient has severe epistaxis or has an associated systemic disease such as a coagulopathy or hematologic malignancy or is on medications that affect clotting, laboratory studies are usually not necessary. If these studies are obtained, a complete blood count and coagulation panel should be ordered. These studies, however, are normal in nearly 80% of patients, including those with systemic conditions that predispose to a coagulopathy. Imaging is also not required in most patients with epistaxis; in patients with recurrent unilateral epistaxis, particularly in those who smoke, a malignant or benign sinonasal neoplasm should be considered as a diagnostic possibility and radiographic imaging should be obtained.

Most anterior nosebleeds do not require any medical treatment and respond to compression of the nasal ala against the septum by the patient for at least 15 minutes. The head position while applying pressure can be either forward or backward depending on which is more comfortable. Vasoconstrictor topical agents may also be useful. If bleeding fails to resolve, cautery can be carried out with chemicals such as silver nitrate or electrical cautery by an otorhinolaryngologist. Anterior nasal packing (which is extremely uncomfortable for patients) for 1 to 3 days can be performed with either nondegradable products or absorbable or biodegradable products. These maneuvers work in 60% to 80% of patients in whom pressure and vasoconstrictor agents do not control bleeding. Patients with posterior epistaxis should be seen by an otorhinolaryngologist who may need to insert posterior packing which will stop 70% of posterior epistaxis. Patients for whom these maneuvers are unsuccessful may require surgical ligation or embolization of persistently bleeding nasal arteries.

Many physicians prescribe topical or oral antibiotics while packing is in place in either the anterior or posterior locations to prevent toxic shock syndrome. The true risk of developing toxic shock syndrome from nasal packing, however, is unknown.

- Most anterior nosebleeds do not require any medical treatment and respond to compression of the nasal ala against the septum for at least 15 minutes.

Oral Health

Various oral conditions can impact the overall health of the patient. Dental disease can cause pain and discomfort and result in nutritional compromise if the ability to chew is impaired. Periodontal disease has been associated with increased prevalence of coronary heart disease. Mucosal lesions can cause pain and discomfort, and oral cancers pose a direct threat to health. Xerostomia, common in elderly patients, is frequently exacerbated by medication adverse effects. Gingival hyperplasia is also strongly associated with exposure to medications: anticonvulsant agents (especially phenytoin), cyclosporine, and nifedipine are most frequently implicated.

The U.S. Preventive Services Task Force concluded in 2004 that the evidence is insufficient to recommend for or against screening adults for oral cancer. Some patients have poor access to dental care, however, and for these patients, and for patients at high risk of oral disease (tobacco, alcohol, or methamphetamine use; bulimia; family history of oral cancer), some groups recommend that screening oral examinations be performed. This examination should include inspection of the teeth and oral mucosa, looking for evidence of caries, periodontal disease, and leukoplakia or ulcerative lesions of the mucosa. Palpation of the neck and submandibular area for masses or lymphadenopathy is also appropriate.

Oral Infections and Ulcers

Oral lesions can be caused by infection, neoplasm, and systemic conditions. Common infectious causes of mucosal lesions include *Candida*, herpes simplex virus, coxsackievirus, HIV (bacillary angiomatosis, Kaposi sarcoma, hairy leukoplakia), and syphilis. The most common malignancy in the oral cavity is squamous cell carcinoma (particularly in tobacco users); melanoma can also occur. Systemic diseases associated with oral findings include lichen planus, bullous pemphigoid and pemphigus vulgaris, erythema multiforme and Stevens-Johnson syndrome, and Behçet syndrome. More information about oral mucosal lesions is provided in MKSAP 16 Dermatology.

Dental Infection

Dental infections may involve either the tooth and underlying bony structures or the gingiva and periodontal tissues. Infections of the tooth structure are typically asymptomatic until they involve the pulp cavity, at which point the patient develops a toothache. Infection frequently extends into the underlying bone, forming a periapical abscess. Definitive treatment of these types of infection requires either endodontic removal of diseased pulp (root canal) or extraction of the infected tooth. In patients without cellulitis or symptoms of systemic infection, antibiotic therapy is not necessary if dental intervention can be performed within several days.

Periodontal disease involves the gum, connective tissue, and bone supporting the teeth. Most periodontal disease is a chronic, indolent condition that poses a long-term risk of tooth loss. Periodontal disease has also been associated with atherosclerotic cardiovascular disease. Oral hygiene (including toothbrushing and flossing) and removal of plaque are the mainstay of therapy. Oral antimicrobial rinses may also be helpful in preventing progression of disease, although evidence is limited.

Halitosis

Eighty percent to 90% of cases of halitosis (bad breath) originate in the mouth. The remainder are attributed to other conditions, including chronic sinusitis, nasal polyps, and tonsillar stones. Some systemic conditions, such as ketoacidosis, advanced kidney failure, and advanced liver disease, can produce characteristic breath odors. Esophageal diverticula and chronic pulmonary infections (abscess, bronchiectasis) may also cause halitosis. A clinician can sometimes differentiate oral, nasal, and other causes of halitosis by positioning his or her nose in front of the patient's face and asking the patient to exhale several breaths through the mouth, then several through the nose. Oral halitosis should have a stronger odor coming from the mouth, and nasal from the nose; if both are equal it raises concern of a systemic, esophageal, or pulmonary cause of halitosis. Treatment for bad breath should focus on oral hygiene, particularly flossing between the teeth and cleaning (and possible scraping) the posterior tongue, both common sites of origin of halitosis. Patients with primary dental disorders (caries, abscesses, periodontal disease) should be referred for appropriate dental care. Chlorhexidine mouthwashes may reduce odor.

Tongue Syndromes

Geographic tongue manifests as patchy areas of atrophy of the filiform papillae, leading to erythematous patches on the tongue with white borders. Lesions typically recur and regress in various areas over time. Patients are usually asymptomatic, although tongue discomfort is occasionally reported.

Atrophic glossitis, a bright red, smooth, sometimes tender tongue without visible taste buds, can be seen in patients with vitamin B_{12} deficiency and has been reported in those with iron deficiency and with celiac disease. Treatment should be directed at the underlying disorder.

Burning Mouth Syndrome

Burning mouth syndrome is characterized by a burning sensation in the mouth or tongue in the absence of an explanatory diagnosis. Patients frequently have other oral symptoms such as dryness or taste alterations. It appears to be most prevalent in postmenopausal women. It is typically managed by addressing xerostomia, if present, and excluding other possible causes, such as atrophic candidiasis, herpes virus infection, post-herpetic neuralgia, local reaction to dental products, and nutritional deficiencies. Medications directed at neuropathic pain, such as anticonvulsant agents and tricyclic antidepressants, may be helpful.

Temporomandibular Disorders

Temporomandibular disorders are a group of pain problems that involve the temporomandibular joint (TMJ) and associated structures. Typical features include jaw pain and headache and clicking, grinding, or grating at the TMJ. Although temporomandibular symptoms are common, most are self-limiting; fewer than 5% of adults with temporomandibular symptoms develop chronic symptoms. Temporomandibular disorders are classified into articular disorders, which include derangements of the intra-articular disk that normally sits between the mandibular condyle and its articulation in the glenoid fossa, and masticatory muscle disorders, which include myofascial pain syndrome.

Diagnostic evaluation of temporomandibular disorders should focus on eliminating alternative diagnoses, such as dental pain, otitis and mastoiditis, salivary gland disorders, temporal arteritis, trigeminal neuralgia, and herpes zoster. Palpation of the TMJ by applying mild anterior pressure with a finger placed posteriorly to each tragus may reveal tenderness, clicking, or crepitus. Side-to-side jaw movement with the fingers palpating the TMJ may also show similar abnormalities or asymmetry in findings. The jaw muscles should also be palpated for evidence of asymmetry or tenderness. Although not indicated in most patients, diagnostic imaging may be helpful in excluding dental disease if suspected and assessing TMJ anatomy to distinguish articular disorders from muscle disorders in complex cases. CT is particularly helpful in the diagnosis of osteoarthritis of the TMJ, whereas MRI provides additional information about the soft tissues, vascularization, and cartilaginous structures. In general, the therapeutic value of imaging is modest, and most patients are managed conservatively regardless of the underlying etiology.

Initial treatment of temporomandibular disorders focuses on noninterventional, nonpharmacologic strategies. Jaw relaxation, heat, and therapeutic exercises may be helpful. For patients with chronic temporomandibular disorders, cognitive-behavioral therapy has been shown to reduce pain, depression, and interference with activities. Biofeedback may also be of value. Jaw appliances and occlusal splints have been a prominent part of temporomandibular disorder therapy for years despite questionable evidence of benefit. Evidence is limited on the benefit of pharmacotherapy, but NSAIDs and tricyclic antidepressants are sometimes used.

Patients with anatomic abnormalities of the TMJ, such as osteoarthritis or disk derangements, may benefit from intra-articular injections of corticosteroids or hyaluronic acid, although neither is recommended for long-term use. Arthrocentesis, arthroscopy, and joint replacement may be helpful, but controlled trials are few and of poor quality.

KEY POINT

- Initial treatment of temporomandibular disorders focuses on noninterventional, nonpharmacologic strategies, such as jaw relaxation, heat, and therapeutic exercises.

Anorectal Disorders

Approach to the Patient with Anorectal Disorders

Patients with anorectal disorders should be questioned regarding bowel frequency and consistency, bleeding, pain,

and itching. Weight loss may suggest underlying inflammatory bowel disease or malignancy. Fever may be associated with abscess. Hard stools can contribute to the formation of hemorrhoids and anal fissures, and history of sharp pain following instrumentation or an unusually hard bowel movement should increase suspicion of anal fissure. Pain with defecation is typical of anal fissures and anorectal abscesses but can also occur with hemorrhoids. A palpable mass on defecation suggests a prolapsed internal hemorrhoid or overt anal prolapse.

Physical examination should include inspection for external masses, thrombosed external hemorrhoids, skin lesions, and excoriations. Having the patient bear down during the examination can sometimes reveal prolapsed internal hemorrhoids. Digital rectal examination is valuable to exclude perirectal abscess and anorectal neoplasia. Anoscopy allows for visualization of internal hemorrhoids, anal fissures, and cancers of the anal canal.

Hemorrhoids and Rectal Bleeding

Hemorrhoids are dilated veins in the hemorrhoidal plexus surrounding the anal canal. They are classified as internal or external depending on whether they are above or below the dentate line. Internal hemorrhoids are more frequently associated with painless bleeding, whereas external hemorrhoids more often cause pain; thrombosed external hemorrhoids are particularly painful. Internal hemorrhoids may prolapse and only be externally visible or palpable during a bowel movement or Valsalva maneuver.

Hemorrhoids are a common cause of bright red blood from the rectum, and further evaluation should be based on risk for colon cancer and other gastrointestinal diseases. Visualizing a hemorrhoid or other source of bleeding in a low-risk patient younger than 40 years without other symptoms to suggest inflammatory bowel disease or colon cancer may spare the patient further endoscopic evaluation as the risk of malignancy is low in this age group. Patients 40 to 50 years old with typical hemorrhoidal symptoms but at low risk for colon cancer should probably have at least sigmoidoscopy. In patients older than 50 years, rectal bleeding should not be considered hemorrhoidal without additional investigation. These patients should undergo colonoscopy to evaluate the source of bleeding provided that routine screening has not been recently performed.

Initial treatment of hemorrhoids should focus on interventions to soften bowel movements, sitz baths, and topical anesthetics or topical corticosteroids to relieve pain and itching. Recurrent hemorrhoids that fail to respond to conservative therapy can be treated with sclerotherapy, banding, photocoagulation, or surgical resection.

KEY POINT

- In patients older than 50 years, rectal bleeding should not be considered hemorrhoidal without additional investigation.

Anal Fissure

Anal fissures are tears in the anal skin distal to the dentate line, and may therefore be exquisitely painful, particularly with defecation. They are most often caused by local trauma such as hard stools or anal instrumentation. High-fiber diets and other measures that soften stools may help to reduce the risk of anal fissures, although the specific causes are poorly understood, particularly of fissures that are persistent or recurrent. Anoscopy typically reveals a small mucosal tear, most often in the posterior midline.

Acute anal fissures often heal spontaneously; treatment should start with warm sitz baths for symptom relief, increased dietary fiber to soften stools, and topical anesthetics to decrease pain with bowel movements. Chronic anal fissures are more challenging to treat. Topical nitroglycerin has the most evidence of benefit but must be compounded at a lower concentration for anorectal use (0.2% instead of 2%, the standard concentration). Topical calcium channel blockers (also compounded) and botulinum toxin injections may also be helpful, but evidence is limited. Internal anal sphincterotomy is occasionally used for refractory anal fissures but carries an increased risk of incontinence.

Anorectal Abscess

Anorectal abscesses typically originate in one of the anal crypt glands surrounding the anal canal at the dentate line. Pain and tenderness to palpation are typical, and fluctuance may be noted either on palpation of the external anus or internally on digital rectal examination.

Definitive management involves surgical drainage, which can often be accomplished in an outpatient setting with local anesthesia. Antibiotics are generally unnecessary unless there are specific risk factors, such as extensive cellulitis, diabetes mellitus, or the patient is immunocompromised.

Chronic Anorectal Pain

Chronic anorectal pain syndromes include chronic proctalgia (levator ani syndrome), characterized by chronic pain or aching, with episodes lasting more than 20 minutes, and proctalgia fugax, characterized by sudden severe pain that disappears completely within seconds or minutes. Neither condition is well understood. The approach to chronic proctalgia is similar to other chronic pain syndromes. Proctalgia fugax rarely requires specific treatment because of the brief nature of symptoms.

Pruritus Ani

Many conditions, including infection, primary skin diseases, local irritants, and malignancy, can cause anal itching. Dietary factors, including caffeine, alcohol, spices, citrus foods, milk products, tomatoes, and peanuts, have been implicated in pruritus ani; dietary modification is frequently recommended, although its effectiveness has not been established.

For some patients, anal itching becomes a primary and self-perpetuating problem. Patients should have a careful external and digital rectal examination; endoscopic evaluation should be considered in patients with a history of rectal bleeding or change in bowel movements. Patients without an apparent underlying cause should be counseled on proper anal hygiene (fecal soiling can cause irritation), including the avoidance of excessive cleaning or astringent cleansers. Protective ointments such as zinc oxide and limited short-term use of topical corticosteroids may be helpful.

Mental and Behavioral Health

Depression

The prevalence of depression in the United States is 15%, and depression is the second most common cause of primary care visits. Patients with chronic medical disorders, such as diabetes mellitus, heart disease, stroke, and cancer, have an increased risk of developing depression, and depression can negatively influence morbidity and mortality outcomes in these patients.

Despite its high prevalence and severe negative effects, depression often goes undiagnosed in the primary care setting. Brief screening tools have been validated, with the simplest being a two-question instrument (see Routine Care of the Healthy Patient). It is imperative to assess the presence of suicidal ideation and level of functional impairment, which may guide treatment decisions. Patients with active suicidal plans warrant urgent referral to a psychiatrist or emergency hospitalization in order to immediately treat their depression.

Diagnosis of Depressive Disorders

A major depressive episode is diagnosed according to the DSM-IV by the presence of five or more of the following symptoms during the same 2-week period, at least one of which is either (1) depressed mood or (2) loss of interest or pleasure:

1. Depressed mood most of the day, nearly every day

2. Loss of interest or pleasure in all or almost all activities most of the day, nearly every day

3. Significant weight loss when not dieting, or weight gain; or decrease or increase in appetite nearly every day

4. Insomnia or hypersomnia nearly every day

5. Psychomotor agitation or retardation nearly every day

6. Fatigue or loss of energy nearly every day

7. Feelings of worthlessness or inappropriate guilt nearly every day

8. Diminished ability to think or concentrate nearly every day

9. Recurrent thoughts of death, recurrent suicidal ideation with or without a specific plan; suicide attempt

The nine-item Patient Health Questionnaire (PHQ-9) is a validated instrument for identifying and assessing severity of depression, with a sensitivity of 80% and specificity of 92%. Each of the nine symptoms is scored from 0 (not bothered by the symptom at all) to 3 (bothered by the symptom nearly every day), for a maximum score of 27. A score of 10 or greater indicates the diagnosis of depression.

Minor (subsyndromal) depression is characterized by the presence in the preceding 2 weeks of two to four depressive symptoms associated with impaired social functioning, mental health, and health perceptions. Dysthymia has a similar level of symptoms as minor depression but symptoms must be present most of the time for a duration of 2 years or more. Depressive symptoms are common after the loss of a loved one; treatment should be considered if the bereaved person meets the criteria for major depression 2 months after the loss.

Seasonal affective disorder is a cyclical depression usually occurring in the fall and winter months with improvement in spring and summer. Lack of exposure to sunlight seems to be the triggering factor.

Premenstrual dysphoric disorder occurs in 3% to 5% of menstruating women. It is characterized by recurrent symptoms of depression, anxiety, or emotional lability within 1 week of menstruation and resolving within 1 week after menstruation. Postpartum depression occurs in up to 15% of women within 6 months of giving birth and can lead to significant negative outcomes in both mother and child, such as decreased effectiveness at home and work, increased risk of maternal suicide, and poorer infant-mother bonding.

Management of Depression

Most patients with mild to moderate depression can be diagnosed and treated by primary care physicians. Before initiating treatment the physician should rule out underlying medical illnesses causing depressive symptoms and evaluate any comorbid conditions. Treatment can be multimodal and may include medication, psychotherapy, or a combination of both. Psychiatric referral is recommended for any patient with (1) suicidal or homicidal ideation, (2) bipolar disorder, (3) psychotic symptoms, or (4) symptoms refractory to at least two medications.

Response rates with cognitive-behavioral therapy (CBT), interpersonal therapy, or psychodynamic therapy are similar to those with medication alone; the best outcomes occur with the combination of medication and formal psychotherapy, which is usually performed by a trained psychotherapist.

There are several classes of antidepressant agents with proven efficacy in relieving depressive symptoms (**Table 49**). The choice of agent is primarily based on side effect profile, cost, prominent symptoms, and patient preference. Treatment should be to full remission of symptoms, and symptoms should be monitored regularly. The American College of Physicians recommends that treatment for a first episode continue for 4 to 9 months after full remission of symptoms, and that patients with recurrent depression consider lifelong therapy.

Antidepressants have been associated with a risk of precipitating suicidal ideation in children, adolescents, and young adults; therefore, close monitoring is required. The risk of suicide in untreated depression, however, is likely much greater.

The most commonly prescribed antidepressants are currently the selective serotonin reuptake inhibitors (SSRIs), which have good efficacy and also treat anxiety syndromes. SSRIs have an excellent safety profile compared with tricyclic antidepressants, but sexual side effects are common. Serotonin-norepinephrine reuptake inhibitors (SNRIs) may be especially helpful in patients with concomitant pain syndromes. Bupropion may be a good alternative for those with sexual side effects on SSRI or SNRI therapy but may lower seizure threshold in higher doses and thus is contraindicated in patients with seizure disorders. Because of potential interactions with other medications, monoamine oxidase inhibitors (MAOIs) are not frequently used relative to other agents. However, a transdermal preparation of selegiline is available that is the only nonoral antidepressant available. All SSRIs, SNRIs, and MAOIs can cause serotonin syndrome, which is characterized by mental status changes, neuromuscular hyperactivity, and autonomic instability and is potentially lethal.

Patients refractory to a single SSRI may respond to a change in therapy, which may include replacement with another antidepressant, either from the same or a different class; addition of a second antidepressant; or a psychotherapeutic intervention. Patients with severe or refractory depressive symptoms (suicidality, poor cognitive functioning, interference with activities of daily living) should be referred to psychiatric providers, who may employ electroconvulsive and other multimodality interventions.

The treatment of seasonal affective disorder involves full-spectrum light therapy in addition to antidepressants and CBT.

Treatment of premenstrual and postpartum depression is similar to that of other forms of depression. There are no contraindications to breastfeeding while on antidepressants; however, SSRIs and SNRIs are FDA pregnancy category C, which warrants consideration of risks and benefits of treating maternal depression versus theoretical risks to the fetus.

TABLE 49.	Characteristics of Selected Antidepressants	
Drug	**Advantages**	**Disadvantages**
SSRIs		
Citalopram	Few drug interactions	Gastrointestinal, sexual side effects
Escitalopram	Few drug interactions	Gastrointestinal, sexual side effects
Fluoxetine	Long half-life reduces risk of withdrawal syndrome; effective for anxiety disorders, OCD, PMDD	Long half-life can lead to accumulation, drug interactions common (cytochrome P-450 inhibitor)
Paroxetine	Effective for anxiety disorders, panic disorder, PTSD, OCD	High risk in pregnancy (class D), drug interactions (cytochrome P-450 inhibitor), weight gain; high risk for withdrawal syndrome
Sertraline	Few drug interactions; effective for panic disorder, PTSD, OCD, PMDD	
SNRIs		
Venlafaxine	Effective in anxiety disorders	Nausea, can increase blood pressure
Desvenlafaxine	Effective in anxiety disorders	Nausea, can increase blood pressure
Duloxetine	Effective in pain conditions, generalized anxiety disorder	Nausea, urinary retention
Tricyclic antidepressants		
Nortriptyline	Drug level monitoring possible, analgesic effect	Cardiac toxicity with overdose, anticholinergic effects
Amitriptyline	Analgesic effect, sedating effect	Cardiac toxicity with overdose, anticholinergic effects, sedation, weight gain
Serotonin antagonist/norepinephrine agonist		
Mirtazapine	Sedating, increased appetite; available as orally disintegrating tablet	Weight gain, sedation
Norepinephrine and dopamine reuptake inhibitor		
Bupropion	Fewer sexual side effects than SSRIs, improved concentration, less weight gain	Seizure risk
MAOIs		Oral formulation can cause hypertensive crisis, serotonin syndrome
Tranylcypromine	Good for atypical symptoms	Dietary restrictions, hypertensive crisis, hypotension, serotonin syndrome
Selegiline transdermal system	Fewer dietary restrictions than other MAOIs, transdermal	Hypotension, serotonin syndrome

GAD = generalized anxiety disorder; MAOI = monoamine oxidase inhibitor; OCD = obsessive-compulsive disorder; PMDD = premenstrual dysphoric disorder; PTSD = posttraumatic stress disorder; SNRI = serotonin-norepinephrine reuptake inhibitor; SSRI = selective serotonin reuptake inhibitor.

KEY POINTS

- Psychiatric referral is recommended for any patient with depression associated with suicidal or homicidal ideation, bipolar disorder, psychotic symptoms, or refractory symptoms.

- In the treatment of depression, the best outcomes are achieved with a combination of medication and psychotherapy.

Anxiety Disorders

Anxiety disorders are among the most common psychiatric disorders in the general population; of these, generalized anxiety disorder (GAD) is the most common, with a prevalence of approximately 4% to 6%. GAD is characterized by excessive anxiety and worry about various events or activities on most days for at least 6 months, with difficulty controlling worrying. Associated symptoms include fatigue, irritability, restlessness, insomnia, and difficulty concentrating. Patients with GAD often have comorbid anxiety disorders, depression, or substance abuse. Patients with GAD often have somatoform symptoms, which can make them high utilizers of health care resources. Most patients with GAD or panic disorder present to their primary care physician or the emergency department rather than a mental health professional. The history should include inquiries into underlying medical conditions that can cause anxiety symptoms as well as any history of comorbid psychiatric disorders, substance abuse, recent stressors, coping skills, and family history of psychiatric disorders.

Panic disorder is a syndrome characterized by sudden panic attacks with the sudden onset of somatic symptoms, which may include chest pain, palpitations, sweating, nausea, dizziness, dyspnea, and numbness. These symptoms usually last from 5 to 60 minutes. The diagnosis of panic disorder requires that an attack be followed by at least 1 month of worry about a recurrence of an attack. The incidence of panic disorder is twice as high in women as in men. About one half of patients with panic disorder also have associated agoraphobia, with fears of being in crowds or in places from which escape would be difficult. Studies have shown higher suicide attempt rates in those with panic disorder compared with the general population. Although not common, medical disorders potentially presenting with anxiety-like symptoms need to be considered, including cardiac disease, thyroid disease, or pheochromocytoma.

Treatment options for GAD and panic disorder include medication and psychotherapy. CBT has been shown to be the most effective psychotherapeutic intervention in controlled trials, appears to be equal in efficacy to pharmacologic interventions, and has a lower relapse rate. SSRIs and SNRIs have been shown to be effective for both GAD and panic disorder. Buspirone is another pharmacologic option, although it may take several weeks to show clinical effect. Benzodiazepines are frequently used, either alone or in conjunction with other treatments, although they carry a risk of dependence and should not be used in those with a history of substance abuse. Panic disorder that is severe or refractory appears to be most amenable to the combination of CBT and pharmacotherapy compared with either treatment alone.

Posttraumatic Stress Disorder

Clinical Presentation
Posttraumatic stress disorder (PTSD) occurs in response to exposure to a traumatic event that involves serious threat to oneself or others. PTSD is characterized by at least 1 month of symptoms that include intrusive thoughts about the trauma, nightmares or flashbacks, avoidance of reminders of the event, and hypervigilance with sleep disturbance. To meet DSM-IV criteria, the symptoms must be in each of three areas: re-experiencing the event, avoiding reminders of the event, and heightened arousal. Risk factors for PTSD include lower socioeconomic status, parental neglect, a family or personal history of a psychiatric condition, poor social support, and initial severity of reaction to the traumatic event. Common events precipitating PTSD include military combat, sexual assault, mass displacement or disaster, and severe physical illness. PTSD most commonly presents within 1 month of the traumatic event, but symptoms can be delayed for more than 6 months. Comorbid psychiatric conditions may include depression, anxiety, and substance abuse. Traumatic brain injury (TBI) and postconcussion syndrome are often coexistent as

well (see MKSAP 16 Neurology). A study of returning U.S. veterans reported that patients with mild TBI had a 6-fold greater prevalence of PTSD versus those without such an injury. Patients with PTSD have a higher incidence of marital and occupational problems and a higher incidence of suicide than the general population.

Treatment
PTSD symptoms are complex and often require multimodal treatments. Early intervention may prevent chronicity of symptoms. No advantage has been identified for either psychotherapy or pharmacotherapy, although, for patients with refractory PTSD, combination therapy may be most useful. Trauma-focused CBT focuses on cognitively reframing distorted thinking patterns while gradually re-exposing the patient to the traumatic experience to allow desensitization of triggered symptoms. Simple stress management interventions can also be helpful in alleviating some symptoms. The most effective medications for PTSD are SSRIs, with positive symptoms (hyperarousal, flashbacks) responding best. Tricyclic antidepressants may also be used. Benzodiazepines have not been shown to be effective despite their anxiolytic effect. Finally, the α-blocker prazosin has been demonstrated to reduce the incidence and severity of nightmares but not other associated symptoms.

Social Anxiety Disorder
Social anxiety disorder is one of the most common anxiety disorders, with a lifetime prevalence estimated at 2.4%. It is characterized by a severe, persistent fear of social or performance situations, such as public speaking, test taking, or parties. In these situations, autonomic symptoms of anxiety occur, including blushing, dyspnea, palpitations, and emotional distress. Social anxiety disorder can be generalized or specific to a single activity. Patients generally realize their fear is excessive and often avoid trigger situations, which may lead to impairment in social function. Effective treatments include CBT as well as SSRI pharmacotherapy. Pharmacotherapy, particularly with an SSRI, has been demonstrated effective for both short- and long-term use. MAOIs have shown efficacy, although to a lesser extent.

Obsessive-Compulsive Disorder
Patients with obsessive-compulsive disorder (OCD) report recurrent obsessions or compulsions sufficiently severe to occupy 1 hour daily or result in marked distress or impaired social function. Obsessions are persistent ideas, thoughts, impulses, or images experienced as intrusive and are associated with significant anxiety or distress. Examples include fears of having left doors unlocked and fears of germ contamination. Compulsions are repetitive behaviors, such as handwashing, checking, ordering, or counting, that are repeated to decrease the anxiety related to the obsessions.

CBT, with exposure and response prevention interventions, is the preferred primary treatment for OCD. Pharmacotherapy is used in conjunction with CBT in patients with severe symptoms or in those with an incomplete response to CBT alone. SSRIs in higher doses are the primary pharmacotherapy, although clomipramine may be effective; some antipsychotic agents may also be useful as adjunctive therapy in severe cases.

KEY POINTS

- Cognitive-behavioral therapy is the most effective nonpharmacologic intervention for generalized anxiety disorder and panic disorder and may be equal in efficacy to pharmacologic interventions and have lower relapse rates.

- Cognitive-behavioral therapy, with exposure and response prevention interventions, is the preferred primary treatment for obsessive-compulsive disorder.

Intermittent Explosive Disorder

Intermittent explosive disorder (IED), an impulse control disorder, may affect 0.3% of the U.S. population. It is characterized by repeated episodes of aggressive violent behaviors grossly out of proportion to the situation. Examples include road rage, severe temper tantrums, and domestic abuse. Explosive episodes may be accompanied by feelings of irritability or rage and by physical symptoms of tingling, tremors, palpitations, or head pressure. Outbursts may result in injury. Persons with IED often later express remorse or embarrassment. Episodes may occur in clusters or be separated in time.

Treatment is achieved through both CBT and pharmacotherapy. Mood stabilizers and anticonvulsant agents (such as carbamazepine, phenytoin, and lithium) may be effective in decreasing aggressive behavior. SSRIs are helpful in treating comorbid depression in these patients.

Bipolar Disorder

Bipolar disorder is characterized by manic or hypomanic mood episodes and depressive episodes and affect up to 2% of the general population. A manic episode is marked by a persistent period of elevated mood, irritability, lack of need for sleep, racing thoughts, high energy levels, increased talkativeness, spending sprees, hypersexuality, and increased self-confidence, with possible delusions of grandeur or psychosis. Bipolar disorder is a leading cause of suicide, and is highly associated with substance abuse problems. Bipolar disorder is thought to be underdiagnosed; many patients presenting with symptoms of major depression are not asked about manic symptoms and are therefore not recognized as having bipolar disease.

Treatment of bipolar disorder is more complex than unipolar depression and is optimally managed in conjunction with a psychiatrist. Treatment is mainly with mood-stabilizing drugs (lithium, valproate, carbamazepine) or lamotrigine and is vital given the high recurrence of both depressive and manic symptoms in the absence of treatment. Although lithium has long been the mainstay of maintenance therapy, it has a narrow therapeutic window with long-term negative effects on the thyroid and kidneys; in addition, it is teratogenic. For acute manic episodes, the combination of either lithium or valproate with an atypical antipsychotic agent such as olanzapine, quetiapine or aripiprazole appears to be more effective than either mood stabilizer alone. Adjunctive psychotherapy may help patients adjust to having this chronic illness and may enhance compliance with maintenance pharmacotherapy. It is important that the history be assessed for manic symptoms in any patient being considered for initiation of pharmacologic treatment for depression, both to identify the presence of the disorder and to avoid triggering a manic episode, which may occur with treatment with SSRIs.

Somatoform Disorders
Clinical Presentation and Evaluation

Somatization refers to the presence of medically unexplained symptoms (MUSs). MUSs are seen in all populations, although they are more common in women, minorities, and those with less education or lower socioeconomic status. MUSs are relatively common in primary care offices, accounting for up to 50% of all symptom-related visits. Although 10% to 20% of patients in primary care practices have four or more unexplained symptoms, only a small number of these patients have a true somatoform disorder. True somatoform disorders are psychiatric diseases that involve persistent medically unexplained symptoms or symptoms that are out of proportion to medically expected findings and significantly affect a patient's ability to function. Somatoform disorders can cause great distress to patients, families, and physicians; in addition, patients suffering from these diseases are often high utilizers of the medical system, subjecting them to batteries of costly and potentially dangerous diagnostic tests.

Somatization disorder requires that multiple MUSs be present for years in multiple organ systems, although each symptom can wax and wane and all need not be present simultaneously. To fulfill the diagnostic criteria, symptoms need to have started before age 30 years and include gastrointestinal, pain, pseudoneurologic, and sexual symptoms. *Undifferentiated somatoform disorder* requires only a single somatic symptom that is present for at least 6 months (for example, nausea). Patients with *conversion disorder* have a single pseudoneurologic symptom that is not explained by a medical evaluation and often follows lay understanding of neurology (for example, hemiparesis that does not follow crossed corticospinal tracts). In *hypochondriasis*, patients misinterpret normal bodily sensations and are afraid these symptoms are manifestations of serious illness. Patients with *body dysmorphic disorder* are preoccupied with a real (usually minor) or imagined physical finding (for example, swelling of the face when examination reveals no edema).

The evaluation of possible somatoform disorders requires the consideration of both a medical and psychiatric differential diagnosis. Even when somatoform disorders are strongly suspected, clinicians should perform a thorough history and physical examination to construct a differential diagnosis that could explain a patient's symptoms medically. Laboratory and other testing should be ordered logically to evaluate plausible medical diagnoses; extensive and elaborate testing to explore unsupported or very unlikely diagnoses should be avoided despite a patient's concerns and requests. Testing should not be ordered to reassure a patient, as tests, even those with normal results, rarely help patients improve their level of function and increase the risk of iatrogenic complications. It is also important to screen for psychiatric comorbidities, including depression, panic disorder, and substance abuse. In addition, clinicians must carefully rule out malingering and factitious disorders. In these conditions, a patient purposely adopts a physical symptom. Patients with malingering do this for external gain (such as avoidance of work), whereas those with a factitious disorder do so in order to remain in the sick role.

Management

Patients with a somatoform disorder are psychologically dependent on potential illness, and unlike conversion or malingering, the symptoms expressed are not consciously fabricated. Treatment for somatoform disorders starts with an honest discussion of the diagnosis. Comorbid medical or psychiatric diseases should be treated. Regular office visits should be scheduled at frequent intervals. Some patients will need limits on visits or between-visit communications. Visits should focus on new or changed symptoms. These should be thoroughly evaluated to exclude new medical problems, although the disorder may require an increased reliance on physical signs rather than symptoms. Otherwise, primary care encounters should focus on functioning with symptoms rather than elimination of the symptoms.

No therapy has been shown to be consistently helpful in treating somatoform disorders. Reassurance can be helpful; however, it rarely leads to a resolution of symptoms. Although antidepressants have shown benefit in patients with medically unexplained symptoms, they have not been consistently shown to benefit patients with somatoform disorders. Several studies have shown a benefit from CBT, and psychiatric evaluation is often appropriate. Such referrals must be handled with care because patients with somatoform disorders can be sensitive to feelings of abandonment.

> **KEY POINT**
>
> - In patients with somatoform disorders, primary care visits should focus on the evaluation of new or changed symptoms and functioning with somatic symptoms rather than elimination of the symptoms.

Eating Disorders

Types of Eating Disorders

Anorexia nervosa is defined by four diagnostic criteria: an abnormally low body weight (<85% of expected) in association with an intense fear of gaining weight, an overemphasis of body weight on self-evaluation, and, in women and girls, amenorrhea for at least three consecutive menstrual cycles. It is classified as either restricting (with regular caloric restriction) or binge-eating/purging (binge eating that may or may not be associated with self-induced vomiting or the misuse of laxatives, diuretics, or enemas). The lifetime prevalence of anorexia nervosa is 1.0% to 3.7%, with adolescent girls and young women disproportionately affected. A family history of eating disorders or a diagnosis of childhood anxiety or OCD increases the risk for developing anorexia nervosa. The SCOFF questionnaire is a brief five-question instrument that can be used in the primary care setting to screen for anorexia nervosa (**Table 50**).

Physical signs of anorexia nervosa may be obvious on general inspection, as patients may present with parotid gland hyperplasia, dry and brittle hair, lanugo, yellowing skin, and

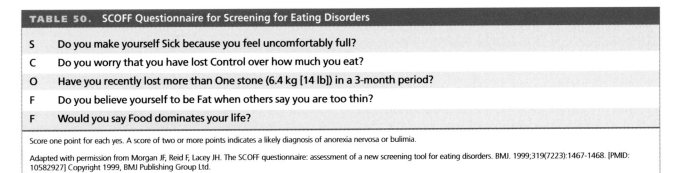

TABLE 50.	SCOFF Questionnaire for Screening for Eating Disorders
S	Do you make yourself **S**ick because you feel uncomfortably full?
C	Do you worry that you have lost **C**ontrol over how much you eat?
O	Have you recently lost more than **O**ne stone (6.4 kg [14 lb]) in a 3-month period?
F	Do you believe yourself to be **F**at when others say you are too thin?
F	Would you say **F**ood dominates your life?

Score one point for each yes. A score of two or more points indicates a likely diagnosis of anorexia nervosa or bulimia.

Adapted with permission from Morgan JF, Reid F, Lacey JH. The SCOFF questionnaire: assessment of a new screening tool for eating disorders. BMJ. 1999;319(7223):1467-1468. [PMID: 10582927] Copyright 1999, BMJ Publishing Group Ltd.

xerosis. Other signs include a low BMI (usually <18.5), bradycardia, orthostatic hypotension, and hypothermia. Cognitive impairment and a depressed or anxious mood are common in patients with anorexia nervosa, and these patients are also at high risk for suicide.

In a study reviewing the prognosis of 5590 patients treated for anorexia nervosa, the mortality rate was 5%. Among survivors, approximately 47% experienced a full recovery, whereas 33% improved and 20% remained chronically ill. Younger age (<19 years) and treatment within 3 years of diagnosis may be associated with improved recovery rates.

Although bulimia nervosa is more common than anorexia nervosa, affecting approximately 1% to 1.5% of women, it may be more difficult to diagnose. This disorder is characterized by recurrent episodes of binge eating with compensatory behavior aimed at preventing weight gain, including self-induced vomiting and misuse of medications (purging type) or fasting and excessive exercise (nonpurging type). Additional diagnostic criteria include the presence of these behaviors at least twice a week for 3 months and the excessive influence of body weight and shape on the patient's self-perception. Patients with bulimia nervosa are usually ashamed of and secretive about their abnormal eating patterns and may not seek medical treatment; nor may bulimia be suspected in typically normal-weight patients. The SCOFF screening tool, as well as subtle physical findings, such as dental caries and enlarged salivary glands, may aid in the diagnosis of bulimia nervosa. Scarring on the dorsum of the hand (Russell sign) caused by repeated abrasions during self-induced vomiting, is highly suggestive. As with anorexia nervosa, additional psychiatric illnesses may accompany bulimia nervosa, including anxiety and depression.

Eating disorder not otherwise specified (EDNOS) is diagnosed in patients who have disordered eating but do not fulfill the diagnostic criteria for anorexia nervosa or bulimia nervosa. The most common subtype of EDNOS is binge-eating disorder, which has a prevalence of about 2% to 3% in the general population; approximately one third of diagnosed patients are male. Characteristic behavior includes consumption of large quantities of food in a 2-hour period with an associated sense of lack of control. Although the binge episodes often occur in secret and patients feels disgust afterward, there is no compensatory behavior after the binge. Characteristic physical findings include an increased BMI; some patients may be severely obese. The Eating Attitudes Test (www.eat-26.com) is a useful screen for binge-eating disorder in the primary care setting.

Medical Complications of Eating Disorders

Hypokalemia, hypomagnesemia, and metabolic alkalosis may be seen in patients with anorexia nervosa or bulimia nervosa. A patient with severe anorexia nervosa may experience significant cardiovascular complications, including bradycardia and orthostatic hypotension; hospitalization is necessary if these

abnormalities are noted. The hypoestrogenic state that is characteristic of anorexia nervosa results in amenorrhea and low bone mineral density, and current guidelines recommend obtaining a dual-energy x-ray absorptiometry scan if menses are absent for more than 6 months. The most worrisome complication of anorexia nervosa is refeeding syndrome, which occurs when a severely malnourished patient receives aggressive oral, enteral, or parenteral nutritional repletion. This syndrome is associated with large volume shifts and sudden changes in electrolyte levels, resulting in edema, hypomagnesemia, hypophosphatemia, hypokalemia, and in rare cases, death. Close monitoring and repletion of electrolytes are essential for avoiding this complication. **H**

Treatment of Eating Disorders

There is limited evidence to indicate the optimal therapeutic approach in patients with anorexia nervosa. Individual psychotherapy may be most beneficial during acute refeeding, and there is weak evidence that CBT is efficacious in preventing relapse after weight has been restored. There is no role for monotherapy with psychotropic medications in anorexia nervosa, although they are indicated to treat comorbid psychiatric disorders and may have an adjunctive role in severely ill patients. As underweight patients are at increased risk for adverse effects, specific agents should be avoided, including bupropion, tricyclic antidepressants, and MAOIs.

In patients with bulimia nervosa and binge-eating disorder, in contrast to those with anorexia nervosa, there is strong evidence to support the use of CBT. Pharmacotherapy is a useful adjunct to CBT, and SSRI antidepressants have been shown to be effective and safe for treatment. Fluoxetine has been FDA-approved for the treatment of bulimia nervosa, and sertraline may also be effective. Topiramate has been shown to reduce binge eating and promote weight loss.

KEY POINTS

- Psychotherapy and nutritional support are the primary treatments for acutely ill patients with anorexia nervosa.
- Cognitive-behavioral therapy is an effective treatment for bulimia nervosa and binge-eating disorder.

Schizophrenia

Schizophrenia has a prevalence of 1% in the general population and affects women and men equally. It usually begins in the teenage years or in the early 20s; the strongest risk factor for its development is family history. First-degree relatives of persons with schizophrenia have a 6% to 17% lifetime incidence of the disease. It is manifested by positive and negative symptoms. Positive symptoms include paranoid delusions, hearing voices, and hallucinations; negative symptoms include flat affect, social withdrawal, and lack of interest or enjoyment in life. Thought tends to be disorganized, with confused speech and rapid shifts in topic. No symptom or sign is pathognomonic for schizophrenia. Diagnosis is based on the presence of signs and symptoms for at least 1 month in duration, with some manifestations of the disease present for at least 6 months. The onset of schizophrenia can be abrupt or insidious. Schizophrenia is thought to have several inciting factors, but genetics appears to play the biggest role in its development. It is important to consider other psychiatric diagnoses (depression with psychotic features, bipolar disorder) or medical diseases (substance abuse and withdrawal, delirium, central nervous system tumors) in the differential diagnosis, as 22% of those initially diagnosed with schizophrenia have their diagnosis changed during subsequent hospitalizations. Patients with schizophrenia should be co-managed with psychiatrists and other mental health professionals whenever possible.

Atypical antipsychotic agents, such as clozapine and olanzapine, have less risk of extrapyramidal side effects than traditional antipsychotic agents, such as haloperidol and chlorpromazine. However, adverse effects of these newer agents confer a higher risk of diabetes, lipid disorders, and weight gain. There is little consensus about the frequency of how often these metabolic parameters should be monitored, but most recommendations suggest monitoring periodically.

KEY POINT

- It is important to consider other psychiatric diagnoses and medical diseases in the differential diagnosis of schizophrenia, as 22% of those initially diagnosed with schizophrenia have their diagnosis changed during subsequent hospitalizations.

Attention-Deficit/Hyperactivity Disorder

Attention-deficit/hyperactivity disorder (ADHD) first manifests in childhood and is characterized by inattention, hyperactivity, and impulsivity accompanied by functional impairment in at least two settings (home, work, school). Although many children with ADHD show improvement as they age, symptoms of inattention may persist into adulthood. Prevalence in adults is estimated at 4%. ADHD is more likely in first-degree relatives of persons with ADHD. It may be associated with neurodevelopmental disorders (cerebral palsy, autism, learning disabilities) and with psychiatric disorders (substance abuse, mood disorders).

There are no diagnostic tests for ADHD. The DSM-IV-TR includes criteria for ADHD in children but may be applicable to adults if adapted. For example, functional impairment manifests differently in adult patients, who can have problems at both work and school. Adults with ADHD are more likely to have traffic infractions, vehicular accidents, and spousal separation and divorce than the general population.

Diagnosing ADHD in an adult patient can be challenging but should be considered in a patient with a history of inattention or impulsive behavior and significant functional impairment beginning in early childhood. About 10% to 20% of adults with substance abuse or mood disorders have ADHD; it is therefore important to review the patient's history for evidence of ADHD in childhood.

The first-line treatment for childhood ADHD is stimulants, such as amphetamine and methylphenidate. These agents may be effective in adults but must be used more cautiously, particularly in patients with hypertension or cardiovascular disease. The increased risk of substance use disorders is also of concern in adults with ADHD, as stimulants are controlled substances with high potential for abuse or diversion. Atomoxetine is a selective norepinephrine reuptake inhibitor specifically approved for treatment of ADHD in adults and has shown benefit. Bupropion and tricyclic antidepressants may also be beneficial. Because the natural history of ADHD usually shows gradual improvement with age, it is important to regularly verify the ongoing need for medication with periodic "drug holidays" in well controlled patients. CBT has been reported to be effective for ADHD but may be most helpful as an adjunct to medications.

KEY POINT

- Because attention-deficit/hyperactivity disorder usually shows gradual improvement with age, it is important to regularly verify the need for medication in adults.

Autism Spectrum Disorders

Autism spectrum disorders are characterized by difficulties in social interactions and repetitive behaviors or narrow interests. Severe autism accompanied by developmental delay is evident in early childhood, while those with milder symptoms and no cognitive deficits may not be diagnosed until later in life. Approximately 0.9% of children have an autism spectrum disorder, according to Centers for Disease Control and Prevention estimates, and autism spectrum disorders are thought to be equally prevalent in adults.

DSM-IV-TR diagnostic criteria for autistic disorder are based on childhood behavior and include impairment in social interaction; impairment in communication; and repetitive patterns of behavior, interests, or activities, with onset before age 3 years. Patients with these symptoms without significant delay in language or cognitive development may meet criteria for Asperger disorder. The current draft version of the DSM-V, however, has eliminated Asperger disorder in favor of a broader definition of autism spectrum disorder that no longer requires the presence of developmental delay but includes impairment of everyday functioning. The new definition also specifies that symptoms must be present in early childhood but may not become fully manifest until later in life, when social demands exceed capacities. Persons with Asperger disorder frequently come to medical attention later than autistic children because of their lesser developmental deficits. Making the formal diagnosis of an autism spectrum disorder in adults is difficult and frequently requires a specialized clinical evaluation using a number of diagnostic tools.

Managing adults with autism spectrum disorders is highly influenced by individual patient characteristics. For those with difficulty with physical contact, physical examination should be limited only to essential maneuvers, performed slowly, and explained in detail before proceeding. Efforts should be made to communicate with patients who are unable to speak as they frequently are able to comprehend and participate in decision making; alternative methods of communication (pen and paper, pictures, assistive devices) should be considered. Repetitive and stereotyped behaviors are calming for many patients with autism and should not be interrupted unless they are harmful or disruptive. The assistance of a caregiver or colleague who is familiar with the individual patient and how best to interact with him or her is invaluable.

KEY POINT

- Because patients with autism generally have difficulty with physical contact, physical examination should be limited only to essential maneuvers, performed slowly, and explained in detail before proceeding.

Difficult Patient Encounters

Several studies indicate that physicians experience about 15% of patient encounters as difficult. Difficult encounters often involve patients who have a depressive or anxiety disorder, poorer functional status, unmet expectations, reduced satisfaction, and greater use of health care services. Physicians often report the most difficulty with patients by whom they feel manipulated or frustrated, patients who are time consuming and have unrealistic demands, patients who do not follow recommendations, patients who express anger, and those who interrupt physician routine and make extra work. Patients who have somatization disorder, chronic pain, substance abuse, or an undiagnosable medical problem are often labeled as difficult. Patients with identifiable personality disorders, such as borderline, dependent, histrionic, obsessive, or antisocial personality disorders, also are frequently labeled as difficult.

Physician characteristics also play a role in generating a difficult patient encounter. Physicians who are fatigued or harried or develop a dislike for a patient are more likely to consider a patient difficult. Additional physician characteristics include having less experience, having a higher perceived workload, and having poor communication skills.

It is vital for a physician to identify the underlying emotion that is creating difficulty in order to best address it. Frequent negative emotions in providers include anger, fear of losing control, fear of displeasing, and fear of harming the patient, as well as those stemming from unique personal issues, such as fear of incompetence, fear of death, or reminders of illnesses in the provider's personal life.

One of the first steps in improving a difficult patient interaction is recognizing the underlying emotion at work in the situation. Often, being open with the patient about any patient behaviors that are eliciting the negative reaction can be helpful in alleviating the underlying tension. It is important that the physician take responsibility for managing his or her own negative emotion rather than expecting the patient to respond, however, as the physician may be better able to overcome the inherent conflicts in the situation.

Depending on the clinical situation, it may be important for the physician to specifically address certain behaviors, such as limit setting with borderline patients or setting expectations for frequency of visits with high utilizers. Being observant of and compassionate about the underlying emotions that drive patients to become "difficult" is one of the best ways to remedy unpleasant interactions. If a complete lack of trust develops or it becomes obvious that a therapeutic relationship is not possible, the physician should consider transferring care of the patient to another provider.

KEY POINT

- Both patient and physician factors contribute to difficult patient encounters.

Geriatric Medicine

Functional Assessment

In older patients, functional status is as important as medical illness in determining overall well-being. Function in geriatric patients is a predictor of independent living as well as the development of future medical illnesses. Therefore, functional assessment and treatment of disorders associated with functional decline must be incorporated into the evaluation and care of elderly patients in both office and hospital settings.

Aids to functional assessment, beyond history and physical examination, may include screening instruments and a multidisciplinary assessment involving occupational and physical therapists as well as physicians trained in geriatric medicine. Activities of daily living (ADLs) are basic self-care activities, including bathing, dressing, and feeding, that help determine a patient's required level of support (**Table 51**). Instrumental activities of daily living (IADLs) are activities that are associated with independent living, including shopping for food, administering one's own medications, and handling finances. To

TABLE 51. Indices to Assess Basic and Instrumental Activities of Daily Living

Index (time to complete)	Functional Activities Assessed
Katz Index of Independence in Activities of Daily Living[a] (5-10 min)	Bathing
	Dressing
	Toileting
	Transferring
	Continence
	Feeding
Barthel Index[b] (5-10 min)	Feeding
	Bathing
	Grooming
	Dressing
	Bowels
	Bladder
	Toilet use
	Transfers
	Mobility
	Stairs
Lawton and Brody Instrumental Activities of Daily Living Scale[c] (5-10 min)	Ability to use a telephone
	Shopping
	Food preparation
	Housekeeping
	Laundry
	Mode of transportation
	Responsibility for own medications
	Ability to handle finances
Direct Assessment of Functional Status[d] (30-35 min)	Time orientation
	Communication
	Transportation
	Finance
	Shopping
	Eating
	Dressing and grooming

[a]The Katz index is scored by assigning a score of 1 to each activity if it can be completed independently, which is defined as having no supervision, direction, or personal assistance; scores are then added for a range of 0 to 6.

[b]Each item on the Barthel index is assigned a 0 to 10 value, resulting in a score of 0 to 100, with higher scores reflecting independence.

[c]The Lawton and Brody scale results in a score of 0 to 8, with a score of 8 representing independence and 0 representing total dependence for activities of daily living.

[d]The Direct Assessment of Functional Status is a more complex 85-item instrument that evaluates individual tasks for each of the skills using direct observation.

ensure accuracy and objectivity, assessment of these activities should include direct observations of patients by health care personnel when possible. Assessing ADLs and IADLs in the hospital can facilitate discharge planning.

Fall Prevention and Home Safety

Falls are a serious problem for older adults and occur in approximately one third of community-dwelling adults who are 65 years or older and half of similarly aged hospitalized adults. Falling is most often related to patient and environmental factors. Those at greatest risk include persons with gait imbalance, stroke, or dementia, or who use an assistive device to walk. Chronic conditions associated with falls include arthritis, depression, orthostatic hypotension, and visual deficits. Leg muscle weakness, Parkinson disease, and peripheral neuropathy also can increase risk. Falls are associated with increased morbidity and mortality, a decline in functional abilities, and a loss of independence.

Because of the high prevalence of falls, as well as the associated burden of illness and cost and the potential to improve outcomes, the Institute of Medicine has identified prevention of falls as a priority area. Screening for fall risk and institution of fall prevention strategies has been proposed as a way to limit the impact of falls in the geriatric population. The American Geriatrics Society recommends that physicians ask adults aged 75 years and older if they have difficulty with walking and balance and if they have fallen in the past year. For patients who have fallen, the history should include a description of the circumstances of the fall as well as a review of current medications. Psychotropic medications increase the risk of falling, and their gradual withdrawal reduces the rate of falls. Educating physicians about modifying medications in the elderly has been shown to reduce the risk of falling.

Physical examination for patients with a history of falling in the past year should include assessment of gait and mobility; this can be facilitated by using the timed "Up & Go" (TUG) test. The patient is asked to rise from a chair, walk 10 feet, turn around, walk back, and sit down again in the same chair. The physician observes the patient for ease of performance, speed, and balance. Patients should perform the task using any routine assistive devices, such as a cane or walker. The average healthy adult can complete the task in less than 10 seconds; those completing the task in more than 14 seconds are considered to be at high risk for subsequent falls. A recent pooled analysis of nine cohort studies including nearly 35,000 community-dwelling adults with a mean age of 73.5 years found that increased gait speed was associated with increased survival. In these studies, patients were asked to walk at their usual pace. The walk distance varied from 2.4 m (8 ft) to 6 m (20 ft), and speed was calculated as meters per second. For men between 75 and 84 years old, mean 10-year survival was 15% for gait speeds slower than 0.4 m/s and 50% for gait speeds 1.4 m/s or faster. For women the same age, the corresponding 10-year survival rates were 35% and 92%, respectively. This model, using age, sex, and gait speed, performed as well in predicting survival as more complex models based on several factors, including chronic conditions, smoking, and blood pressure.

Physical examination should also include assessment for visual deficits and lower extremity joint examination to detect arthritis. Cardiovascular evaluation should include assessment for orthostatic hypotension, arrhythmia, and, when syncope or presyncope is suspected, for carotid sinus hypersensitivity. Neurologic examination should include evaluation of cognitive function, lower extremity weakness, and peripheral neuropathy.

Finally, the home environment should be evaluated for falling hazards. Environmental hazards are responsible for 25% to 66% of falls in the home, and hazards can be found in two thirds or more of homes. Common environmental hazards include throw rugs; low toilet seats; no grab bar for bathtub, shower, or toilet; no nightlight in the bedroom, kitchen, or living room; uneven lighting of stairway or poorly visible step edges; and difficult-to-reach kitchen storage. Other hazards include slippery bathing areas, general clutter, difficult-to-reach light switches, and unsafe handrails. Recommendations to improve home safety include installing nonslip stripping to noncarpeted steps, removing all unevenness in floors (thresholds) and changing chair seat height so that the patient's upper and lower legs are at 90-degree angles when sitting. If the physician or family member has a concern about the patient's living environment, a home nurse evaluation for home safety should be arranged. The USPSTF, however, was not able to find sufficient evidence for or against home hazard modification.

Persons with a history of falls should undergo the assessment detailed above followed by individually tailored interventions to reduce the risk for future falling. Evidence-based interventions include prescribing gait, exercise, and balance training. A Cochrane Database review of interventions to prevent falls in elderly persons living in the community also found evidence for use of anti-slip shoes in icy conditions, pacemaker installation in patients with carotid sinus hypersensitivity, and cataract surgery in the first eye affected.

A recent systematic review and meta-analysis recommends prescribing vitamin D at a dose of 800 IU daily for elderly patients who have vitamin D deficiency, for those residing in long-term care facilities, and potentially for all elderly adults at increased risk for falling. The Institute of Medicine recommends a vitamin D intake of 600 units/d for all men and women aged 51 to 70 years old and 800 units/d for men and women older than 70 years. In a meta-analysis of adults aged 60 years or older, vitamin D supplementation for at least 6 months resulted in a 14% relative risk reduction for falls (number needed to treat = 15). The proposed mechanism of action of vitamin D is its beneficial effect on muscle strength and function and on gait. The USPSTF recommends exercise or physical therapy and vitamin D supplementation to prevent falls in community-dwelling adults aged 65 years or older who are at increased risk for falls.

Mild Cognitive Impairment and Dementia

Mild cognitive impairment (MCI), or cognitive impairment without dementia, is associated with decreased quality of life and functional status, loss of independence, and increased health care costs. MCI is present in about one fifth of patients older than 70 years and may be present in nearly one third of hospitalized patients older than 75 years. The most common subtypes include prodromal Alzheimer disease, vascular cognitive impairment, and MCI due to medical conditions and stroke. (In vascular cognitive impairment, cardiovascular or cerebrovascular disease is present, but the cognitive impairment is not temporally linked to a single stroke). MCI may be more common in older patients with depression, neurologic conditions, alcohol abuse, and low baseline intellect. Patients who develop essential tremor after age 65 years may be more likely to have MCI than either those without essential tremor or those who develop tremor before age 65 years. Progression from MCI to dementia is about 12% annually but is higher (17%-20%) in those with stroke and prodromal Alzheimer disease. Researchers are evaluating cerebrospinal fluid markers and genetic markers as predictors for progression to Alzheimer disease. A recent study found that a genetic variation in the caspase-1 gene predicted accelerated progression from MCI to Alzheimer disease over a 2-year period, but the clinical utility of this genetic test is unknown at this time.

The Mini–Mental State Examination (MMSE) has been the standard screening instrument for cognitive function, with a sensitivity of 76% and specificity of 88% for detecting cognitive impairment. Scores of 24 to 25 out of 30 suggest mild impairment, scores of 19 to 24 suggest mild dementia, and scores of 10 to 19 suggest moderate dementia. The MMSE may under-diagnose those with high intellect and may over-diagnose those with low intellect or with delirium. A briefer screening tool, the Mini-Cog (sensitivity 76%, specificity 89%), performs comparably to the MMSE and employs a three-item recall test followed by the clock-drawing test if any one of the three items is missed. If all three items are recalled, no further testing is necessary. The Sweet 16 (sensitivity 80%, specificity 70%) is a newer instrument that is easier to administer than the MMSE and can be completed in 2 to 3 minutes. The 16 items include eight orientation items, three immediate-recall and three delayed-recall items, and two backward digit span items. When screening for dementia, it is also extremely important to ask a family member or caregiver about memory loss, personality change, word-finding difficulties, changes in activity level, getting lost, and difficulty in performing ADLs to place testing results into a clinical context.

Although there is no widely accepted treatment for MCI, cognitive rehabilitation has been shown to have some effectiveness in improving functioning in some patients. Cognitive rehabilitation is performed by neuropsychologists and occupational therapists and involves using external memory aids as well as teaching patients organizational and attention skills. A randomized trial of cognitive rehabilitation for patients with MCI with a mean age of 79 years demonstrated improved memory at 2 weeks and 4 months.

Depression

Depression is common in older adults, with major depressive disorder being present in 6% to 9% of patients older than 60 years presenting to physicians' offices and some form of depression in 25% of persons older than age 60 years. Depression in older adults may present with somatic and vegetative symptoms rather than dysphoria. Depression is more common in patients residing in institutions and in those with acute or chronic illnesses, including cardiovascular and cerebrovascular disease, cognitive decline and dementia, and bereavement. Medical conditions associated with depression include hypothyroidism, hyperthyroidism ("apathetic hyperthyroidism"), chronic pain, Parkinson disease, cancer, diabetes mellitus, vitamin B_{12} deficiency, alcohol abuse, and use of corticosteroids or interferon. Depressed patients presenting with cognitive decline (pseudodementia) may display delayed responses to cognitive test questions compared with patients with true dementia. Treatment of the depression improves cognitive function in these patients. Because depression in older adults is often perceived as an expected consequence of chronic illness, it is frequently undiagnosed and untreated.

The PHQ-9 (see Mental and Behavioral Health) can be used to identify and assess severity of depression in older adults. When tested in adults aged 65 years and older, its sensitivity and specificity for diagnosing major depressive disorder were 100% and 77%, respectively. The Geriatric Depression Scale consists of 15 questions, and a score of 5 or greater indicates depression. Its sensitivity is 80% to 90% and its specificity is 70% to 85%.

The USPSTF has found good evidence that treatment of depression in older adults who are identified through screening in primary care settings decreases clinical morbidity. Treatment may include antidepressants, psychotherapy, or both. Relapse may occur more frequently in older compared with younger adults. Patients older than 70 years receiving selective serotonin reuptake inhibitor (SSRI) therapy may have fewer recurrences of depression if treated for 2 years. Evidence is fair that SSRI use is associated with an increased risk for upper gastrointestinal bleeding in older patients, with risk increasing with age. SSRIs can also cause the syndrome of inappropriate antidiuretic hormone secretion (SIADH). The use of stimulants can be considered for some older patients with apathetic major depressive illness. For elderly patients with insomnia and weight loss, mirtazapine may be preferred because of its beneficial effect on these symptoms. For patients with refractory severe depression, electroconvulsive therapy (ECT) can be considered in medically stable patients.

Hearing

Hearing loss is present in one third of patients aged 65 years and older and in 80% of those 80 years or older. The most common cause of hearing loss is presbycusis, or age-related hearing loss. Presbycusis results in high-frequency hearing loss, which typically impairs sound localization and hearing the spoken voice (particularly in noisy environments). Hearing impairment can lead to depression, limited activity, and social isolation. Among the available screening tests, the whispered voice test, in which the examiner stands 2 feet behind a seated patient and assesses the ability of the patient to repeat a whispered combination of numbers and letters, or a single question about whether the patient has hearing difficulty seem to be nearly as accurate as hand-held audiometry or a detailed hearing loss questionnaire. The USPSTF concludes that evidence is insufficient to weigh the benefits and harms of screening for hearing loss in older adults. The Canadian Task Force on the Periodic Health Examination has recommended screening older adults for hearing impairment using single-question screening, the whispered voice test, or audiometry. The use of hearing aids does not result in normal hearing but can improve communication abilities. Only 20% of patients who could potentially benefit from using a hearing aid actually use one. Cochlear implants can be considered for patients who are not able to distinguish more than 50% of words in a test sentence using the worst ear with a hearing aid in place.

Vision

Visual impairment, defined as best corrected vision worse than 20/40, is present in 1% of persons aged 65 to 69 years and increases to 17% in those older than 80 years. The most common causes of visual impairment in older persons are refractive errors, cataracts, and age-related macular degeneration (AMD). Diabetic retinopathy and glaucoma are also important causes of visual impairment.

The USPSTF found insufficient evidence to recommend for or against screening adults for glaucoma and also concluded that the current evidence is insufficient to recommend for or against screening for visual acuity in older adults. Although evidence was adequate that early treatment of refractive error, cataracts, and AMD improves or prevents loss of visual acuity, evidence that these improvements would enhance functional outcomes was inadequate. The American Academy of Ophthalmology recommends comprehensive eye examinations every 1 to 2 years for persons 65 years or older who have no risk factors. When screening is performed by primary care physicians, use of a visual acuity test (such as the Snellen eye chart) is recommended.

Some evidence suggests that the use of multifocal lenses may increase risk for falls in older adults, probably because looking down through the reading segment of the lens causes the ground to be out of focus.

The Older Driver

The risk for automobile accidents is increased among older drivers, and both patients and physicians have a responsibility to reduce this risk. Although patients often self-restrict their driving as they become aware of driving difficulties, "low mileage" drivers may be at the greatest risk. Medical conditions most likely to cause problems include those affecting vision, motor function, and cognition. Specific medical conditions that increase risk include cataract, arthritis, dizziness, history of falls, arrhythmia, and seizure disorders, as well as substance abuse and use of sedating medications. Dementia is associated with a two-fold risk for driving accidents. Although some studies have shown impaired driving in older adults with MCI, there are not enough data to make clear recommendations regarding assessing or restricting drivers with MCI. The American Medical Association (AMA) recommends that physicians assess patients for physical or mental impairments that might adversely affect driving abilities. In addition, older drivers can be evaluated by driver rehabilitation specialists (associated with hospital occupational therapy departments) who can also make recommendations for safer driving. State-specific physician reporting requirements, along with tools for patients and physicians, can be found in the AMA's *Physician's Guide to Assessing and Counseling Older Drivers* (available at www.ama-assn.org/ama/pub/physician-resources/public-health/promoting-healthy-lifestyles/geriatric-health/older-driver-safety/assessing-counseling-older-drivers.page).

KEY POINTS

- Adults aged 75 years and older should be assessed for fall risk by asking if they have difficulty with walking and balance and if they have fallen in the past year.
- Evidence-based interventions to reduce falls in older adults include supplemental vitamin D; modification of risk factors in the home; reducing or eliminating psychoactive medications; and prescribing gait, exercise, and balance training to patients with abnormal gait or balance.
- Depression in older adults may present with somatic and vegetative symptoms rather than dysphoria.

Levels of Care

For patients who cannot live independently at home, either following a hospitalization or as a result of progressive decline, various care options may be available. Levels of care can be divided into postacute and long-term care. Postacute care options following hospitalization include inpatient rehabilitation (for patients with stable medical issues able to participate in ≥3 hours/d of therapy); skilled nursing facilities, for patients requiring care that must be administered by trained nursing personnel or needing rehabilitation services but are unable to participate in at least 3 hours/day of therapy (sometimes called subacute rehabilitation); long-term acute care hospitals (LTACHs), which provide long-term complex care following hospital discharge, including ventilator care and weaning; advanced health care services provided in the home (home health care); and hospice or palliative care. Long-term care options include supportive home care, which includes assistance in performing ADLs; assisted living, which provides institution-based care in semi-independent units with variable levels of assistance available; nursing homes, which provide ongoing nursing-level care; and adult day care, in which care services are provided during the day. It is not uncommon, particularly in elderly patients being discharged from the hospital, for patients to receive postacute care but ultimately require a higher level of chronic care than before admission. It is, therefore, imperative that physicians have a basic understanding of various care options so that they can help patients or their representatives make the best possible decisions for both long-term and transitional care.

Pressures to discharge patients as soon as medical conditions requiring hospitalization are resolved may interfere with the process of determining the best long-term living situation for a patient. Primary care physicians are particularly important advocates for their patients and can provide valuable input to hospitalists to ensure optimal post-discharge planning. Care managers, funded either privately or through public agencies, can also be valuable assets in configuring the best living situation for a patient.

Polypharmacy

Polypharmacy refers to the use of many medications together, and it tends to be a term used almost exclusively in the context of elderly patients. Ninety percent of noninstitutionalized patients older than 65 years take at least one medication, and approximately 50% take five or more medications each week. Twelve percent of patients older than 65 years take ten or more medications each week. As more medications are prescribed, rates of adverse drug reactions and medication errors rise. More drugs being taken together increases the risk of drug-drug interactions.

Many drugs used in the elderly have been studied primarily in younger patients with significantly longer life expectancies, and their safety and efficacy in older patients are not well established. Drug metabolism may be altered in the elderly owing to decreased glomerular filtration or underlying illness as well as to altered pharmacokinetics related to aging. A recent study found that four medications were responsible for two thirds of emergency hospitalizations for adverse drug events. Hospitalizations involving three of them (warfarin, insulin, and oral hypoglycemic agents) were related to unintentional overdose. Warfarin was implicated most frequently, accounting for one third of emergency hospitalizations. The fourth class of drugs, oral antiplatelet agents, were implicated by acting alone or by interacting with warfarin.

Frequent, routine review to verify need for medication and appropriate dosing is an important aspect of optimal geriatric care. Many strategies have been studied to monitor and reduce polypharmacy. Biannual review (or more frequently for higher numbers of medications taken) of medication lists helps to prevent duplication of medication classes. The "Good Palliative–Geriatric Practice" (GP-GP) algorithm for drug discontinuation (available at http://archinte.jamanetwork.com/article.aspx?doi=10.1001/archinternmed.2010.355) has been shown to be effective in reducing polypharmacy and improving mortality and morbidity in nursing home inpatients and has been studied in smaller populations of community-dwelling outpatients and found to be effective. **H**

KEY POINTS

- Altered pharmacodynamics, multiple medications, and increased susceptibility to adverse effects make polypharmacy a major problem in geriatric patients.

- Frequent, routine review to verify need for medication and appropriate dosing is an important aspect of optimal geriatric care.

Urinary Incontinence

Epidemiology
Urinary incontinence, or involuntary urine leakage, affects one third of middle-aged and older women and 20% of older men. These numbers likely underestimate its true prevalence, however, as many patients do not report incontinence to their physician. In addition to female sex, risk factors include age, diabetes mellitus, obesity, history of vaginal childbirth, history of gynecologic surgery, pelvic floor muscle weakness, high caffeine intake, tobacco use, menopause, and impairment in cognition or mobility. Urinary incontinence in men may result from benign prostatic hyperplasia (overflow incontinence) or from surgery or radiation therapy for prostate cancer.

Urinary incontinence is associated with excess health care expenditures. It increases the risk of falls and may lead to social isolation, embarrassment, decreased quality of life, functional decline, and admission to a nursing home. Effective treatment is available and improves quality of life. Although much of the evidence regarding management of incontinence comes from studies enrolling only women, most principles can be generalized to men.

Evaluation
Urinary incontinence is categorized as (1) urge incontinence (loss of urine accompanied by sense of urgency; caused by detrusor overreactivity); (2) stress incontinence (loss of urine with effort, coughing, or sneezing; caused by sphincter incompetence); (3) mixed urge and stress incontinence; and (4) overflow incontinence (caused by outlet obstruction).

Functional incontinence, defined as simply not getting to the toilet quickly enough, may occur in patients with significant mobility and cognitive impairments. Determining the type (or types) of incontinence guides management.

Because patients may not report incontinence spontaneously, the Agency for Healthcare Research and Quality recommends routine screening for all frail older men and women; some groups also recommend screening women aged 65 years and older for incontinence. Standardized questionnaires can distinguish urge from stress incontinence, including the 3 Incontinence Questions (3IQ) (**Figure 27**). For urge incontinence, the 3IQ has a sensitivity of 75%, specificity of 77%, positive likelihood ratio of 3.29, and negative likelihood ratio of 0.32. The 3IQ's metrics for stress incontinence are similar (86%, 60%, 2.13, and 0.24, respectively).

The evaluation should include a targeted history, including surgeries, instrumentations, and other relevant interventions; medication review; and physical examination, including a pelvic examination in women and a digital rectal examination in men. Men should be asked about prostate symptoms. Reversible causes should be noted, including delirium, urinary tract infection, atrophic vaginitis, medications, depression, hyperglycemia, impaired mobility, and fecal impaction. Urinalysis should be performed. Unless there is high clinical suspicion for neurologic disease or bladder outlet obstruction, a post-void residual urine volume determination is not necessary.

Treatment
General recommendations for all patients with urinary incontinence include caffeine restriction and, if overweight or obese, weight reduction. Excess fluid intake should be avoided, especially at nighttime, but not at the expense of adequate hydration. Any underlying causes should be addressed. Further treatment depends on the type of urinary incontinence.

Behavioral Therapy
Pelvic floor muscle training (PFMT, or Kegel exercises) and bladder training/urge suppression techniques are the two most effective behavioral therapies. PFMT is considered first-line therapy for patients with stress incontinence and is of likely benefit in patients with mixed urge and stress incontinence. PFMT exercises, if performed correctly and diligently, strengthen the pubococcygeus muscles that form the pelvic floor and enhance urinary retention by increasing the tone of the supporting structures of the urethra. The patient is instructed to contract the pelvic muscles as if trying to interrupt urination. In women, correct technique may be assessed by inserting a finger into the vagina and feeling the circumvaginal muscles tighten and the pelvic floor move upward. Patients should work up to three or four sets of ten contractions daily, with contractions lasting 10 seconds. Bladder

1. During the last 3 months, have you leaked urine (even a small amount)?

❑ Yes   ❑ No

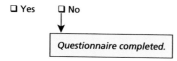

Questionnaire completed.

2. During the last 3 months, did you leak urine:
(Check all that apply.)

❑ a. When you were performing some physical activity, such as coughing, sneezing, lifting, or exercise?
❑ b. When you had the urge or the feeling that you needed to empty your bladder, but you could not get to the toilet fast enough?
❑ c. Without physical activity and without a sense of urgency?

3. During the last 3 months, did you leak urine *most often*:
(Check only one.)

❑ a. When you were performing some physical activity, such as coughing, sneezing, lifting, or exercise?
❑ b. When you had the urge or the feeling that you needed to empty your bladder, but you could not get to the toilet fast enough?
❑ c. Without physical activity and without a sense of urgency?
❑ d. About equally as often with physical activity as with a sense of urgency?

Definitions of type of urinary incontinence are based on responses to question 3:

Response to Question 3	Type of Incontinence
a. Most often with physical activity	Stress only or stress predominant
b. Most often with the urge to empty the bladder	Urge only or urge predominant
c. Without physical activity or sense of urgency	Other cause only or other cause predominant
d. About equally with physical activity and sense of urgency	Mixed

FIGURE 27. The 3 Incontinence Questions (3IQ) for evaluation of urinary incontinence.

Reprinted with permission from Brown JS, Bradley CS, Subak LL, et al; Diagnostic Aspects of Incontinence Study (DAISy) Research Group. The sensitivity and specificity of a simple test to distinguish between urge and stress urinary incontinence. Ann Intern Med. 2006;144:715-723. [PMID: 16702587] Copyright 2006, American College of Physicians.

training and suppressive therapy are indicated for urge and mixed incontinence. Patients are instructed to void regularly throughout the day, regardless of urge, and progressively increase the interval between voids. Urge to void outside of the schedule is managed by suppression techniques. The patient is instructed to contract pelvic floor muscles quickly three or four times, use a distraction technique (counting backwards from 100), and, when the urge passes, walk to the bathroom to urinate.

A systematic review of 96 randomized controlled trials of nonsurgical treatments for urinary incontinence concluded that PFMT alone improved stress incontinence compared with usual care. The pooled relative risk ratio for continence was 7.1. Individual therapy, biofeedback, and use of skilled therapists improved outcomes. Bladder training alone improved symptoms but not continence rates. In studies of stress and urge incontinence, PFMT coupled with bladder training increased continence rates (pooled relative risk ratio, 13).

Prompted voiding (periodically asking the patient about incontinence, reminding and assisting the patient to go to the toilet, and providing positive reinforcement for continence) is effective in elderly nursing home residents with functional incontinence.

Pharmacologic Therapy

Effective pharmacologic therapy is available for treatment of incontinence. Data on long-term continence rates are lacking, however, and adverse effects may limit long-term tolerability.

In patients with stress incontinence for whom PFMT has not been successful, duloxetine, a serotonin and norepinephrine reuptake inhibitor, is an option. In a systematic review of randomized, controlled trials, duloxetine improved incontinence rates and quality of life but did not cure incontinence.

For urge incontinence, anticholinergic antimuscarinic medications are first-line therapy. Options include oxybutynin, tolterodine, fesoterodine, darifenacin, solifenacin, and trospium. High-quality head-to-head trials comparing individual antimuscarinics are limited. However, all of these drugs appear to provide similar small benefits in continence rates without clear superiority of newer agents relative to older medications, except for a slightly lower incidence of anticholinergic side effects. Anticholinergic agents are contraindicated in patients with angle-closure glaucoma.

Treatment of prostate-related lower urinary tract symptoms is addressed in further detail in Men's Health.

Medications that have been found to be ineffective for incontinence are pseudoephedrine (an α-agonist), oral estrogens (may worsen incontinence), and transdermal and vaginal estrogens. Conclusive long-term data for imipramine, a tricyclic antidepressant with α-agonist and anticholinergic properties, are lacking.

Combined use of behavioral therapy with pharmacologic therapy has not been shown to be more effective than medication alone in women with urge incontinence. Although behavioral therapy may reduce incontinence frequency during active treatment, it does not improve ability to stop the medication.

Devices, Injectable Bulking Agents, and Surgery
For stress incontinence, medical devices (pessaries, intravaginal devices, urethral plugs, vaginal cones) are available. Pessaries are most effective but require fitting by experienced practitioners. The most effective surgeries for stress incontinence are sling procedures for intrinsic sphincter deficiency (success rate, 80%-90%), retropubic suspension, needle bladder neck suspension, and anterior vaginal repair with plication of the bladder neck (success rates 79%, 74%, and 65%, respectively). Although increasingly used, results of studies of periurethral injection of bulking agents (collagen, porcine dermal implant, myoblasts, fibroblasts, and dextran) for treatment of stress incontinence have been variable.

For urge incontinence, studies of intradetrusor botulinum toxin injection report complete continence in 32% to 86% of patients, with mean duration of 6 months. Variable cure rates are seen with sacral nerve stimulation and augmentation cystoplasty.

Condom or indwelling (Foley) urinary catheters increase risk of urinary tract infections. Their use, except as palliative or temporizing measures, is not advised.

KEY POINTS
- Pelvic floor muscle training and bladder training/urge suppression techniques are effective behavioral therapies for stress urinary incontinence.
- Pharmacologic options for urinary incontinence treatment include oxybutynin or tolterodine for urge incontinence and duloxetine for stress incontinence.

Pressure Ulcers
Clinical Presentation
Pressure ulcers are a common condition, particularly in persons who are acutely hospitalized, admitted to nursing homes, or receiving home health care. More than 2.5 million pressure ulcers are reported nationally in acute care settings alone. Annual treatment costs are estimated at $11 billion. They result from continuous pressure, friction, and shearing forces to the skin. Risk factors include increased age, reduced mobility, reduced level of consciousness, malnutrition, peripheral vascular disease, incontinence, and poor skin condition.

Pressure ulcers most commonly occur on bony prominences, usually on the hips and lower extremities. One study reported that 36% of patients with hip fractures developed pressure ulcers. It is important to differentiate pressure ulcers from ulcers related to diabetic neuropathy or venous or arterial insufficiency, as treatments for these conditions vary.

Prevention and Management
Preventive interventions are much more cost effective than the prolonged and intensive efforts required to treat pressure ulcers. Patients should be assessed at each hospital or nursing home admission for risks of development of ulcers. Skin inspection of those at high risk should be conducted regularly. Preventive efforts should focus on avoiding friction, shear, and heavy moisture, which are often a result of wound drainage or incontinence. Various types of support surfaces, including beds, mattresses and overlays, have been studied to evaluate their ability to prevent pressure ulcers. Foam mattresses that distribute pressure over a larger area (relative risk [RR], 0.40; 95% CI, 0.21 to 0.74) and medical grade sheepskin (RR, 0.56; 95% CI, 0.32 to 0.97) are beneficial in preventing ulcers in hospitalized patients compared with standard mattresses. The effectiveness of alternating and constant low-pressure mattresses and overlays is not clear. Scientific evidence for nutritional supplements, seat cushions, and lotions is minimal.

Treatment of existing ulcers can be informed by staging (**Table 52**). Treatment should be provided by interdisciplinary teams, with a focus on addressing predisposing and exacerbating factors that initially led to the ulcer. In general, a wide variety of dressings, barriers, and gels may be used, with a focus on maintaining a clean and moist wound environment and managing exudates. Higher-stage ulcers with eschar may require surgical or nonsurgical debridement. Attention to superinfection, frank cellulitis, and potential underlying osteomyelitis is vital. The presence of infectious complications is an indication for systemic antibiotic therapy.

Stage I ulcers can generally be treated with transparent films and do not require debriding. Emphasis should be placed on prevention of further progression. Stage II ulcers can be treated using an occlusive dressing to keep the area moist. Wet-to-dry dressings should be avoided because debridement is usually unnecessary at this stage. Stage III and IV ulcers generally require surgical or nonsurgical debridement, treatment of wound infection, and appropriate dressings based on the wound environment. For nonhealing wounds that are stage III or higher, imaging to rule out underlying osteomyelitis is indicated. Surgical wound intervention may be necessary in severe or nonhealing ulcers if conservative measures fail.

Although often used, there is no evidence that supplementation with either vitamin C or zinc is helpful in the absence of deficiency. Adequate nutrition to maintain a positive anabolic balance should be provided. Negative-pressure

TABLE 52.	Classification of Pressure Ulcers
Stage	**Description**
Suspected deep tissue injury	Purple or maroon localized area of discolored, intact skin or blood-filled blister due to damage of underlying soft tissue from pressure and/or shear. May be difficult to detect in persons with dark skin tones.
Stage I	Intact skin with nonblanchable redness of a localized area, usually over a bony prominence. Darkly pigmented skin may not have visible blanching; its color may differ from the surrounding area.
Stage II	Partial-thickness loss of dermis presenting as a shallow open ulcer with a red-pink wound bed, without slough. May also present as an intact or open/ruptured serum-filled blister.
Stage III	Full-thickness tissue loss. Subcutaneous fat may be visible but bone, tendon, or muscle is not exposed. Slough may be present but does not obscure the depth of tissue loss. May include undermining and tunneling. Depth varies by anatomic location and may be extremely deep in areas of significant adiposity.
Stage IV	Full-thickness tissue loss with exposed bone, tendon, or muscle. Slough or eschar may be present on some parts of the wound bed. Often includes undermining and tunneling.
Unstageable	Full-thickness tissue loss in which the base of the ulcer is covered by slough (yellow, tan, gray, green, or brown) and/or eschar (tan, brown, or black) in the wound bed.

Adapted with permission from National Pressure Ulcer Advisory Panel. Pressure ulcer stages revised by NPUAP. http://npuap.org/pr2.htm. Published February 2007. Accessed October 6, 2011. Copyright 2007, National Pressure Ulcer Advisory Panel.

wound therapy using a vacuum-assisted closure device has been shown to enhance patient comfort and is less labor intensive than standard therapy, but in three controlled trials, it has not been shown to improve objective measures of wound healing.

KEY POINTS

- Skin inspection should be conducted regularly in patients at high risk of pressure ulcer.
- Foam alternatives to standard mattresses and medical grade sheepskin support surfaces are effective in preventing pressure ulcers.
- Staging of existing pressure ulcers is helpful in guiding appropriate therapy.

Perioperative Medicine

General Recommendations

The preoperative risk assessment allows the internist to identify and mitigate, if possible, complications from surgery for which the patient is at higher-than-baseline risk. In addition, the preoperative risk assessment can serve an important patient safety role by aiding with medication reconciliation, noting baseline abnormalities in physical examination, and, if appropriate, outlining goals of care. Although there is no set time to perform a preoperative risk assessment, scheduling a visit 3 to 4 weeks before a proposed procedure allows time to complete a diagnostic evaluation and implement preoperative management without delaying surgery.

Internists are also consulted to assist in the postoperative care of patients; these internists may be hospitalists or other consultants who did not perform the preoperative evaluation.

However, preoperative and in-hospital management should ideally be linked through close communication, particularly in complex, high-risk patients, in whom coordination and consistency of care may lead to avoidance of unexpected problems and improved transition from inpatient to outpatient settings.

Perioperative Testing

Patients undergoing even minor surgeries are often asked to obtain a comprehensive battery of laboratory and other testing. However, results of up to 5% of tests can be abnormal given chance alone, and this prevalence is increased in older, medically ill patients who often undergo surgery. Thus, this approach uncovers a relatively high number of abnormal test results that are of no clinical significance or are falsely positive. Each abnormal test typically requires further testing, which delays surgery, adds expense, rarely influences perioperative care, and may lead to potentially dangerous and low-value care. For example, comprehensive preoperative testing has not been shown to be helpful in cataract surgery and is not endorsed by any major specialty society or payer.

Preoperative tests should be based on known or suspected comorbidities and should only be ordered when a result will alter management. For example, pregnancy testing should be conducted in women of reproductive age, cervical spine radiographs should be ordered to assess for odontoid-axial stability in patients with rheumatoid arthritis, serum creatinine and calculated glomerular filtration rate should be measured in patients with or at risk for chronic kidney disease, and serum potassium level should be obtained in patients taking diuretics. In each case, the test is performed to evaluate for evidence of a condition that can have a silent presentation or assess an important physiologic variable likely to be abnormal.

Perioperative Medication Management

The preoperative evaluation should explicitly address perioperative medication management. The internist should collect a comprehensive medication list that includes herbal and over-the-counter medications. This list is essential for both perioperative management and medication reconciliation.

Medication reconciliation, or ensuring continuity of medications from the preoperative period until full recovery, is an important component of perioperative management. Alterations in medication associated with surgery or other interventions are a source of potential medication errors but also represent an opportunity to review a patient's medication regimen for need and for appropriate dosing.

There is a relative paucity of either evidence or consensus regarding perioperative medication use. Specific recommendations exist for the management of aspirin, clopidogrel, anticoagulants, antihypertensive agents, oral hypoglycemic agents, and short-acting insulins (see individual sections and **Table 53**). For other medications, management is usually based on an individualized assessment of the need for the treatment and the potential consequences of either continuing, stopping, or adjusting the dose of the medication in the perioperative period.

Patients are routinely advised to fast on the morning of surgery. The true risk of perioperative aspiration in nonfasting patients, however, is unclear, and medications deemed necessary can be taken with a small amount of water on the day of surgery. **H**

KEY POINTS

- Preoperative imaging and laboratory tests should be ordered only when an abnormal result is suspected on the basis of known or suspected comorbidities and when such a result would alter management.

- As part of the preoperative evaluation, a list of all medications taken by the patient should be generated; those for which risk outweighs benefit during the perioperative period should be temporarily discontinued.

Cardiovascular Perioperative Management

Unexpected perioperative myocardial infarction in patients undergoing noncardiac surgery is a much feared complication, although it impacts less than 5% of patients. Searching for undiagnosed coronary artery disease (CAD) in unselected patients, therefore, is a costly and low-yield strategy that places patients at risk for delayed surgery and complications from diagnostic procedures. Prevention of perioperative myocardial infarction now emphasizes cardiac evaluation in patients at highest risk for these complications.

Although a number of risk stratification schemas have been developed, the Revised Cardiac Risk Index (RCRI) is the most widely used. This risk score was developed in 1999 based on a cohort of patients undergoing noncardiac surgery. Clinicians can quickly calculate a RCRI score based on history and easily available laboratory testing (**Table 54**, page 128). The RCRI is considered to be the best available prognostic scoring system to distinguish low- versus high-risk patients.

Recommendations from the American College of Cardiology/American Heart Association (ACC/AHA) regarding perioperative cardiovascular evaluation for noncardiac surgery are presented in **Figure 28** (page 127). Regardless of their cardiac risk, patients who need emergent surgery should not delay surgery for preoperative testing. Consultation for these patients will necessarily focus on managing postoperative complications. Conversely, patients with "active cardiac conditions" (see Figure 28) are at extremely high risk for perioperative cardiac complications. Elective surgery for these patients, including minor surgery, should be deferred until these conditions have been treated.

ACC/AHA recommendations highlight three groups of patients in whom the risk of perioperative cardiac complications is low enough that preoperative cardiac evaluation is rarely, if ever, warranted: patients undergoing low-risk surgery, those who have at least moderate exercise capacity (>4 metabolic equivalents [METs]), and those who have low exercise capacity but no RCRI risk factors. However, preoperative noninvasive cardiac testing should be considered in patients with poor or unknown exercise tolerance based on the presence and number of RCRI risk factors and the nature of the surgery, provided that the results will impact management. For patients in whom cardiac testing is pursued, exercise stress testing is preferred. In general, exercise stress tests provide additional information, specifically exercise tolerance, compared with pharmacologic stress tests. However, many patients requiring preoperative stress testing have limited exercise tolerance and thus require a pharmacologic stress test. Although both nuclear stress tests and dobutamine stress echocardiograms can predict perioperative cardiac events, data from meta-analyses suggest that dobutamine stress echocardiography is superior.

Coronary revascularization is not routinely recommended for patients with CAD before noncardiac surgery. Coronary artery bypass grafting has considerable risks (which may be more than the proposed surgery) and should be reserved for patients who already meet criteria for revascularization, including those with stable angina with high-risk lesions, such as left main or three-vessel disease. Similarly, percutaneous coronary intervention (PCI) generally is reserved for patients already meeting criteria for PCI, such as those with unstable angina, and mostly has not been shown to be helpful preoperatively in patients without such conditions. If PCI is performed preoperatively, the choice of intervention (balloon angioplasty, bare metal stent, drug-eluting stent) should take into account both the nature of the atherosclerotic lesion and urgency of the surgery, as

TABLE 53. Suggested Perioperative Medication Management

Medication Class	Recommendation	Comments
Anticoagulant	Continue for minor surgery. Discontinue before major surgery: 6 h for intravenous heparin; 12-24 h for LMWH; 3-5 d for warfarin; 1-2 d (normal kidney function), 3-5 d (creatinine clearance <50 mL/min) for dabigatran.	Bridging with heparin indicated for high-risk patients and possibly moderate-risk patients (see text, Table 57, and Table 58).
Antiplatelet	Clopidogrel: discontinue 5-7 d before surgery; patients with cardiac stent may require continuation.	Aspirin and clopidogrel use in patients with cardiac stent and/or at high risk is controversial.
	Aspirin: continue if minor surgery. Continue if indication is recent myocardial infarction (up to 6 months), cardiac stent, or high risk for coronary event; otherwise, discontinue 7-10 d before major surgery (other than CABG)	Aspirin should be started before CABG.
Cardiovascular	Continue β-blockers, calcium channel blockers, nitrates, antiarrhythmia agents. ACEIs and ARBs should be used with caution. Diuretics optional (usually withheld).	ACEIs and ARBs can promote intraoperative hypotension, especially in patients with hypovolemia; perioperative use, especially in persons with left ventricular dysfunction, is controversial.
Lipid lowering	Continue statins; hold cholestyramine.	
Pulmonary	Continue controller and rescue inhalers as well as systemic corticosteroids (if used). Probably continue leukotriene antagonists and lipoxygenase inhibitors.	
Gastrointestinal	Continue H_2 receptor blockers and proton pump inhibitors.	
Hypoglycemic agents	Oral hypoglycemic agents: discontinue 12-72 h before surgery depending upon half-life of the drug and risk of hypoglycemia.	Hypoglycemia is more dangerous than hyperglycemia; caution to always have some basal insulin in patients with type 1 diabetes.
	Short-acting insulin: hold morning of surgery; may need dose reduction preoperatively if modified diet (e.g., gastrointestinal surgery).	
	Long-acting insulin: reduce dose, typically to one-half to two-thirds of usual dose.	
Thyroid	Continue thyroid replacement, propylthiouracil, methimazole.	
Corticosteroids	Continue; increase to stress doses if indicated.	Stress-dose corticosteroids for patients taking >10 mg/d prednisone for >3 weeks.
Estrogen	Discontinue several weeks before surgery. May continue oral contraceptives and increase level of deep venous thrombosis prophylaxis.	
Psychiatric	Discontinue MAOIs 10-14 d before surgery; SSRIs and TCAs can either be continued or tapered 2-3 weeks before surgery. Continue antipsychotic medications. Can continue lithium, although some experts taper and discontinue several days before surgery.	Paucity of evidence, although most agents confer at least some theoretical risk. Risk of serotonin syndrome with some anesthetic agents. Must weigh risks of continuing vs. stopping. May wish to consult with psychiatrist.
Neurologic	Continue anticonvulsants. May continue antiparkinsonian agents, although some experts may discontinue the night before surgery. Discontinue Alzheimer drugs.	
Herbal	Discontinue up to 1 week before surgery.	
Analgesic	NSAIDs and COX-2 inhibitors are usually discontinued 7 d before surgery. Long-acting narcotics continued or dose reduced.	
Immunomodulators	Methotrexate should be continued; other agents have not been studied but are usually continued.	Paucity of data; risk of disease flare balanced against risk of adverse reaction from medication.

ACEI = angiotensin-converting enzyme inhibitor; ARB = angiotensin receptor blocker; CABG = coronary artery bypass grafting; COX-2 = cyclooxygenase-2; LMWH = low-molecular-weight heparin; MAOI = monoamine oxidase inhibitor; SSRI = selective serotonin reuptake inhibitor; TCA = tricyclic antidepressant.

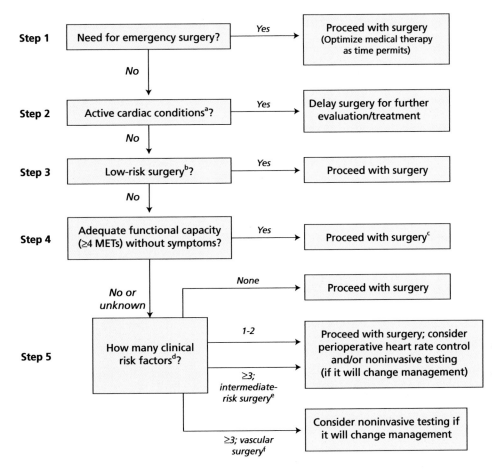

FIGURE 28. Perioperative cardiac evaluation and care for noncardiac surgery. MET = metabolic equivalent.

[a]Active cardiac conditions: unstable coronary syndromes (myocardial infarction <30 days ago, unstable or severe angina), decompensated heart failure, significant arrhythmia, severe valvular disease.

[b]Low-risk surgical procedure examples: endoscopic, superficial, breast, cataract, ambulatory.

[c]Consider noninvasive testing in patients undergoing vascular surgery with ≥1-2 risk factors if it will change management.

[d]Clinical risk factors: (1) history of heart disease, (2) history of compensated or prior heart failure, (3) history of cerebrovascular disease, (4) kidney insufficiency, (5) diabetes mellitus. Unlike the Revised Cardiac Risk Index (RCRI), the ACC/AHA guidelines do not limit diabetes to insulin-requiring to be considered a risk factor.

[e]Intermediate-risk surgery: intraperitoneal, intrathoracic, endovascular aortic aneurysm repair, carotid endarterectomy, head/neck, orthopedic, prostate.

[f]Vascular surgery: aortic or other major vascular surgery; peripheral vascular surgery.

Recommendations from Fleisher LA, Beckman JA, Brown KA, et al. 2009 ACCF/AHA focused update on perioperative beta blockade incorporated into the ACC/AHA 2007 guidelines on perioperative cardiovascular evaluation and care for noncardiac surgery: a report of the American College of Cardiology Foundation/American Heart Association Task Force on Practice Guidelines. Circulation. 2009;120(21):e180. [PMID: 19884473]

stenting requires postprocedural antiplatelet therapy that will likely delay surgery (see Hematologic Perioperative Management, below).

β-Blockers have been studied extensively in the context of perioperative care, with sometimes conflicting results. According to recommendations from the ACC/AHA, patients who are already using a β-blocker should not stop this medication preoperatively. The ACC/AHA recommends β-blocker use for patients with CAD who are undergoing vascular surgery. It also recommends β-blockers in patients undergoing intermediate or higher risk surgeries, including vascular surgeries, who have more than one RCRI risk factor. If used, β-blockers should ideally be started a few weeks before surgery at a low dose, and then titrated to control heart rate and blood pressure without hypotension or bradycardia. Although there are no recommendations on the duration of β-blocker therapy started in the perioperative period, most of these patients have other reasons to be on β-blockers and should be continued on these medications indefinitely.

Preoperative heart failure is an independent risk factor for perioperative cardiac morbidity even in the absence of CAD. In general, patients with decompensated heart failure should have surgery deferred if possible. Beyond this there are no specific consensus recommendations for the perioperative management of patients with heart failure. **H**

TABLE 54. Revised Cardiac Risk Index (RCRI)

Assign 1 point each for:

History of ischemic heart disease

Compensated or prior chronic heart failure

Diabetes mellitus requiring insulin

Chronic kidney disease (creatinine >2.0 mg/dL [176.8 µmol/L])

History of cerebrovascular disease

Higher risk surgery (intrathoracic, intraperitoneal, supra-inguinal vascular)

Risk by RCRI Score[a]

Number of Points	Risk
0	0.4%
1	1.0%
2	2.4%
≥3	5.4%

[a]Risk of perioperative cardiac death, nonfatal myocardial infarction, or nonfatal cardiac arrest.

Adapted from Devereaux PJ, Goldman L, Cook DJ, Gilbert K, Leslie K, Guyatt GH. Perioperative cardiac events in patients undergoing noncardiac surgery: a review of the magnitude of the problem, the pathophysiology of the events and methods to estimate and communicate risk. CMAJ. 2005;173(6):627-634. [PMID: 16157727]

TABLE 55. Risk factors for Perioperative Pulmonary Complications

Patient-Related	Surgery-Related
Major	**Major**
Older age	Intrathoracic, intra-abdominal surgeries
COPD	
Chronic heart failure	Surgeries lasting >3 hours
Poor general health status and/or functional dependence	Emergency surgery
Smoking	
Low serum albumin level	
Kidney dysfunction	
Minor or Possible	**Minor or Possible**
Obesity	General anesthesia
Sleep apnea	

KEY POINTS

- Preoperative cardiac stress testing should be reserved for patients with reduced exercise tolerance and multiple cardiovascular risk factors.

- In patients not already on a β-blocker, perioperative β-blocker use is recommended only for those with coronary artery disease who are undergoing vascular surgery and for those undergoing other intermediate or higher risk surgery who have more than one cardiac risk factor.

Pulmonary Perioperative Management

Perioperative pulmonary complications, including prolonged and unexpected intubation, occur after 3% to 13% of surgical procedures. Many risk factors are associated with perioperative pulmonary complications (**Table 55**). Patients with COPD are two to five times more likely to experience such complications, and patients with more severe COPD are likely at higher risk.

The type of surgery is an extremely important predictor of perioperative pulmonary complications. The highest-risk surgeries are thoracic surgeries, abdominal aortic aneurysm repairs, and abdominal surgeries, especially open procedures near the diaphragm. General anesthesia may slightly increase the risk of pulmonary complications compared with spinal anesthesia. However, the added risk is small and not apparent in every study, and the risk of pulmonary complications should not drive the selection of type of anesthesia. There is no correlation between FEV_1 or FVC and perioperative pulmonary complications. Therefore, preoperative spirometry should be reserved for patients with unexplained dyspnea.

Few interventions have been shown to reduce the risk of perioperative pulmonary complications. Pre- and postoperative lung volume expansion, either via deep breathing or incentive spirometry, reduces the risk for pulmonary complications. In patients with poorly controlled asthma, systemic corticosteroids can be used perioperatively. Patients with suboptimally controlled COPD should be treated aggressively with inhaled bronchodilators and probably systemic corticosteroids. Patients should have adequate pain control postoperatively to minimize atelectasis. Smoking is clearly associated with postoperative complications, including both pulmonary and nonpulmonary complications. However, there is mixed evidence regarding the benefit of smoking cessation less than 2 months before surgery, with some studies suggesting recent quitters may have higher rates of perioperative pulmonary complications. Smoking cessation at least 8 weeks before surgery, however, is clearly beneficial. In patients at highest risk for perioperative pulmonary complications, the internist, surgeon, and anesthesiologist should collaborate closely to assess the risk/benefit ratio for surgery and consider alternative surgical or nonsurgical interventions for the patient.

Obstructive sleep apnea (OSA) is associated with difficult intubation and an increased risk of postoperative apnea. The importance of OSA in the perioperative period may be underappreciated, in part because of the high prevalence of undiagnosed OSA in the community. The STOP-BANG questionnaire, a series of eight yes-or-no questions, is an easy-to-use screening tool for OSA (**Table 56**). Three or more positive responses have a sensitivity of 92% and specificity of 63% for predicting perioperative pulmonary complications. In patients with known or suspected OSA, this information should be made known to the anesthesiologist preoperatively and the patient monitored closely postoperatively, possibly with extended observation in an intensive care or step-down unit. These patients may also require continuous or bilevel positive airway pressure. ▣

KEY POINTS

- Preoperative spirometry should be reserved for patients with unexplained dyspnea.
- Pre- and postoperative lung volume expansion, either via deep breathing or incentive spirometry, reduces the risk for pulmonary complications.
- Obstructive sleep apnea (OSA) is associated with perioperative pulmonary complications, and preoperative screening for OSA is warranted because of the high prevalence of undiagnosed OSA in the community and its potential for causing perioperative pulmonary complications.

Hematologic Perioperative Management

Venous Thromboembolism Prophylaxis

Perioperative venous thromboembolism (VTE) is a major preventable surgical complication. The risk of VTE is related to clinical risk factors and proposed surgery (**Table 57**). Preoperative evaluation should focus on assessing for clinical risk factors.

Early ambulation is often sufficient postoperative prophylaxis in patients with a low risk of VTE. In patients with a high risk of bleeding or for whom postoperative bleeding could be catastrophic (for example, neurosurgery patients), postoperative mechanical prophylaxis with pneumatic compression devices can be used alone; elastic graduated compression stockings are not recommended owing to lack of clear efficacy and risk for lower extremity skin damage. For the remainder of patients, drug prophylaxis for VTE with low-molecular-weight heparin (LMWH), fondaparinux, subcutaneous unfractionated heparin (UFH), or warfarin should be provided unless the assessed risk of bleeding outweighs the likely benefits (see MKSAP 16 Hematology and Oncology). Prophylactic anticoagulants should be withheld until the risk of postoperative bleeding is low, at least 12 hours after surgery. In general, prophylaxis should be continued until discharge. Patients with orthopedic surgeries, abdominal or gynecologic surgery for malignancy, or previous VTE should receive prophylaxis for up to 5 weeks after surgery.

Inferior vena cava (IVC) filters have been used for VTE prophylaxis in selected patients at high risk of VTE, especially those who have had a VTE within 1 to 3 months before surgery and for whom anticoagulants will be contraindicated postoperatively. Removable IVC filters are reasonable for these patients. There is no evidence supporting the use of prophylactic IVC filters in other populations, including patients undergoing bariatric surgery, and their routine use is discouraged.

Perioperative Management of Warfarin Therapy

Depending on the patient's thrombotic risk and the type of procedure, perioperative management options for patients using warfarin are to stop the warfarin during the perioperative period, stop the warfarin and bridge with a parenteral anticoagulant, or continue the warfarin throughout the perioperative period. Patients undergoing procedures considered low risk for bleeding, including cataract surgery, dental procedures, and biopsy of nonmajor organs, should continue warfarin during the perioperative period, with a target INR of 1.3 to 1.5 at the time of surgery. In patients using warfarin who are undergoing other surgeries, management of anticoagulant therapy is guided by the patient's risk of perioperative thrombosis (**Table 58**). Patients at low risk for thrombosis should usually discontinue warfarin 4 to 5 days preoperatively without bridging therapy. In patients at intermediate or high risk for perioperative thrombosis, warfarin also should be discontinued 4 to 5 days preoperatively; intermediate-risk patients should be considered for bridging,

---

TABLE 56.	STOP-BANG Screening Tool for Obstructive Sleep Apnea
Parameter	**Question**
Snoring	Do you snore loudly (louder than talking or loud enough to be heard through closed doors)?
Tired	Do you often feel tired, fatigued, or sleepy during daytime?
Observed	Has anyone observed you stop breathing during your sleep?
Blood pressure	Do you have or are you being treated for high blood pressure?
BMI	BMI more than 35?
Age	Age over 50 years?
Neck circumference	Neck circumference greater than 40 cm?
Gender	Gender male?

Scoring: High risk of obstructive sleep apnea: answering *yes* to three or more items; low risk of OSA: answering *yes* to less than three items.

Adapted with permission from Chung F, Yegneswaran B, Liao P, et al. STOP questionnaire: a tool to screen patients for obstructive sleep apnea. Anesthesiology. 2008;108(5):812-821. [PMID: 18431116] Copyright 2008, Lippincott Williams & Wilkins.

TABLE 57. Surgical Risk Stratification and Associated VTE Incidence

Patient Risk	Risk Factor Stratification	VTE Incidence Without Prophylaxis
Low	Minor surgery in patients younger than 40 years with no additional risk factors[a]	Calf vein DVT: 2% Proximal vein DVT: 0.4% Clinical PE: 0.2% Fatal PE: 0.002%
Moderate	Nonmajor surgery in patients aged 40-60 years with no clinical risk factors Minor surgery lasting <30 min in patients with clinical risk factors Major surgery in patients younger than 40 years with no clinical risk factors	Calf vein DVT: 10%-20% Proximal DVT: 2%-4% Clinical PE: 1%-2% Fatal PE: 0.1%-0.4%
High	Nonmajor surgery in patients older than 60 years or with clinical risk factors Major surgery in patients older than 40 years or with clinical risk factors	Calf vein DVT: 20%-40% Proximal DVT: 4%-8% Clinical PE: 2%-4% Fatal PE: 0.4%-1%
Very high	Major surgery in patients older than 40 years with history of VTE, cancer, or certain hypercoagulable states Hip or knee arthroplasty Hip fracture surgery Major trauma Spinal cord injury	Calf vein DVT: 40%-80% Proximal DVT: 10%-20% Clinical PE: 4%-10% Fatal PE: 0.2%-5%

DVT = deep venous thrombosis; PE = pulmonary embolism; VTE = venous thromboembolism.

[a]Potential risk factors include heart failure, nephrotic syndrome, pregnancy, estrogen use, use of general anesthesia, acute respiratory failure, active cancer, stroke with paresis, history of VTE, acute infectious illness, age >60 years, thrombophilia, acute rheumatic disease, inflammatory bowel disease, obesity, trauma, institutionalization, and immobility.

Adapted from PIER. Venous thromboembolism prophylaxis in the surgical patient. http://pier.acponline.org/physicians/diseases/periopr830/periopr830.html. Accessed 8 December 2011.

and high-risk patients should be bridged with either LMWH at therapeutic doses or UFH. Bridging should be started 1 to 2 days after the last dose of warfarin. For patients at intermediate thrombotic risk, LMWH at prophylactic doses is an option, especially for patients with intermediate risk of thrombosis. The decision of which agent to use and at what dosage should be based on patient-specific risks and benefits.

Bridging therapy with LMWH should be stopped 24 hours preoperatively and UFH 4 to 6 hours preoperatively. Patients with an intermediate thrombotic risk who are receiving LMWH for bridging can be given a half dose for the last injection before surgery to minimize the risk of intraoperative bleeding. LMWH or UFH can be resumed as early as 12 to 24 hours after surgery, although the exact timing should depend on the patient's indication for anticoagulation and bleeding risk. Patients at intermediate risk for thrombosis can restart LMWH at prophylactic doses; those at high risk should be treated at therapeutic doses. Warfarin should be restarted once the patient is at low risk for bleeding, and bridging therapy is stopped once the INR is therapeutic.

Perioperative Management of Antiplatelet Medications, Coagulopathies, and Thrombocytopenia

Patients undergoing surgeries with low risk for bleeding can continue aspirin and/or clopidogrel therapy. Patients receiving antiplatelet therapy for recent myocardial infarction or cardiac stent placement should not have this therapy interrupted for 6 weeks for a bare metal stent or myocardial infarction or for 1 year for a drug-eluting stent. Low-risk surgery can usually be performed while the patient is on antiplatelet therapy, whereas most other surgeries should be delayed if possible. Antiplatelet therapy is usually avoided in patients undergoing neurosurgery or other surgeries in which the sequelae of postoperative hemorrhage could be catastrophic. Conversely, aspirin therapy is recommended before coronary artery bypass grafting (CABG), although other antiplatelet agents should be discontinued before elective CABG. There is little evidence or consensus regarding antiplatelet therapy in other instances, and decisions regarding clinical care should be based on a patient's individualized risks and benefits. Aspirin therapy may be safe in patients undergoing other surgeries, although it is often stopped 7 to 10 days before

TABLE 58. Perioperative Bridging Strategies for Patients Using Warfarin

Risk	Conditions	Bridging Strategy
Low	VTE >12 months ago and no additional risk factors	Discontinue warfarin; no bridging
	Atrial fibrillation with CHADS$_2$ score ≤2 without prior CVA	
Intermediate	VTE within 3-12 months or history of recurrent VTE	Discontinue warfarin; consider bridging with LMWH (therapeutic or prophylactic dose) or UFH based on assessment of individual patient and surgery-related factors
	Active malignancy (treated within 6 months or palliatively)	
	Known hypercoagulable state	
	Atrial fibrillation with CHADS$_2$ score of 3 or 4 without prior CVA	
	Newer mechanical heart valve in nonmitral position	
High	VTE <3 months ago or VTE with thrombophilia	Discontinue warfarin; bridge with LMWH (therapeutic dose) or UFH
	CVA <6 months ago	
	Atrial fibrillation with CHADS$_2$ score >4 or prior CVA	
	Mechanical heart valve in mitral position or older aortic prosthesis	

CVA = cerebrovascular accident; LMWH = low-molecular-weight heparin; UFH = unfractionated heparin; VTE = venous thromboembolism.

elective surgery. Antiplatelet therapy is usually restarted 24 hours after surgery unless there is evidence of or elevated risk for postoperative bleeding.

All patients should be carefully screened preoperatively for signs or symptoms of underlying bleeding disorders and anemia. Laboratory testing should be reserved for patients in whom there is a reasonable probability of an abnormal test, and is not required as a routine component of preoperative evaluation. A complete blood count, and possibly coagulation studies, can be obtained in patients undergoing surgery with a high risk for significant bleeding as well as in patients with known or suspected hepatic dysfunction. A preoperative pro-thrombin time may also be reasonable in Ashkenazi Jews, approximately 3% of whom have low factor XI levels from a hereditary deficiency.

In patients with known quantitative platelet deficiencies, the platelet count should be increased to above 50,000/μL (50 × 10^9/L) before elective surgery, if possible. Patients with immune thrombocytopenic purpura should receive corticosteroids, intravenous immune globulin, or Rho(D) immune globulin preoperatively. Patients with thrombotic thrombocytopenic purpura (TTP) should receive plasmapheresis. Platelet transfusion is unlikely to be helpful in patients with TTP; however, other patients with persistent thrombocytopenia are typically transfused with platelets just before surgery. Patients with qualitative platelet dysfunction (for example, from kidney or liver disease) can be given desmopressin acetate 1 hour preoperatively for lower-risk procedures for bleeding. Patients undergoing higher-risk procedures should receive a platelet transfusion. Hematology consultation is often helpful in the perioperative management of these patients.

Perioperative Management of Anemia

Patients with a preoperative hemoglobin concentration below 6 g/dL (60 g/L) or a postoperative hemoglobin concentration below 7 g/dL (70 g/L) have worse outcomes than those with higher hemoglobin levels. Patients with either known anemia or anemia discovered as part of the preoperative evaluation should be evaluated for an underlying cause. Patients who require iron, vitamin B$_{12}$, or folic acid supplements should receive these therapies perioperatively. Patients with anemia of kidney disease or other anemias that are potentially responsive to exogenous erythropoietin should be treated preoperatively only if blood losses are expected to be large and transfusion is contraindicated.

Transfusion is reserved for patients with symptomatic anemia, a preoperative hemoglobin concentration below 6 g/dL (60 g/L), postoperative hemoglobin concentration below 7 g/dL (70 g/L), or patients with symptomatic cardiovascular disease and hemoglobin concentrations between 6 and 10 g/dL (60 and 100 g/L). Transfusing asymptomatic patients with known CAD to achieve a hemoglobin level of greater than 10 g/dL (100 g/L) is frequently done, although the data supporting this practice remain controversial. Patients with sickle cell disease are at high risk for perioperative sickle cell crisis, which can be reduced by reducing the percentage of sickle-cell variant erythrocytes in total blood volume. Consultation with an experienced hematologist is advisable to determine the extent of transfusion needed for these patients.

- Patients on chronic warfarin undergoing low-risk procedures, including cataract surgery, dental procedures, and biopsy of nonmajor organs, can continue warfarin, with a target INR of 1.3 to 1.5 perioperatively.

- Patients on chronic warfarin undergoing intermediate- or high-risk procedures should discontinue warfarin 4 to 5 days before surgery; patients with a low thrombotic risk typically do not require bridging anticoagulant therapy, whereas those with an intermediate or high thrombotic risk should receive heparin bridging therapy perioperatively.

- Aspirin and/or clopidogrel should be continued in patients undergoing low-risk surgery and in patients with recent cardiac stent placement or myocardial infarction; in most other patients, antiplatelet therapy can be safely discontinued 7 to 10 days preoperatively.

Perioperative Management of Endocrine Diseases

Diabetes Mellitus

Patients with diabetes mellitus are at higher risk for perioperative complications, although many of these are related to end-organ damage from the diabetes rather than hypo- or hyperglycemia. Patients with type 1 diabetes mellitus will need to have some insulin continued at all times to prevent the development of diabetic ketoacidosis; this warning should be emphasized in preoperative consultations and in communications with the surgeon and anesthesiologist.

Hyperglycemia increases the risk of infectious and other postoperative complications. Hemoglobin A_{1c} and kidney function should be measured preoperatively in patients with diabetes if these have not been measured recently. Patients found to have poorly controlled diabetes should usually have elective surgeries delayed until their glycemic control is improved, ideally to a fasting plasma glucose level below 220 mg/dL (12.21 mmol/L).

Diabetes medications require adjustment on the morning of surgery. Metformin is usually discontinued at least the night before surgery; other oral hypoglycemic medications should be withheld on the morning of surgery. In general, short-acting insulins should be withheld the morning of surgery. Long-acting insulins are usually dose adjusted, although the exact amount depends on the patient's baseline control and regimen. Typically one-half to two-thirds of the usual dose of long-acting insulin is given in the 12 hours before surgery, with a lesser reduction in patients who are poorly controlled at baseline or who are taking corticosteroids or other agents expected to raise glucose levels. Given the complexities of preoperative medication adjustment, a patient's plasma glucose level should be measured the morning of surgery, and insulin or dextrose may be needed to keep the patient euglycemic.

Oral agents are challenging to use perioperatively because of risk of hypoglycemia given their long half-lives and variable oral intake in the postoperative patient. In addition, metformin confers a risk of lactic acidosis while thiazolidinediones promote fluid retention. Thus, many patients with diabetes, even those who have previously been well controlled with diet or oral medications, may need insulin during the perioperative period. Intensive insulin therapy (IIT) using continuous insulin infusions has been extensively investigated in the postoperative setting with mixed results. Current evidence does not support IIT as part of routine postoperative care. Approaches to glycemic management in hospitalized patients are discussed in MKSAP 16 Endocrinology and Metabolism.

Thyroid Disease

Patients with thyroid disease who have not had recent thyroid function testing and those in whom thyroid disease is suspected should have thyroid function tested preoperatively. Hyperthyroidism can predispose patients to perioperative complications, including atrial fibrillation, cardiomyopathy, respiratory failure, and thrombocytopenia. These risks are highest in patients undergoing thyroid surgery. Patients with hyperthyroidism should be made euthyroid prior to surgery, typically with antithyroid drugs. In patients whose surgery cannot be delayed, β-blockers, iodine, and corticosteroids can be added, although the risks of these medications should be balanced by the degree of thyroid dysfunction and nature of the surgery. In contrast, for patients with hypothyroidism, surgery should be delayed only for severe hypothyroidism; mild or subclinical hypothyroidism does not significantly increase the risk of perioperative complications.

Adrenal Insufficiency

The incidence of acute adrenal insufficiency is relatively low in the perioperative period, even in patients treated with chronic corticosteroids. Patients using chronic low-dose corticosteroids (prednisone ≤10 mg/d), short-term corticosteroids, or inhaled corticosteroids have a low risk for adrenal crisis and do not need preoperative testing or treatment. Patients who chronically use higher doses of corticosteroids (>10 mg/d prednisone for at least 3 weeks) or who have known adrenal insufficiency should take their usual daily dose on the day of surgery. These patients should be well hydrated and can receive supplemental hydrocortisone on the day of surgery, with low doses (for example, 25 mg) for minor surgery and higher doses (up to 150 mg) for major surgery. These doses should be

CONT.
tapered rapidly back to baseline over the first 2 postoperative days unless signs or symptoms of adrenal crisis develop. Adrenocorticotropic hormone stimulation testing should be reserved for patients in whom primary adrenal insufficiency is suspected or in whom empiric supplemental corticosteroids could be harmful. H

KEY POINTS

- Many patients with diabetes mellitus, even those who have previously been well controlled with diet or oral medications, need insulin during the perioperative period.
- For patients with hypothyroidism, surgery should be delayed only for severe hypothyroidism; mild or subclinical hypothyroidism does not significantly increase the risk of perioperative complications.

Perioperative Management of Kidney Disease

Patients with chronic kidney disease (CKD) have a higher incidence of perioperative complications than those without, although many of these complications are attributable to cardiovascular disease. Preoperative evaluation of patients with CKD should include laboratory testing to assess the stage of kidney disease. Patients with significant anemia may benefit from preoperative exogenous erythropoietin if more than minimal blood loss is expected as these patients are unable to physiologically respond to acute blood loss. ACE inhibitors and angiotensin receptor blockers, commonly used in patients with CKD, can cause intraoperative hypotension and may be withheld on the day of surgery.

No agents have been shown to be protective against intraoperative acute kidney injury. In general, patients with CKD should be adequately hydrated perioperatively with anesthetic and other agents selected specifically to avoid hypotension. Intraoperative urine output is not a good predictor of postoperative acute kidney injury, and fluid intake should not be titrated to urine output.

Postoperatively, patients with CKD are at risk for volume overload, electrolyte imbalance, and acute kidney injury. NSAIDs and other nephrotoxic agents should be avoided. Care should be taken that all medications are adjusted for the patient's glomerular filtration rate. Patients with uremia are at risk for platelet dysfunction and postoperative bleeding. In patients on dialysis, the timing of dialysis perioperatively should be coordinated between anesthesiologist, surgeon, and nephrologist. H

KEY POINT

- In patients with chronic kidney disease, care should be taken that all medications are adjusted for the patient's glomerular filtration rate.

Perioperative Management of Liver Disease

Both acute hepatitis and chronic liver disease with cirrhosis are associated with an elevated risk of perioperative complications and death. Surgery can worsen liver disease because of hepatic ischemia and hepatic hypoxemia. The half-life of many medications, including sedatives, opioids, and anesthetic agents, may be prolonged in patients with hepatic dysfunction, causing further hypoxia and hypotension. Poor liver function predisposes to hepatic failure, bleeding, poor wound healing, and infections. The internist should be alert for signs and symptoms of hepatic dysfunction, especially in patients who have risk factors for liver disease. Patients whose history and physical examination suggest ongoing liver disease should receive preoperative liver chemistry tests.

Elective surgery should be deferred to evaluate newly diagnosed liver disease and postponed in patients with acute hepatitis from any cause. Patients with chronic liver disease without evidence of cirrhosis appear to be at no excess perioperative risk. Patients with hemochromatosis should be carefully evaluated for cardiomyopathy. In patients being treated for hepatitis B, the danger of temporary cessation of antiretroviral therapy causing a disease flare should be emphasized to the surgeon.

In patients with chronic liver disease with evidence of cirrhosis, surgical risk is based on both the extent of liver disease and the type of surgery. The Child-Turcotte-Pugh (CTP) score has been used to assess risk: patients with CTP class A liver disease have a 10% risk of death after general surgery; those with class B disease have a 30% risk; and those with class C disease have a 75% to 80% risk. The Model for End-stage Liver Disease (MELD) score, American Society of Anesthesia (ASA) risk score, and patient age are all independent predictors of mortality. These variables have been linked into a single calculator that can be used to estimate postoperative mortality risk (www.mayoclinic.org/meld/mayomodel9.html).

Intraabdominal surgeries, especially hepatic surgery and gallbladder surgery, are high risk in patients with cirrhotic liver disease associated with portal hypertension. The combination of coagulopathy and internal varices makes these surgeries technically challenging. Estimating operative risk in biliary surgery is especially difficult as the jaundice in these patients is multifactorial, confounding the risk prediction models. Coronary artery bypass grafting is also higher risk in patients with cirrhotic liver disease. Herniorrhaphy, in contrast, is average risk.

Preoperative management of cirrhotic liver disease involves optimizing liver function. Patients with coagulopathy are typically treated with oral vitamin K to reverse any nutritional deficiencies. Vitamin K, however, does not typically normalize these patients' coagulopathy, and they may need fresh frozen plasma, cryoprecipitate, or activated factor VIIa. Ascites predisposes to perioperative pulmonary complications, poor wound healing of abdominal surgeries, and excess death. Ascites should primarily be managed with diuretics, as large-volume paracentesis is effective only for a short period of time. Placement of a transjugular intrahepatic portosystemic shunt (TIPS) may be indicated preoperatively in patients with refractory ascites. TIPS may also be appropriate for patients with known esophageal varices undergoing major surgery.

Perioperative management should focus on preventing complications of chronic liver disease. Blood pressure and volume status should be carefully monitored to minimize a renal insult that could precipitate a hepatorenal syndrome. Sedatives and narcotics that are hepatically metabolized should be dosed carefully. Patients with ileus or other causes of slowed intestinal transit should be observed closely for signs of hepatic encephalopathy. If encephalopathy develops, the patient should receive lactulose orally or, if on NPO status (nothing by mouth), via retention enema. Patients with advanced liver disease are at risk for hypoglycemia postoperatively because of impaired gluconeogenesis.

KEY POINT

- Patients with examination findings suggesting ongoing liver disease should receive preoperative liver chemistry tests; elective surgery should be deferred to evaluate newly diagnosed liver disease.

Perioperative Management of Neurologic Disease

Patients with neurologic diseases present specific challenges in the perioperative period. Patients with neuromuscular diseases, including amyotrophic lateral sclerosis, muscular dystrophy, and myasthenia gravis, are at high risk for respiratory failure. Preoperative pulmonary function testing is sometimes done in these patients, although there are no specific risk prediction models for respiratory failure. Close consultation among surgeon, anesthesiologist, internist, and neurologist is essential in safely managing patients with neuromuscular diseases.

Patients with a seizure disorder should have their therapy optimized preoperatively, and anticonvulsant drug levels should be therapeutic. Patients should continue the anticonvulsant drugs through the morning of surgery. The presence of a seizure disorder will usually influence an anesthesiologist's choice of agents. Postoperatively, patients with a seizure disorder may require parenteral medication.

Patients with multiple sclerosis may experience an acute exacerbation after anesthesia. Interferon is typically continued for these patients perioperatively, while baclofen, which is only available orally, may need to be transitioned to a benzodiazepine to prevent postoperative withdrawal seizures.

Patients with Parkinson disease should continue antiparkinsonian agents through the morning of surgery.

Perioperative management of patients who use short-acting dopamine agonists is challenging, as abrupt withdrawal of these agents can produce severe muscle rigidity that can interfere with ventilation and mimic neuroleptic malignant syndrome. Patients with Parkinson disease are also at risk for aspiration secondary to hypersalivation and poor respiratory mechanics.

Perioperative stroke impacts 0.3% to 0.8% of postsurgical patients and is further discussed in MKSAP 16 Neurology. Risk factors for delirium in the postoperative setting are similar to those in medically hospitalized patients and include pain, immobilization, anemia, hypoxemia, and sedative and opioid use. Early consultation by an internist or geriatrician for patients at risk for postoperative delirium may be helpful. Delirium is further discussed in MKSAP 16 Pulmonary and Critical Care Medicine.

Bibliography

Interpretation of the Medical Literature

Guyatt G, Rennie D, Meade MO, Cook DJ, eds. Users' Guides to the Medical Literature: A Manual for Evidence-Based Clinical Practice. 2nd ed. New York, NY: McGraw-Hill; 2008.

Ho PM, Peterson PN, Masoudi FA. Evaluating the evidence: is there a rigid hierarchy? Circulation. 2008;118(16):1675-1684. [PMID: 18852378]

Lin KW, Slawson DC. Identifying and using good practice guidelines. Am Fam Physician. 2009;80(1):67-70. [PMID: 19621847]

Sox HC, Greenfield S. Comparative effectiveness research: a report from the Institute of Medicine. Ann Intern Med. 2009;151(3):203-205. [PMID: 19567618]

Routine Care of the Healthy Patient

2008 PHS Guideline Update Panel, Liasons, and Staff. Treating tobacco use and dependence: 2008 update U.S. Public Health Service Clinical Practice Guideline executive summary. Respir Care. 2008;53(9):1217-1222. [PMID: 18807274]

Berg AO, Baird MA, Botkin JR, et al. National Institutes of Health State-of-the-Science Conference Statement: Family History and Improving Health. Ann Intern Med. 2009;151(12):872-877. [PMID: 19884615]

Fiore MC, Baker TB. Clinical practice. Treating smokers in the health care setting. N Engl J Med. 2011;365(13):1222-1231. [PMID: 21991895]

Heshka JT, Palleschi C, Howley H, Wilson B, Wells PS. A systematic review of perceived risks, psychological and behavioral impacts of genetic testing. Genet Med. 2008;10(1):19-32. [PMID: 18197053]

Kahn JA. HPV vaccination for the prevention of cervical intraepithelial neoplasia. New Engl J Med. 2009;361(3):271-278. [PMID: 19605832]

Lambert LC, Fauci AS. Influenza vaccines for the future. New Engl J Med. 2010;363(21):2036-2044. [PMID: 21083388]

Lin JS, O'Connor E, Whitlock EP, Beil TL. Behavioral counseling to promote physical activity and a healthful diet to prevent cardiovascular disease in adults: a systematic review for the U.S. Preventive Services Task Force. Ann Intern Med. 2010;153(11):736-750. [PMID: 21135297]

Long EF, Brandeau ML, Owens DK. The cost-effectiveness and population outcomes of expanded HIV screening and antiretroviral treatment in the United States. Ann Intern Med. 2010;153(12):778-789. [PMID: 21173412]

Porter ME. What is value in health care? N Engl J Med. 2010;363(26):2477-2481. [PMID: 21142528]

Powers BJ, Olsen MK, Smith VA, Woolson RF, Bosworth HB, Oddone EZ. Measuring blood pressure for decision making and quality reporting: where and how many measures? Ann Intern Med. 2011;154(12):781-788. [PMID: 21690592]

Rollnick S, Butler CC, Kinnersley P, Gregory J, Mash B. Motivational interviewing. BMJ. 2010;340:c1900. [PMID: 20423957]

Saitz R, Alford DP, Bernstein J, Cheng DM, Samet J, Palfai T. Screening and brief intervention for unhealthy drug use in primary care settings: randomized clinical trials are needed. J Addict Med. 2010;4(3):123-130. [PMID: 20936079]

Schousboe J, Kerlikowski K, Loh A, Cummings SR. Personalizing mammography by breast density and other risk factors for breast cancer: analysis of health benefits and cost-effectiveness. Ann Intern Med. 2011;155(1):10-20. [PMID: 21727289]

Smith PC, Schmidt SM, Allensworth-Davies D, Saitz R. A single-question screening test for drug use in primary care. Arch Intern Med. 2010;170(13):1155-1159. [PMID: 20625025]

Thompson SG, Ashton HA, Gao L, Scott RA; Multicentre Aneurysm Screening Study Group. Screening men for abdominal aortic aneurysm: 10 year mortality and cost effectiveness results from the randomised Multicentre Aneurysm Screening Study. BMJ. 2009;338:b2307. [PMID: 19553269]

U.S. Preventive Services Task Force. Behavioral counseling to prevent sexually transmitted infections: U.S. Preventative Services Task Force recommendation statement. Ann Intern Med. 2008;149(7):491-496, W95. [PMID: 18838729]

Zolotor AJ, Denham AC, Weil A. Intimate partner violence. Prim Care. 2009;36(1):167-179, x. [PMID: 19231608]

Patient Safety

Chassin MR, Loeb JM, Schmaltz SP, Wachter RM. Accountability measures—using measurement to promote quality improvement. N Engl J Med. 2010;363(7):683-688. [PMID: 20573915]

Schiff GD, Bates DW. Can electronic clinical documentation help prevent diagnostic errors? N Engl J Med. 2010;362(12):1066-1069. [PMID: 20335582]

Swensen, SJ, Meyer GS, Nelson EC, et al. Cottage industry to postindustrial care—the revolution in health care delivery. N Engl J Med. 2010;362(5):e12. [PMID: 20089956]

Professionalism and Ethics

Braddock CH 3rd, Edwards KA, Hasenberg NM, Laidley TL, Levinson W. Informed decision making in outpatient practice: time to get back to basics. JAMA. 1999;282(24):2313-2320. [PMID: 10612318]

Castillo LS, Williams BA, Hooper SM, Sabatino CP, Weithorn LA, Sudore RL. Lost in translation: the unintended consequences of advance directive law on clinical care. Ann Intern Med. 2011;154(2):121-128. [PMID: 21242368]

DesRoches CM, Rao SR, Fromson JA, et al. Physicians' perceptions, preparedness for reporting, and experiences related to impaired and incompetent colleagues. JAMA. 2010;304(2):187-193. [PMID: 20628132]

Gallagher TH, Studdert D, Levinson W. Disclosing harmful medical errors to patients. N Engl J Med. 2007;356(26):2713-2719. [PMID: 17596606]

Localio AR. Patient compensation without litigation: a promising development. Ann Intern Med. 2010;153(4):266-267. [PMID: 20713794]

Owens DK, Qaseem A, Chou R, Shekelle P; Clinical Guidelines Committee of the American College of Physicians. High-value, cost-conscious health care: concepts for clinicians to evaluate the benefits, harms, and costs of medical interventions. Ann Intern Med. 2011;154(3):174-180. [PMID: 21282697]

Quill T, Arnold RM. Evaluating requests for hastened death #156. J Palliat Med. 2008;11(8):1151-1152. [PMID: 18980457]

Snyder L; American College of Physicians Ethics, Professionalism, and Human Rights Committee. American College of Physicians Ethics Manual: sixth edition. Ann Intern Med. 2012;156(1 Pt 2):73-104. [PMID: 22213573]

Palliative Care

Bakitas M, Lyons KD, Hegel MT, et al. Effects of a palliative care intervention on clinical outcomes in patients with advanced cancer: the Project ENABLE II randomized controlled trial. JAMA. 2009;302(7):741-749. [PMID: 19690306]

Lorenz KA, Lynn J, Dy SM, et al. Evidence for improving palliative care at the end of life: a systematic review. Ann Intern Med. 2008;148(2):147-159. [PMID: 18195339]

Morrison RS, Penrod JD, Cassel JB, et al. Cost savings associated with US hospital palliative care consultation programs. Arch Intern Med. 2008;168(16):1783-1790. [PMID: 18779466]

Reville B, Axelrod D, Maury R. Palliative care for the cancer patient. Prim Care. 2009;36(4):781-810. [PMID: 19913186]

Swetz KM, Kamal AH. Palliative care. Ann Intern Med. 2012;156(3):ITC21. [PMID: 22312158]

Temel JS, Greer JA, Muzikansky, et al. Early palliative care for patients with metastatic non-small-cell lung cancer. N Engl J Med. 2010;363(8):733-742. [PMID: 20818875]

Common Symptoms

American Geriatrics Society Panel on the Pharmacologic Management of Persistent Pain in Older persons. Pharmacologic management of persistent pain in older persons. J Am Geriatr Soc. 2009;57(8):1331-1346. [PMID: 19573219]

Anderson JL, Adams CD, Antman EM, et al; American College of Cardiology; American Heart Association Task Force on Practice Guidelines (Writing Committee to Revise the 2002 Guidelines for the Management of Patients With Unstable Angina/Non-ST-Elevation Myocardial Infarction); American College of Emergency Physicians; Society for Cardiovascular Angiography and Interventions; Society of Thoracic Surgeons; American Association of Cardiovascular and Pulmonary Rehabilitation; Society for Academic Emergency Medicine. ACC/AHA 2007 guidelines for the management of patients with unstable angina/non-ST-Elevation myocardial infarction: a report of the American College of Cardiology/American Heart Association Task Force on Practice Guidelines (Writing Committee to Revise the 2002 Guidelines for the Management of Patients With Unstable Angina/Non-ST-Elevation Myocardial Infarction) developed in collaboration with the American College of Emergency Physicians, the Society for Cardiovascular Angiography and Interventions, and the Society of Thoracic Surgeons endorsed by the American Association of Cardiovascular and Pulmonary Rehabilitation and the Society for Academic Emergency Medicine. J Am Coll Cardiol. 2007;50(7):e1-e157. [PMID: 17692738]

Bittner ML, Marcus DA, Tenzer P, Romito K. Using Opioids in the Management of Chronic Pain Patients: Challenges and Future Options. American Academy of Family Physicians. 2010.

Bohnert AS, Valenstein M, Bair MJ, et al. Association between opioid prescribing patterns and opioid overdose-related deaths. JAMA. 2011;305(13):1315-1321. [PMID: 21467284]

Cooper PN, Westby M, Pitcher DW, Bullock I. Synopsis of the National Institute for Health and Clinical Excellence Guideline for management of transient loss of consciousness. Ann Intern Med. 2011;155(8):543-549. [PMID: 21930835]

Dunn KM, Saunders KW, Rutter CM, et al. Opioid prescriptions for chronic pain and overdose: a cohort study. Ann Intern Med. 2010;152(2):85-92. [PMID: 20083827]

Eccleston C, Williams AC, Morley S. Psychological therapies for the management of chronic pain (excluding headache) in adults. Cochrane Database Syst Rev. 2009;(2):CD007407. [PMID: 19370688]

Fife TD, Iverson DJ, Lempert T, et al; Quality Standards Subcommittee, American Academy of Neurology. Practice parameter: therapies for benign paroxysmal positional vertigo (an evidence based review): report of the Quality Standards Subcommittee of the American

Academy of Neurology. Neurology. 2008;70(22):2067-2074. [PMID: 18505980]

Gilron I, Bailey JM, Tu D, Holden RR, Jackson AC, Houlden RL. Nortriptyline and gabapentin, alone and in combination for neuropathic pain: a double-blind, randomised controlled crossover trial. Lancet. 2009;374(9697):1252-1261. [PMID: 19796802]

Gonzales R, Bartlett JG, Besser RE, et al; American Academy of Family Physicians; American College of Physicians-American Society of Internal Medicine; Centers for Disease Control; Infectious Diseases Society of America. Principles of appropriate antibiotic use for treatment of uncomplicated acute bronchitis: background. Ann Intern Med. 2001;134(6):521-529. [PMID: 11255532]

Hess EP, Dipti A, Chandra S, et al. Diagnostic accuracy of the TIMI risk score in patients with chest pain the emergency department: a meta-analysis. CMAJ. 2010;182(10):1039-1044. [PMID: 20530163]

Hotson JR, Baloh RW. Acute vestibular syndrome. N Engl J Med. 1998;339(10):680-685. [PMID: 9725927]

Irwin RS, Baumann MH, Bolser DC, et al; American College of Chest Physicians (ACCP). Diagnosis and management of cough executive summary: ACCP evidence-based clinical practice guidelines. Chest. 2006;129(1 suppl):1S-23S. [PMID: 16428686]

Moore RA, Straube S, Wiffen PJ, Derry S, McQuay HJ. Pregabalin for acute and chronic pain in adults. Cochrane Database Syst Rev. 2009;(3):CD007076. [PMID: 19588419]

Moya A, Sutton R, Ammirati F, et al; Task Force for the Diagnosis and Management of Syncope; European Society of Cardiology (ESC); European Heart Rhythm Association (EHRA); Heart Failure Association (HFA); Heart Rhythm Society (HRS). Guidelines for the diagnosis and management of syncope (version 2009). Eur Heart J. 2009;30(21):2631-2671. [PMID: 19713422]

Nijrolder I, van der Horst H, van der Windt D. Prognosis of fatigue: a systematic review. J Psychosom Res. 2008;64(4):335-349. [PMID: 18374732]

Ouyang H, Quinn J. Diagnosis and evaluation of syncope in the emergency department. Emerg Med Clin North Am. 2010;28(3):471-485. [PMID: 20709239]

Parry SW, Tan MP. An approach to the evaluation and management of syncope in adults. BMJ. 2010;340:c880. [PMID: 20172928]

Schroeder K, Fahey T. Over-the-counter medications for acute cough in children and adults in ambulatory settings. Cochrane Database Syst Rev. 2004;(4):CD001831. [PMID: 15495019]

Schutte-Rodin S, Broch L, Buysse D, Dorsey C, Sateia M. Clinical guideline for the evaluation and management of chronic insomnia in adults. J Clin Sleep Med. 2008;4(5):487-504. [PMID: 18853708]

Sloane PD, Coeytaux RR, Beck RS, Dallara J. Dizziness: state of the science. Ann Intern Med. 2001;134(9 Pt 2):823-832. [PMID: 11346317]

Swap CJ, Nagurney JT. Value and limitations of chest pain history in the evaluation of patients with suspected acute coronary syndromes. JAMA. 2005;294(20):2623-2629. [PMID: 16304077]

Wilson JF. In the clinic. Insomnia. Ann Intern Med. 2008;148(1):ITC13-1-ITC13-16. [PMID: 18166757]

Musculoskeletal Pain

Chou R, Qaseem A, Snow V, et al; Clinical Efficacy Assessment Subcommittee of the American College of Physicians; American College of Physicians; American Pain Society Low Back Pain Guidelines Panel. Diagnosis and treatment of low back pain: a joint clinical practice guideline from the American College of Physicians and the American Pain Society. Ann Intern Med. 2007;147(7):478-491. [PMID: 17909209]

Chou R, Shekelle P. Will this patient develop persistent disabling low back pain? JAMA. 2010;303(13):1295-1302. [PMID: 20371789]

Coombes BK, Bisset L, Vicenzino B. Efficacy and safety of corticosteroid injections and other injections for management of tendinopathy: a systematic review of randomised controlled trials. Lancet. 2010;376(9754):1751-1767. [PMID: 20970844]

Gaujoux-Viala C, Dougados M, Gossec L. Efficacy and safety of steroid injections for shoulder and elbow tendonitis: a meta-analysis of randomised controlled trials. Ann Rheum Dis. 2009;68(12):1843-1849. [PMID: 19054817]

Jarvik JG, Comstock BA, Kliot M, et al. Surgery versus non-surgical therapy for carpal tunnel syndrome: a randomised parallel-group trial. Lancet. 2009;374(9695):1074-1081. [PMID: 19782873]

Kuijper B, Tans JTJ, Beelen A, Nollet F, de Visser M. Cervical collar or physiotherapy versus wait and see policy for recent onset cervical radiculopathy: randomised trial. BMJ. 2009;339:b3883. [PMID: 19812130]

Nikolaidis I, Fouyas IP, Sandercock PA, Statham PF. Surgery for cervical radiculopathy or myelopathy. Cochrane Database Syst Rev. 2010;(1):CD001466. [PMID: 20091520]

Ottenheijm RP, Jansen MJ, Staal JB, et al. Accuracy of diagnostic ultrasound in patients with suspected subacromial disorders: a systematic review and meta-analysis. Arch Phys Med Rehabil. 2010;91(10):1616-1625. [PMID: 20875523]

Seida JC, LeBlanc C, Schouten JR, et al. Systematic review: nonoperative and operative treatments for rotator cuff tears. Ann Intern Med. 2010;153(4):246-255. [PMID: 20621893]

Young C. In the clinic. Plantar fasciitis. Ann Intern Med. 2012;156(1 Pt 1):ITC1-1-ITC1-16. [PMID: 22213510]

Dyslipidemia

Ginsberg HN, Elam MB, Lovato MC, et al; ACCORD Study Group. Effects of combination lipid therapy in type 2 diabetes mellitus. N Engl J Med. 2010;362(17):1563-1574. [PMID: 20228404]

Blaha MJ, Bansal S, Rouf R, Golden SH, Blumenthal RS, Defilippis AP. A practical "ABCDE" approach to the metabolic syndrome. Mayo Clin Proc. 2008;83(8):932-941. [PMID: 18674478]

Calderon RM, Cubeddu LX, Goldberg RB, Schiff ER. Statins in the treatment of dyslipidemia in the presence of elevated liver aminotransferase levels: a therapeutic dilemma. Mayo Clin Proc. 2010;85(4):349-356. [PMID: 20360293]

Egan A, Colman E. Weighing the benefits of high-dose simvastatin against the risk of myopathy. N Engl J Med. 2011;365(4):285-287. [PMID: 21675881]

Hayward RA, Krumholz HM, Zulman DM, Timbie JW, Vijan S. Optimizing statin treatment for primary prevention of coronary artery disease. Ann Intern Med. 2010;152(2):69-77. [PMID: 20083825]

Joy TR, Hegele RA. Narrative review: statin-related myopathy. Ann Intern Med. 2009;150(12):858-868. [PMID: 19528564]

Kromhout D, Giltay EJ, Geleijnse JM; Alpha Omega Trial Group. n-3 fatty acids and cardiovascular events after myocardial infarction. N Engl J Med. 2010;363(21):2015-2026. [PMID: 20929341]

Mottillo S, Filion KB, Genest J, et al. The metabolic syndrome and cardiovascular risk a systematic review and meta-analysis. J Am Coll Cardiol. 2010;56(14):1113-1132. [PMID: 20863953]

Ray KK, Seshasai SRK, Erqou S, et al. Statins and all-cause mortality in high-risk primary prevention: a meta-analysis of 11 randomized controlled trials involving 65,229 participants. Arch Intern Med. 2010;170(12):1024-1031. [PMID: 20585067]

Taylor AJ, Villines TC, Stanek EJ, et al. Extended-release niacin or ezetimibe and carotid intima-media thickness. N Engl J Med. 2009;361(22):2113-2122. [PMID: 19915217]

Tota-Maharaj R, Defilippis AP, Blumenthal RS, Blaha MJ. A practical approach to the metabolic syndrome: review of current concepts and management. Curr Opin Cardiol. 2010;25(5):502-512. [PMID: 20644468]

Obesity

Adams TD, Gress RE, Smith SC, et al. Long-term mortality after gastric bypass surgery. N Engl J Med. 2007;357(8):753-761. [PMID: 17715409]

Foster GD, Wyatt HR, Hill JO, et al. Weight and metabolic outcomes after 2 years on a low-carbohydrate versus low-fat diet: a randomized trial. Ann Intern Med. 2010;153(3):147-157. [PMID: 20679559]

Lang IA, Llewellyn DJ, Alexander K, Melzer D. Obesity, physical function, and mortality in older adults. J Am Geriatr Soc. 2008;56:1474-1478. [PMID: 18662211]

Leblanc ES, O'Connor E, Whitlock EP, Patnode CD, Kapka T. Effectiveness of primary care-relevant treatments for obesity in adults: a systematic evidence review for the U.S. Preventive Services Task Force. Ann Intern Med. 2011;155(7):434-477. [PMID: 21969342]

Li Z, Maglione M, Tu W, et al. Meta-analysis: pharmacologic treatment of obesity. Ann Intern Med. 2005;142(7):532-546. [PMID: 15809465]

Maciejewski ML, Livingston EH, Smith VA, et al. Survival among high-risk patients after bariatric surgery. JAMA. 2011;305(23):2419-2526. [PMID: 21666276]

Maggard MA, Shugarman LR, Suttorp M, et al. Meta-analysis: surgical treatment of obesity. Ann Intern Med. 2005;142(7):547-559. [PMID: 15809466]

Silk AW, McTigue KM. Reexamining the physical examination for obese patients. JAMA. 2011;305(2):193-194. [PMID: 21191004]

Men's Health

Greco KA, McVary KT. The role of combination medical therapy in benign prostatic hyperplasia. Int J Impot Res. 2008;20(suppl 3):S33-S43. [PMID: 19002123]

Gupta BP, Murad MH, Clifton MM, Prokop L, Nehra A, Kopecky SL. The effect of lifestyle modification and cardiovascular risk factor reduction on erectile dysfunction: a systematic review and meta-analysis. Arch Intern Med. 2011;171(20):1797-1803. [PMID: 21911624]

Qaseem A, Snow V, Denberg TD, et al; Clinical Efficacy Assessment Subcommittee of the American College of Physicians. Hormonal testing and pharmacologic treatment of erectile dysfunction: a clinical practice guideline from the American College of Physicians. Ann Intern Med. 2009;151(9):639-649. [PMID: 19884625]

Rosen RC, Cappelleri JC, Smith MD, et al. Development and evaluation of an abridged, 5-item version of the International Index of Erectile Function (IIEF-5) as a diagnostic tool for erectile dysfunction. Int J Impot Res. 1999;11(6):319-326. [PMID: 10637462]

Shah NR, Mikami DJ, Cook C, et al. A comparison of outcomes between open and laparoscopic surgical repair of recurrent inguinal hernias. Surg Endosc. 2011;25(7):2330-2337. [PMID: 21298523]

Touma NJ, Nickel JC. Prostatitis and chronic pelvic pain in men. Med Clin North Am. 2011;95(1):75-86. [PMID: 21095412]

Traish AM, Miner MM, Morgentaler A, Zitzmann M. Testosterone deficiency. Am J Med. 2011;124(7):578-587. [PMID: 21683825]

Tsertsvadze A, Fink HA, Yazdi F, et al. Oral phosphodiesterase-5 inhibitors and hormonal treatments for erectile dysfunction: a systematic review and meta-analysis. Ann Intern Med. 2009;151(9):650-661. [PMID: 19884626]

Wampler SM, Llanes M. Common scrotal and testicular problems. Prim Care. 2010;37(3):613-626. [PMID: 20705202]

Women's Health

Amy JJ, Tripathi V. Contraception for women: an evidence based overview. BMJ. 2009;339:b2895. [PMID: 19666684]

Berghella V, Buchanan E, Pereira L, Baxter JK. Preconception care. Obstet Gynecol Surv. 2010;65(2):119-131. [PMID: 20100361]

Casablanca Y. Management of dysfunctional uterine bleeding. Obstet Gynecol Clin North Am. 2008;35(2):219-234. [PMID: 18486838]

Chlebowski RT, Andersonn GL, Gass M, et al; WHI Investigators. Estrogen plus progestin and breast cancer incidence and mortality in postmenopausal women. JAMA. 2010;304(15):1684-1692. [PMID: 20959578]

Harel Z. Dysmenorrhea in adolescents and young adults: from pathophysiology to pharmacological treatments and management strategies. Expert Opin on Pharmacother. 2008;9(15):2661-2672. [PMID: 18803452]

Kingsberg S, Althof SE. Evaluation and treatment of female sexual disorders. Int Urogynecol J Pelvic Floor Dysfunct. 2009;(20)(suppl 1):S33-S43. [PMID: 19440781]

Lanston A. Emergency contraception: update and review. Semin Reprod Med. 2010;28(2):95-102. [PMID: 20352558]

Martin KA, Manson JE. Approach to the patient with menopausal symptoms. J Clin Endocrinol Metab. 2008;93(12):4567-4575. [PMID: 19056840]

Nappi RE, Martini E, Terreno E, et al. Management of hypoactive sexual desire disorder in women: current and emerging therapies. Int J Womens Health. 2010;2:167-175. [PMID: 21072309]

Rossouw JE, Prentice RL, Manson JE, et al. Postmenopausal hormone therapy and risk for cardiovascular disease by age and years since menopause. JAMA. 2007;297(13):1465-1477. [PMID: 17405972]

Rungruang B, Kelley JL 3rd. Benign breast diseases: epidemiology, evaluation, and management. Clin Obstet Gynecol. 2011;54(1):110-124. [PMID: 21278510]

Santen RJ, Mansel R. Benign breast disorders. N Engl J Med. 2005;353(3):275-285. [PMID: 16034013]

Vercellini P, Somigliana E, Viganò P, Abbiati A, Barbara G, Fedele L. Chronic pelvic pain in women: etiology, pathogenesis, and diagnostic approach. Gynecol Endocrinol. 2009;25(3):149-158. [PMID: 19347704]

Wilson, JF. In the clinic. Vaginitis and cervicitis. Ann Intern Med. 2009;151(5):ITC3-1-ITC3-15; Quiz ITC3-16. [PMID: 19721016]

Eye Disorders

Ahmed R, Foroozan R. Transient monocular visual loss. Neurol Clin. 2010;28(3):619-629. [PMID: 20637992]

Arroyo JG. A 76-year-old man with macular degeneration. JAMA. 2006;295(20):2394-2406. [PMID: 16720825]

Asbell PA, Dualan I, Mindel J, Brocks D, Ahmad M, Epstein S. Age-related cataract. Lancet. 2005;365(9459):599-609. [PMID: 15708105]

Cronau H, Kankanala RR, Mauger T. Diagnosis and management of red eye in primary care. Am Fam Physician. 2010;81(2):137-144. [PMID: 20082509]

Hollands H, Johnson D, Brox AC, Almeida D, Simel DL, Sharma S. Acute-onset floaters and flashes: is this patient at risk for retinal detachment? JAMA. 2009;302(20):2243-2249. [PMID: 19934426]

Magauran B. Conditions requiring emergency ophthalmologic consultation. Emerg Med Clin North Am. 2008;26(1):233-238, viii. [PMID: 18249265]

Weinreb RN, Khaw PT. Primary open-angle glaucoma. Lancet. 2004;363(9422):1711-1720. [PMID: 15158634]

Ear, Nose, Mouth, and Throat Disorders

Calderon MA, Alves B, Jacobson M, Hurwitz B, Sheikh A, Durham S. Allergen injection immunotherapy for seasonal allergic rhinitis. Cochrane Database Syst Rev. 2007;(1):CD001936. [PMID: 17253469]

Chow AW, Benninger MS, Brook I, et al. IDSA clinical practice guideline for acute bacterial rhinosinusitis in children and adults. Clin Infect Dis. 2012;54(8):e72-e112. [PMID: 22438350]

Coco A, Vernacchio L, Horst M, Anderson A. Management of acute otitis media after publication of the 2004 AAP and AAFP clinical practice guideline. Pediatrics. 2010;125(2):214-220. [PMID: 20100746]

Douglass AB, Gonsalves W, Maier R, et al. Smiles for Life: A National Oral Health Curriculum for Family Medicine. A model for curriculum development by STFM groups. Fam Med. 2007;39(2):88-90. [PMID: 17273948]

Friedewald VE, Kornman KS, Beck JD, et al; American Journal of Cardiology; Journal of Periodontology. The American Journal of Cardiology and Journal of Periodontology Editors' Consensus: periodontitis and atherosclerotic cardiovascular disease. Am J Cardiol. 2009;104(1):59-68. [PMID: 19576322]

Hobson J, Chisholm E, El Refaie A. Sound therapy (masking) in the management of tinnitus in adults. Cochrane Database Syst Rev. 2010;(12):CD006371. [PMID: 21154366]

Osguthorpe DJ, Nielsen DR. Otitis externa: Review and clinical update. Am Fam Physician. 2006;74(9):1510-1516. [PMID: 17111889]

Powers JH. Diagnosis and treatment of acute otitis media: evaluating the evidence. Infect Dis Clin North Am. 2007;21(2):409-426, vi. [PMID: 17561076]

Roland PS, Smith TL, Schwartz SR, et al. Clinical practice guideline: Cerumen impaction. Otolayngol Head Neck Surg. 2008;139(3)(suppl 2):S1-S21. [PMID: 18707628]

Schlosser RJ. Clinical practice. Epistaxis. N Engl J Med. 2009;360(8):784-789. [PMID: 19228621]

Schreiber BE, Agrup C, Haskard DO, Luxon LM. Sudden sensorineural hearing loss. Lancet. 2010;375(9721):1203-1211. [PMID: 20362815]

Scrivani SJ, Keith DA, Kaban LB. Temporomandibular disorders. N Engl J Med. 2008;359(25):2693-2705. [PMID: 19092154]

Stachler RJ, Chandrasekhar SS, Archer SM, et al; American Academy of Otolaryngology-Head and Neck Surgery. Clinical practice guideline: sudden hearing loss. Otolaryngol Head Neck Surg. 2012;146(3 suppl):S1-35. [PMID: 22383545]

Young J, De Sutter A, Merenstein D, et al. Antibiotics for adults with clinically diagnosed acute rhinosinusitis: a meta-analysis of individual patient data. Lancet. 2008;371(9616):908-914. [PMID: 18342685]

Anorectal Disorders

Schubert MC, Sridhar S, Schade RR, Wexner SD. What every gastroenterologist needs to know about common anorectal disorders. World J Gastroenterol. 2009;15(26):3201-3209. [PMID: 19598294]

Mental and Behavioral Health

American Psychiatric Association Work Group on Eating Disorders. Practice guideline for the treatment of patients with eating disorders (revision). Am J Psychiatry. 2000;157(1 suppl):1-39. [PMID: 10642782]

Belmaker RH. Treatment of bipolar depression. N Engl J Med. 2007;356(17):1771-1773. [PMID: 17392296]

Brugha TS, McManus S, Bankart J, et al. Epidemiology of autism spectrum disorders in adults in the community in England. Arch Gen Psychiatry. 2011;68(5):459-465. [PMID: 21536975]

Bulik CM, Berkman ND, Brownley KA, Sedway JA, Lohr KN. Anorexia nervosa treatment: a systematic review of randomized controlled trials. Int J Eat Disord. 2007;40(4):310-320. [PMID: 17370290]

Fancher TL, Kravitz RL. In the clinic. Depression. Ann Intern Med. 2010;152(9):ITC51-15; quiz ITC5-16. [PMID: 20439571]

Franklin ME, Foa EB. Treatment of obsessive compulsive disorder. Annu Rev Clin Psychol. 2011;7:229-243. [PMID: 21443448]

Gammicchia C, Johnson C. Autism Information for Paramedics and Emergency Room Staff. Autism Society. Available at www.autism-society.org/about-us/publications/resource-materials.html. Accessed July 9, 2012.

Gartlehner G, Hansen RA, Morgan LC, et al. Comparative benefits and harms of second-generation antidepressants for treating major depressive disorder: an updated meta-analysis. Ann Intern Med. 2011;155(11):772-785. [PMID: 22147715]

Gartlehner G, Hansen RA, Morgan LC, et al. Second-Generation Antidepressants in the Pharmacologic Treatment of Adult Depression: An Update of the 2007 Comparative Effectiveness Review [Internet]. Rockville (MD): Agency for Healthcare Research and Quality (US); 2011 Dec. (Comparative Effectiveness Reviews, No. 46.) Peer Reviewers. Available at www.effectivehealthcare.ahrq.gov/index.cfm/search-for-guides-reviews-and-reports/?pageaction=displayproduct&productid=862. Accessed July 9, 2012.

Jones RM, Arlidge J, Gillham R, Reagu S, van den Bree M, Taylor PJ. Efficacy of mood stabilisers in the treatment of impulsive or repetitive aggression: systematic review and meta-analysis. Br J Psychiatry. 2011;198(2):93-98. [PMID: 21282779]

Kroenke K, Spitzer RL, Williams JB, Monahan PO, Löwe B. Anxiety disorders in primary care: prevalence, impairment, comorbidity, and detection. Ann Intern Med. 2007;146(5):317-325. [PMID: 17339617]

Kroenke K. Unburdening the difficult clinical encounter. Arch Intern Med. 2009;169(4):333-334. [PMID: 19237715]

Schultz SH, North SW, Shields CG. Schizophrenia: a review. Am Fam Physician. 2007;75(12):1821-1829. [PMID: 17619525]

Sim LA, McAlpine DE, Grothe KB, Himes SM, Cockerill RG, Clark MM. Identification and treatment of eating disorders in the primary care setting. Mayo Clin Proc. 2010;85(8):746-751. [PMID: 20605951]

Stein MB, Goin MK, Pollack MH, et al. Practice guideline for the treatment of patients with panic disorder. Arlington, VA: American Psychiatric Association, 2009.

Wilens TE, Faraone SV, Biederman J. Attention-deficit/hyperactivity disorder in adults. JAMA. 2004;292(5):619-623. [PMID: 15292088]

Geriatric Medicine

Budnitz DS, Lovegrove MC, Shehab N, Richards CL. Emergency hospitalizations for adverse drug events in older Americans. N Engl J Med. 2011;365:2002-2012. [PMID: 22111719]

Burgio KL, Kraus SR, Menefee S, et al; Urinary Incontinence Treatment Network. Behavioral therapy to enable women with urge incontinence to discontinue drug treatment: a randomized trial. Ann Intern Med. 2008;149(3):161-169. [PMID: 18678843]

Carr DB, Ott BR. The older adult driver with cognitive impairment: "It's a very frustrating life". JAMA. 2010;303(16):1632-1641. [Erratum in: JAMA. 2010;303(23):2357]. [PMID: 20424254]

Fong TG, Jones RN, Rudolph JL, et al. Development and validation of a brief cognitive assessment tool: the sweet 16. Arch Intern Med. 2011;171(5):432-427. [PMID: 21059967]

Garfinkel D, Mangin D. Feasibility study of a systematic approach for discontinuation of multiple medications in older adults: addressing polypharmacy. Arch Intern Med. 2010;170(18):1648-1654. [PMID: 20937924]

Gillespie LD, Robertson MC, Gillespie WJ, et al. Interventions for preventing falls in older people living in the community. Cochrane Database Syst Rev. 2009;(2):CD007146. [PMID: 19370674]

Hayes BD, Klein-Schwartz W, Barrueto F. Polypharmacy and the geriatric patient. Clin Geriatr Med. 2007;23:371-390. [PMID: 17462523]

Kalyani RR, Stein B, Valiyil R, Manno R, Maynard JW, Crews DC. Vitamin D treatment for the prevention of falls in older adults: systematic review and meta-analysis. J Am Geriatr Soc. 2010;58(7):1299-1310. [PMID: 20579169]

Kane RL. Finding the right level of posthospital care: "We didn't realize there was any other option for him". JAMA. 2011;305(3):284-293. [PMID: 21245184]

Kinsella GJ, Mullaly E, Rand E, et al. Early intervention for mild cognitive impairment: a randomised controlled trial. J Neurol Neurosurg Psychiatry. 2009;80(7):730-736. [PMID: 19332424]

Li C, Friedman B, Conwell Y, Fiscella K. Validity of the Patient Health Questionnaire 2 (PHQ-2) in identifying major depression in older people. J Am Geriatr Soc. 2007;55(4):596-602. [PMID: 17397440]

McInnes E, Dumville JC, Jammali-Blasi A, Bell-Syer SE. Support surfaces for treating pressure ulcers. Cochrane Database Syst Rev. 2011;(12):CD009490. [PMID: 22161450]

McInnes E, Jammali-Blasi A, Bell-Syer SE, Dumville JC, Cullum N. Support surfaces for pressure ulcer prevention. Cochrane Database Syst Rev. 2011;(4):CD001735. [PMID: 21491384]

Panel on Prevention of Falls in Older Persons; American Geriatrics Society and British Geriatrics Society. Summary of the Updated American Geriatrics Society/British Geriatrics Society clinical practice guideline for prevention of falls in older persons. J Am Geriatr Soc. 2011;59(1):148-157. [PMID: 21226685]

Plassman BL, Langa KM, Fisher GG, et al. Prevalence of cognitive impairment without dementia in the United States. Ann Intern Med. 2008;148(6):427-434. [PMID: 18347351]

Reddy M, Gill SS, Kalkar SR, Wu W, Anderson PJ, Rochon PA. Treatment of pressure ulcers: a systematic review. JAMA. 2008;300(22):2647-2662. [PMID: 19066385]

Shamliyan T, Wyman JF, Ramakrishnan R, Sainfort F, Kane RL. Systematic Review: Benefits and Harms of Pharmacologic Treatment for Urinary Incontinence in Women. Ann Intern Med. 2012 Apr 9 [Epub ahead of print] [PMID: 22492633]

Studenski S, Perera S, Patel K, et al. Gait speed and survival in older adults. JAMA. 2011:305(1):50-58. [PMID: 21205966]

Wyman JF, Croghan CF, Nachreiner NM, et al. Effectiveness of education and individualized counseling in reducing environmental hazards in the homes of community-dwelling older women. J Am Geriatr Soc. 2007;55(10):1548-1556. [PMID: 17908058]

Perioperative Medicine

Carson JL, Grossman BJ, Kleinman S, et al; for the Clinical Transfusion Medicine Committee of the AABB. Red Blood Cell Transfusion: A Clinical Practice Guideline From the AABB*. Ann Intern Med. 2012;157(1):49-58. [PMID: 22751760]

Douketis JD, Berger PB, Dunn AS, et al; American College of Chest Physicians. The perioperative management of antithrombotic therapy: American College of Chest Physicians Evidence-Based Clinical Practice Guidelines (8th Edition). Chest. 2008;133(6 suppl):299S-339S. [PMID: 18574269]

Douketis JD, Spyropoulos AC, Spencer FA, et al; American College of Chest Physicians. Perioperative management of antithrombotic therapy: Antithrombotic Therapy and Prevention of Thrombosis, 9th ed: American College of Chest Physicians Evidence-Based Clinical Practice Guidelines. Chest. 2012;141(2 suppl):e326S-e350S. [PMID: 22315266]

Eilers H, Liu KD, Gruber A, Niemann CU. Chronic kidney disease: implications for the perioperative period. Minerva Anestesiol. 2010;76(9):725-736. [PMID: 20820151]

Ford MK, Beattie WS, Wijeysundera DN. Systematic review: prediction of perioperative cardiac complications and mortality by the revised cardiac risk index. Ann Intern Med. 2010;152(1):26-35. [PMID: 20048269]

Hepner DL. The role of testing in the preoperative evaluation. Cleve Clin J Med. 2009;76(suppl 4):S22-S27. [PMID: 19880831]

Lieb K, Selim M. Preoperative evaluation of patients with neurological disease. Semin Neurol. 2008;28(5):603-610. [PMID: 19115168]

Lipshutz AK, Gropper MA. Perioperative glycemic control: an evidence-based review. Anesthesiology. 2009;110(2):408-421. [PMID: 19194167]

Marik PE, Varon J. Requirement of perioperative stress doses of corticosteroids: a systematic review of the literature. Arch Surg. 2008;143(12):1222-1226. [PMID: 19075176]

O'Leary JG, Yachimski PS, Friedman LS. Surgery in the patient with liver disease. Clin Liver Dis. 2009;13(2):211-231. [PMID: 19442915]

Patel MS, Carson JL. Anemia in the preoperative patient. Med Clin North Am. 2009;93(5):1095-1104. [PMID: 19665622]

Qaseem A, Humphrey LL, Chou R, Snow V, Shekelle P; Clinical Guidelines Committee of the American College of Physicians. Use of intensive insulin therapy for the management of glycemic control in hospitalized patients: a clinical practice guideline from the American College of Physicians. Ann Intern Med. 2011;154(4):260-267. [PMID: 21320941]

Smetana GW, Lawrence VA, Cornell JE; American College of Physicians. Preoperative pulmonary risk stratification for noncardiothoracic surgery: systematic review for the American College of Physicians. Ann Intern Med. 2006;144(8):581-595. [PMID: 16618956]

Vasu TS, Doghramji K, Cavallazzi R, et al. Obstructive sleep apnea syndrome and postoperative complications: clinical use of the STOP-BANG questionnaire. Arch Otolaryngol Head Neck Surg. 2010;136(10):1020-1024. [PMID: 20956751]

General Internal Medicine Self-Assessment Test

This self-assessment test contains one-best-answer multiple-choice questions. Please read these directions carefully before answering the questions. Answers, critiques, and bibliographies immediately follow these multiple-choice questions. The American College of Physicians is accredited by the Accreditation Council for Continuing Medical Education (ACCME) to provide continuing medical education for physicians.

The American College of Physicians designates MKSAP 16 General Internal Medicine for a maximum of 24 *AMA PRA Category 1 Credits*™. Physicians should claim only the credit commensurate with the extent of their participation in the activity.

Earn "Same-Day" CME Credits Online

For the first time, print subscribers can enter their answers online to earn CME credits in 24 hours or less. You can submit your answers using online answer sheets that are provided at mksap.acponline.org, where a record of your MKSAP 16 credits will be available. To earn CME credits, you need to answer all of the questions in a test and earn a score of at least 50% correct (number of correct answers divided by the total number of questions). Take any of the following approaches:

> ➢ Use the printed answer sheet at the back of this book to record your answers. Go to mksap.acponline.org, access the appropriate online answer sheet, transcribe your answers, and submit your test for same-day CME credits. There is no additional fee for this service.

> ➢ Go to mksap.acponline.org, access the appropriate online answer sheet, directly enter your answers, and submit your test for same-day CME credits. There is no additional fee for this service.

> ➢ Pay a $10 processing fee per answer sheet and submit the printed answer sheet at the back of this book by mail or fax, as instructed on the answer sheet. Make sure you calculate your score and fax the answer sheet to 215-351-2799 or mail the answer sheet to Member and Customer Service, American College of Physicians, 190 N. Independence Mall West, Philadelphia, PA 19106-1572, using the courtesy envelope provided in your MKSAP 16 slipcase. You will need your 10-digit order number and 8-digit ACP ID number, which are printed on your packing slip. Please allow 4 to 6 weeks for your score report to be emailed back to you. Be sure to include your email address for a response.

If you do not have a 10-digit order number and 8-digit ACP ID number or if you need help creating a username and password to access the MKSAP 16 online answer sheets, go to mksap.acponline.org or email custserv@acponline.org.

CME credit is available from the publication date of December 31, 2012, until December 31, 2015. You may submit your answer sheets at any time during this period.

Directions

*Each of the numbered items is followed by lettered answers. Select the **ONE** lettered answer that is **BEST** in each case.*

Item 1

A 32-year-old man is evaluated during a routine examination. He is in good health, has no concerning symptoms, and takes no medications. He does not smoke, seldom drinks alcohol, and exercises 30 minutes daily 5 days per week. He ingests a heart-healthy diet. All of his immunizations are up to date. The patient has no symptoms or health problems.

Which of the following is the most reasonable next screening step for genetic disease in this patient?

(A) Obtain a family history of disease
(B) Obtain a three-generation pedigree
(C) Refer for genetic counseling
(D) Screen for common genetic mutations

Item 2

A 58-year-old woman is evaluated for a 7-week history of tingling pain involving the first, second, and third digits of the left hand. The pain is worse at night and radiates into the thenar eminence. The pain does not radiate into the proximal forearm. She has hypothyroidism and her only current medication is levothyroxine.

On physical examination, the patient reports pain with plantar flexion at the wrist with the elbow extended. She also reports pain with percussion over the median nerve at the level of the wrist. There is no thenar or hypothenar eminence atrophy. Strength is 5/5 with thumb opposition. A hand diagram is completed (shown) demonstrating the location of the patient's paresthesia.

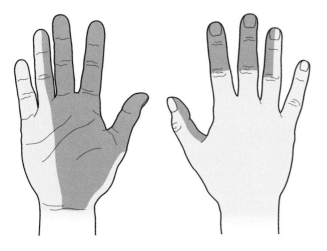

In addition to avoidance of repetitive wrist motions, which of the following is the most appropriate initial treatment?

(A) Local corticosteroid injection
(B) Oral ibuprofen
(C) Surgical intervention
(D) Wrist splinting

Item 3

A 40-year-old woman is evaluated for having difficulty at work. She is a nurse, and over the past 6 months she has become very zealous about avoiding infection. She washes her hands six or seven times before entering patients' rooms and then again afterwards. She is having difficulty completing tasks on time. She showers multiple times daily and has scrubbed her skin raw in several areas. She recognizes that these actions are unreasonable but she no control over them. She has no history of psychiatric disease, bipolar disorder, or schizophrenia.

On physical examination, vital signs are normal. Both hands are raw and there are several areas of denuded skin on her arms and legs.

In addition to cognitive-behavioral therapy, which of the following is the most appropriate pharmacologic treatment?

(A) Fluoxetine
(B) Haloperidol
(C) Lorazepam
(D) Quetiapine

Item 4

A 24-year-old man is evaluated for a 2-hour history of epistaxis, which began after blowing his nose. The bleeding is controlled by placing pressure on the anterior portion of the nose for 3 minutes but then recurs. The bleeding is from the left nostril only. He has severe seasonal rhinitis that has been active recently. He has no history of bleeding, bruising, or clotting, and there is no family history of bleeding disorders. Current medications are loratadine and an intranasal corticosteroid.

On physical examination, he is afebrile, blood pressure is 138/88 mm Hg, and pulse rate is 82/min. Blood pressure and pulse are without significant change from supine to standing positions. He is holding a tissue against his nose. Examination of the left naris with a nasal speculum after the removal of dried blood reveals a small oozing vessel in the septum in the Kiesselbach area. The right naris is clear of blood, and a skin examination demonstrates no petechiae or bruises.

Which of the following is the most appropriate management of this patient?

(A) Arterial embolization
(B) Cauterization and nasal packing
(C) Complete blood count and coagulation studies
(D) Uninterrupted nasal pressure for 15 to 30 minutes
(E) Urgent otorhinolaryngology evaluation

Item 5

A 54-year-old woman is evaluated during a routine examination. She is very concerned by her lack of interest in sexual intercourse. The patient feels like she "just doesn't want to be touched." She used to enjoy intercourse and does not know why she feels this way now, but she acknowledges that it is causing tremendous stress in her marriage. She has been menopausal for the past 2 years. She uses lubrication for intercourse, which is successful in reducing discomfort. She has no previous history of menstrual irregularities, pelvic surgeries, sexual trauma, or sexually transmitted infections. She currently takes calcium and vitamin D supplements daily.

On physical examination, external genitalia are normal, with no pain with vulvar palpation or with speculum insertion. The vaginal walls are pale with decreased rugae and petechial hemorrhages. Decreased vaginal lubrication is noted. The remainder of the physical examination is normal.

Which of the following is the most likely diagnosis?

(A) Dyspareunia
(B) Hypoactive sexual desire disorder
(C) Sexual aversion disorder
(D) Vaginismus

Item 6

An 88-year-old man in hospice care is evaluated for dyspnea. He has advanced dementia, severe COPD, and coronary artery disease. Based on prior discussions with his family regarding the goals of care, it was decided that his treatment should consist of comfort care measures only. All of his medications except as-needed albuterol and ipratropium have been discontinued.

On physical examination, he is afebrile, blood pressure is 108/76 mm Hg, pulse rate is 110/min, and respiration rate is 26/min. Oxygen saturation is satisfactory. He is cachectic and tachypneic and is disoriented and in moderate respiratory distress. Heart sounds are distant and tachycardic but an S_3 is not present. Chest examination reveals decreased breath sounds as well as diffuse, fine inspiratory crackles consistent with prior examinations. Extremities are warm and dry.

In addition to continuing his bronchodilator therapy, which of the following is the most appropriate next step in the treatment of this patient?

(A) Ceftriaxone and azithromycin
(B) Lorazepam
(C) Methylprednisolone
(D) Morphine

Item 7

A 55-year-old woman is evaluated for fatigue for the past 9 months. She used to be an avid runner, but now can only walk 1 mile before experiencing severe muscle aches, joint pain and fatigue for the next several days. She reports no insomnia but describes her 8 hours of nightly sleep as unrefreshing. She does not smoke, drink, or use illicit drugs. She describes tender lymph nodes in her neck and axillae. She reports having "the flu" last winter and believes her fatigue

began after that. She has undergone several comprehensive medical evaluations with no explanation for her symptoms. Recent records from previous physicians reveal normal complete blood count, comprehensive metabolic panel, and thyroid function studies.

On physical examination, vital signs are normal. BMI is 24. There is no lymphadenopathy, but the patient notes tenderness when lymph node areas are palpated. There is tenderness to joint movement but no evidence of synovitis or restricted movement. There is generalized tenderness to muscle palpation; strength is normal. The remainder of the physical examination is unremarkable. Mini–Mental State Examination score is 29/30; a two-question depression screen is negative.

Which of the following should be done next to help diagnose this patient's symptoms?

(A) Epstein-Barr virus titer
(B) Erythrocyte sedimentation rate
(C) Parvovirus B19 titer
(D) No additional testing

Item 8

A 29-year-old woman is evaluated preoperatively before elective breast reduction and liposuction. She feels well and has no symptoms or pertinent medical history. She exercises regularly. Her last menstrual period was 3 weeks ago. She drinks alcohol socially and does not smoke cigarettes. She has no family history of premature heart disease or abnormal bleeding. The procedure will be done under general anesthesia. She takes no medications or supplements. Results of the physical examination are normal.

Which of the following is the most appropriate preoperative test to perform next?

(A) Chest radiography
(B) Coagulation studies
(C) Electrocardiography
(D) Pregnancy testing
(E) No further testing

Item 9

A 66-year-old woman is evaluated for several months of a "whistling" or "swishing" sound in her right ear. She notes that it gets faster and louder when she exercises and thinks it is timed to her heartbeat. She does not notice any hearing loss, dizziness, or vertigo.

On physical examination, temperature is 37.4 °C (99.3 °F), blood pressure is 138/84 mm Hg, and pulse rate is 84/min. Auditory acuity to normal conversation appears normal, and otoscopic examination is unremarkable bilaterally. Neurologic examination is normal.

Which of the following is the most appropriate next step in the management of this patient?

(A) Audiometry
(B) Auscultation over the right ear, eye, and neck

(C) Trial of a sound-masking device

(D) Trial of a nasal corticosteroid spray

Item 10

A 46-year-old woman is evaluated during a routine examination. Her 72-year-old mother was just diagnosed with lung cancer, so the patient asks you for help with quitting smoking. She has a 27-pack-year smoking history. She made one previous quit attempt several years ago using over-the-counter nicotine gum, but she was unable to quit for more than a few days. Medical history is significant for seizure disorder. Review of systems discloses mild shortness of breath with exertion and occasional wheezing. Medications are a multivitamin and phenytoin.

On physical examination, vital signs are normal. Lung examination reveals occasional wheezing and a prolonged expiratory phase. The rest of the examination is normal.

In addition to counseling regarding tobacco use, which of the following is an appropriate adjunct to increase her likelihood of successful smoking cessation?

(A) A benzodiazepine

(B) Bupropion

(C) Electronic smokeless cigarette use

(D) Nicotine replacement therapy

Item 11

A 23-year-old man is evaluated for a 3-day history of redness and itchiness of the right eye. He had an upper respiratory tract infection 3 days before the eye symptoms began. Each morning he has awoken with crusting over the lids. He is otherwise healthy, with no ocular trauma or recent medical problems.

On physical examination, he is afebrile, blood pressure is 122/72 mm Hg, pulse rate is 66/min, and respiration rate is 16/min. Right eye conjunctival injection is present, with some crusting at the lids. Bilateral vision is 20/20. Pupils are equally round and reactive to light.

Which of the following is the most appropriate management of this patient?

(A) Cool compresses to the affected eye

(B) Oral antihistamine

(C) Topical antibiotics

(D) Topical corticosteroids

Item 12

A 67-year-old man is evaluated for right groin pain. The pain began spontaneously 2 days ago. Yesterday, he was evaluated in the emergency department and was diagnosed with groin strain and discharged home. He is reevaluated today because the groin pain has continued without improvement. He has well-controlled hypertension and a 30-pack-year smoking history. Medications are hydrochlorothiazide and aspirin.

On physical examination, he is afebrile. Blood pressure is 100/62 mm Hg and pulse rate is 104/min. Respiration rate is 16/min. The abdomen is slightly distended but nontender. There is no focal tenderness over the hip or pelvis. Active and passive range of motion testing of his right hip does not exacerbate his groin pain. The patient is reassured that a groin muscle strain is the likely cause of his discomfort. He is advised to take more fluids and rest.

12 hours later he is brought to the emergency department because of diffuse severe abdominal pain. A CT scan of the abdomen shows a rupturing 8.2-cm abdominal aortic aneurysm.

Which of the following categories of diagnostic error is responsible for missing the correct diagnosis at the follow-up examination?

(A) Anchoring heuristic

(B) Availability heuristic

(C) No-fault error

(D) Representativeness heuristic

Item 13

A 32-year-old man is evaluated for a 3-day history of productive cough, sore throat, coryza, rhinorrhea, nasal congestion, generalized myalgia, and fatigue. His sputum is slightly yellow. His two children (ages 3 years and 1 year) had similar symptoms 1 week ago. He is a nonsmoker and has no history of asthma.

On physical examination, temperature is 37.5 °C (99.4 °F), blood pressure is 128/76 mm Hg, pulse rate is 92/min, and respiration rate is 14/min. There is bilateral conjunctival injection. The nasal mucosa is boggy, with clear drainage. The oropharynx is erythematous without tonsillar enlargement or exudates. The tympanic membranes and external auditory canals are normal. Lungs are clear to auscultation. There is no rash or lymphadenopathy.

Which of the following is the most appropriate treatment?

(A) Albuterol

(B) Amoxicillin

(C) Chlorpheniramine

(D) Codeine

Item 14

A 48-year-old man is evaluated for a 2-day history of episodic dizziness with nausea. He noted the onset abruptly and compares the feeling to "being on a roller coaster." His most severe episodes occurred while arising from bed and when parallel parking his car. The symptoms lasted 30 to 40 seconds and were followed by two episodes of emesis. He has no recent fever, headache, tinnitus, hearing loss, double vision, dysarthria, weakness, or difficulty walking. He had a similar episode 5 years ago. Medical history is significant for depression. His only medication is citalopram.

On physical examination, vital signs are normal. Results of cardiac and neurologic examinations are normal. The

Dix-Hallpike maneuver precipitates severe horizontal nystagmus after about 20 seconds. With repeated maneuvers, the nystagmus is less severe.

Which of the following is the most likely diagnosis?

(A) Benign paroxysmal positional vertigo
(B) Cerebellar infarction
(C) Meniere disease
(D) Vestibular neuronitis

Item 15

A 47-year-old woman is evaluated for an abnormal complete blood count obtained as part of a life insurance physical examination. She has no active medical problems. She underwent Roux-en-Y gastric bypass surgery 10 years ago and has successfully kept off the weight she lost after the surgery. She has not seen a physician for more than 7 years. She has no family history of hematologic disorders or colon cancer.

On physical examination, temperature is normal, blood pressure is 124/80 mm Hg, and pulse rate is 78/min. BMI is 24. Cardiovascular, pulmonary, and neurologic examinations are all normal. There is no thyromegaly. Abdominal examination shows a well-healed surgical scar. The remainder of the examination is unremarkable. A stool sample is guaiac-negative. The laboratory results obtained by the patient are shown.

Laboratory studies:

Leukocyte count	4200/µL (4.2 × 10⁹/L)
Hemoglobin	10.9 g/dL (109 g/L)
Mean corpuscular volume	107 fL
Platelet count	122,000/µL (122 × 10⁹/L)
Reticulocyte count	1.5%

Which of the following is the most appropriate test to establish the diagnosis?

(A) Bone marrow biopsy
(B) Colonoscopy
(C) Serum thyroid-stimulating hormone level
(D) Serum vitamin B_{12} level

Item 16

A 28-year-old woman is evaluated during a routine examination. Her 52-year-old mother was recently diagnosed with Huntington disease. The patient has no symptoms. She is planning on starting a family. Physical examination, including complete neurologic examination, is normal.

Which of the following should be done next?

(A) Obtain genetic testing for Huntington disease
(B) Order brain MRI
(C) Reassure the patient that she is unlikely to develop Huntington disease
(D) Refer for genetic counseling

Item 17

An 85-year-old man is admitted to a nursing home. He has diabetes mellitus, coronary artery disease, chronic heart failure, and dementia. On physical examination, vital signs are normal. He has a full thickness 5 × 8 cm pressure ulcer on his left buttock covered with a thick eschar. There is visible subcutaneous fat beneath the eschar; no bone or tendon is exposed. His skin is dry and there is evidence of mild dehydration and malnutrition. He has urinary but not fecal incontinence. His current medications are lisinopril, metformin, hydrochlorothiazide, glipizide, and carvedilol.

Which of the following is the most appropriate management of this patient's ulcer?

(A) Debridement
(B) Hyperbaric oxygen therapy
(C) Negative-pressure wound vacuum therapy
(D) Oral vitamin C and zinc supplementation
(E) Surgical flap therapy

Item 18

An 80-year-old man is evaluated for a 1-year history of progressive urinary symptoms including weak stream, hesitancy, and nocturia four times nightly. He has coronary artery disease and chronic heart failure. His current medications are lisinopril, isosorbide dinitrate, aspirin, and metoprolol.

On physical examination, vital signs are normal. He has mild suprapubic tenderness and a symmetrically enlarged prostate without nodules or tenderness. The remainder of the physical examination is normal.

Which of the following is the most appropriate diagnostic test to perform next?

(A) Postvoid residual urinary volume measurement
(B) Plasma glucose level
(C) Prostate-specific antigen testing
(D) Transrectal ultrasound
(E) Urinalysis

Item 19

A 58-year-old man recently diagnosed with multiple myeloma with bony metastases is evaluated before hospital discharge. He is being discharged today on hospice care after receiving melphalan and prednisone and having a poor response to therapy. He is currently on intravenous morphine as needed for pain and has requested 10 mg every 4 hours over the last 24 hours. On physical examination, vital signs are normal.

Which of the following is the most appropriate treatment of this patient's pain?

(A) Fentanyl transdermal patch
(B) Methadone
(C) Short-acting hydromorphone
(D) Sustained-release morphine

Item 20

A 29-year-old man is evaluated for the gradual onset of right-sided hearing loss. He reports a continuous high-pitched ringing in his right ear that has been present for 3 to 4 months.

On physical examination, vital signs are normal. When a vibrating 512 Hz tuning fork is placed on the top of his head, it is louder in the left ear. When placed adjacent to his right ear, it is heard better when outside the ear canal than when touching the mastoid bone. Otoscopic examination is normal bilaterally. Neurologic examination is normal other than right-sided hearing loss.

Which of the following is the most appropriate management of this patient?

(A) Biofeedback therapy
(B) Immediate treatment with oral corticosteroids
(C) MRI of the posterior fossa and internal auditory canal
(D) Otolith repositioning maneuver

Item 21

A 72-year-old woman is evaluated in the emergency department after an episode of syncope. While watching a movie, the patient felt palpitations; the next thing she remembers is being on the floor. She experienced a similar episode about 1 month ago. History is significant for hypertension, hypothyroidism, osteoporosis, and chronic kidney disease. Medications are amlodipine, lisinopril, levothyroxine, and calcium supplements. She currently feels well.

On physical examination, temperature is normal, blood pressure is 148/78 mm Hg, pulse rate is 84/min and regular, and respiration rate is 12/min. Oxygen saturation on ambient air is normal. There is no thyromegaly, carotid upstrokes are +2 without bruits, and there is no jugular venous distention. Cardiac auscultation reveals a grade 2/6, early peaking, crescendo-decrescendo systolic murmur at the right upper sternal border with occasional extra beats. The remainder of the physical examination is normal.

A resting electrocardiogram and rhythm strip show a sinus rate of 85/min with occasional premature ventricular contractions but no sustained arrhythmia, normal axis and intervals, and no ischemic changes.

Which of the following is the most likely cause of this patient's syncope?

(A) Aortic stenosis
(B) Cardiac arrhythmia
(C) Myocardial ischemia
(D) Transient ischemic attack

Item 22

A 56-year-old woman is evaluated for a 6-month history of symmetric bilateral lower extremity edema. She notices no leg swelling upon arising in the morning; her symptoms appear by midday and worsen thereafter. She does not have pain but notes her legs feel heavy and her shoes leave indentations in her skin with prolonged standing. She has no periorbital or upper extremity edema, chest pain, shortness of breath, paroxysmal nocturnal dyspnea, orthopnea, change in urinary habits, or abdominal fullness. She has no history of malignancy, immobility, or hormone replacement therapy.

On physical examination, vital signs are normal. BMI is 34. Results of the cardiovascular examination and abdominal examination are normal. The lungs are clear. There is no inguinal lymphadenopathy, lower extremity rash, or erythema. There is 1+ pitting ankle edema bilaterally.

Laboratory studies:

Creatinine	0.8 mg/dL (70.7 μmol/L)
Albumin	4.1 g/dL (41 g/L)
Alanine aminotransferase	28 units/L
Aspartate aminotransferase	24 units/L
Bilirubin	1.1 mg/dL (18.8 μmol/L)
Sodium	140 meq/L (140 mmol/L)
Potassium	3.9 meq/L (3.9 mmol/L)

Results of thyroid function testing are normal. Urinalysis shows no protein or blood.

Which of the following is the most appropriate next step in management?

(A) Compression stockings
(B) CT scan of abdomen and pelvis
(C) Furosemide
(D) Lower extremity venous duplex ultrasonography

Item 23

A 29-year-old man is evaluated for a 1-day history of left shoulder pain. He was throwing a football approximately 30 yards when the pain began. The pain is located over the left lateral deltoid muscle. He notes weakness with abduction. He has no previous history of shoulder problems, no history of trauma, and no paresthesia. He has been taking ibuprofen as needed for pain.

On physical examination, he is afebrile, blood pressure is 126/80 mm Hg, and pulse rate is 96/min. There is pain in the left shoulder with active abduction beginning at approximately 60 degrees, and he has difficulty actively abducting the left arm beyond 60 degrees. The patient is unable to slowly lower his left arm to his waist (positive drop-arm test). He has no pain with his left arm in full flexion (negative Neer test). When the patient is asked to hold the arm extended anteriorly at 90 degrees with the forearm bent to 90 degrees (at 12 o'clock), he does not have pain with the arm internally rotated to cross in front of the body (negative Hawkins test). There is no pain with forward elevation of the left arm to 90 degrees with active adduction of the arm (negative cross-arm test). Strength (other than during abduction) is intact.

Which of the following is the most appropriate next step in management?

(A) MRI of the left shoulder
(B) NSAID therapy
(C) Physical therapy
(D) Subacromial corticosteroid injection

Item 24

A 70-year-old man is admitted to the hospital for peritonitis. He has Alzheimer disease, hypertension, type 2 diabetes mellitus, cirrhosis, and ascites. He has been falling frequently at home. His current medications are metformin, donepezil, lisinopril, and propranolol.

On physical examination, temperature is 38.5 °C (101.3 °F), blood pressure is 130/70 mm Hg, pulse rate is 80/min, and respiration rate is 12/min. He is oriented to person and is in no acute distress. There is shifting dullness on abdominal examination and diffuse abdominal tenderness with palpation. There are areas of blanching erythema on the lower back and buttocks. There is no ulceration or skin breakdown. Laboratory studies show serum albumin level of 2.8 g/dL (28 g/L).

Which of the following interventions is most appropriate for preventing pressure ulcers in this patient?

(A) Doughnut-type device
(B) Free ambulation
(C) Indwelling urinary catheter
(D) Pressure-distributing mattress

Item 25

A 56-year-old woman is evaluated for severe vaginal itching and discomfort. Her symptoms have progressively worsened for the past 4 months. There is no associated vaginal discharge or vaginal odor. She is experiencing significant vaginal dryness and intercourse has become painful despite the use of lubricants. She has been menopausal since age 53 years. Her only medications are calcium and vitamin D.

On physical examination, vital signs are normal. BMI is 29. She has pale, dry vaginal walls with decreased rugae and petechial hemorrhages. There is scant vaginal discharge. Vaginal pH is 6.0. Wet mount shows occasional leukocytes. "Whiff" test is negative. There are no clue cells and no hyphae on potassium hydroxide preparation.

Which of the following is the most appropriate management of this patient?

(A) Oral conjugated estrogen with medroxyprogesterone acetate
(B) Oral metronidazole
(C) Vaginal clotrimazole
(D) Vaginal estradiol

Item 26

A 58-year-old man is evaluated for an 8-month history of slowly progressive right shoulder pain. The pain is located over the anterior shoulder and is worse with moving his arm across his chest and also when he fully abducts his arm. His only medication is acetaminophen.

On physical examination, vital signs are normal. He has pain when he forward elevates his right arm to 90 degrees and actively adducts his arm across his chest wall (positive cross-arm test). There is pain with shoulder abduction beyond 120 degrees. He exhibits normal shoulder internal and external range of motion. There is pain with palpation of the acromioclavicular joint. He has no pain with his left arm in full flexion (negative Neer test). He is able to slowly lower his right arm to his waist (negative drop-arm test).

Which of the following is the most likely diagnosis?

(A) Acromioclavicular joint degeneration
(B) Adhesive capsulitis
(C) Rotator cuff tear
(D) Rotator cuff tendinitis

Item 27

A 59-year-old man is evaluated during a follow-up examination. He has COPD and hypertension. He has an 80-pack-year history of cigarette use, but has recently decreased his smoking to a half pack of cigarettes daily. Medications are ipratropium and amlodipine.

On physical examination, temperature is 37.3 °C (99.2 °F), blood pressure is 138/92 mm Hg, pulse rate is 96/min, and respiration rate is 22/min. BMI is 29. He is barrel-chested with diffuse wheezing on lung examination. The remainder of the physical examination is normal.

Which of the following is the most appropriate management regarding this patient's tobacco use?

(A) Assess his interest in smoking cessation
(B) Prescribe bupropion
(C) Prescribe nicotine replacement therapy
(D) Refer for smoking cessation counseling

Item 28

A 45-year-old woman is evaluated in the hospital after radical hysterectomy for cervical carcinoma. Aside from postoperative pain, she has no symptoms. She has no history of venous thromboembolism or excessive bleeding. Her only current medication is morphine as needed.

On physical examination, temperature is normal, blood pressure is 110/72 mm Hg, and pulse rate is 84/min. There is trace edema in the legs. Prothrombin time, activated partial thromboplastin time, and INR are normal.

In addition to early ambulation, which of the following interventions is the most appropriate in this patient for thromboembolism prophylaxis?

(A) Enoxaparin for 5 weeks
(B) Inferior vena cava filter placement
(C) Unfractionated heparin until discharge
(D) Warfarin for 3 months

Item 29

A 55-year-old man is evaluated for a 1-day history of seeing flashing lights, "squiggly" lines, and floating objects in his left eye followed by loss of vision at the outer periphery of the eye shortly after having breakfast this morning. He now describes seeing what looks like a curtain coming down in that location. He has myopia requiring prescription glasses.

On physical examination, vital signs are normal. Vision in the right eye is 20/100 uncorrected and 20/40 with glasses. Vision in the left eye is 20/100 uncorrected and 20/40 with glasses. Pupils are equally reactive to light and accommodation. There is no conjunctival injection. Findings on funduscopic examination are shown.

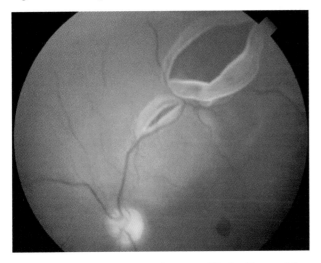

Which of the following is the most likely diagnosis?

(A) Central retinal artery occlusion
(B) Central retinal vein occlusion
(C) Ocular migraine
(D) Retinal detachment
(E) Temporal arteritis

Item 30

A 73-year-old woman is admitted to the hospital for drug-related hypersensitivity syndrome. She was hospitalized 2 weeks ago for a right ankle fracture and subsequently underwent open reduction and internal fixation. On the day of discharge she was noted to have a urinary tract infection and was prescribed trimethoprim-sulfamethoxazole despite a previously documented allergy to this agent in her internist's office chart, which was paper based and not linked to the hospital's electronic order entry system and drug allergy alert system.

After admitting the patient to the hospital and stopping her antibiotic, which of the following is the most appropriate immediate next step to reduce the likelihood of future similar errors?

(A) Discuss with the patient's internist the need to emphasize to patients the importance of communicating medication allergies with other caregivers
(B) Emphasize to the patient the importance of knowing and communicating her known allergies with caregivers
(C) Encourage hospital administration to consider implementation of an electronic health record
(D) Plan an intervention to improve communication of medication allergies from outpatient to inpatient records

Item 31

A 30-year-old woman is evaluated during a follow-up examination. She has had recurrent episodes of presyncope and syncope over the past few months. She continues to have an episode every 3 to 4 weeks, with no discernible pattern or trigger. She reports becoming light-headed and feeling faint, without other associated symptoms, followed by transient loss of consciousness for several seconds followed by spontaneous recovery without residual symptoms. On previous evaluation, an electrocardiogram (ECG) and echocardiogram were normal. Results of 24-hour continuous ambulatory ECG monitoring were unremarkable, and a cardiac event recorder showed no arrhythmia associated with presyncopal symptoms. History is significant for anxiety and intermittent insomnia; the patient takes no medications for these conditions. There is no history of prior head trauma. She does not use drugs or alcohol.

On physical examination, temperature is normal. Blood pressure is 122/68 mm Hg and pulse rate is 72/min while supine. After three minutes of standing, blood pressure is 112/84 mm Hg and pulse rate is 88/min, without reproduction of syncope or symptoms. The remainder of the examination is normal. Serum electrolytes, kidney function, and thyroid function studies are normal.

Which of the following is the most appropriate next step in the evaluation of this patient?

(A) Electroencephalography
(B) Exercise cardiac stress test
(C) Signal-averaged electrocardiogram
(D) Tilt-table testing

Item 32

A 32-year-old woman is evaluated as a new patient. She is planning to attempt conception with her partner. She has a history of systemic lupus erythematosus complicated by chronic kidney disease that has been inactive for several years off of treatment. She has had borderline blood pressure elevations since the diagnosis of kidney disease. She was also diagnosed with impaired fasting glucose and mild hyperlipidemia 2 years ago, both of which have been treated with dietary changes. Her current medications are calcium and vitamin D supplements.

On physical examination, blood pressure is 156/92 mm Hg and her vital signs are otherwise normal. BMI is 26. The remainder of the physical examination, including a gynecologic examination, is normal.

Laboratory studies:

Electrolytes	Normal
Blood urea nitrogen	12 mg/dL (4.2 mmol/L)
Creatinine	1.2 mg/dL (106.0 µmol/L)
Total cholesterol	250 mg/dL (6.4 mmol/L)
LDL cholesterol	160 mg/dL (4.1 mmol/L)
HDL cholesterol	34 mg/dL (0.8 mmol/L)
Triglycerides	200 mg/dL (2.26 mmol/L)
Spot urine albumin/ creatinine ratio	300 mg/g
Hemoglobin A$_{1c}$	7.5%

In addition to a daily prenatal vitamin, which of the following is the most appropriate treatment?

(A) Aspirin
(B) Lisinopril
(C) Metformin
(D) Simvastatin

Item 33

A 78-year-old woman living in a nursing home is evaluated for incontinence. Over the past year, she has had progressive decline in her cognitive status and now spends most of the day in bed. She requires coaxing to join the other residents in their communal meals and requires assistance for eating and bathing. When accompanied by an aide or family member, she is able to walk slowly to the bathroom without leakage and to urinate. Medical history is significant for dementia and depression treated with citalopram.

She is a frail, elderly woman in no acute distress. On physical examination, temperature is normal, blood pressure is 132/88 mm Hg, and pulse rate is 68/min. BMI is 23. Her score on the Mini–Mental State Examination is 14/30. Her gait is slow and she requires assistance. Abdominal examination is without suprapubic fullness. Rectal examination reveals normal sphincter tone. Results of urinalysis are normal.

Which of the following is the most appropriate management of this patient?

(A) Cystoscopy
(B) Indwelling Foley catheter
(C) Pelvic floor muscle training
(D) Prompted voiding
(E) Tolterodine

Item 34

A 31-year-old woman is evaluated during a routine office visit. She is married and in a monogamous relationship with her husband of 10 years. She has been getting annual Pap smears since the age of 20 years, all of which have been within normal limits, including the most recent, 1 year ago. She has no family history of cervical cancer. On physical examination, vital signs are normal.

Which of the following is the most appropriate management of this patient?

(A) Obtain human papillomavirus DNA testing
(B) Obtain Pap smear in 2 years
(C) Obtain Pap smear now
(D) Discontinue Pap smears

Item 35

A 78-year-old man is evaluated for a 1-year history of forgetfulness and not being able to remember names. He is a retired attorney. He reports no problems with performing activities of daily living, planning his day, or managing his finances. He is frustrated but not depressed and is still able to enjoy life. He has hypertension and hyperlipidemia, controlled with hydrochlorothiazide and simvastatin.

On physical examination, he is afebrile, blood pressure is 140/82 mm Hg, and pulse rate is 78/min. Mini–Mental State Examination score is 25. The lungs are clear. The heart is without murmur. Neurologic, motor, and sensory examinations are normal.

Which of the following is the most likely diagnosis?

(A) Alzheimer disease
(B) Mild cognitive impairment
(C) Pseudodementia
(D) Vascular dementia

Item 36

A 76-year-old woman was evaluated 10 days ago for weight loss and occasional hemoptysis. Non–small cell lung cancer was subsequently diagnosed. In addition to a 4 × 5 cm single lesion in the left upper lobe of her lung, there are metastatic lesions in the left humerus, as well as a single lesion in the left lobe of the liver. She does all of her own activities of daily living and is able to walk 1 mile before stopping because of fatigue. Her only medications are a daily multivitamin and a calcium supplement.

On physical examination, vital signs are normal. She appears comfortable and in no distress and is interested in life-prolonging therapy.

Which of the following is the most appropriate time to begin palliative care discussions with this patient?

(A) After she develops symptoms
(B) At the current visit
(C) When admitted to hospice care
(D) When she no longer desires active treatment

Item 37

A 58-year-old woman is evaluated for a 2-day history of burning, stinging pain in her posterior neck that radiates down her left arm and began after she spent several hours painting the ceiling of her home. She reports no trauma or other symptoms. She feels mild numbness and paresthesias on the back of her left hand.

On physical examination, vital signs are normal. Neck range of motion is limited by pain, especially in extension. Axial loading of the neck increases pain. There is slightly diminished sensation on the back of the left hand. There are no motor deficits. Reflexes are symmetric.

Which of the following is the most appropriate management of this patient?

(A) Analgesics and avoidance of provocative activities
(B) Cervical traction
(C) Electromyography/nerve conduction study
(D) MRI of cervical spine

Item 38

A 55-year-old man is evaluated during a follow-up appointment for a 6-month history of nonproductive cough. The cough predictably comes after meals, at bedtime, or any time he lies down, but it can occur at other times as well. He experiences heartburn throughout the day. He has no shortness of breath, dyspnea on exertion, fever, chills, postnasal drip, recent upper respiratory tract infection, or wheezing. Omeprazole was prescribed 2 weeks ago but he reports no change in his cough or heartburn symptoms. He is a nonsmoker, does not drink alcohol, and takes no other medications.

Vital signs are normal, as is the remainder of the physical examination. Chest radiograph is normal.

Which of the following is the most appropriate treatment?

(A) Amoxicillin-clavulanate
(B) Continue omeprazole
(C) Inhaled albuterol
(D) Loratadine with pseudoephedrine

Item 39

A 42-year-old woman is evaluated for chest pain that started a few days ago. It is midsternal, sharp, constant, and worsens with deep inspiration and recumbency. It does not radiate to the back and does not worsen with physical activity. The pain has increased slightly over the past day. She has no recent fevers or chills, cough, joint pain, or rash. Two weeks ago, she had symptoms consistent with acute tracheobronchitis.

On physical examination, temperature is 37.5 °C (99.5 °F), blood pressure is 122/80 mm Hg, pulse rate is 88/min, and respiration rate is 17/min. BMI is 32. She is uncomfortable lying down and prefers to sit forward for the examination. Cardiac auscultation demonstrates normal heart sounds with no murmur or rub. The remainder of the examination is normal.

Electrocardiogram is shown. Chest radiograph is normal.

Which of the following is the most likely diagnosis?

(A) Acute coronary syndrome
(B) Acute pericarditis
(C) Acute pleuritis
(D) Acute pulmonary embolism

Item 40

A 60-year-old man is evaluated for a 1-year history of generalized fatigue and lack of energy. He has had erectile dysfunction for the past 9 months. He has chronic low back pain and hypertension. Current medications are metoprolol, hydrochlorothiazide, hydrocodone, and naproxen.

On physical examination, vital signs are normal. Cardiac, lung, and thyroid examinations are all normal. Laboratory studies show a morning total serum testosterone level of 180 ng/dL (6.2 nmol/L). Complete blood count, metabolic panel, and thyroid-stimulating hormone level are all normal.

Which of the following is the most appropriate next step in the management of this patient?

(A) Discontinue hydrocodone
(B) Discontinue metoprolol
(C) Recheck testosterone level
(D) Start testosterone replacement therapy

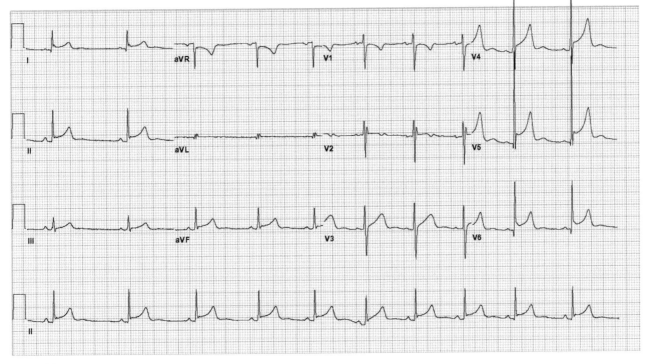

ITEM 39

Item 41

A 67-year-old man is evaluated during a routine examination. He has hypertension and obesity. He also has a history of gout, but has not had an attack in more than 1 year. His current medications are lisinopril and a daily aspirin.

On physical examination, blood pressure is 140/82 mm Hg; vital signs are otherwise normal. BMI is 32. His waist circumference is 107 cm (42 in). There is no hepatomegaly.

Laboratory studies:

Total cholesterol	192 mg/dL (4.97 mmol/L)
HDL cholesterol	27 mg/dL (0.70 mmol/L)
LDL cholesterol (directly measured)	68 mg/dL (1.76 mmol/L)
Triglycerides	554 mg/dL (6.26 mmol/L)
Glucose	100 mg/dL (5.5 mmol/L)
Creatinine	1.1 mg/dL (97.2 µmol/L)

In addition to recommending weight loss and exercise, which of the following is the most appropriate treatment for his lipid abnormalities?

(A) Colesevelam
(B) Extended-release nicotinic acid
(C) Fenofibrate
(D) Omega-3 fatty acids

Item 42

A 65-year-old man is evaluated for a 3-day history of scrotal pain. He notes some pain with urination and tenderness in the left testicular region. He has felt febrile at home with some nausea and generalized weakness. He has not had similar symptoms before and has not had any trauma. He has no nocturia, urinary frequency, or weak urinary stream. He takes no medications.

On physical examination, temperature is 38.7 °C (101.6 °F), blood pressure is 140/80 mm Hg, pulse rate is 90/min, and respiration rate is 14/min. He is in moderate distress. The left scrotum shows erythema with mild fullness. The testicle itself is nontender, but there is fullness superior to it that is extremely tender to palpation, with some discomfort to palpation over the posterior aspect of the testicle. The left testicle is lower in the scrotum than the right testicle. The prostate is normal in size and nontender. Leukocyte count is 14,000/µL (14 × 10⁹/L) with 18% band forms.

Which of the following is the most likely diagnosis?

(A) Acute prostatitis
(B) Epididymitis
(C) Indirect hernia
(D) Orchitis
(E) Testicular torsion

Item 43

An 82-year-old man was admitted to the hospital 2 days ago with pneumonia, sepsis, and acute kidney injury. Medical history is significant for recurrent lung cancer, for which he previously underwent lobectomy, now with adrenal metastases. He has remained anuric since admission. This morning his serum potassium level was 7.2 meq/L (7.2 mmol/L) with electrocardiographic changes. It is clear that dialysis is indicated. The patient is unable to give consent, and his wife is his surrogate decision maker. She says that he was aware of the poor prognosis from his lung cancer and expressed a desire not to be kept alive on machines for a long period of time. However, he was looking forward to his great-grandson's graduation from college in 3 weeks and hoped that he could be able to attend. The wife is willing to consent to dialysis.

On physical examination, temperature is 38.1 °C (100.5 °F), blood pressure is 110/64 mm Hg, pulse rate is 112/min, and respiration rate is 28/min.

Which of the following is the most appropriate management of this patient?

(A) Start long-term hemodialysis
(B) Start temporary hemodialysis
(C) Withdraw all life-sustaining treatment
(D) Withhold dialysis and continue medical treatment

Item 44

A 38-year-old woman is evaluated for gritty, burning eyes that worsen over the course of the day. She reports her eyes are often dry and are worse on windy days. She also reports dry mouth with difficulty salivating at times. She has no other symptoms.

On physical examination, vital signs are normal. The conjunctiva is irritated. She has normal vision by Snellen chart. Fundi are normal. Decreased tear production is documented with the Schirmer test. The remainder of the physical examination is normal.

The antinuclear antibody test, rheumatoid factor, and anti-Ro/SSA and anti-La/SSB tests are positive.

Which of the following is the most likely diagnosis?

(A) Meibomianitis
(B) Primary Sjögren syndrome
(C) Rheumatoid arthritis
(D) Systemic lupus erythematosus

Item 45

A 28-year-old woman is evaluated for a painful lump in her left breast of 6 weeks' duration. There is neither discharge from the nipple nor skin changes over the area. Her last normal menstrual period was 3 weeks ago and she thinks that the lump became slightly larger right before and during her menses. She is on low-dose oral contraceptives. She has no history of breast disease or breast biopsy. Menarche was at age 12 years. She has never been pregnant. A maternal aunt had breast cancer.

On physical examination, vital signs are normal. BMI is 24. There is a 1.5-cm mobile, soft, slightly tender mass in the lower mid quadrant of the left breast. There is no nipple discharge and no abnormalities of the overlying skin. The right breast has no masses. There is no axillary lymphadenopathy. The remainder of the examination is unremarkable.

Which of the following is the most appropriate management of this patient?

(A) Core needle biopsy

(B) Mammography

(C) Repeat clinical breast examination in 6 months

(D) Ultrasonography

Item 46

A 94-year-old woman is brought to the emergency department by her daughter for a 5-day history of progressive weakness, anorexia, dizziness, and mild confusion. She was hospitalized 2 weeks ago for an acute exacerbation of chronic heart failure that was treated with intravenous diuretics and an increase in her daily oral diuretic dose. She initially did well following discharge, and a follow-up appointment with her primary care physician is scheduled for next week. She has a history of chronic atrial fibrillation, upper gastrointestinal bleeding owing to a duodenal ulcer 18 months ago, COPD, hypertension, post-herpetic neuralgia, chronic kidney disease, depression, anxiety, and seasonal rhinitis. Medications are furosemide, potassium chloride, aspirin, omeprazole, ipratropium and albuterol inhalers, metoprolol, gabapentin, loratadine, and as-needed lorazepam.

On physical examination, she is a pleasant but frail-appearing woman who is arousable but mildly confused. Temperature is 37.3 °C (99.1 °F), blood pressure is 108/56 mm Hg, pulse rate is 95/min, and respiration rate is 16/min. Oxygen saturation is 94% on ambient air. The mucous membranes are dry. The pupils are symmetric and reactive. Heart examination is significant for an irregularly irregular rate and a grade 3/6 crescendo-decrescendo murmur at the right upper sternal border. The lungs are clear to auscultation. The abdomen is scaphoid without hepatosplenomegaly. There is no peripheral edema. Her neurologic examination is nonfocal except for her cognitive deficits.

Laboratory studies show normal serum electrolytes and a plasma glucose level of 110 mg/dL (6.1 mmol/L). Her serum creatinine level is 1.4 mg/dL (123.8 μmol/L), increased from 1.2 mg/dL (106.1 μmol/L) at the time of hospital discharge. Her complete blood count reveals a leukocyte count of 7500/μL (7.5×10^9/L) with a normal differential, a hematocrit of 35%, and normal platelet count. A urinalysis shows trace ketones but no cells. A chest radiograph is significant for severe kyphoscoliosis and changes consistent with emphysema, but not pneumonia or heart failure.

Which of the following is the most likely cause of the patient's clinical presentation?

(A) Acute kidney injury

(B) Medication effect

(C) Occult infection

(D) Recent stroke

Item 47

A 60-year-old man is admitted to the hospital with a traumatic hip fracture. A total hip arthroplasty under general anesthesia is planned. He has COPD and reports that he is significantly limited in his exercise tolerance because of dyspnea, although his functional capacity has remained stable over the past 4 to 6 months. He has a cough with occasional white sputum, unchanged for the past 6 months. He has no other acute respiratory symptoms. He smokes 1 pack per day of cigarettes. Current medications are tiotropium, albuterol, and fluticasone/salmeterol.

On physical examination, temperature is normal, blood pressure is 108/72 mm Hg, pulse rate is 78/min, and respiration rate is 18/min. Oxygen saturation is 96% on ambient air. Pulmonary examination demonstrates scattered crackles and wheezing, unchanged from his baseline findings. Cardiac examination shows regular rate and rhythm and a normal S_1 and S_2.

Which of the following should be recommended before surgery?

(A) Nocturnal continuous positive airway pressure

(B) Chest radiograph

(C) Incentive spirometry

(D) Pulmonary function testing

Item 48

A 46-year-old man is evaluated for a 3-week history of occasional painless bright red rectal bleeding. He has no fatigue, lightheadedness, weight loss, or abdominal pain. His stools are frequently firm, occasionally hard, and there is no change in the frequency or consistency of his bowel movements. He has never been screened for colorectal cancer.

On physical examination, temperature is 37.2 °C (98.9 °F), blood pressure is 132/78 mm Hg, and pulse rate is 84/min. Digital rectal examination yields a stool sample that is positive for occult blood; the examination is otherwise normal. Anoscopy reveals a few internal hemorrhoids without active bleeding. Laboratory studies show a blood hemoglobin level of 14 g/dL (140 g/L).

Which of the following is the most appropriate management of this patient?

(A) Banding of hemorrhoids

(B) Colonoscopy

(C) Fiber supplementation without further evaluation

(D) Home fecal occult blood testing

Item 49

A 52-year-old man is evaluated during a periodic health examination. He has benign prostatic hyperplasia, and his father died of prostate cancer at the age of 74 years. His only current medication is tamsulosin. He has no urinary symptoms. Vital signs are normal, as is the remainder of the physical examination.

Which of the following is the most appropriate management?

(A) Discuss the risks and benefits of prostate cancer screening
(B) Obtain a prostate-specific antigen level
(C) Perform a digital rectal examination
(D) Perform a digital rectal examination and obtain a prostate-specific antigen level

Item 50

A 72-year-old man is evaluated in the emergency department for a 12-hour episode of dizziness, described as a "spinning sensation" when he opens his eyes. He has nausea without vomiting, has had no loss of consciousness, no palpitations, and no other neurologic symptoms. He requires assistance to walk. He prefers to keep his eyes closed but has no diplopia. He has hypertension, hyperlipidemia, and type 2 diabetes mellitus. He had an upper respiratory tract infection 2 weeks ago. Medications are hydrochlorothiazide, lisinopril, simvastatin, and metformin.

On physical examination, vital signs are normal. There are no orthostatic changes. Results of a cardiovascular examination are normal. He has no focal weakness. He cannot stand without assistance. Vertical nystagmus occurs immediately with the Dix-Hallpike maneuver. It persists for 90 seconds and does not fatigue. Electrocardiogram is consistent with left ventricular hypertrophy and shows no acute changes.

Which of the following is the most appropriate next step in management?

(A) CT scan of the head without contrast
(B) MRI with angiography of the brain
(C) Otolith repositioning
(D) Trial of vestibular suppressant medication

Item 51

A 48-year-old woman is evaluated during a routine examination. She is concerned about her gradual weight gain over the years and requests counseling on how she can most effectively lose weight.

Over 8 years, she has gained approximately 18 kg (40 lb). With several commercial diets, she has lost weight but always gains it back. She has a sedentary job, and often skips breakfast or eats dinner on the run. She states she cannot fit exercise into her busy day. She takes no medications and has no allergies.

On physical examination, temperature is normal, blood pressure is 132/70 mm Hg, pulse rate is 80/min, and respiration rate is 12/min. BMI is 32. There is no thyromegaly. The abdomen is obese, soft, nontender, and without striae. Fasting plasma glucose level is 106 mg/dL (5.9 mmol/L) and thyroid function test results are normal.

Which of the following is the most appropriate next step to help this patient achieve long-term weight reduction?

(A) Exercise 15-30 minutes 5 days/week
(B) Laparoscopic adjustable band surgery

(C) Orlistat
(D) Reduce current caloric intake by 500-1000 kcal/d

Item 52

A 75-year-old woman is evaluated during a follow-up examination for recently diagnosed symptomatic peripheral arterial disease. The patient has hypothyroidism, hypertension, atrial fibrillation, and smokes cigarettes (30-pack-year history). Her current medications are diltiazem, warfarin, hydrochlorothiazide, levothyroxine, calcium, and vitamin D.

On physical examination, she is afebrile, blood pressure is 140/82 mm Hg, pulse rate is 66/min, and respiration rate is 12/min. BMI is 21. Posterior tibialis and dorsalis pedis pulses are diminished bilaterally (1+); the skin on the anterior aspect of the lower legs is shiny and hairless. Heart rhythm is irregularly irregular and without murmurs. Neurologic and musculoskeletal examinations are normal.

Laboratory studies:

Total cholesterol	238 mg/dL (6.16 mmol/L)
HDL cholesterol	36 mg/dL (0.93 mmol/L)
LDL cholesterol	165 mg/dL (4.27 mmol/L)
Triglycerides	205 mg/dL (2.32 mmol/L)
Serum creatinine	0.9 mg/dL (79.6 µmol/L)

In addition to strongly recommending smoking cessation, which of the following is the safest treatment for this patient?

(A) Atorvastatin
(B) Pravastatin
(C) Rosuvastatin
(D) Simvastatin

Item 53

A 42-year-old woman is evaluated for a 6-month history of heavy menstrual bleeding. She has been menstruating for the last 8 days and is still going through 10 pads or more daily with frequent clots. She has fatigue but no dizziness. Previous evaluation for this problem has included normal thyroid function and prolactin testing. She has no other medical problems and takes no medications. Pelvic ultrasonography has demonstrated a large posterior submucosal fibroid. A surgical treatment is planned in 2 weeks.

On physical examination, vital signs are normal. Abdominal examination is benign, and the pelvic examination reveals a moderate amount of blood in the vaginal vault.

Hemoglobin level is 10.5 g/dL (105 g/L). Pregnancy test is negative.

Which of the following is the most appropriate next management step?

(A) Estrogen/progesterone multiphasic oral contraceptive
(B) Intravenous estrogen
(C) Oral medroxyprogesterone acetate
(D) Reevaluation in 1 week

Item 54

A 31-year-old woman is evaluated for a 4-week history of anterior knee pain. It developed insidiously and has progressively worsened. The pain worsens with prolonged sitting and with walking up and down stairs. There is no morning stiffness. She has no history of trauma. She is taking acetaminophen as needed for the pain.

On physical examination, vital signs are normal. The pain is reproduced by applying pressure to the surface of the patella with the knee in extension and moving the patella both laterally and medially. There is no effusion, swelling, or warmth. Range of knee motion is normal, without crepitus or pain.

Which of the following is the most likely diagnosis?

(A) Knee osteoarthritis
(B) Patellofemoral pain syndrome
(C) Pes anserine bursitis
(D) Prepatellar bursitis

Item 55

An 87-year-old woman is evaluated for dizziness of 1 year's duration. She describes feeling lightheaded and unsteady when she walks but has not fallen. She denies vertigo, tinnitus, headache, loss of consciousness, chest pain, palpitations, or focal weakness. Medical history is significant for hypertension, glaucoma, and left eye cataract. Current medications are lisinopril and latanoprost ophthalmic drops.

On physical examination, blood pressure is 142/72 mm Hg supine and 136/66 mm Hg standing, pulse rate is 72/min supine and 76/min standing. BMI is 22. On neurologic examination, she has 20/50 vision, decreased auditory acuity, and 4+/5 motor strength throughout. Vibration and position sensation are normal. There is no tremor, cogwheeling, or bradykinesia, and her gait is not ataxic, although she feels safer holding on to the wall. There is no nystagmus. The lungs are clear. Cardiovascular examination is normal.

Laboratory studies, including a metabolic profile and complete blood count, are normal.

Which of the following is the most appropriate management of this patient?

(A) Physical therapy with gait evaluation
(B) Replace latanoprost with timolol
(C) Replace lisinopril with losartan
(D) Vestibular rehabilitation therapy

Item 56

A 50-year-old woman is evaluated during a follow-up appointment for moderate depression. Eight weeks ago, she was started on bupropion; 4 weeks ago, the dose was increased to the maximal dose. At this time, her PHQ-9 score has not improved over baseline, and she confirms that her symptoms have not improved. She has no suicidal ideation and does not have hallucinations or other psychotic features. She has no previous episodes of high energy, spending sprees, lack of need of sleep, or previous psychiatric problems. She is not interested in psychotherapy at this time.

Which of the following is the most appropriate next step in treatment?

(A) Add buspirone
(B) Continue bupropion at current dose for an additional 8 weeks
(C) Discontinue bupropion, begin sertraline
(D) Refer for electroconvulsive therapy

Item 57

A 44-year-old man is evaluated during a routine examination. He is concerned about his general health and risk of diabetes mellitus. He has no medical problems. Both parents and his sister have type 2 diabetes mellitus.

On physical examination, temperature is normal, blood pressure is 130/79 mm Hg, pulse rate is 66/min, and respiration rate is 14/min. BMI is 28. The remainder of the physical examination is normal.

Laboratory studies:

Glucose (fasting)	104 mg/dL (5.8 mmol/L)
Total cholesterol	247 mg/dL (6.40 mmol/L)
HDL cholesterol	50 mg/dL (1.30 mmol/L)
LDL cholesterol	177 mg/dL (4.58 mmol/L)
Triglycerides	100 mg/dL (1.13 mmol/L)

Which of the following interventions is the most appropriate initial strategy to decrease this patient's chance of developing type 2 diabetes mellitus?

(A) Acarbose
(B) Metformin
(C) Pioglitazone
(D) Weight loss and exercise

Item 58

A physician is asked to advise the Pharmacy and Therapeutics Committee of the hospital regarding a new drug to prevent deep venous thrombosis (DVT), drug "Z." The physician reviews a recent randomized controlled trial of 5000 patients that compared drug Z with drug C, which is commonly used and is on the hospital's formulary. The following data are abstracted from the trial:

Study results:

Drug	DVT Cases
Drug Z (n = 2500)	25
Drug C (n = 2500)	50

Based on these data, how many patients need to be treated (number needed to treat, NNT) with drug Z, compared with drug C, to prevent one extra case of DVT?

(A) 1
(B) 2
(C) 25
(D) 100
(E) 167

Item 59

A 21-year-old man is evaluated in the emergency department for left ankle pain that began 6 hours ago when he inverted his left ankle while playing soccer. He was unable to bear weight immediately after the injury, but is now able to bear weight with some difficulty.

There is ecchymosis and swelling around the entire ankle joint, with tenderness to palpation of the anterior talofibular ligament. He is able to bear weight but finds it painful to do so. There is no tenderness to palpation of bony structures (lateral and medial malleolus, base of fifth metatarsal) or the Achilles tendon. There is no ankle instability. Compression of the distal tibia and fibula does not cause any discomfort (negative squeeze test).

Which of the following is the most appropriate management for this patient?

(A) Ankle joint corticosteroid injection
(B) Ankle MRI
(C) Ankle radiograph
(D) Ankle splinting
(E) Urgent surgical evaluation

Item 60

A 61-year-old woman is evaluated for hot flushes, which have been persistent for the last 10 years. They occur at least 7 times per day, last for approximately 60 seconds, and are associated with severe sweating, palpitations, and occasional nausea. She is awakened several times per night. She has tried herbal medications, including soy and black cohosh, but has not experienced any benefit. She has hypertension, type 2 diabetes mellitus, and hyperlipidemia. Five years ago, she developed deep venous thrombosis after hip replacement surgery. Her current medications are ramipril, metformin, atorvastatin, calcium, and vitamin D.

On physical examination, vital signs are normal. BMI is 29. The remainder of the examination is normal.

Which of the following is the most appropriate treatment?

(A) Citalopram
(B) Oral estrogen therapy
(C) Oral estrogen/progesterone therapy
(D) Topical (vaginal) estrogen
(E) Venlafaxine

Item 61

A 60-year-old man is evaluated for new-onset monocular cloudy vision of the left eye that began 4 hours ago. He has type 2 diabetes mellitus and coronary artery disease. His current medications are aspirin, simvastatin, lisinopril, metoprolol, and metformin.

On physical examination, vital signs are normal. When a light is shined into his left eye it is not reactive, but shining a light in his right eye causes his left pupil to contract (left afferent pupillary defect). The visual acuity of the right eye is 20/30, that of the left eye is 20/120. Retinal findings are shown. The remainder of the examination is normal.

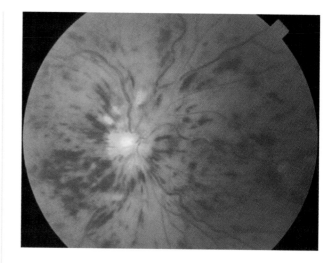

Which of the following is the most likely diagnosis?

(A) Acute angle closure glaucoma
(B) Central retinal artery occlusion
(C) Central retinal vein occlusion
(D) Retinal detachment

Item 62

A 62-year-old man is evaluated before elective total hip arthroplasty. He reports no prior medical problems aside from hip osteoarthritis. His only medications are ibuprofen and oxycodone. He drinks 1 pint of liquor daily.

On physical examination, temperature is normal, blood pressure is 100/62 mm Hg, and pulse rate is 92/min. He is alert and oriented. He has gynecomastia and multiple spider angiomata. He is jaundiced. There is ascites but no hepatomegaly or splenomegaly.

Laboratory studies:

Platelet count	52,000/µL (52 × 10⁹/L)
Bilirubin (total)	2.3 mg/dL (39.3 µmol/L)
Alanine aminotransferase	68 units/L
Aspartate aminotransferase	90 units/L
INR	1.8

Abdominal ultrasound shows a cirrhotic liver and ascites. The patient's Child-Turcotte-Pugh (CTP) score is class C.

Which of the following is the best management of this patient?

(A) Administer prednisolone for 1 week prior to surgery
(B) Administer vitamin K for 3 days prior to surgery
(C) Nonoperative management
(D) Proceed with surgery

Item 63

A 52-year-old man is evaluated during a routine examination. He is asymptomatic but is concerned about his weight. Medical history is significant for prediabetes and elevated cholesterol levels. He smokes one or two cigars a week. He drinks one or two alcoholic beverages a few nights each week. He does not get any regular exercise.

On physical examination, vital signs are normal. BMI is 33. The examination is otherwise unremarkable. The patient indicates he is ready to make important lifestyle changes to improve his health.

Which of the following is the best initial management?

(A) Assess the patient's confidence in making lifestyle changes
(B) Determine which lifestyle change the patient believes is most important
(C) Inform the patient he needs to lose weight
(D) Provide advice on smoking cessation

Item 64

A 56-year-old woman is evaluated during a follow-up visit after presenting as a new patient 2 weeks ago. At that time, her blood pressure was found to be elevated (156/88 mm Hg) and follow-up laboratory tests were ordered. She has had no major illnesses. Her father had type 2 diabetes mellitus and died at age 52 years of a myocardial infarction. She is currently taking no medications.

On physical examination, blood pressure is 156/92 mm Hg in the left arm and 160/90 mm Hg in the right arm. Pulse rate is 86/min and respiration rate is 16/min. BMI is 34. Waist circumference is 39 in (99 cm). Results of a funduscopic examination are normal.

Laboratory studies:

Blood urea nitrogen	16 mg/dL (5.7 mmol/L)
Creatinine	0.9 mg/dL (79.6 µmol/L)
LDL cholesterol (fasting)	162 mg/dL (4.19 mmol/L)
HDL cholesterol (fasting)	32 mg/dL (0.83 mmol/L)
Triglycerides (fasting)	148 mg/dL (1.67 mmol/L)
Glucose (fasting)	98 mg/dL (5.4 mmol/L)
Urinalysis	Trace protein, no glucose

In addition to hypertension and obesity, which of the following is the most likely diagnosis?

(A) Hypertriglyceridemia
(B) Impaired fasting glucose
(C) Metabolic syndrome
(D) No additional diagnoses

Item 65

An 85-year-old man is evaluated following a recent diagnosis of non–small cell lung cancer with metastatic disease to the liver, spine, multiple ribs, and sternum. He has declined treatment. The patient describes pain in his ribs that is present throughout the day and wakes him from sleep. He rates his pain as a 2 or 3 on a 10-point pain scale. His only medication is acetaminophen, 1000 mg every 6 hours, but this is not entirely effective in relieving his pain. Palpation of the right anterior chest and sternum reproduces his pain.

Which of the following is the most appropriate treatment?

(A) Gabapentin
(B) Ibuprofen
(C) Meperidine, orally
(D) Morphine, intramuscularly

Item 66

A 52-year-old man presents for routine care. Several years ago he was told that his cholesterol level was borderline. He is a vegetarian and a marathon runner, does not smoke, and drinks alcohol only socially. He takes a daily multivitamin. His father had a myocardial infarction at the age of 42 years.

On physical examination, vital signs are normal. BMI is 22. The remainder of the examination is normal.

Laboratory studies:

Total cholesterol	325 mg/dL (8.42 mmol/L)
HDL cholesterol	50 mg/dL (1.30 mmol/L)
LDL cholesterol	196 mg/dL (5.08 mmol/L)
Triglycerides	185 mg/dL (2.09 mmol/L)
Glucose	72 mg/dL (3.9 mmol/L)
Thyroid-stimulating hormone	0.52 µU/mL (0.52 mU/L)

Which of the following is the most appropriate management?

(A) Calculate the non-HDL cholesterol level
(B) Measure high-sensitivity C-reactive protein
(C) Initiate fibrate therapy
(D) Initiate statin therapy

Item 67

A 72-year-old woman is evaluated for a fall three nights ago. She lives in a single-floor apartment. At about 2 AM, she got up to go to the bathroom and fell after bumping into a wall. She had no lightheadedness or loss of consciousness and has not fallen before. Her home has no rugs and no thresholds between rooms. She normally has no problems walking and does not use an assistive device.

On physical examination, vital signs are normal. BMI is 23. She is alert and oriented. There are no orthostatic blood pressure changes or pulse changes. Visual testing using a Snellen chart reveals 20/20 distance vision in both eyes. The remainder of the physical examination, including a motor examination, is normal. In the Timed "Up & Go" test, she walks 10 feet in 10 seconds (normal, ≤14 sec).

Which of the following is the most appropriate next step in this patient's management?

(A) Ask about use of night lights
(B) Begin an individualized exercise program
(C) Ophthalmology evaluation
(D) Provide patient with a walker

Item 68

A 28-year-old woman is evaluated after being brought to the office by her boyfriend. He reports that she has been hearing voices and exhibiting increasingly paranoid behavior, believing that the mailman is trying to poison her. She has not gone to work in 4 weeks and spends most of her day alone in her bedroom wearing head phones and listening to heavy metal rock music. Her boyfriend reports that she has had several other episodes of paranoid behavior over the past 8 months but none as bad as the current one. The patient is minimally interactive. She previously drank two beers daily (none recently) and smoked marijuana at parties. Her father was diagnosed with schizophrenia at age 18 years. Her mother died of breast cancer 2 years ago after a long illness.

On physical examination, vital signs are normal. She appears disheveled and withdrawn. She is a thin woman, staring straight ahead and not making eye contact. She declines to talk to the physician or undress to be examined. A urine toxicology screen is positive for cannabinoids. A complete blood count and basic chemistry panel are normal.

Which of the following is the most likely diagnosis?

(A) Bipolar disorder
(B) *Cannabis* abuse with psychosis
(C) Major depressive disorder with psychotic features
(D) Schizophrenia

Item 69

A 20-year-old woman presents for a gynecologic examination and discussion of contraception. She has been sexually active for the past 3 years and has been using condoms. However, she finds condom use inconvenient, although she admits she is bad about remembering to take pills. She has had four partners in the past, currently has a new partner, has no history of sexually transmitted infection, and has never been pregnant. Medical history and family history are noncontributory. She drinks 2 to 4 beers on the weekends and does not smoke cigarettes.

Physical examination, including pelvic examination, is normal.

Which of the following is the most appropriate contraceptive recommendation for this patient?

(A) Condom use with combination estrogen-progesterone pills
(B) Condom use with subcutaneous progesterone implants
(C) Depot medroxyprogesterone acetate
(D) Estrogen-progesterone vaginal ring

Item 70

A 68-year-old man is evaluated for continuing urinary frequency and nocturia. His symptoms have been slowly progressive over the past 1 to 2 years with a weak urinary stream and hesitancy. He was started on doxazosin 6 months ago, which he tolerates well and initially provided some improvement. However, his symptoms have continued and are beginning to interfere with his quality of life, particularly the urinary frequency and nocturia. His only other medical problem is hypertension, for which he takes lisinopril and metoprolol.

On physical examination, he is afebrile, blood pressure is 140/85 mm Hg, pulse rate is 70/min, and respiration rate is 14/min. BMI is 25. He has a symmetric moderately enlarged prostate gland with no prostate nodules or areas of tenderness. A urinalysis is normal.

Which of the following is most appropriate next step in treatment of this patient's benign prostatic hyperplasia?

(A) Add finasteride
(B) Change doxazosin to finasteride
(C) Change doxazosin to tamsulosin
(D) Prescribe a fluoroquinolone antibiotic for 4 weeks

Item 71

A 30-year-old woman is evaluated during a routine examination in November. She received a routine tetanus, diphtheria, and acellular pertussis (Tdap) booster 5 years ago. She is sexually active with a single lifetime sexual partner. She has had no history of sexually transmitted infection. She was born in the United States and reports getting "routine shots" in childhood. She has had regular Pap smears without any abnormal results; her most recent was 3 years ago. She does not smoke cigarettes. She works as an attorney in a large corporate law firm. Findings on physical examination are unremarkable.

Which of the following vaccinations should be administered?

(A) Hepatitis B vaccine series
(B) Human papillomavirus vaccine series
(C) Influenza vaccine
(D) Tetanus and diphtheria (Td) vaccine

Item 72

A 32-year-old woman is evaluated following a diagnosis of chronic fatigue syndrome. She has a several-year history of chronic disabling fatigue, unrefreshing sleep, muscle and joint pain, and headache. A comprehensive evaluation has not identified any other medical condition, and a screen for depression is normal. Her only medications are multiple vitamins and dietary supplements. Physical examination is normal.

Which of the following is the most appropriate management for this patient's symptoms?

(A) Acyclovir
(B) Evening primrose oil
(C) Graded exercise program
(D) Growth hormone
(E) Sertraline

Item 73

A 36-year-old woman comes for her fifth visit in the past 3 months. She has a history of chronic abdominal pain and reports continued excruciating, diffuse, chronic abdominal pain and bloating. She has intermittent diarrhea and constipation, but reports no weight loss or other localizing symptoms. She is able to carry out routine activities of daily living. She has tried multiple over-the-counter medications as well as previous prescriptions for omeprazole, psyllium fiber supplements, dicyclomine, loperamide, and NSAIDs, all of which she states "do not touch" her pain. She states that she tried her friend's acetaminophen-oxycodone and had good relief. A previous workup (including complete blood count, comprehensive metabolic panel, amylase, lipase, anti-transglutaminase antibodies, and abdominal CT scan) was negative. She reports several episodes of abuse as a child and has been in a number of difficult and disruptive relationships as an adult. Although she smokes cigarettes, she denies any past or present alcohol or drug use. She is currently on no medications.

Results of the physical examination are normal. When her request for acetaminophen-oxycodone is denied, she becomes angry and upset, stating that all she needs is a medicine that works.

Which of the following is the most appropriate approach to this patient?

(A) Initiate an ongoing discussion of the causes and significance of her pain
(B) Prescribe a limited number of acetaminophen-oxycodone tablets
(C) Refer to a gastroenterologist
(D) Request that her care be transferred to another physician

Item 74

A 58-year-old man is evaluated as a new patient. A review of his previous records shows he received a pneumococcal vaccination 6 years ago when he was admitted to the hospital with community-acquired pneumonia. He feels well with no acute symptoms. He has type 2 diabetes mellitus, hypertension, and hyperlipidemia. Medications are insulin glargine, metformin, lisinopril, and simvastatin. Results of the physical examination are unremarkable.

When should this patient receive an additional pneumococcal vaccination?

(A) Today
(B) Today and repeat every 5 years
(C) Today and at age 65 years
(D) At age 65 years
(E) No further pneumococcal vaccinations are required

Item 75

A 30-year-old woman is evaluated for hyperlipidemia. Medical history is significant for type 1 diabetes mellitus, hypothyroidism, and hypertension. She is planning pregnancy. Her father was diagnosed with coronary artery disease at the age of 47 years. Her current medications are levothyroxine, hydrochlorothiazide, insulin glargine, and insulin aspart.

On physical examination, vital signs and the remainder of the physical examination are normal.

Laboratory studies:

Hemoglobin A_{1c}	8.1%
Total cholesterol	223 mg/dL (5.78 mmol/L)
HDL cholesterol	67 mg/dL (1.74 mmol/L)
LDL cholesterol	140 mg/dL (3.63 mmol/L)
Triglycerides	90 mg/dL (1.02 mmol/L)

In addition to recommending therapeutic lifestyle changes, which of the following is the most appropriate management of this patient's lipid levels?

(A) Colesevelam
(B) Ezetimibe
(C) Gemfibrozil
(D) Simvastatin

Item 76

A 67-year-old woman is admitted to the hospital with shortness of breath and is found to have a pulmonary embolus. She is begun on low-molecular-weight heparin. Upon further evaluation, a large left breast mass is found along with a malignant left-sided pleural effusion. Biopsy of the breast mass reveals poorly differentiated adenocarcinoma. Although she has a limited social support system and minimal understanding of her disease, she is interested in evaluating possible treatment options for her condition. She continues to have mild shortness of breath and marked anxiety related to her newly diagnosed condition, but otherwise feels well.

In addition to oncology and surgery consultations, which of the following is the most appropriate next step in this patient's care?

(A) Antidepressant therapy
(B) Hospice care referral
(C) Long-acting morphine
(D) Palliative care consultation

Item 77

A 32-year-old woman is evaluated for a 6-month history of nonproductive cough. She has no history of recurrent upper respiratory tract infections and has never smoked cigarettes. She has no fever, dyspnea on exertion, hemoptysis, heartburn, or wheezing. She has worked in the same office for 7 years and has lived in the same house for the past 20 years. She has not traveled out of the area for more than 2 years. She has no pets at home, no occupational or other exposure to toxic chemicals, and no family history of pulmonary disease. She takes no medications.

The vital signs and results of the physical examination are normal.

A complete blood count with differential is normal. Chest radiograph is normal. Pulmonary function tests are normal and a methacholine challenge test is negative.

Which of the following is the most appropriate diagnostic test to perform next?

(A) Bronchoscopy
(B) 24-hour esophageal pH manometry
(C) Sinus imaging
(D) Sputum testing for eosinophils

Item 78

A 78-year-old woman is evaluated after she tripped while carrying a garbage bag to the trash bin in her kitchen. She remembers falling but did not injure herself. She has had no previous falls. She reports no loss of consciousness, light-headedness, or dizziness. She has no history of seizures. She lives in a one-floor apartment with no steps, no loose rugs, and good lighting. She has a history of hypertension. Her daughter heard the fall and immediately came into the kitchen; when she entered, her mother was already getting back up and was not confused. Her only current medication is lisinopril.

On physical examination, blood pressure is 138/85 mm Hg, without orthostatic changes. There are no ecchymoses or tenderness over the hips and no pain on ambulation. The physical examination is otherwise normal.

Which of the following is the most appropriate management of this patient?

(A) Assess gait and mobility
(B) Discontinue lisinopril
(C) Prescribe an exercise program
(D) Provide a standard walker

Item 79

A 38-year-old woman is evaluated for left knee pain. The pain has been present for the past 3 weeks. Before onset, she had been preparing for a 5-kilometer race by running approximately 2 miles per day, 6 days per week, for the past 6 months. Walking up steps makes the pain worse; she also notes pain at night. She has never had this pain before.

On physical examination, vital signs are normal. There is tenderness to palpation located near the anteromedial aspect of the proximal tibia. A small amount of swelling is present at the insertion of the medial hamstring muscle. There is no medial or lateral joint line tenderness.

Which of the following is the most likely diagnosis?

(A) Iliotibial band syndrome
(B) Patellofemoral pain syndrome
(C) Pes anserine bursitis
(D) Prepatellar bursitis

Item 80

A 32-year-old woman at 30 weeks' gestation is evaluated for a 1-week history of thick, white vaginal discharge as well as severe vaginal itching and discomfort. She was diagnosed with vulvovaginal candidiasis 8 weeks ago, treated, and had symptom resolution at that time. Her only medication is a prenatal vitamin.

On physical examination, vital signs are normal. There is vulvar edema, erythema, and excoriations with a thick, white, "cottage cheese" discharge present in the vaginal vault. There is no cervical motion or adnexal tenderness. Vaginal pH is 4.5; potassium hydroxide preparation shows yeast and hyphae. There are no clue cells or motile trichomonads on saline microscopy.

Which of the following is the most appropriate treatment?

(A) Boric acid, topically
(B) Clotrimazole, topically
(C) Fluconazole, orally
(D) Voriconazole, orally

Item 81

A 56-year-old woman is evaluated for an 8-week history of persistent nonproductive cough. The cough is paroxysmal and is preceded by a tickle in the back of her throat. She has no shortness of breath, hemoptysis, fever, chills, sore throat, myalgia, otalgia, wheezing, or rhinorrhea. Approximately 3 months ago, she was diagnosed with type 2 diabetes mellitus and hypertension and was started on metformin, hydrochlorothiazide, lisinopril, and atorvastatin. She has a 10-pack-year history of tobacco use, but stopped smoking 5 years ago.

On physical examination, vital signs are normal. There is no conjunctival injection, oropharyngeal erythema, or cobblestoning. The lungs are clear and cardiovascular examination is unremarkable. Chest radiograph is normal.

Which of the following is the most appropriate treatment?

(A) Albuterol inhaler
(B) Discontinue lisinopril
(C) Loratadine
(D) Omeprazole

Item 82

A 70-year-old man is evaluated before elective cataract surgery. Aside from decreased vision he has no symptoms. He has coronary artery disease and a seizure disorder. He does not have chest pain, dyspnea, or recent seizures. He had a myocardial infarction 6 months ago and was treated with a drug-eluting stent placed in the left anterior descending coronary artery. Current medications are aspirin, clopidogrel, simvastatin, metoprolol, and phenytoin.

On physical examination, temperature is normal, blood pressure is 142/88 mm Hg, and pulse rate is 64/min. The remainder of the examination is normal.

Which of the following is the best perioperative management of this patient's medications?

(A) Continue all medications
(B) Discontinue clopidogrel 1 week before surgery
(C) Hold metoprolol the morning of surgery
(D) Hold phenytoin on the morning of surgery

Item 83

A 54-year-old man is evaluated for a long-standing history of COPD. Although he had previously done well, his lung function has progressively declined over the past year. He is oxygen dependent and is unable to perform even minor physical activity without severe dyspnea. He is not a transplant candidate and is unhappy with his quality of life and prognosis. He requests a prescription that he can take that will cause him to die at the time of his choosing.

Which of the following is the most appropriate next step in management of this patient's request?

(A) Assess the adequacy of his current treatment
(B) Consult legal counsel about state law in such cases
(C) Decline the request
(D) Prescribe sedating medication that could ensure a comfortable death

Item 84

A 37-year-old woman is evaluated for right forefoot pain on the plantar surface. She describes the pain as burning in character and worsening with standing. She feels as if she is "walking on a marble." The pain began 2 to 3 months ago. She has never had this problem before. She frequently wears high heels.

On physical examination, there is tenderness to palpation on the plantar surface of the foot in the space between the third and fourth toes. There is no tenderness to palpation of the plantar surface of the metatarsal head, no tenderness to palpation of the metatarsophalangeal joint, and no dorsal metatarsal tenderness to palpation.

Which of the following is the most likely diagnosis?

(A) Hammer toe
(B) Metatarsal stress fracture
(C) Morton neuroma
(D) Tarsal tunnel syndrome

Item 85

A 25-year-old woman presents as a new patient for re-evaluation of an abdominal mass. She reports finding a right lower quadrant mass 9 months ago. She reports that the mass has been stable in size, does not vary with meals or a Valsalva maneuver, and is not tender. She has had no change in bowel habits. A review of her chart reveals that she has been seen by two internists, a gastroenterologist, and a general surgeon since her initial presentation. All reported normal physical examination findings. She has no history of colorectal cancer. She has been unable to work because of the mass.

On physical examination, her affect is normal, with no evidence of delusional thinking or hallucinations. Vital signs are normal. Abdominal examination shows no masses or hernia. Results of a metabolic panel are normal. An abdominal ultrasound 5 months ago and a CT scan of the abdomen and pelvis 3 months ago both were normal.

Which of the following is the most appropriate management?

(A) Cognitive-behavioral therapy
(B) Diazepam
(C) MRI of the abdomen
(D) Olanzapine

Item 86

A 42-year-old woman is evaluated in the emergency department after fainting earlier in the evening. She was at a dinner party and reports having two glasses of wine. After standing for approximately 35 minutes, she felt warm, diaphoretic, and anxious; as she moved toward a chair, she lost consciousness. She recovered spontaneously within 2 minutes and has been completely lucid ever since. Medical history is significant only for hypothyroidism and perennial allergies; medications are levothyroxine and fexofenadine.

On physical examination, she is alert and oriented. Vital signs are normal without orthostatic changes. Thyroid is normal. The remainder of the physical examination is normal. A 12-lead electrocardiogram is normal.

Which of the following is the most appropriate next step in the management of this patient?

(A) Admit to hospital for observation and telemetry
(B) Head CT scan
(C) Obtain echocardiography
(D) Perform tilt-table testing
(E) No further testing

Item 87

A 78-year-old-woman is evaluated in the emergency department after she fell at home last night. She has long-standing sleeping difficulties and last night got out of bed and fell in her hallway. She had no loss of consciousness and notes left hip pain. She has hypertension, hyperlipidemia, and gastroesophageal reflux disease. Her current medications are lisinopril, simvastatin, and omeprazole.

On physical examination, she is afebrile. Blood pressure is 142/82 mm Hg supine and 138/76 mm Hg standing, and pulse rate is 76/min supine and 78/min standing. She appears frail with generalized weakness. There is mild tenderness in the left lateral hip and weakness of the quadriceps muscles bilaterally. There are no ecchymoses in the left hip area. She is slow getting up from a chair and has a slow walking speed but no ataxia. Distance vision using glasses without bifocal lenses evaluated with a Snellen chart is normal. There is mild difficulty with near vision evaluated using a near-vision testing card. Lungs are clear. The heart rhythm is regular with no murmur. There is no focal neurologic deficit. Radiograph of the left hip and femur reveals no fracture.

Acetaminophen is prescribed for pain. Arrangements are made for home physical therapy and for a visiting nurse to perform a home safety evaluation.

Which of the following is the most appropriate additional management of this patient?

(A) Discontinue lisinopril
(B) Prescribe vitamin D
(C) Prescribe zolpidem at bedtime
(D) Refer for prescription glasses with bifocal lenses

Item 88

A 69-year-old woman is evaluated for involuntary leakage of urine with coughing, sneezing, laughing, or when lifting heavy boxes at work. She has no dysuria, frequency, or urgency and she has no mobility problems. She is gravida 4, para 4, and underwent a total abdominal hysterectomy 20 years ago for uterine fibroids. She has type 2 diabetes mellitus. Medications are metformin and lisinopril. She has no known drug allergies.

On physical examination, vital signs are normal. BMI is 31. There is bulging of the anterior vaginal wall when the patient is asked to cough, accompanied by leakage of urine. Bimanual examination is unremarkable. The remainder of her examination is normal.

Laboratory studies show fasting plasma glucose level of 89 mg/dL (5.0 mmol/L) with hemoglobin A$_{1c}$ of 6.5%. Urinalysis is normal.

Which of the following is the most appropriate treatment?

(A) Pelvic floor muscle training
(B) Prompted voiding
(C) Pubovaginal sling
(D) Tolterodine

Item 89

A 97-year-old woman was hospitalized with jaundice, abdominal pain, weight loss, nausea, and intermittent vomiting 1 week ago. She was found to have poorly differentiated metastatic pancreatic adenocarcinoma. She lives with her daughter. Current medications are morphine, a stool softener, and a laxative. On physical examination, vital signs are normal. She is a depressed-appearing woman in no distress who appears cachectic but comfortable.

During bedside discussions, the patient has deferred all medical decision-making to her family. They have asked that "everything be done" and have declined to place the patient on do-not-resuscitate status. They have requested that a surgeon be consulted to remove the cancer and that an oncologist be consulted for initiation of chemotherapy. The health care team has arranged a family meeting to address end-of-life care.

Which of the following is the best initial communication strategy for the family meeting?

(A) Ask the patient's opinion about an advanced directive
(B) Explain that curative therapy is futile
(C) Explain the diagnosis and the prognosis
(D) Explore the family's understanding about the patient's condition

Item 90

A 62-year-old woman is evaluated for a 3-month history of a palpable nonpainful breast mass. She has no nipple discharge. She underwent menarche at age 14 years and menopause at age 55 years. She has no history of previous breast biopsies and no family history of breast, ovarian, or colorectal cancer. Her current medications are calcium and vitamin D. She took hormone replacement therapy for 1 year after menopause because of vasomotor symptoms.

On physical examination, temperature is 37.4 °C (99.3 °F), blood pressure is 135/80 mm Hg, pulse rate is 80/min, and respiration rate is 14/min. There is a firm, nontender mass in the upper outer quadrant of the right breast, approximately 2 cm at its largest dimension. There is no nipple discharge or change in or fixation to the overlying skin. There is no axillary lymphadenopathy. A diagnostic mammogram obtained 2 days before the visit revealed no masses or calcifications.

Which of the following is the most appropriate management of this patient?

(A) Breast MRI
(B) Breast ultrasonography
(C) Core needle biopsy
(D) Reassurance

Item 91

A 44-year-old man is evaluated for low back pain. Five days ago he was playing racquetball when he felt a popping sensation in his back and felt a shooting pain down his leg. The pain worsened over the next 2 to 3 days, causing some difficulty with sleeping. He started taking ibuprofen on day 2, and has improved slightly since then. He currently rates his pain as 5 or 6 out of 10. He has no numbness, weakness, or bladder/bowel incontinence.

On physical examination, vital signs are normal. BMI is 31. Straight leg raise test on both the left and right sides reproduces pain in the left leg. The ankle reflex is diminished on the left side compared with the right side. He is able to walk with some discomfort. No motor or sensory deficits are observed. Saddle anesthesia is not present. Rectal tone is normal.

Which of the following is the most appropriate management of this patient?

(A) Analgesics and mobilization as tolerated
(B) Complete blood count and erythrocyte sedimentation rate
(C) Epidural corticosteroid injection
(D) Lumbar spine MRI
(E) Lumbar spine radiograph

Item 92

A 75-year-old man is hospitalized with sepsis leading to multi-organ failure. A meeting with family members is convened to discuss goals of care for the patient. The treatment team, including infectious disease and critical care consultants, has indicated that the patient is deteriorating despite optimized therapy, and the prognosis is poor. The daughter brings an Internet printout of a trial of a new medication for sepsis. The abstract states "We gave drug 'X' to 100 consecutive patients with refractory sepsis in our five intensive care units located in the same geographic region. Eight percent were alive at 30 days." Although drug "X" is marketed in the United States, it is not FDA-approved for treatment of sepsis. A quick literature search reveals no other studies of drug "X" in the treatment of sepsis.

Which of the following is the main reason that it is difficult to determine the effectiveness of drug "X" based on the published study?

(A) No comparison group

(B) Outcome assessment not blinded

(C) Patients not randomly assigned to treatment

(D) Small study size

Item 93

A 37-year-old man is seen as a new patient. He requests a refill of dexamphetamine, which he takes for attention-deficit/hyperactivity disorder (ADHD). He was diagnosed in childhood when he had difficulty in school and has been on the medication ever since. His symptoms are generally well controlled with occasional impulsive behavior (traffic ticket 3 years ago, confrontation with his boss 5 years ago). He has had no problems over the past 2 years. He is otherwise healthy and drinks three or four beers per week. He smokes socially, less than one pack per week. He does not use illicit drugs. His only medication is dexamphetamine.

On physical examination, temperature is 36.6 °C (97.8 °F), blood pressure is 149/92 mm Hg, pulse rate is 96/min, and respiration rate is 14/min. BMI is 23. The remainder of the physical examination is normal.

Which of the following is the most appropriate management?

(A) Continue dexamphetamine

(B) Switch to atomoxetine

(C) Switch to fluoxetine

(D) Switch to methylphenidate

(E) Stop medications and reassess

Item 94

An 85-year-old woman is evaluated before hospital discharge after a 2-week hospitalization for a traumatic right hip fracture treated with open reduction and internal fixation complicated by a pulmonary embolism, catheter-associated urosepsis, and acute delirium. She has improved steadily but continues to require low-level supplemental oxygen, remains significantly debilitated, and is able to participate in only 30 minutes of physical therapy daily. Medical history is significant for type 2 diabetes mellitus, hypertension, depression, and obesity. Her daughter meets with the treating internist to discuss discharge planning. She feels her mother has been failing for several years and

is no longer able to live independently as she had before hospitalization. She asks that the patient be transferred back to the hospital or emergency department if she develops more acute medical issues following discharge, and requests that the patient receive everything short of aggressive resuscitation with cardiopulmonary resuscitation and intubation if this situation were to arise. The treating internist meets separately with the patient and she agrees that these are her preferences.

Based on the patient's medical status and the wishes of the patient and her family, which of the following postdischarge care options is most appropriate?

(A) Inpatient rehabilitation facility

(B) Long term acute care hospital

(C) Residential hospice facility

(D) Skilled nursing facility

Item 95

A 76-year-old woman is evaluated for a 1-day history of headache, left eye pain, nausea and vomiting, seeing halos around lights, and decreased visual acuity of the left eye. She has type 2 diabetes mellitus, hypertension, and atrial fibrillation. Medications are metformin, digoxin, metoprolol, hydrochlorothiazide, and warfarin.

On physical examination, temperature is 36.8 °C (98.2 °F), blood pressure is 148/88 mm Hg, pulse rate is 104/min, and respiration rate is 16/min. Visual acuity wearing glasses is 20/40 (right eye) and 20/100 (left eye). The left eye has conjunctival erythema. The right pupil is reactive to light, the left pupil is sluggish and constricts in response to light from 6 mm to 4 mm. On palpation of the ocular globe, the left globe feels firm as compared with the right.

Which of the following is the most likely diagnosis?

(A) Acute angle-closure glaucoma

(B) Central retinal artery occlusion

(C) Ocular migraine

(D) Temporal arteritis

Item 96

A 28-year-old man is evaluated for pain on the radial aspect of the right wrist that occurs with use of the thumb. The pain has been present for 2 weeks. He has never had this pain before and has not had any trauma. He works as a computer programmer and plays video games for 3 to 4 hours each night when he gets home from work.

On physical examination, vital signs are normal. Localized tenderness to palpation is present over the distal radial styloid; pain is present with resisted thumb abduction and extension, and the patient has pain on the radial side of the thumb when he is asked to make a fist over the fully flexed thumb and then to ulnar deviate the hand (positive Finkelstein test). There are no palpable masses; there is no joint pain, bogginess, or swelling; sensation is intact throughout the wrist and hand, strength is 5/5 throughout.

Which of the following is the most likely diagnosis?

(A) Carpometacarpal arthritis

(B) de Quervain tenosynovitis

(C) Flexor carpi radialis ganglion cyst

(D) Scaphoid fracture

Item 97

A 32-year-old woman is evaluated for a 3-month history of left-sided jaw pain and clicking below her left ear when she chews. She reports no joint problems elsewhere, no visual changes, and no headache other than the jaw pain. She has some trouble sleeping at night, but the pain is more likely to affect her at work. Once or twice a month she goes home early because of jaw pain.

On physical examination, temperature is 37.3 °C (99.1 °F), blood pressure is 118/72 mm Hg, and pulse rate is 60/min. There is mild tenderness and palpable crepitus over the left temporomandibular joint. Otoscopy is normal bilaterally. She has no lymphadenopathy, rash, or salivary gland masses. Oropharynx is normal. Thyroid is normal. She has no tooth pain when teeth are tapped with a tongue blade.

Which of the following is the most appropriate next step in management?

(A) Fluoxetine

(B) Ibuprofen

(C) Jaw MRI

(D) Jaw relaxation, heat, and therapeutic exercises

(E) Radiography of the teeth

Item 98

A 49-year-old woman is evaluated for vertigo of 1 week's duration. She was seen 1 week ago in the emergency department. During that visit, she described severe vertigo that predictably occurred while abruptly turning her head to the right and lasted less than 1 minute. She had no antecedent viral illness, headache, hearing loss, tinnitus, diplopia, dysarthria, dysphagia, or weakness. She was diagnosed with benign paroxysmal positional vertigo and given instructions for head tilting exercises (Epley maneuver). Her symptoms improved but have not abated. She is afraid to drive because of the symptoms. She has no history of hypertension, diabetes mellitus, hyperlipidemia, or tobacco use.

On physical examination, vital signs are normal. With the Dix-Hallpike maneuver, she develops horizontal nystagmus and nausea after 15 seconds. The nystagmus lasts approximately 1 minute. The Epley maneuver is unsuccessful in relieving symptoms. The remainder of the examination is normal, including the neurologic examination.

Which of the following is the most appropriate management?

(A) Brain MRI

(B) Hydrochlorothiazide

(C) Meclizine

(D) Vestibular rehabilitation

Item 99

An 84-year-old man who resides in a skilled nursing facility is brought to the office by his daughter, who reports that he has become less active in the past few months. The patient does not have a change in mood. He has multiple somatic symptoms including headache, scalp pain, and constipation, all of which are long-standing, intermittent, of brief duration, and not associated with any positive physical examination or laboratory test findings. There has been no weight loss. He has osteoarthritis but has no difficulty with ambulation and has had no falls. His wife died 4 months ago. His only medication is acetaminophen.

On physical examination, he is afebrile, blood pressure is 148/92 mm Hg, and pulse rate is 68/min. He is slow to respond but answers questions appropriately. He is alert and oriented. His gait is slow but otherwise unremarkable. The remainder of the physical examination is normal.

Complete blood count, comprehensive metabolic profile, and serum thyroid-stimulating hormone level are normal.

Which of the following is the most appropriate diagnostic test to perform next?

(A) Dix-Hallpike maneuver

(B) Mini–Mental State Examination

(C) PHQ-9 depression assessment

(D) Timed "Up & Go" test

Item 100

A 60-year-old woman is evaluated for increased irritability and anxiety. She was in an automobile accident 3 months ago in which she was rear-ended by a car at a stop light. Since that time she has nightmares about the incident and states she has not returned to driving for fear of being in another accident. Her sleep is poor and her husband states she is becoming more socially isolated since she has stopped driving. She has continued to perform her usual hobbies at home. She has no suicidal thoughts. On physical examination, all vital signs are normal.

Which of the following is the most likely diagnosis?

(A) Generalized anxiety disorder

(B) Major depressive disorder

(C) Obsessive-compulsive disorder

(D) Posttraumatic stress disorder

Item 101

A 59-year-old woman is evaluated in the emergency department for midsternal chest pain. The pain began several hours ago as a vague ache in her left upper sternal region that progressed in intensity and severity. The pain abated spontaneously after approximately 45 minutes. She had no further chest pain until several hours later, when it recurred unprovoked by exertion. She has no shortness of breath, nausea or vomiting, syncope, previous history of chest pain, or known cardiac disease or risk factors for venous thromboembolism. Medical history is significant for hyperlipidemia and hypertension. She does not smoke cigarettes. Medications are simvastatin, aspirin, lisinopril, and hydrochlorothiazide.

On physical examination, she is afebrile, blood pressure is 110/70 mm Hg, pulse rate is 68/min, and respiration rate is 22/min. BMI is 28. Oxygen saturation on ambient air is 97%. Estimated central venous pressure is 8 cm H_2O and carotid pulses are without bruits. Lungs are clear. Heart sounds are normal. There is a grade 2/6 holosystolic murmur at the left sternal border with radiation to the apex. There is no lower extremity edema. The remainder of the examination is normal.

Electrocardiogram is shown. Chest radiograph is normal.

Which of the following is the most appropriate initial management of this patient?

(A) Adenosine stress test
(B) Admit to the coronary care unit
(C) CT pulmonary angiography
(D) Ibuprofen administration

Item 102

A 36-year-old man is evaluated during a routine health examination. He has no family history of hypertension, hyperlipidemia, or cardiovascular disease. He has never used tobacco, drinks approximately two beers each week, and does not use illicit drugs. He is fairly sedentary but feels well and is without cardiovascular or other symptoms.

On physical examination, he is afebrile, blood pressure is 112/70 mm Hg, and pulse rate is 76/min. BMI is 25.

Laboratory studies:

Total cholesterol	148 mg/dL (3.83 mmol/L)
LDL cholesterol	96 mg/dL (2.48 mmol/L)
HDL cholesterol	44 mg/dL (1.14 mmol/L)
Triglycerides	88 mg/dL (0.99 mmol/L)

Which of the following is the recommended interval for follow-up screening for hypertension in this patient?

(A) 1 year
(B) 2 years
(C) 3 years
(D) 4 years
(E) 5 years

Item 103

A 72-year-old woman is evaluated for short-term memory loss. She has trouble remembering names, where she placed certain items such as her keys, and occasionally, what she did earlier in the day. She avoids some social situations and feels lower self esteem because of memory problems and decreased social contact, but notes no depression, low energy, or sleep disturbance, and she still enjoys playing cards with her husband. She does not need help with eating, dressing, or bathing. She has hypertension, well controlled with hydrochlorothiazide. She has no history of stroke. She is concerned about her condition and wants to know if anything can be done about it.

On physical examination, temperature is 37.2 °C (98.9 °F), blood pressure is 135/84 mm Hg, and pulse rate is 72/min. She is conversant, with a normal range of affect. Neurologic examination is without focal deficit. The remainder of the physical examination is normal. Mini–Mental State Examination score is 26.

Which of the following is the most appropriate management of this patient?

(A) Anticholinesterase inhibitor
(B) Cognitive rehabilitation

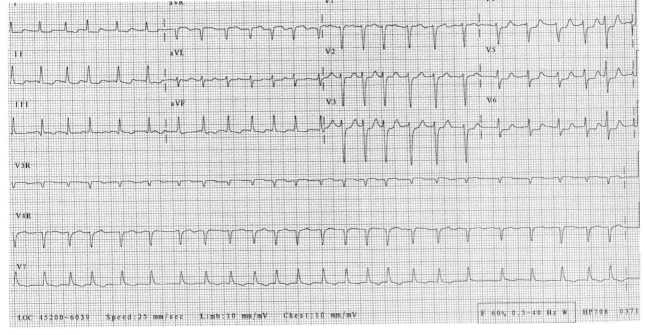

ITEM 101

(C) PET scan

(D) Reassurance that progression to dementia is unlikely

Item 104

A 70-year-old man is evaluated for sharp left-sided pleuritic chest pain and shortness of breath that began suddenly 24 hours ago. The pain has been persistent over the past 24 hours and does not worsen or improve with exertion or position. History is significant for severe COPD, hypertension, and hyperlipidemia. He is a current smoker with a 52-pack-year history of smoking. Medications are ipratropium, albuterol, lisinopril, simvastatin, and aspirin.

On physical examination, temperature is normal, blood pressure is 128/80 mm Hg, pulse rate is 88/min, and respiration rate is 18/min. BMI is 24. Oxygen saturation on ambient air is 89%. Cardiac examination reveals distant heart sounds but no S_3. Lung examination reveals hyperresonance, decreased chest wall expansion, and decreased breath sounds on the left. The trachea is midline.

Which of the following is the most appropriate diagnostic test to perform next?

(A) Chest CT

(B) Chest radiography

(C) Echocardiography

(D) Electrocardiography

Item 105

A 28-year-old man is evaluated for a 6-week history of intractable nausea. He states he is nauseated all day although he is able to eat if he forces himself. He has had no vomiting, weight loss, or change in stool pattern. He went to an emergency department last week because of his symptoms, and the results of laboratory testing at that time were normal.

He reports a 1-year history of intermittent episodes of severe right upper quadrant abdominal pain and bloating, as well as separate episodes of intermittent numbness of the right side of his face and body. He says that he has had neck and back pain, dysuria, intermittent odynophagia, and loss of libido for the past 3 years. He does not have sleep disturbance, anhedonia, or crying spells. Prior laboratory testing, upper endoscopy, colonoscopy, CT scan of the abdomen and pelvis, and MRI of the cervical and lumbar spine were normal. Current medications are acetaminophen, odansetron, and tramadol. He is currently unemployed.

On physical examination, vital signs are normal. The abdomen shows diffuse tenderness to palpation but is otherwise normal. Neurologic examination is normal. A two-question depression screen is normal.

Which of the following is the most likely diagnosis?

(A) Celiac disease

(B) Malingering

(C) Multiple sclerosis

(D) Somatization disorder

Item 106

A 28-year-old man is evaluated for a 6-month history of pelvic pain, urinary frequency, and painful ejaculation. He has been treated with antibiotics for urinary tract infections three times in the past 6 months, each time with temporary relief of symptoms but recurrence shortly after completion of antibiotics.

On physical examination, vital signs are normal. There is minimal suprapubic tenderness with palpation. The prostate is of normal size with minimal tenderness and no nodules. Urinalysis shows multiple leukocytes, bacteria, and no erythrocytes.

Which of the following is the most appropriate treatment of this patient?

(A) 1-week course of trimethoprim-sulfamethoxazole

(B) 1-month course of ciprofloxacin

(C) Cognitive-behavioral therapy

(D) Finasteride

Item 107

A 28-year-old woman is evaluated for headache, purulent nasal discharge, and left unilateral facial and maxillary tooth pain present for 4 days.

On physical examination, temperature is 37.3 °C (99.1 °F); vital signs are otherwise normal. There is mild tenderness to palpation over the maxillary sinus on the left. Nasal examination shows inflamed turbinates bilaterally with a small amount of purulent discharge. Maxillary transillumination is darker on the left than on the right. Otoscopic examination is normal bilaterally. There is no lymphadenopathy in the head or neck.

Which of the following is the most appropriate next step in management?

(A) Amoxicillin

(B) Chlorpheniramine

(C) Nasal culture

(D) Sinus CT

(E) Systemic corticosteroids

Item 108

A 72-year-old woman is evaluated for sudden hearing loss in the left ear with moderate ringing that started yesterday. She has no vertigo or dizziness.

On physical examination, vital signs are normal. Otoscopic examination is initially obscured by cerumen bilaterally. Once cerumen is removed, the tympanic membranes appear normal and there is some redness in the canals bilaterally. When a 512 Hz tuning fork is placed on top of the head, it is louder in the right ear. When placed adjacent to the left ear, it is heard better when outside the ear canal than when touching the mastoid bone. Neurologic examination is normal other than left-sided hearing loss.

Which of the following is the most appropriate management of this patient?

(A) Acyclovir
(B) Neomycin, polymyxin B, and hydrocortisone ear drops
(C) Triethanolamine ear drops
(D) Urgent audiometry and referral

Item 109

A 78-year-old man is brought to the emergency department with a 1-hour history of vomiting bright red blood. Despite profuse hematemesis, he clearly states that he does not want a blood transfusion for religious reasons. Four minutes after he arrives, he starts to have new severe substernal chest pain and 2 minutes later loses consciousness. His wife, who he appointed his agent with durable power of attorney for health care, confirms his long-standing religious beliefs against transfusion. Medical history is significant for coronary artery disease, hypertension, and hyperlipidemia. There is no history of cognitive decline or impaired judgment. His current medications are aspirin, simvastatin, and amlodipine.

On physical examination, temperature is 36.8 °C (98.2 °F), blood pressure is 80/40 mm Hg, pulse rate is 156/min, and respiration rate is 24/min. His skin is pale, clammy, and cool to touch. The chest is clear to auscultation. Cardiac examination reveals tachycardia but is otherwise normal. The abdomen is soft and nondistended.

Complete blood count shows a hemoglobin level of 6 g/dL (60 g/L) and hematocrit of 18%. Electrocardiogram shows 2- to 3-mm ST-segment depression in leads V_3 through V_6.

Which of the following is the most appropriate management?

(A) Immediate blood transfusion
(B) Obtain an emergency court-appointed guardian
(C) Seek permission from the patient's wife to transfuse
(D) Treat without transfusion

Item 110

A 24-year-old man is evaluated in the emergency department for a 6-hour history of acute scrotal pain. The pain occurred suddenly while mowing the lawn. The patient is not sexually active and has no recent trauma, history of penile discharge, urinary urgency, frequency, or dysuria.

On physical examination, he is afebrile, blood pressure is 160/100 mm Hg, pulse rate is 100/min, and respiration rate is 12/min. The right testicle rides high in the scrotum and is exquisitely tender. The cremasteric reflex is absent on the right side. There is no abnormal mass in the scrotum or inguinal area. There is no penile discharge. A urinalysis is normal.

Which of the following is the most likely diagnosis?

(A) Epididymitis
(B) Strangulated inguinal hernia
(C) Orchitis
(D) Testicular torsion

Item 111

A 25-year-old woman is evaluated for a 1-week history of malodorous vaginal discharge associated with vulvar itching and burning. She is sexually active and has had three partners in the past 6 months. She has no history of sexually transmitted infection.

On physical examination, vital signs are normal. BMI is 22. There is a thin, gray, homogeneous discharge coating the vaginal walls. There are no external genital lesions and no vulvar erythema or excoriations. The cervix appears normal. There is no cervical motion tenderness or adnexal tenderness. Vaginal pH is 6.0, "whiff" test is positive. Results of saline microscopy are shown. Microscopy after the addition of potassium hydroxide does not show hyphae or pseudohyphae. A urine pregnancy test is negative.

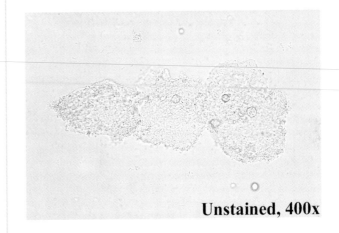

Unstained, 400x

Which of the following is the most appropriate treatment?

(A) Clotrimazole cream, 7-day topical regimen
(B) Fluconazole, single-dose oral regimen
(C) Metronidazole, 7-day oral regimen
(D) Metronidazole, single-dose oral regimen

Item 112

A 56-year-old man is evaluated for a 7-month history of difficulty maintaining erections. He has difficulty with sexual intercourse and achieving orgasm. He reports that sexual desire is good. He does not have penile curvature, genital pain, depressed mood, or anxiety. He has not tried anything for this problem. He is active, jogging for 30 minutes 4 to 5 times per week. He has type 2 diabetes mellitus, which is diet controlled, and hyperlipidemia. He does not use alcohol, tobacco, or illicit drugs. Current medications are aspirin and simvastatin.

On physical examination, he is afebrile, blood pressure is 124/70 mm Hg, and pulse rate is 76/min. BMI is 24. The testes are bilaterally descended and normal in size and consistency, the penis is normal in appearance, and there is normal distribution of male secondary hair. Rectal examination reveals a normal-sized prostate. Posterior tibialis and dorsalis pedis pulses are palpable bilaterally and the neurologic examination is normal.

Serum thyroid-stimulating hormone level is 2.95 μU/mL (2.95 mU/L) and early morning serum total testosterone level is 320 ng/dL (11 nmol/L).

Which of the following is the most appropriate treatment?

(A) Intracavernosal alprostadil
(B) Penile pump
(C) Sildenafil
(D) Testosterone therapy

Item 113

A 78-year-old woman was recently admitted to the hospital for an acute exacerbation of chronic heart failure. She has coronary artery disease and hypertension. During that admission she was treated with intravenous diuretics, with reduction of her weight to slightly below her established optimal weight goal and resolution of her heart failure symptoms. Upon discharge her dosages of lisinopril and oral furosemide were increased from their preadmission level, and spironolactone was started. She was scheduled for a follow-up appointment with her internist in 1 week.

Four days after discharge she presents to the emergency department because of worsening shortness of breath since hospital discharge and is readmitted for further treatment. She has no chest pain but has noticed increased swelling in her lower extremities. She states that she has been taking her medications as directed.

On physical examination, temperature is 37.4 °C (99.3 °F), blood pressure is 115/78 mm Hg, and respiration rate is 18/min. Oxygen saturation on ambient air is 89%. The chest examination reveals mild bilateral crackles at the lung bases. Heart examination shows a regular rate without murmur. There is trace lower extremity edema. The remainder of the examination is unremarkable.

Laboratory studies are significant for normal serum electrolyte levels and a serum creatinine level of 1.2 mg/dL (106 μmol/L) (unchanged from discharge). A chest radiograph shows bilateral hilar infiltrates consistent with pulmonary edema.

Which of the following is the most likely cause of her readmission?

(A) Diuretic resistance
(B) Inadequate hospital follow-up
(C) Medication nonadherence
(D) Spironolactone intolerance

Item 114

An 84-year-old man is evaluated for a 5-day history of rhinitis, nasal congestion, sneezing, and nonproductive cough. The symptoms began with a sore throat, which resolved after 24 hours. He has mild ear pain when blowing his nose or coughing. He has a history of coronary artery disease and hypertension. Medications are aspirin, metoprolol, and hydrochlorothiazide.

On physical examination, temperature is 36.5 °C (97.7 °F), blood pressure is 130/72 mm Hg, pulse rate is 82/min, and respiration rate is 16/min. He has nasal congestion and has an occasional cough. There is mild clear nasal discharge with no sinus tenderness. The oropharynx is without injection or exudate. There is no lymphadenopathy. External auditory canals are normal. The tympanic membranes are dull bilaterally but without injection. A small left middle ear effusion is noted.

Which of the following is the most appropriate management?

(A) Amoxicillin
(B) Erythromycin
(C) Referral to an otorhinolaryngologist
(D) Reassurance and observation

Item 115

A 32-year-old man is evaluated for daytime fatigue of 9 months' duration. He has never fallen asleep at the wheel, but falls asleep at other times during the day. He does not think he snores, but his wife is unavailable to confirm this. He reports no leg symptoms. He has no significant medical history and takes no medications. He does not smoke. He drinks two or three beers on Friday and Saturday nights. He does not exercise regularly, and has gained 9.1 kg (20 lb) since getting married 18 months ago.

On physical examination, temperature is normal, blood pressure is 128/76 mm Hg, and pulse rate is 82/min. BMI is 32. Neck circumference is 43 cm (17 in). Pharynx is normal. The thyroid is difficult to palpate owing to the patient's large neck size. The lungs are clear, and the cardiovascular and neurologic examinations are normal.

In addition to counseling regarding sleep hygiene and weight loss, which of the following is the most appropriate management for this patient?

(A) Advise alcohol abstinence
(B) Initiate therapy with zolpidem
(C) Order iron studies
(D) Refer for polysomnography

Item 116

A 46-year-old man is evaluated for dull, aching, right groin pain. He says it has been present for the past 3 months. The pain was initially severe, improved for a few weeks, but slowly has been worsening since that time. He is now walking with a limp. He has no history of trauma. He drinks six beers a day and has done so for the past 25 years. He is a current smoker, with a 30-pack-year history.

On physical examination, vital signs are normal. He has limited internal and external rotation of the right hip. Internal rotation is limited to a greater degree than external rotation and pain is present with rotating the thigh medially and laterally (log-rolling). Radiographs of the right hip are normal.

Which of the following is the most likely diagnosis?

(A) Hip osteoarthritis
(B) L1 radiculopathy

(C) Osteonecrosis of the hip

(D) Septic arthritis of the hip

Item 117

A 33-year-old woman is evaluated for chronic pain. She has a history of fibromyalgia and reports widespread musculoskeletal pain involving her hips, knees, back, and neck with significant worsening in recent weeks. The pain in her neck and back is 7/10 in intensity and is constant. She participated in a 3-month course of physical therapy with little improvement in her symptoms. The patient reports that she is sleeping about 3 to 4 hours per night because her pain is keeping her awake. Previously she had been able to work, but now she has difficulty getting out of bed every day. Her current medications are gabapentin and duloxetine.

On physical examination, vital signs are normal. BMI is 28. She has several tender trigger points. Her neck has limited range of motion secondary to pain. There is tenderness to palpation over the paravertebral muscles of the lower lumbar spine. Strength is 5/5 in all extremities, reflexes are 2+ and symmetric, sensation to light touch and pinprick is normal throughout, and a straight leg raise test is negative. Her affect is flat.

Which of the following is the most appropriate management?

(A) Electromyogram/nerve conduction velocity study

(B) Evaluate for intimate partner violence

(C) High-dose ibuprofen

(D) Oxycodone/acetaminophen

Item 118

A 78-year-old man is evaluated for routine follow up of hypertension. He reports that he is able to perform all activities of daily living and that he only drives in the neighborhood and to nearby stores. He has used a cane while walking since he fell 3 months ago. His only medication is chlorthalidone.

On physical examination, vital signs are normal. His corrected vision with glasses is 20/20 in both eyes. His gait is somewhat slow and he needs some assistance getting on to the examination table. The remainder of the physical examination is normal. He scores 25/30 on the Mini–Mental State Examination.

Which of the following is the most appropriate management of this patient?

(A) Advise the patient that he should no longer drive

(B) Advise the patient to continue to drive only locally

(C) Ask about any driving difficulties

(D) Report the patient to the state department of transportation

Item 119

A 24-year-old man is evaluated for a 6-month history of episodic substernal chest pain. Episodes occur four to seven times per week and are accompanied by palpitations and sweating, as well as a "sense of doom." They resolve spontaneously after approximately 30 minutes. His symptoms are unrelieved with antacids, can occur at rest or with exertion, and are nonpositional. There are no specific precipitating factors. He is a nonsmoker. His lipid levels, which were checked recently at a school wellness fair, are normal. He has no personal or family history of coronary artery disease, diabetes mellitus, hyperlipidemia, or hypertension. He is not taking any medications.

On physical examination, vital signs are normal. He has no cardiac murmurs and no abdominal pain. Complete blood count, serum thyroid-stimulating hormone level, and electrocardiogram are all normal.

Which of the following is the most appropriate management of this patient?

(A) Cardiac event monitor

(B) Cardiac stress test

(C) Empiric trial of proton pump inhibitor

(D) Selective serotonin reuptake inhibitor

Item 120

A 47-year-old woman is evaluated during a follow-up appointment. She had been hospitalized for acute pancreatitis secondary to alcohol abuse. She has had no previous primary medical care. She takes no medications and is currently unemployed. She has been arrested one time for driving while intoxicated, but no longer drives. She smokes one pack of cigarettes daily and does not currently use illicit drugs; she did use marijuana when she was younger. She tells you she only drinks when she can afford it, which may be once a week or less, and usually has 6 or 7 drinks when she does. She has never had withdrawal symptoms.

Physical examination reveals a thin woman in no apparent distress; vital signs are normal. Sclera and skin are anicteric. The liver edge is felt 4 cm below the right costal margin. There is mild epigastric tenderness but no ascites or other stigmata of chronic liver disease.

Which of the following is the most appropriate management for this patient?

(A) Connect her drinking habits with the negative consequences

(B) Identify that she is an alcoholic and needs to abstain from drinking

(C) Initiate therapy with disulfiram

(D) Initiate therapy with naltrexone

Item 121

A 54-year-old man is evaluated after urgent transfer to the intensive care unit following an elective hemicolectomy. His surgery was performed under general anesthesia and he was extubated before leaving the operating room. After several hours of observation in the postanesthesia care unit, he was reported by nursing staff to be drowsy but awake and responsive with stable vital signs, and was transferred to a general surgical ward.

A few hours later he was noted to be in respiratory distress, was intubated, and placed on mechanical ventilation. He is currently awake and alert while being ventilated. His wife reports that he is a nonsmoker, has hypertension but no known lung or heart problems, and had been doing well prior to surgery except for chronic tiredness.

On physical examination, temperature is normal, blood pressure is 150/90 mm Hg, pulse rate is 98/min, and respiration rate is 12/min. BMI is 39. Oxygen saturation by pulse oximetry is 99% on 40% FIO_2. Heart and lung examinations are normal. There is no lower extremity edema.

Laboratory studies performed just before intubation included an arterial blood gas measurement with a pH of 7.24 and a PCO_2 of 75 mm Hg (10 kPa). Serum bicarbonate level was 28 meq/L (28 mmol/L). CT angiogram shows no pulmonary embolism and normal lungs. Electrocardiogram shows sinus tachycardia with no ST- or T-wave changes.

Which of the following is the most likely cause of his respiratory failure?

(A) Myocardial ischemia
(B) Obstructive sleep apnea
(C) Premature extubation
(D) Sepsis

Item 122

A 42-year-old woman is evaluated for a 10-day history of right shoulder pain, located posteriorly and superiorly, that becomes worse with overhead activities. She has no history of trauma. She recently painted her basement ceiling. She has no weakness or paresthesia of her right arm and has never had this problem before. She has been taking ibuprofen as needed for the pain.

On physical examination, vital signs are normal. There is no shoulder asymmetry and no tenderness to palpation of bony structures or soft tissue structures. There is full range of motion (other than with internal rotation, which is limited by pain) and strength is 5/5 throughout the right arm, with sensation intact. She is able to slowly lower her extended arm from over her head to her side (negative drop-arm test). There is pain with abduction of the right arm between 60 and 120 degrees. The patient is asked to hold the arm extended anteriorly at 90 degrees with the forearm bent to 90 degrees (at 12 o'clock), as if holding a shield. When the arm is internally rotated to cross in front of the body, the patient feels pain in the shoulder (positive Hawkins test).

Which of the following is the most likely diagnosis?

(A) Acromioclavicular joint degeneration
(B) Adhesive capsulitis
(C) Rotator cuff impingement
(D) Rotator cuff tear

Item 123

A 30-year-old man is evaluated during a routine examination. He is asymptomatic. He is a nonsmoker and has no history of illicit drug use. He has had two lifetime female sexual partners and is sexually active in a monogamous relationship with a woman for the past 5 years. His father is 58 years old and has hypertension; his mother is 57 years old and has hyperlipidemia. Results of the physical examination, including vital signs, are normal. Results of a fasting lipid panel 4 years ago were normal.

Which of the following is the most appropriate screening test to obtain?

(A) Fasting lipid panel
(B) Fasting plasma glucose
(C) HIV enzyme immunoassay antibody testing
(D) Thyroid-stimulating hormone level

Item 124

A physician unexpectedly encounters a colleague at a pub on a Friday night. They enjoy four or five drinks together while watching the first hour of a baseball game. Suddenly, the colleague's pager goes off. Annoyed, she looks at it, and says, slurring her words, "It's the hospital. I have to go admit a patient." When he tries to stop her, she gets angry and shakes him off.

Which of the following is the most appropriate course of action for this physician to take regarding his colleague?

(A) Contact the hospital chief of staff and report his concerns immediately
(B) Report his concerns to state authorities on Monday
(C) Take his colleague aside later and discuss his concerns with her
(D) No obligation to intervene

Item 125

A 55-year-old man is evaluated before scheduled endoscopic sinus surgery. In addition to symptoms of chronic sinusitis, he has chronic knee pain that limits his activity to below 4 metabolic equivalents (METs). He has no chest pain, dyspnea, or lower extremity edema. He has type 2 diabetes mellitus, coronary artery disease, chronic kidney disease, hypertension, hyperlipidemia, osteoarthritis, and chronic sinusitis. He had a myocardial infarction 5 years ago and was treated with a single bare metal stent. Medications are insulin glargine, metoprolol, aspirin, simvastatin, lisinopril, and acetaminophen.

On physical examination, temperature is normal, blood pressure is 142/84 mm Hg, and pulse rate is 56/min. The electrocardiogram is consistent with a previous lateral myocardial infarction and is unchanged from 1 year ago. Serum creatinine level is 2.1 mg/dL (186 µmol/L).

Which of the following is the most appropriate preoperative management of this patient?

(A) Discontinue metoprolol
(B) Obtain dobutamine stress echocardiogram
(C) Refer for cardiac catheterization
(D) Proceed to surgery without further testing

Item 126

A 32-year-old woman presents for emergency department follow-up. She was seen 1 week ago for a facial laceration. She tells you she cannot remember the incident. She had a humeral fracture 1 year ago, and has had bruising on her arms and legs on several visits. History is significant for depression and recurrent urinary tract infection. Her only current medication is citalopram. Upon questioning about intimate partner violence, the patient admits that her husband often beats her.

Physical examination is significant for normal vital signs; a healing, sutured, 4-cm laceration across the left zygomatic arch; and several 5- to 6-cm ecchymoses on her upper extremities.

Which of the following is the most appropriate next step in management?

(A) Advise the patient to leave her current living situation immediately

(B) Ask her to bring her husband to her next appointment

(C) Assess her immediate safety and develop a safety plan

(D) Report the husband to the police

(E) Request psychiatry consultation

Item 127

A 50-year-old woman is evaluated for nonischemic cardiomyopathy. Her exercise tolerance is not limited. She takes an ACE inhibitor daily. She took a β-blocker briefly but discontinued because of fatigue. Results of the physical examination are normal.

The patient inquires whether she should receive drug "H". Drug H was studied in 2000 patients ages 40 to 80 years (mean age 63 years) with New York Heart Association functional class III or IV heart failure. Patients were randomized to receive drug H or a placebo in addition to usual medications. Eighty percent of patients in the trial also took a β-blocker and 70% an ACE inhibitor. At the end of 3 years, patients taking drug H had a significantly reduced rate of a composite outcome of death or heart failure exacerbations. Approximately 5% of the patients taking drug H had serious adverse events, compared with 2% in the placebo group.

Which of the following is the main reason why this patient should not be treated with drug H?

(A) Her heart failure is too mild

(B) She is too young

(C) She should be treated with a β-blocker first

(D) The drug's adverse event rate is too high

Item 128

A 16-year-old patient is brought to the office by his mother for an evaluation. His mother notes that he has been "strange" since a very young age. He did not start speaking until age 3 years. Since that time, he has been home-schooled but has avoided other children and adults in social contexts. He is prone to emotional outbursts, and frequently repeats back what is said to him many times over. Currently he spends most of his time in his room, and is unwilling to help with routine chores at home. However, he is fascinated by trains, and when he is engaged will recite numerous details about trains.

Which of the following is the most likely diagnosis?

(A) Autism spectrum disorder

(B) Obsessive-compulsive disorder

(C) Schizophrenia

(D) Social anxiety disorder

Item 129

A 25-year-old woman is evaluated in October before starting a certified nursing assistant degree program. She was diagnosed with HIV infection 3 months ago. She reports having received "all my shots as a child," and specifically recalls having chickenpox as a child. Before starting school she needs to provide proof of her immunization status. Her only medication is an oral contraceptive. Findings on physical examination are unremarkable.

Which of the following is the most appropriate next step in this patient's immunization management?

(A) Administer a single measles, mumps, and rubella booster now

(B) Administer live, attenuated, intranasal influenza vaccine now

(C) Begin hepatitis B immunization series

(D) Certify her as immune to varicella given her clinical history

(E) Obtain a CD4 cell count

Item 130

A 38-year-old man is evaluated in the emergency department for a 2-week history of nonpleuritic, sharp, anterior chest pain. Each episode of pain lasts 3 to 10 hours. He states that the pain is to the left of the sternum but at times it radiates across the entire chest. It does not radiate to the shoulders, arms, or back. The pain can be present at rest. It is worsened with lateral movement of the trunk. He does not notice any change in intensity with walking or other activity. He has no other symptoms and no other medical problems. He does not use drugs and takes no medications.

On physical examination, temperature is 37.0 °C (98.6 °F), blood pressure is 132/70 mm Hg, pulse rate is 90/min, and respiration rate is 14/min. BMI is 26. There is reproducible point tenderness along the sternum. The remainder of the examination, including the cardiovascular examination, is normal.

Which of the following is the most likely diagnosis?

(A) Acute pericarditis

(B) Aortic dissection

(C) Costochondritis

(D) Unstable angina

Item 131

A 19-year-old woman is evaluated for painful menses. She usually misses one or two days of school each month owing to these symptoms, which include cramps and nausea. Menarche occurred at age 12 years. Menses have been regular for the past 2 years, occurring every 29 days. The patient is not sexually active, and her medical history is noncontributory. She takes no medications.

Physical examination, including external pelvic examination, is normal.

Which of the following is the most appropriate management option for this patient?

(A) Combined estrogen-progesterone contraceptive
(B) Depot medroxyprogesterone acetate
(C) Ibuprofen
(D) Measurement of follicle-stimulating hormone and luteinizing hormone levels
(E) Pelvic ultrasound

Item 132

A 42-year-old man is evaluated for a 4-month history of left elbow pain. The pain radiates to his hand and is worse at night, with flexion of the arm at the elbow, and with wrist flexion. The pain is accompanied by an intermittent tingling sensation in the fourth and fifth fingers. He has no weakness and has never had this problem before.

On physical examination, vital signs are normal. Pain is elicited in the left elbow with flexion of the arm at the elbow. There is decreased light touch sensation involving both palmar and dorsal surfaces of the fourth and fifth fingers to the level of the wrist. No tenderness to palpation of any of the structures of the elbow is elicited.

Which of the following is the most likely diagnosis?

(A) Lateral epicondylitis
(B) Medial epicondylitis
(C) Olecranon bursitis
(D) Ulnar nerve entrapment

Item 133

A 48-year-old man is evaluated for watery bowel movements. The patient is having 8 to 12 watery bowel movements daily. Several days before the diarrhea began, the patient went to an urgent care clinic with a sinus headache. He was diagnosed with bacterial sinusitis and given a 7-day course of antibiotics. He was asked to return to the urgent care center if he experienced any problems or did not improve. He says there was no discussion of adverse effects or alternatives to antibiotic therapy. Stool assay is positive for *Clostridium difficile* toxin.

Which of the following can be concluded about informed consent in this case?

(A) Acceptance of the antibiotics fulfilled requirements for informed consent

(B) Informed consent is only needed for invasive procedures
(C) Informed consent only applies when signing a consent form
(D) Informed consent was not properly obtained

Item 134

A 47-year-old man is evaluated for follow-up of left-sided cervical radiculopathy. He presented 2 weeks ago with severe arm and hand pain that developed shortly after doing yard work; no trauma was noted. He was treated with NSAIDs and rest. Although his pain symptoms have improved, he has developed progressive difficulty opening jars because he has trouble holding onto the lid. On two occasions over the past several days, he has dropped a coffee cup without intending to.

On physical examination, vital signs are normal. There is normal bulk and tone of the trapezius muscle on the left. Triceps strength is normal on the left, although the biceps muscle group shows 4/5 strength relative to the right. There are also diminished biceps and brachioradialis reflexes on the left. The remainder of the examination is unremarkable.

An MRI of the cervical spine shows herniation of the C5-C6 disk with compression of the left C6 nerve root and increased signal in the area of compression.

Which of the following is the most appropriate next step in management?

(A) Continued analgesics and rest
(B) Epidural corticosteroid injection
(C) Physical therapy for strengthening
(D) Surgical evaluation

Item 135

A 33-year-old woman is evaluated for chronic lower pelvic pain. It has been persistent for the past year but has worsened in recent months. She describes it as a constant, aching discomfort centered over her lower pelvis that persists during her menstrual cycle and has prevented her from being sexually active with her partner. She also reports a 4-month history of urinary urgency and frequency. She has been empirically treated twice for urinary tract infections, but her urinary symptoms improve for only a few days and then recur. She has no history of pelvic surgeries or pelvic infections and has never been pregnant. She has no associated constipation, diarrhea, abdominal distention, or flank pain. She currently takes ibuprofen as needed for pain.

On physical examination, vital signs are normal. BMI is 24. There is mild tenderness to palpation over the pelvic floor muscles with significant tenderness over the anterior vaginal wall. External genitalia are normal in appearance; there is no tenderness to palpation over the vulva. There is no cervical motion tenderness, adnexal tenderness, or discomfort with palpation of the uterus.

Laboratory studies show normal electrolytes, kidney function, and a complete blood count. Erythrocyte sedimentation rate is 4 mm/h. Urinalysis is without erythrocytes or leukocytes and is negative for nitrite and leukocyte esterase. Urine culture is negative. Tests for chlamydial infection and gonorrhea are negative.

Transvaginal/transabdominal ultrasonography is negative for endometrial or ovarian masses and no abnormalities are noted.

Which of the following is the most likely diagnosis?

(A) Endometriosis
(B) Interstitial cystitis
(C) Irritable bowel syndrome
(D) Pelvic adhesions

Item 136

A 66-year-old man with diabetic neuropathy is evaluated for increasing pain in his lower extremities. The pain is 7/10 in intensity, constant, and keeps him awake at night. He has been treated with trials of NSAIDs, amitriptyline, pregabalin, gabapentin, and duloxetine, both individually and in various combinations, without significant control of his symptoms. He presented to an outside emergency department 3 weeks ago and was prescribed oxycodone-acetaminophen 5 mg/325 mg. He has been taking 2 tablets every 6 hours as recommended and has experienced good relief of his pain, although his symptoms worsen with late or missed doses. Medical history is also significant for hypertension, hyperlipidemia, and ischemic cardiomyopathy. He has no personal or family history of drug or alcohol abuse. Current medications are gabapentin, amitriptyline, insulin glargine, insulin aspart, lisinopril, aspirin, simvastatin, carvedilol, and oxycodone-acetaminophen.

On physical examination, temperature is 36.7 °C (98.2 °F), blood pressure is 122/76 mm Hg, pulse rate is 64/min, and respiration rate is 12/min. BMI is 28. He has decreased sensation to light touch and pinprick in a stocking-glove distribution, and reflexes are 1+ and symmetric. Romberg test is positive. There is no hepatomegaly, scleral icterus, or jaundice.

Laboratory studies are significant for normal electrolytes, liver chemistry studies, vitamin B_{12} level, and complete blood count. The serum creatinine level is 1.3 mg/dL (115 μmol/L).

A previous resting electrocardiogram showed first-degree atrioventricular block and small Q waves in an anterolateral distribution without active ischemia.

Which of the following is the most appropriate treatment for this patient's neuropathic pain?

(A) Continue oxycodone-acetaminophen at the current dose
(B) Discontinue oxycodone-acetaminophen and start tramadol
(C) Transition to methadone
(D) Transition to sustained-release morphine

Item 137

An 81-year-old man is evaluated for a 3-week history of shortness of breath, chest pain, palpitations, difficulty sleeping, early morning awakening, and lack of interest in getting out of bed in the morning. The patient's wife died of cancer 9 months ago. He says that he has been seeing her face at night when he closes his eyes and frequently awakes at night thinking that she is next to him in bed. Medical history is significant for hypertension and hyperlipidemia. Medications are hydrochlorothiazide, atorvastatin, and diphenhydramine at bedtime as needed for sleep. Results of the physical examination are normal.

Chemistry panel and complete blood count are normal. Electrocardiogram reveals normal sinus rhythm with left ventricular hypertrophy without ischemic changes. Chest radiograph is normal. Exercise treadmill test is negative for cardiac ischemia.

Which of the following is the most likely diagnosis?

(A) Anticholinergic drug side effect
(B) Complicated grief
(C) Generalized anxiety disorder
(D) Major depression with psychotic features

Item 138

A 34-year-old woman is evaluated for a 6-month history of allergies that have not responded to treatment. She normally has hay fever in the spring, but it typically subsides after 1 to 2 months and the symptoms can be controlled with antihistamines and decongestants. Now she reports intractable nasal congestion and rhinorrhea present for months. She does not have sinus pain or dental pain. She lives in a 10-year old house with no known mold problems and has no pets. She does not think her symptoms are worse or better when she leaves the house or travels. She notes no sneezing or itchy eyes. Current medications are oxymetazoline nasal spray, pseudoephedrine, cetirizine, and diphenhydramine at bedtime. She has no other medical problems.

On physical examination, temperature is 36.8 °C (98.2 °F), blood pressure is 124/72 mm Hg, pulse rate is 96/min, and respiration rate is 16/min. BMI is 23. Nasal mucosa is hyperemic and slightly edematous with clear nasal drainage. The pharynx is normal without tonsillar enlargement or cobblestoning.

Which of the following is the most likely diagnosis?

(A) Chronic rhinosinusitis
(B) Chronic vasomotor rhinitis
(C) Granulomatosis with polyangiitis (Wegener granulomatosis)
(D) Rhinitis medicamentosa

Item 139

A 34-year-old woman is evaluated for significant breast pain. She says her breasts are generally very "sensitive" but she develops more pronounced discomfort shortly before she has her menstrual period, when both breasts seem to ache and throb. She has not noticed any associated skin discoloration, nipple discharge, or breast masses. She is obese and has gastroesophageal reflux disease. She does not use tobacco or alcohol. She otherwise feels well and has increased her exercise level to help her lose weight. She has no shortness of breath, nausea, vomiting, difficulty swallowing, or recent rashes. Her menses are regular and occur every 28 days. Her mother was diagnosed with breast cancer at age 53 years and her sister had a benign breast biopsy. Her current medications are omeprazole and a daily multivitamin.

On physical examination, vital signs are normal. BMI is 32. Her breasts are symmetric in shape and appearance. There are no palpable masses in either breast, and there is no supraclavicular or axillary lymphadenopathy. There is no nipple discharge or skin discoloration or dimpling. There is diffuse tenderness to palpation over both breasts, most prominent in the upper outer quadrants. Cardiovascular, pulmonary, and abdominal examinations are normal. There is no tenderness to palpation over the chest wall.

Which of the following is the most appropriate management?

(A) Danazol
(B) Diagnostic mammography
(C) Support bra
(D) Tamoxifen

Item 140

A 26-year-old man is evaluated for a 2-month history of depressed mood, lack of energy, and increased sleep. He has had less interest in his usual hobby of woodworking and has found it more difficult to perform well at his job at a law firm. In the past, he has had periods of high energy requiring little sleep without getting tired. During these periods he recalls going on spending sprees and having many sexual partners. He does not have any suicidal ideation. His mother has a history of alcohol abuse. The physical examination, including the mental status examination, is normal.

Which of the following is the most appropriate treatment?

(A) Duloxetine
(B) Lamotrigine
(C) Lorazepam
(D) Sertraline

Item 141

A 55-year-old woman is evaluated during a follow-up appointment. She has hypertension and hyperlipidemia. She does not use alcohol. Review of systems is notable for fatigue and occasional constipation. She is menopausal. Her family history is noncontributory. Her medications are simvastatin (40 mg/d), aspirin, and lisinopril.

On physical examination, she is afebrile, blood pressure is 140/82 mm Hg, pulse rate is 66/min, and respiration rate is 12/min. BMI is 25. She has mildly dry skin. There is no evidence of xanthomas and no hepatomegaly.

Laboratory studies:

Total cholesterol	284 mg/dL (7.36 mmol/L)
LDL cholesterol	231 mg/dL (5.98 mmol/L)
HDL cholesterol	55 mg/dL (1.42 mmol/L)
Triglycerides	113 mg/dL (1.28 mmol/L)
Glucose (fasting)	100 mg/dL (5.5 mmol/L)

Additional laboratory results reveal normal kidney and liver function.

In addition to recommending diet and exercise therapy, which of the following is the most appropriate management?

(A) Add gemfibrozil
(B) Increase simvastatin to 80 mg/d
(C) Measure hemoglobin A_{1c} level
(D) Measure thyroid-stimulating hormone level

Item 142

A 54-year-old woman is evaluated before an elective cholecystectomy. Medical history is significant for atrial fibrillation, type 2 diabetes mellitus, chronic heart failure, hypertension, and a transient ischemic attack 2 months ago. Medications are warfarin, insulin glargine, insulin lispro, metoprolol, lisinopril, furosemide, and simvastatin.

On physical examination, temperature is normal, blood pressure is 142/88 mm Hg, and pulse rate is 88/min and irregularly irregular. The remainder of the physical examination is normal. INR is 2.5.

Which of the following is the most appropriate treatment?

(A) Administer half the usual dose of warfarin for 5 days before surgery
(B) Continue warfarin
(C) Discontinue warfarin 5 days before surgery
(D) Discontinue warfarin 5 days before surgery and administer enoxaparin until the morning of surgery

Item 143

A 22-year-old woman is evaluated during a routine examination. She has a history of anorexia nervosa but has been in remission for the past 2 years. She has recently been under significant stress related to her parents' divorce, and has started restricting her caloric intake because she is worried about gaining weight. She has not had a menstrual period for 4 months (previously she had regular menses) and she has lost 13.6 kg (30 lb) in the last 12 weeks. Medical history is significant for depression and osteopenia. Current medications are calcium and vitamin D.

On physical examination, temperature is 36.4 °C (97.6 °F), blood pressure is 100/60 mm Hg, pulse rate is 60/min, and respiration rate is 12/min. There is no orthostasis. BMI is 16. There is fine, soft hair covering the arms, chest, and abdomen. The heart rate is slow with a regular rhythm. The abdomen is scaphoid. The skin is pale and there is no edema. Pulmonary, abdominal, and musculoskeletal examinations are normal. Blood chemistry studies are normal except for a sodium level of 132 meq/L (132 mmol/L) and a phosphorus level of 2.5 mg/dL (0.81 mmol/L). A pregnancy test is negative.

In addition to referring the patient for nutritional rehabilitation, which of the following is the most appropriate treatment?

(A) Amitriptyline
(B) Bupropion
(C) Cognitive-behavioral therapy
(D) Megestrol acetate
(E) Oral contraceptive pills

Item 144

A 75-year-old man is evaluated for low back pain. The pain began several months ago and is getting worse. Its intensity is now 6 or 7 (on a scale of 1-10) most days. It worsens with activity and improves with sitting. He has been unable to walk or exercise because of the pain and has gained 9.0 kg (20 lb) in the past year. He has not experienced any bowel or bladder incontinence or lower extremity numbness or tingling, and has not had fevers or chills. Medical history is significant for hypertension, hyperlipidemia, and peptic ulcer disease. He does not use tobacco or alcohol. His current medications are hydrochlorothiazide, lisinopril, simvastatin, omeprazole, and aspirin. He has been taking additional aspirin, which has been providing modest pain relief.

On physical examination, vital signs are normal. BMI is 34. There is mild tenderness to palpation over the lower lumbar paravertebral muscles. Patellar and ankle jerk reflexes are 1+ and symmetric. Sensation to light touch and pinprick is symmetric, and strength is 5/5 in the lower extremities. Complete blood count and metabolic panel are normal.

A radiograph of the lumbar spine shows degeneration of the L4 and L5 vertebrae, osteophyte formation, and facet arthropathy with narrowing of the spinal canal.

Which of the following is the most appropriate treatment for this patient's symptoms?

(A) Acetaminophen
(B) Amitriptyline
(C) Cyclobenzaprine
(D) Ibuprofen

Item 145

A 60-year-old woman is evaluated during a routine examination. She has hyperlipidemia. She has a 5-pack-year smoking history but is not actively using tobacco and has no history of illicit drug use. She is married and in a monogamous relationship with her husband of 25 years. She has no family history of breast, colon, or cervical cancer. Her only medication is simvastatin.

On physical examination, she is afebrile, blood pressure is 118/76 mm Hg, and pulse rate is 74/min. BMI is 25. Pap smear and mammography, both performed 11 months ago, were within normal limits.

Which of the following conditions should also be screened for in this patient?

(A) Abdominal aortic aneurysm
(B) Depression

(C) Hepatitis B virus infection
(D) Osteoporosis

Item 146

A 38-year-old woman is evaluated for a 2-year history of irritability and frequent headaches, accompanied by nausea and sweating. She is a housecleaner and has had increasing difficulty concentrating at work over the past year, and it takes her much longer to clean houses lately. She has a difficult time getting to sleep and frequently arises after 2 to 3 hours of fitful sleep in bed. Her mood is good. She worries frequently about her ability to pay her bills and what she will do for retirement. She has cut back on activities with friends and does not like to go out in social situations anymore. She has asthma, and her only current medication is albuterol as needed.

On physical examination, she is afebrile, blood pressure is 130/72 mm Hg, pulse rate is 98/min, and respiration rate is 14/min. BMI is 22. Serum thyroid-stimulating hormone level, complete blood count, and urinalysis are normal.

Which of the following is the most likely diagnosis?

(A) Attention-deficit/hyperactivity disorder
(B) Bipolar disorder
(C) Generalized anxiety disorder
(D) Major depressive disorder

Item 147

A 56-year-old woman is evaluated during a routine examination. On review of systems, she reports a 2-year history of decreased interest in sexual intercourse. Her lack of interest is gradually worsening and starting to cause problems in her marriage. She has no history of sexual trauma, sexually transmitted infection, or pelvic surgery. Her last menstrual period was 2 years ago.

On physical examination, vital signs are normal. Gynecologic examination shows pink, well-lubricated vaginal walls; there is no cervical motion or adnexal tenderness and no discomfort with speculum insertion.

Which of the following is the most appropriate treatment of this patient?

(A) Sex therapy
(B) Sildenafil
(C) Systemic estrogen and progesterone therapy
(D) Systemic testosterone therapy

Item 148

A 70-year-old woman is evaluated for a 3-month history of vision problems. She reports that objects may appear blurry or distorted, particularly in the central field. She has difficulty reading and recognizing faces. She has no eye pain or recent eye trauma. She is a smoker. Her only medication is tiotropium.

On physical examination, vital signs are normal. Funduscopic findings are shown (see next page). The remainder of the eye examination is normal.

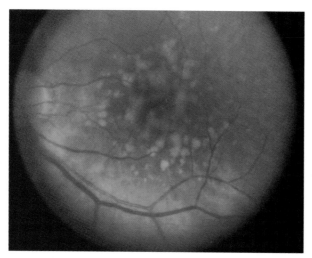

ITEM 148

Which of the following is the most likely diagnosis?

(A) Age-related macular degeneration
(B) Cataracts
(C) Primary open angle glaucoma
(D) Retinal detachment

Item 149

A 70-year-old man is evaluated preoperatively before elective total hip arthroplasty. He is able to ambulate on a level surface slowly but is unable to carry laundry or groceries up stairs because of his hip pain. He has had no recent chest pain or pressure. He has no orthopnea. Other than his hip pain, he feels well. He has hypertension and hyperlipidemia. Current medications are metoprolol, losartan, and simvastatin.

On physical examination, temperature is 36.8 °C (98.3 °F), blood pressure is 132/78 mm Hg, pulse rate is 64/min, and respiration rate is 14/min. Results of the remainder of the examination are normal. Serum creatinine level is 1.3 mg/dL (115 μmol/L). An electrocardiogram shows sinus rhythm with no ST- or T-wave abnormalities.

Which of the following is the most appropriate diagnostic test to perform next?

(A) Cardiac catheterization
(B) CT coronary angiography
(C) Dobutamine stress echocardiography
(D) No further testing needed before surgery

Item 150

A 42-year-old-man is evaluated for obesity. His weight has gradually increased over the past two decades and is currently 168.2 kg (370 lb). Five years ago, he was diagnosed with type 2 diabetes mellitus, hypertension, and hyperlipidemia. Over the past 6 months, he has unsuccessfully tried diet and exercise therapy for his obesity. He tried over-the-counter orlistat but could not tolerate the gastrointestinal side effects. Medications are metformin, lisinopril, and simvastatin. His total weight loss goal is 45.4 kg (100 lb).

On physical examination, temperature is normal, blood pressure is 130/80 mm Hg, pulse rate is 80/min, and respiration rate is 14/min. BMI is 48. Waist circumference is 121.9 cm (48 in). There is no thyromegaly. Heart sounds are normal with no murmur. There is no lower extremity edema.

Results of complete blood count, thyroid studies, and urinalysis are unremarkable.

Which of the following is the most appropriate management of this patient?

(A) Bariatric surgery evaluation
(B) Prescribe phentermine
(C) Reduce caloric intake to below 800 kcal/d
(D) Refer to an exercise program

Item 151

A 66-year-old man is evaluated during a routine examination. He is asymptomatic and walks for 2 miles on the treadmill three times a week. He has hypertension. He drinks three or four beers three times per week and has done so for the past 30 years. He is a former smoker, smoking one pack per day for 2 years between the ages of 20 and 25 years. Current medications are hydrochlorothiazide and aspirin.

On physical examination, he is afebrile, blood pressure is 124/76 mm Hg, and pulse rate is 72/min. BMI is 23. The examination is otherwise unremarkable. A fasting lipid profile last year was within normal limits. His most recent colonoscopy was performed 5 years ago and was negative for any polyps.

Which of the following is the most appropriate screening test?

(A) Abdominal ultrasonography
(B) Chest radiography
(C) Coronary artery calcium score determination
(D) Fasting lipid profile
(E) No additional testing

Item 152

A 44-year-old man is evaluated for chronic back pain. Six months ago he underwent decompressive spinal laminectomy for treatment of refractory pain secondary to spinal stenosis. He was discharged on oxycodone-acetaminophen, 5 mg/325 mg, and despite taking 2 tablets every 6 hours, he continues to report severe discomfort. He has been taking ibuprofen and cyclobenzaprine to help with the pain and has been using hot compresses intermittently. His surgeon has been satisfied with his operative treatment and has recommended that he start a physical therapy program, but the patient reports that he is in too much pain to exercise. Medical history is significant for mild depression and tobacco use. His father abused alcohol and his mother has COPD secondary to smoking.

On physical examination, vital signs are normal. BMI is 32. There is mild tenderness to palpation over the lumbar paravertebral muscles. A complete neurologic examination of the lower extremities and a straight leg raise test cannot be performed because of patient discomfort, although there are no abnormalities noted on limited testing.

In addition to starting the patient on a good bowel regimen, which of the following is the most appropriate management?

(A) Amitriptyline
(B) Change analgesic to extended-release morphine
(C) Evaluate for opioid dependency
(D) MRI of the lumbar spine

Item 153

A 42-year-old man is evaluated for difficulty sleeping the past several months. He reports trouble both falling asleep and staying asleep. He has not tried any over-the-counter medications. He drinks two or three beers on the weekends only and this has not changed; he also drinks two cups of coffee in the mornings. His wife, who is present, has not heard any snoring, gasping, or other breathing problems at night. He reports no leg symptoms. They have recently moved to a new apartment; he reports that the bedroom may be hotter than the previous one, although his wife reports feeling comfortable.

Results of the physical examination are unremarkable. Vital signs are normal, BMI is 26, and mood and mental status are normal.

Which of the following is the best initial management for this patient?

(A) Advise alcohol abstinence
(B) Benzodiazepine
(C) Counseling regarding sleep hygiene
(D) Over-the-counter antihistamine

Item 154

A 28-year-old woman is evaluated for a 3-month history of fatigue and muscle cramps. She states that she is eating well, drinking plenty of fluids, and exercising regularly, but the fatigue is starting to interfere with her ability to complete her daily 3-mile run. She has a previous history of anorexia nervosa diagnosed at age 16 years requiring two inpatient hospitalizations. She has had a normal weight and menstrual cycle for the last 4 years. She currently takes daily calcium and vitamin D supplements.

On physical examination, temperature is 36.6 °C (98.0 °F), blood pressure is 106/64 mm Hg, pulse rate is 66/min, and respiration rate is 12/min. BMI is 22. She has poor dentition with multiple dental caries. The remainder of the examination is normal. Pregnancy test is negative.

Laboratory studies:

Complete blood count	Normal
Electrolytes	
Sodium	132 meq/L (132 mmol/L)
Potassium	3.2 meq/L (3.2 mmol/L)
Chloride	95 meq/L (95 mmol/L)
Bicarbonate	31 meq/L (31 mmol/L)
Blood urea nitrogen	6 mg/dL (2.1 mmol/L)
Creatinine	0.8 mg/dL (70.7 µmol/L)
Thyroid-stimulating hormone	2.5 µU/mL (2.5 mU/L)

Which of the following is the most likely diagnosis?

(A) Anorexia nervosa, binge-eating/purging subtype
(B) Binge-eating disorder
(C) Bulimia nervosa, purging subtype
(D) Night-eating syndrome

Item 155

A 48-year-old man is evaluated for pain located on his lateral thigh. He describes the pain as a burning sensation that has been present for 3 weeks. He has never had this pain before and has no associated leg weakness or back pain.

On physical examination, vital signs are normal. BMI is 34. Dysesthesia is present in the anterolateral thigh. There is no tenderness to palpation of the lateral femoral epicondyle. Knee and hip examinations are normal. A straight leg raising test is negative bilaterally and strength is 5/5 in both extremities.

Which of the following is the most likely diagnosis?

(A) Greater trochanteric bursitis
(B) Iliotibial band syndrome
(C) L5 radiculopathy
(D) Meralgia paresthetica

Item 156

A 78-year-old man is evaluated in the emergency department after a witnessed episode of syncope. The patient reports that, while eating dinner, he experienced a pounding in his chest and then fell to the floor. His wife estimates he was unconscious for approximately 30 seconds, had no head trauma, and was oriented and alert upon regaining consciousness. He has not experienced any similar episodes in the past, although he has felt the pounding previously. Medical history is significant for hypertension, COPD, osteoarthritis, and benign prostatic hyperplasia. Medications are chlorthalidone, lisinopril, celecoxib, ipratropium-albuterol inhaler, and tamsulosin. He currently feels well except for pain in his right thigh where he fell.

On physical examination, temperature is normal. Blood pressure is 138/88 mm Hg and pulse rate is 82/min, without orthostatic changes. Respiration rate is 16/min. Oxygen saturation on ambient air is normal. Carotid upstrokes are +2 without bruits, and there is no jugular venous distention. Cardiac examination is normal, with the exception of occasional extra beats. The remainder of the examination, including neurologic examination, is normal. 12-Lead electrocardiogram shows a few premature ventricular contractions without evidence of ischemia.

Which of the following is the most appropriate next step in this patient's management?

(A) Carotid Doppler ultrasonography
(B) Echocardiography
(C) Inpatient cardiac monitoring
(D) Noncontrast CT of head

Item 157

A 26-year-old woman is evaluated in the emergency department for an 8-day history of sore throat, fever, and neck pain. She has severe pain on the left side of her neck with swallowing. She has had fevers for the past week with rigors starting today. Over the past 3 to 4 days she has had increasing cough. She was previously healthy and takes no medications.

On physical examination, temperature is 39.1 °C (102.3 °F), blood pressure is 108/68 mm Hg, pulse rate is 116/min, and respiration rate is 20/min. BMI is 19. She is toxic-appearing. The neck is tender to palpation along the left side without lymphadenopathy. The pharynx is erythematous with tonsillar enlargement and no exudates. The chest is clear to auscultation. Other than tachycardia, the cardiac examination is normal.

Chest radiograph is shown. Leukocyte count is 18,400/µL (18.4×10^9/L) with 17% band forms. Serum creatinine level is 0.8 mg/dL (70.7 µmol/L).

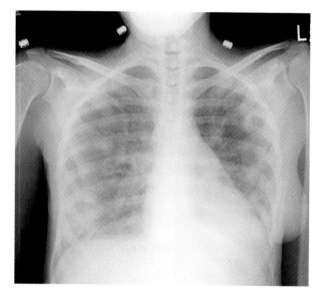

Which of the following tests is most likely to establish the diagnosis?

(A) CT of the chest with contrast
(B) CT of the neck with contrast
(C) Radiography of the pharyngeal soft tissues
(D) Transthoracic echocardiography

Item 158

A 56-year-old man presents for evaluation of elevated liver chemistry test results that were obtained during an application for life insurance. At an office visit 12 weeks ago, he was started on simvastatin for dyslipidemia. He has not experienced any side effects with this medication and specifically does not have nausea, vomiting, or abdominal pain.

On physical examination today, blood pressure is 140/80 mm Hg; vital signs are otherwise normal. BMI is 29. There is no scleral icterus, hepatomegaly, or abdominal tenderness.

Laboratory studies:

	12 Weeks Ago	Current
Alanine aminotransferase	28 units/L	76 units/L
Aspartate aminotransferase	21 units/L	63 units/L
Total bilirubin	0.8 mg/dL (13.6 µmol/L)	1 mg/dL (17.1 µmol/L)

Which of the following is the most appropriate management?

(A) Discontinue simvastatin
(B) Measure serum antibodies to hepatitis B and C
(C) Order liver ultrasonography
(D) No change in management

Item 159

A 30-year-old man was admitted to the hospital 2 days ago with an acute exacerbation of asthma. He was placed on a regimen of corticosteroids and inhaled β-agonists. He has responded well and is ready for discharge today with plans for a short course of oral corticosteroids as well as inhaled corticosteroids and β-agonists. He reports receiving "all his shots" while growing up. He does not smoke cigarettes. He is in a monogamous relationship with his wife and reports no illicit drug use.

Which of the following vaccines should this patient receive?

(A) Hepatitis B
(B) Human papillomavirus
(C) Meningococcal
(D) Pneumococcal

Item 160

A 66-year-old woman is evaluated in the hospital 12 hours after a total knee arthroplasty. She is experiencing anorexia and some nausea and is not eating. She has a history of type 2 diabetes mellitus treated with glimepiride.

On physical examination, vital signs are normal. BMI is 35. Her preoperative hemoglobin A_{1c} concentration was 6.9%, and plasma glucose level 6 hours postoperatively is 250 mg/dL (13.9 mmol/L).

Which of the following is the most appropriate treatment of her diabetes?

(A) Glimepiride
(B) Long- and short-acting insulin
(C) Sliding scale insulin
(D) No treatment at this time

Item 161

A 19-year-old man is evaluated for a 2-day history of sore throat, cough, fever, and chills. On physical examination, temperature is 38.9 °C (102.0 °F), blood pressure is 122/82 mm Hg, pulse rate is 88/min, and respiration rate is 14/min. The pharynx is erythematous with tonsillar enlargement and exudates bilaterally. There is no cervical lymphadenopathy.

Which of the following is the most appropriate management?

(A) Obtain throat culture and start penicillin therapy

(B) Perform rapid antigen detection testing

(C) Start penicillin therapy

(D) No further testing or treatment indicated

Item 162

A 42-year-old man is seen for follow-up of hepatitis C. Three years ago, serologic tests were positive for hepatitis A virus and negative for hepatitis B virus. He received a single dose of hepatitis B vaccine but was lost to follow-up. He feels well today without specific symptoms. Findings on physical examination are unremarkable.

Which of the following is the most appropriate management of this patient's hepatitis B vaccination?

(A) Complete the hepatitis B vaccine series

(B) Measure hepatitis B surface antibody

(C) Restart the hepatitis B vaccine series

(D) No further vaccination or serologic testing for hepatitis B is needed

Item 163

A 19-year-old woman is evaluated for a 1-week history of left ear canal pruritus, redness, and pain. She swims 1 mile each day and has recently started wearing plastic ear plugs to keep water out of her ears while swimming.

On physical examination, she is afebrile, blood pressure is 98/66 mm Hg, pulse rate is 62/min, and respiration rate is 16/min. She appears healthy and in no distress. There is pain with tugging on the pinna and compression or movement of the tragus. The left ear canal is shown. With irrigation,

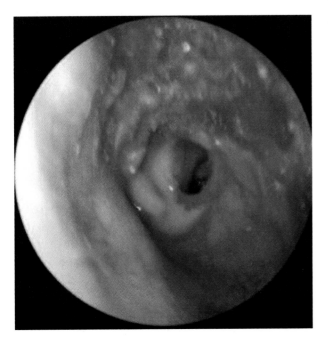

the left tympanic membrane appears normal. There is no preauricular or cervical lymphadenopathy.

Which of the following is the most likely diagnosis?

(A) Acute otitis externa

(B) Delayed-type hypersensitivity reaction to ear plugs

(C) Malignant otitis externa

(D) Otitis media

Item 164

A 38-year-old woman is evaluated during a routine examination. She has recently divorced and is interested in some form of hormonal contraception, as her ex-husband had a vasectomy after their last child, and she does not want to use condoms. She has no history of deep venous thrombosis, hypertension, or heart disease. She drinks one glass of wine 4 or 5 nights per week, and smokes a pack of cigarettes daily. Family history is significant for stroke in her mother at age 72 years. All previous Pap smears have been negative.

Physical examination, including pelvic examination, is normal. A Pap smear is obtained.

Which of the following is the most appropriate hormonal contraceptive option for this patient?

(A) Estrogen patch

(B) Estrogen-progesterone combination

(C) Progesterone contraceptive

(D) No hormonal-based method

Item 165

A 70-year-old man is evaluated for a 6-month history of low energy and decreased libido. He is not in a depressed mood and is still interested in daily activities. He has glaucoma and hypertension. Over the past year his vision has decreased and his ophthalmologist has adjusted his medications repeatedly. His current medications are timolol drops, latanoprost drops (a prostaglandin analogue), dorzolamide drops (a topical carbonic anhydrase inhibitor), lisinopril, and amlodipine.

On physical examination, temperature is 37.6 °C (99.7 °F), blood pressure is 138/84 mm Hg, pulse rate is 48/min and regular, and respiration rate is 12/min. BMI is 28. Other than bradycardia, the results of the physical examination are normal. An electrocardiogram shows only sinus bradycardia.

Which of this patient's medications should be discontinued?

(A) Amlodipine

(B) Dorzolamide

(C) Latanoprost

(D) Lisinopril

(E) Timolol

Item 166

A 65-year-old man is evaluated for a 6-month history of inability to achieve a successful erection. He is otherwise asymptomatic. He has coronary artery disease and hyperlipidemia. A bare metal stent was placed 5 years ago to his mid–left anterior descending coronary artery after he experienced exertional chest pain. Currently, he exercises in the form of brisk walking 3 to 4 times per week. He does not smoke. His current medications are aspirin, metoprolol, and simvastatin. He has no family history of early coronary artery disease.

On physical examination, he is afebrile, blood pressure is 114/80 mm Hg, pulse rate is 84/min, and respiration rate is 16/min. BMI is 29. Results of the cardiac examination are normal. He has no gynecomastia, the testes are normal in size, and sensation is intact in both lower extremities. The dorsalis pedis and posterior tibialis pulses are palpable bilaterally.

An electrocardiogram is normal. Laboratory investigation reveals a serum thyroid-stimulating hormone level of 2.75 μU/mL (2.75 mU/L) and an 8 AM total testosterone level of 425 ng/dL (15 nmol/L).

Which of the following is the most appropriate management for this patient?

(A) Begin sildenafil
(B) Begin testosterone replacement therapy
(C) Perform exercise stress testing
(D) Stop metoprolol

Item 167

A 22-year-old woman is evaluated during a follow-up appointment for plantar fasciitis. She has been doing appropriate stretching exercises for the past 8 weeks and has been using acetaminophen, 1000 mg every 8 hours, with some improvement in pain. The pain is still present, however, and interferes with her job. She has never had pain like this before.

On physical examination, there is tenderness to palpation of the plantar medial calcaneal tuberosity and 1 to 2 cm distally along the plantar fascia. Passive dorsiflexion of the toes increases the patient's pain. Pes planus is present. There is no ecchymosis, tenderness, or swelling over the plantar fascia and no tenderness of the calcaneus with medial or lateral pressure. The calcaneal tuberosity is neither prominent nor tender. Sensation is intact on the plantar surface of the foot.

Which of the following is the most appropriate treatment?

(A) Arch supports
(B) Corticosteroid injection
(C) Extracorporeal shock wave therapy
(D) Plantar fascia release surgery

Item 168

A 60-year-old woman is admitted to the hospital for abdominal pain. A subsequent evaluation has revealed a large cecal mass, and hemicolectomy is planned. She is able to walk her dog at a brisk pace, actively garden, and shovel light snow. She has had no chest pain or dyspnea on exertion. She has type 2 diabetes mellitus, hypertension, hyperlipidemia, and chronic kidney disease. Current medications are insulin, lisinopril, and simvastatin.

On physical examination, temperature is normal, blood pressure is 132/88 mm Hg, and pulse rate is 78/min. Heart rate and rhythm are regular with no murmurs or gallops. Laboratory studies show a serum creatinine level of 2.4 mg/dL (212 μmol/L). Electrocardiogram shows normal sinus rhythm without ST- or T-wave abnormalities.

Which of the following is the most appropriate diagnostic test to perform prior to surgery?

(A) Adenosine thallium stress test
(B) Cardiac catheterization
(C) Exercise stress test
(D) Proceed to surgery without further testing

Answers and Critiques

Item 1   Answer: A

Educational Objective: Identify appropriate genetic counseling strategies.

The most appropriate screening step for genetic diseases in this patient is to inquire about any diseases that "run in the family" and, specifically, to inquire about family history of the more common and important inherited diseases, including breast, ovarian, prostate, and colon cancer, as well as early cardiovascular disease. A detailed family history should follow for those conditions identified through this preliminary questioning. Patient-reported family histories for first-degree relatives have been shown to be accurate and valuable for breast and colon cancer, but a negative family history for ovarian and endometrial cancer is less accurate. Although few diseases follow strict Mendelian genetics that allow for a relatively certain prediction of disease, knowledge regarding the frequency of disease occurrence in a given family cohort is helpful in assessing individual risk for developing specific disorders with a genetic predisposition.

Genetic counseling with the option for testing should be offered when: (1) the patient has a personal or family history suggestive of a genetic susceptibility condition; (2) the genetic test can be adequately interpreted; and (3) the test results will aid in diagnosis or influence the medical or surgical management of the patient or family at hereditary risk. It is premature to refer for genetic counseling without first determining if there is concern for a genetic disorder.

The process of taking a family history typically employed by medical genetics professionals is both labor- and time-intensive. It typically involves a three-generation pedigree and may require hours to complete. Given the multiple demands on the internist during the clinical encounter, this degree of detail is not feasible.

Although it is standard of care to perform genetic testing for certain mutations in unselected preconception, prenatal, and newborn populations, and direct-to-consumer genomic kits are commercially available, at least three important issues make it unwise to perform genetic testing in unselected populations seen by internists: (1) the clinical validity of such a test may be lacking, (2) there may be a high likelihood of false-positive tests, and (3) the harms of performing a genetic test may outweigh any benefits.

> **KEY POINT**
> - The most appropriate first screening step for genetic diseases is to inquire about any diseases that "run in the family" and to inquire specifically about family history of the more common and important inherited diseases, including breast, ovarian, prostate, and colon cancer, as well as early cardiovascular disease.

Bibliography

Berg AO, Baird MA, Botkin JR, et al. National Institute of Health State-of-the-Science Conference Statement: Family History and Improving Health. Ann Intern Med. 2009; 151(12):872-877. [PMID: 19884615]

Item 2   Answer: D

Educational Objective: Treat carpal tunnel syndrome.

This patient has carpal tunnel syndrome, and the most appropriate initial treatment, in addition to the avoidance of repetitive wrist motions, is wrist splinting. Wrist splinting appears to be most effective when done in the neutral position compared with 20 degrees of extension. In one prospective study, full-time splinting was superior to nocturnal splinting at 6 weeks in terms of nerve latencies, although there was significant cross-over of patients between groups in this study. Nocturnal splinting has the advantage of being more convenient to patients in comparison with full-time splinting.

Local corticosteroid injection has been shown to provide short-term (up to 3 months) pain relief, although the effect does not appear to be durable. Contraindications to local corticosteroid injections include thenar weakness and atrophy, profound sensory loss, and acute carpal tunnel syndrome.

Owing to possible adverse effects, drug therapy should be reserved for patients in whom wrist splinting has failed. Although NSAIDs are frequently used as first-line therapy, evidence is lacking as to their effectiveness.

Surgical intervention should be reserved for patients in whom both nonpharmacologic and pharmacologic conservative therapies have failed. Other indications include progressive sensory or motor deficits and moderate to severe findings on electrodiagnostic studies. In one randomized controlled trial of 116 patients, those with carpal tunnel syndrome who underwent surgical intervention had better outcomes (function and symptoms) than those who underwent nonsurgical management, although clinically, the benefit was modest.

> **KEY POINT**
> - Initial therapy for carpal tunnel syndrome is wrist splinting and avoidance of repetitive wrist motions.

Bibliography

Jarvik JG, Comstock BA, Kliot M, et al. Surgery versus non-surgical therapy for carpal tunnel syndrome: a randomised parallel-group trial. Lancet. 2009;374(9695):1074-1081. [PMID: 19782873]

Item 3   Answer: A

Educational Objective: Treat obsessive-compulsive disorder.

In addition to cognitive-behavioral therapy (CBT), the pharmacologic treatment of choice for this patient is a selective serotonin reuptake inhibitor (SSRI) such as fluoxetine. She has the hallmark features of obsessive-compulsive disorder (OCD), including recurrent obsessions or compulsions sufficiently severe to occupy 1 hour daily or result in marked distress or impaired social function. Obsessions are persistent ideas, thoughts, impulses, or images experienced as intrusive and are associated with significant anxiety or distress. Examples include fears of having left doors unlocked and fears of germ contamination. Compulsions are repetitive behaviors, such as handwashing, checking, ordering, or counting, that are repeated to decrease the anxiety related to the obsessions. Cognitive-behavioral therapy (CBT) with an exposure therapy element is the treatment of choice for OCD. SSRIs are the most effective pharmacotherapy and should be used in patients who are resistant or only partially responsive to CBT and in those with more severe OCD or in whom a rapid response is critical. Higher SSRI doses are often needed to treat OCD as compared with depression, and the dose may be escalated at 2- to 4-week intervals. Adjunctive use of antipsychotics has some evidence of benefit.

Haloperidol, a typical antipsychotic agent, has been shown to be effective in combination with an SSRI for OCD in patients who are refractory to initial treatment. Haloperidol has many serious adverse effects, including QT-interval prolongation and extrapyramidal symptoms that further limit its use as a first-line agent.

Benzodiazepines, such as lorazepam, are not effective for treating OCD and should be avoided given their lack of efficacy and high risk for dependence.

Quetiapine is an atypical antipsychotic agent that has not been shown to improve OCD symptoms in patients who are refractory to serotonin reuptake inhibitor monotherapy.

KEY POINT

- **Cognitive-behavioral therapy (CBT) with an exposure element is the treatment of choice for obsessive-compulsive disorder (OCD); high-dose selective serotonin reuptake inhibitors should be used in patients who are resistant or only partially responsive to CBT and in those with more severe OCD or in whom a rapid response is critical.**

Bibliography

Soomro GM, Altman D, Rajagopal S, Oakley-Browne M. Selective serotonin re-uptake inhibitors (SSRIs) versus placebo for obsessive compulsive disorder (OCD). Cochrane Database Syst Rev. 2008;(1):CD001765. [PMID: 18253995]

Item 4   Answer: D

Educational Objective: Manage epistaxis.

This patient should be told to apply uninterrupted nasal pressure for 15 to 30 minutes, to not remove the clot or blow his nose, and to temporarily discontinue nasal corticosteroids. More than 90% of epistaxis cases occur at the anterior nasal septum in the Kiesselbach area, the anteroinferior aspect of the nasal septum where multiple arteries anastomose to form a plexus. These episodes of bleeding almost always stop with consistent pressure for at least 15 minutes. Direct causes of epistaxis include nose picking, dry air during winter months, intranasal corticosteroids and decongestants, bacterial or viral rhinosinusitis, and less commonly tumors.

Nasal arterial embolization is reserved for severe refractory epistaxis, which this patient does not have.

The patient would not require cauterization and anterior nasal packing unless the bleeding fails to resolve with at least 15 to 30 minutes of pressure. Nasal packing with or without nasal constrictive agents is effective (60%-80%) but uncomfortable for the patient given that the packing is left in for 1 to 3 days.

Based upon the patient's history, it is unlikely that he has a bleeding disorder as a systemic cause of his epistaxis and is unlikely to have developed a significant anemia from 2 hours of epistaxis. Laboratory studies are rarely helpful in healthy patients with epistaxis. Even in patients with known bleeding disorders, laboratory studies and coagulation studies are normal in 80% of patients.

It is not necessary to consult an otorhinolaryngologist because the patient reports that the bleeding stops with pressure and the examiner has identified an oozing vessel in the anterior nasal septum. Posterior bleeds warrant referral because they can be difficult to control by application of direct external pressure.

KEY POINT

- **Anterior nosebleeds almost always stop with consistent pressure for at least 15 minutes.**

Bibliography

Schlosser R. Epistaxis. N Engl J Med. 2009;360(8):784-789. [PMID: 19228621]

Item 5   Answer: B

Educational Objective: Diagnose hypoactive sexual desire disorder.

The most likely diagnosis is hypoactive sexual desire disorder (HSDD). Female sexual dysfunction, defined as sexual difficulties that are persistent and personally distressing to the patient, affects up to 35% of sexually active women and is common among middle-aged women. HSDD is defined as a persistent lack of desire for or receptiveness to sexual activity or a persistent lack of sexual thoughts. HSDD is one of the most common causes of female sexual dysfunction, and prevalence ranges from 12% to 19%. Natural and surgical menopause may contribute to the development of HSDD, as the associated decline in testosterone levels may decrease sexual motivation and desire. There is no FDA-approved medication for the treatment of female HSDD; individual and couples sex therapy or psychotherapy may be beneficial.

Dyspareunia is persistent urogenital pain that occurs around intercourse and is not related exclusively to inadequate lubrication or vaginismus. Several conditions may cause dyspareunia, including interstitial cystitis, pelvic adhesions, infections, endometriosis, pelvic venous congestion, and vulvodynia. Treatment is aimed at correcting the underlying abnormality. This patient's absence of sexual pain, history of previously normal sexual intercourse, and lack of symptoms and signs associated with any of the aforementioned conditions (no urinary symptoms, no history of pelvic surgeries or sexually transmitted infections) make dyspareunia an unlikely etiology for her current sexual problems.

Sexual aversion disorder is a persistent or recurrent aversive response to any genital contact with a sexual partner. Physiologic responses often accompany these feelings, with associated nausea and shortness of breath. Frequently there is a history of a painful or traumatic sexual event. Although this patient is avoiding intercourse, this is related to low sexual desire and motivation. Patients with sexual aversion disorder avoid intercourse because of feelings of revulsion and disgust.

Vaginismus is involuntary and recurrent spasm of the outer third of the vaginal musculature that interferes with vaginal penetration. Pain may accompany this involuntary spasm, and there is often associated avoidance and anticipatory fear of penetration. Prevalence ranges between 1% and 6%. On examination, this patient easily tolerated insertion of the vaginal speculum without any evidence of muscular spasm, although it should be noted that some women experience vaginismus only during sexual activity (situation-specific).

KEY POINT

- Hypoactive sexual desire disorder, a common cause of female sexual dysfunction, is defined as a persistent lack of desire for or receptiveness to sexual activity or a persistent lack of sexual thoughts.

Bibliography
Kingsberg S, Althof SE. Evaluation and treatment of female sexual disorders. Int Urogynecol J Pelvic Floor Dysfunct. 2009;20(suppl 1):S33-S43. [PMID: 19440781]

Item 6   Answer: D
Educational Objective: Treat dyspnea at the end of life.

This patient on comfort care should be given morphine. Dyspnea is one of the most common symptoms encountered in palliative care. It is most often the result of direct cardiothoracic pathology, such as pleural effusion, heart failure, COPD, pulmonary embolism, pneumonia, or lung metastases. Dyspnea can also be caused by systemic conditions, such as anemia, muscle weakness, or conditions causing abdominal distention. Patients with underlying lung disease on bronchodilator therapy should have this therapy continued to maintain comfort. Opioids are effective in reducing dyspnea in patients with underlying cardiopulmonary disease and malignancy. In patients already receiving opioids, using the breakthrough pain dose for dyspnea and increasing this dose by 25% if not fully effective may be helpful. A 5-mg dose of oral morphine given four times daily has been shown to help relieve dyspnea in patients with end-stage heart failure. Low-dose (20 mg) extended-release morphine given daily has been used to relieve dyspnea in patients with advanced COPD.

Antibiotics and corticosteroids are appropriately used in patients with exacerbations of severe COPD. However, neither would be expected to provide immediate relief of the patient's respiratory distress and would also be inconsistent with care focusing primarily on comfort measures at the end of life.

In contrast to opioids, benzodiazepines have not demonstrated consistent benefit in treating dyspnea. However, they may be useful in specific patients who have significant anxiety associated with their dyspnea.

KEY POINT

- Opioids are effective in reducing dyspnea in patients with underlying cardiopulmonary disease and malignancy.

Bibliography
Swetz KM, Kamal AH. Palliative care. Ann Intern Med. 2012;156(3):ITC21. [PMID: 22312158]

Item 7   Answer: D
Educational Objective: Diagnose chronic fatigue syndrome.

This patient requires no additional testing. Chronic fatigue syndrome (CFS) is defined as medically unexplained fatigue that persists for 6 months or more, accompanied by at least four of the following symptoms: subjective memory impairment, sore throat, tender lymph nodes, muscle or joint pain, headache, unrefreshing sleep, and postexertional malaise lasting longer than 24 hours.

There is no diagnostic test for CFS. An appropriate history and physical examination should include an assessment for common causes of fatigue, including a sleep history; those with a history of loud snoring, apneic spells, or frequent limb movements during sleep should undergo a sleep study to evaluate for sleep apnea or restless legs syndrome. All patients with fatigue should be assessed for depression and anxiety disorders. Patients with hypothyroidism may present with fatigue in the absence of other findings; it is reasonable to order a thyroid-stimulating hormone level. If significant weight loss, lymphadenopathy, or fever is found, assessment for malignancy and chronic infections should ensue. A complete blood count should be obtained to rule out anemia and to look for evidence of lymphoma or leukemia. A metabolic panel is reasonable to rule out diabetes mellitus, kidney disease, and liver disease. An erythrocyte sedimentation rate can help assess for an active inflammatory process. Additional studies may be warranted in selected patients based on the history and physical examination findings. This patient, however, has no findings on physical examination that warrant additional testing and her previous laboratory evaluation was appropriate and normal; repeating previously normal laboratory tests is not indicated.

Although CFS has been associated with certain viruses, such as Epstein-Barr virus and parvovirus B19, these associations have not been reproduced consistently in studies. Thus, obtaining titers for these viruses would neither definitely identify etiology nor result in a treatable diagnosis.

KEY POINT

- There is no test that is diagnostic for chronic fatigue syndrome; in addition to a complete history and physical examination, reasonable tests to consider are a complete blood count, comprehensive metabolic panel, and thyroid-stimulating hormone level.

Bibliography

Holgate ST, Komaroff AL, Mangan D, Wessely S. Chronic fatigue syndrome: understanding a complex illness. Nat Rev Neurosci. 2011;12(9):539-544. [PMID: 21792218]

Item 8   Answer: D
Educational Objective: Manage preoperative testing in a patient without comorbidities.

The only diagnostic test appropriate to perform preoperatively in this young woman is a pregnancy test. A preoperative pregnancy test is recommended in all women for whom pregnancy is still possible. Any additional preoperative testing should be selective, based on the likelihood of finding an abnormality and, more importantly, that the result will change management. The results of most screening tests will be normal, and any abnormalities found usually do not affect management. Additionally, patients with previously normal laboratory studies in the 4 months prior to surgery and no change in their clinical condition rarely warrant repeat testing. However, most hospital policies continue to require preoperative screening tests despite the evidence to the contrary. This approach is not endorsed by any major physician groups and, owing to chance alone, will yield 1 abnormal result for every 20 tests ordered, which are typically either false-positive results or of no clinical significance.

This patient has no symptoms or signs of pulmonary disease. In the absence of this, chest radiography has a low

pretest probability of abnormality and should not be ordered.

In the absence of a personal or family history of abnormal bleeding, liver disease, significant alcohol use, malabsorption, or anticoagulation therapy, the likelihood of a bleeding disorder is low, and no further preoperative testing is required.

This patient is young, has no signs or symptoms of cardiac disease, and no risk factors for early or silent myocardial infarction. Preoperative electrocardiography should be limited to patients in whom a silent or previously unrecognized myocardial infarction is possible.

KEY POINT

- Perioperative testing should be limited to tests that have a reasonable pretest probability of being abnormal, and whose abnormal result would directly impact perioperative care.

Bibliography

Hepner DL. The role of testing in the preoperative evaluation. Cleve Clin J Med. 2009;76 (suppl 4):S22-7. [PMID: 19880831]

Item 9   Answer: B
Educational Objective: Evaluate pulsatile tinnitus.

Tinnitus that is timed with the patient's pulse (pulsatile tinnitus) is concerning for an intracranial vascular anomaly, such as stenosis, arteriovenous malformation, or glomus tumor, although patients with middle ear congestion may report a pulsatile sensation as part of their symptom complex. It is valuable to listen over the patient's ears, eyes, and neck, because if a vascular abnormality is present, the bruit causing tinnitus may sometimes be detected externally (objective tinnitus). If a bruit is present, or there is other significant concern for a vascular cause of tinnitus, imaging of the cranial vasculature (Doppler ultrasonography or magnetic resonance angiography) is the definitive study to rule out these diagnoses.

Audiometry would be appropriate if the patient had decreased auditory acuity, but this patient's physical examination findings do not suggest hearing loss.

External noise generators to mask the sound of tinnitus are helpful for some patients and may be reasonable to consider in this patient if no reversible cause is found. Evidence supporting their efficacy is sparse, however. The mainstay of therapy for tinnitus is neurocognitive interventions to help patients cope with the problem and diminish dysfunctional cognitive processes associated with the experience of tinnitus.

Nasal corticosteroid sprays can be helpful in patients with eustachian tube dysfunction, although this is an uncommon cause of tinnitus associated with conductive hearing loss. This patient does not demonstrate conductive hearing loss and has no evidence of middle ear congestion on examination. Thus, nasal corticosteroids are not indicated as the next step in management.

KEY POINT

- Patients with pulsatile tinnitus should be evaluated for the possible presence of an intracranial vascular anomaly, such as stenosis, arteriovenous malformation, or glomus tumor as a cause of their symptoms.

Bibliography

Liyanage SH, Singh A, Savundra P, Kalan A. Pulsatile tinnitus. J Laryngol Otol. 2006;120(2):93-97. [PMID: 16359136]

Item 10   Answer: D

Educational Objective: Counsel a patient regarding methods for smoking cessation.

Although both counseling and pharmacotherapy are effective strategies for smoking cessation, the combination of counseling with medication use is more effective than either intervention alone. Nicotine replacement is effective for smoking cessation; its availability in multiple formulations (gum, lozenge, patch, aerosol) allows for alternative options in patients who have not benefited from one type of therapy, as in this patient. Although centrally acting agents (bupropion, varenicline) are also effective treatment options, bupropion would be contraindicated in this patient with an underlying seizure disorder. The choice of cessation method is less important than that an effective method is used correctly by the patient; the array of treatment options allows for individualization based on patient preference, previous experience, cost, and potential side effects. Counseling may be brief or intensive; the two most effective counseling components include practical problem-solving skills and social support.

Many smokers indicate that stress reduction is a primary reason for their tobacco use. Although selected individuals with true anxiety disorders may benefit from anxiolytic therapy, the use of benzodiazepines as a smoking cessation medication has not been documented.

Electronic smokeless cigarettes deliver a warmed aerosol through a cigarette-like device that bears the appearance, physical sensation, and possibly the taste of tobacco smoke, with the intention of helping smokers maintain the activities associated with smoking but without the harmful effects. However, their use in smoking cessation has not been established.

KEY POINT

- Smoking cessation is achieved more effectively with a combination of counseling and anti-smoking medication use than with either intervention alone.

Bibliography

2008 PHS Guideline Update Panel, Liasons, and Staff. Treating tobacco use and dependence: 2008 update U.S. Public Health Service

Clinical Practice Guideline executive summary. Respir Care. 2008;53(9):1217-1222. [PMID: 18807274]

Item 11   Answer: A

Educational Objective: Manage viral conjunctivitis.

The most appropriate management is the application of cool compresses to the affected eye. This patient has symptoms and signs most consistent with viral conjunctivitis. Onset is usually acute, with unilateral redness, watery discharge, itching, crusting, a diffuse foreign body sensation, and mild photophobia. This patient's preceding upper respiratory tract infection, normal vision, and unilateral eye involvement are supportive of this diagnosis. Viral conjunctivitis is managed conservatively with cool compresses. The patient should be told not to share towels or other personal items with family members and should wash his hands frequently throughout the day. He should also be warned that the infection may spread to the other eye before resolving.

Allergic conjunctivitis may be recurrent and seasonal and presents with itching, conjunctival edema, and cobblestoning under the upper lid. It usually responds to topical antihistamines, short-course topical NSAIDs (3 days maximum), and compresses. Oral antihistamines have no role in the treatment of viral conjunctivitis.

Bacterial conjunctivitis usually has a mucopurulent discharge, in contrast to the clear, watery discharge seen in viral conjunctivitis. Topical antibiotics are not efficacious for viral conjunctivitis and can be associated with adverse effects, including the development of contact dermatitis and antibiotic resistance. If a lubricant is required, non-antibacterial lubricating agents may be used.

Topical corticosteroids are not indicated despite the patient's discomfort and should rarely, if ever, be used by physicians other than ophthalmologists. If used inappropriately for herpes simplex, fungal, or bacterial conjunctivitis, topical corticosteroids can lead to corneal scarring, melting, and perforation.

KEY POINT

- Viral conjunctivitis, characterized by acute onset and unilateral redness, watery discharge, itching, crusting, a diffuse foreign body sensation, and mild photophobia, is managed conservatively with cool compresses.

Bibliography

Galor A, Jeng BH. Red eye for the internist: when to treat, when to refer. Clev Clin J Med. 2008;75(2):137-144. [PMID: 18290357]

Item 12   Answer: A

Educational Objective: Identify anchoring as a source of diagnostic error.

This case illustrates an error resulting from an anchoring heuristic. Heuristics are cognitive shortcuts that clinicians employ in an attempt to efficiently reach a diagnosis. Anchoring occurs when a diagnostician latches onto a diagnosis and fails to consider other possibilities for the presenting symptoms. The physician in this case settled on a diagnosis because another physician previously diagnosed the patient. Despite the fact that there are other pieces of data that do not fit the diagnosis—tachycardia, relative hypotension, abdominal distention, and lack of reproducibility of pain with musculoskeletal examination contrary to the diagnosis of "groin strain"—the clinician remains anchored to the diagnosis established in the emergency department. This type of error can be avoided by explicitly looking for findings that do not fit the diagnosis as well as by using a "worst case scenario" approach to patient care—considering the diagnoses that would be most life-threatening to the patient, such as an abdominal aortic aneurysm in a patient with risk factors for this condition.

The availability heuristic is used when a clinician attempts to make a diagnosis based upon what is available in the physician's mind rather than what is most probable. For example, if the physician had seen a similar patient with a groin strain from physical activity the previous week and decided that this was the most likely diagnosis, the clinician would be missing the diagnosis because of the availability heuristic.

A no-fault error is one in which the presentation is misleading and the clinician has little opportunity to pick up clues based on any data that there is an underlying problem.

The representativeness heuristic is used when the clinician applies pattern recognition in making a diagnosis. This source of diagnostic error occurs when the patient's clinical presentation appears to fit a typical case with similar features but the clinician fails to consider other disease processes that may also present in this manner.

KEY POINT

- **Anchoring heuristic errors occur when a clinician holds to an initial impression, such as might occur when a referring physician has provided a diagnosis that is then accepted at face value.**

Bibliography

Trowbridge RL. Twelve tips for teaching avoidance of diagnostic errors. Med Teach. 2008;30(5):496-500. [PMID: 18576188]

Item 13   Answer: C

Educational Objective: Treat acute rhinosinusitis.

Treatment with chlorpheniramine may be considered for this patient. The common cold, or rhinosinusitis, presents with acute cough, nasal congestion, rhinorrhea, and occasionally, low-grade fever. Targeted treatment is aimed at symptom relief. Antihistamines, such as chlorpheniramine, and antihistamine-decongestant combinations have been shown to decrease congestion and rhinorrhea with variable

effects on cough suppression. Second-generation nonsedating antihistamines are generally ineffective for rhinosinusitis symptoms.

Albuterol does not relieve symptoms of rhinosinusitis unless wheezing is present. The patient did not report wheezing or shortness of breath, and wheezes were not heard on examination.

Because rhinosinusitis is caused by viruses, routine antibiotic treatment in immunocompetent hosts is not recommended. Antibiotics do not improve symptoms, illness duration, or patient satisfaction with medical care. Contrary to common belief, purulent sputum does not reliably predict bacterial infection or superinfection. Therefore, sputum purulence should not be used as a criterion for antibiotic administration. Evidence-based guidelines from the Infectious Diseases Society of America suggest that if bacterial rhinosinusitis is highly suspected, based on the presence of persistent symptoms or signs lasting more than 10 days without evidence of clinical improvement, onset with severe symptoms (fever >39.0 °C [102.2 °F]), or onset with worsening symptoms or signs (new fever, headache, or upper respiratory tract infection symptoms that were initially improving), the antibiotic of choice is amoxicillin-clavulanate.

Multiple studies have found little if any improvement in acute cough associated with acute upper respiratory tract infections by using codeine, dextromethorphan, or moguisteine antitussive therapy. The American College of Chest Physicians does not recommend treatment with these medications. Codeine may be effective in patients with chronic cough; however, it is not indicated in this patient with acute rhinosinusitis.

Other treatments that may relieve symptoms of rhinosinusitis include intranasal ipratropium (rhinorrhea and sneezing), intranasal cromolyn (rhinorrhea, cough, throat pain), and short-term topical nasal decongestants (nasal obstruction). Consistent high-quality data on the use of zinc, echinacea, and vitamin C do not support the use of these over-the-counter products for the treatment or prevention of rhinosinusitis.

KEY POINT

- **Antibiotics are not recommended for the treatment of acute rhinosinusitis.**

Bibliography

Siamasek M, Blandino DA. Treatment of the common cold. Am Fam Physician. 2007;75(4):515-520. [PMID: 17323712]

Item 14   Answer: A

Educational Objective: Diagnose benign paroxysmal positional vertigo.

This patient has benign paroxysmal positional vertigo (BPPV). The first step in the evaluation of the patient with dizziness is to distinguish among its major causes: vertigo, presyncope, dysequilibrium, and other nonspecific causes.

This patient describes classic vertigo, a sensation that his stationary environment is spinning around him (or that one is spinning around in one's environment).

There are two major categories of vertigo, peripheral and central. Peripheral causes of vertigo include BPPV, vestibular neuronitis, Meniere disease, aminoglycoside toxicity, and herpes zoster. Patients with all causes of peripheral vertigo have similar findings on the Dix-Hallpike maneuver, in which the examiner supports the patient's head in 20 degrees of extension while sitting, then assists the patient rapidly to the supine position with the head turned to one side and hanging over the edge of the examining table; the test is repeated with the head turned to the other side. A positive test results in horizontal nystagmus with latency of 2 to 40 seconds and duration less than 1 minute, with reproduction of symptoms that will fatigue and habituate. Patients with BPPV describe episodes of vertigo lasting less than 1 minute that occur with a rapid change in head position, as in this patient. Nervous system imaging or other testing is not required for diagnosis in patients with classic findings and an otherwise normal neurologic examination.

Central vertigo may result from ischemia, infarction, or hemorrhage of the brainstem or cerebellum. It is accompanied by diplopia, dysarthria, dysphagia, focal weakness, numbness, or gait abnormalities, depending on the involved area of the brain. On the Dix-Hallpike maneuver, the induced nystagmus has no latency, lasts more than 1 minute, and can have a vertical direction. The Dix-Hallpike maneuver findings in this patient are consistent with peripheral, not central, vertigo. As he has neither cardiovascular risk factors nor focal neurologic abnormalities, cerebellar infarction is unlikely.

The classic triad of Meniere disease is vertigo, unilateral hearing loss, and tinnitus. The vertigo in Meniere disease is usually not positional, as in this patient, and he does not have hearing loss or tinnitus.

Vestibular neuronitis is frequently associated with a viral infection. Symptoms generally last much longer than they do in BPPV (days) but can be more severe. Although symptoms typically resolve within 1 week, residual dizziness can last for months. The recurrent, intense, and brief nature of this patient's episodes of vertigo makes BPPV a more likely diagnosis.

KEY POINT

- **Benign paroxysmal positional vertigo is characterized by brief episodes of severe vertigo brought on by a rapid change in head position and Dix-Hallpike maneuver findings of delayed horizontal nystagmus with a rotatory component concurrent with symptoms of vertigo.**

Bibliography

Bhattacharyya N, Baugh RF, Orvidas L, et al. Clinical practice guideline: benign paroxysmal positional vertigo. Otolaryngol Head Neck Surg. 2008;139(5)(suppl 4):S47-81. [PMID: 18973840]

Item 15   Answer: D

Educational Objective: Diagnose vitamin B_{12} deficiency in a patient who has undergone gastric bypass surgery.

This patient's serum vitamin B_{12} level should be measured. Macrocytic anemia, thrombocytopenia, mild neutropenia, and an inappropriately low reticulocyte count are the hallmark hematologic findings in vitamin B_{12} deficiency. Vitamin B_{12} deficiency is one the most common nonoperative complications of Roux-en-Y gastric bypass surgery. It results from decreased absorption of vitamin B_{12}, mainly through lack of intrinsic factor production from the bypassed gastric mucosa. It is essential for patients who undergo a roux-en-Y gastric bypass procedure to participate in postoperative monitoring of vitamin B_{12} levels and to maintain lifelong adequate vitamin B_{12} supplementation (500-1000 micrograms/d orally or 1000 micrograms intramuscularly monthly). Recent guidelines recommend that serum vitamin B_{12} levels, along with ferritin, folate, vitamin D, and calcium, be monitored twice yearly for the first 2 years after Roux-en-Y gastric bypass surgery and yearly thereafter.

A bone marrow biopsy, a relatively invasive and costly test, is premature at this point. Bone marrow biopsy is indicated for unexplained anemia, leukopenia, thrombocytopenia, or pancytopenia. The patient has a high likelihood of vitamin B_{12} deficiency that can explain the patient's hematologic findings, and a performing a bone marrow biopsy prior to measuring the serum vitamin B_{12} level would be inappropriate.

With no gastrointestinal symptoms, no family history of colorectal cancer, a benign abdominal examination, guaiac-negative stool, and a macrocytic (not microcytic) anemia with neutropenia and thrombocytopenia, the suspicion for gastrointestinal malignancy or other lower gastrointestinal tract disease is very low. Therefore, a colonoscopy is not indicated at this point.

Based on history and physical examination, there is no strong clinical suspicion for thyroid disease. Although hypothyroidism can be associated with mild macrocytosis, the presence of neutropenia and thrombocytopenia is inconsistent with this diagnosis. Therefore, measuring the serum thyroid-stimulating hormone level is not indicated.

KEY POINT

- **Vitamin B_{12} deficiency is common after Roux-en-Y gastric bypass surgery.**

Bibliography

Buchwald H, Ikramuddin S, Dorman RB, Schone JL, Dixon JB. Management of the metabolic/bariatric surgery patient. Am J Med. 2011;124(12):1099-1105. [PMID: 22014789]

Item 16   Answer: D

Educational Objective: Manage a patient's request for genetic testing.

This patient should be referred for genetic counseling. Huntington disease is an autosomal dominant disorder caused by a CAG repeat within the gene on chromosome 4. Because of the potential harms from genetic test information and the need for patients and their families to receive appropriate information for decision-making, patients with possible inherited diseases should undergo genetic testing only in the context of genetic counseling. Genetic counseling should include discussion of possible risks and benefits of early detection and prevention modalities. Genetic counseling with the option for testing should be offered when: (1) the patient has a personal or family history suggestive of a genetic susceptibility condition; (2) the genetic test can be adequately interpreted; and (3) the test results will aid in diagnosis or influence the medical or surgical management of the patient or family at hereditary risk.

Brain MRI in patients with well-defined findings of Huntington disease demonstrates caudate atrophy. Such imaging is unlikely to be helpful in an asymptomatic patient and is not preferred to genetic counseling in estimating the likelihood of disease.

Symptoms of Huntington disease typically begin in the fourth and fifth decades, but 10% of patients have symptoms in the second decade. It is premature to reassure the patient, considering her young age and absence of genetic test data.

> **KEY POINT**
> - Patients with possible inherited diseases should be referred for genetic testing only in the context of genetic counseling.

Bibliography

Berg AO, Baird MA, Botkin JR, et al. National Institute of Health State-of-the-Science Conference Statement: Family History and Improving Health. Ann Intern Med. 2009; 151(12):872-877. [PMID: 19884615]

H **Item 17   Answer: A**
Educational Objective: Manage a pressure ulcer.

This patient has a stage III or IV pressure ulcer, and debridement is the most appropriate management. Both stage III and stage IV pressure ulcers include full-thickness tissue loss. In stage III ulcers, subcutaneous fat may be visible but bone, tendon, and muscle are not exposed, whereas in stage IV ulcers, bone, tendon, or muscle is exposed and undermining and tunneling are often present. The eschar covering this patient's wound precludes the definitive differentiation of a stage III from a stage IV ulcer.

Treatment of pressure ulcers is best managed with an interdisciplinary team approach, with a care plan directed toward addressing the factors that predisposed to the development of the ulcer. Dressings should be chosen to maintain a moist wound environment and manage exudates. When present, infection should be controlled with topical therapies and the addition of systemic antibiotics

when cellulitis is present. The possibility of underlying osteomyelitis should be considered. Surgical or nonsurgical debridement of eschar and nonviable tissue may be needed. Wet-to-dry dressings may aid in debridement but caution must be used to avoid removing excessive viable tissue with dressing changes.

Cochrane reviews do not support a role for electromagnetic therapy, ultrasound therapy, or hyperbaric oxygen therapy in pressure ulcer treatment.

Negative-pressure wound vacuum healing has been used for stage IV ulcers. However, three clinical trials have not shown superiority to standard therapy. Wound vacuum therapy may be more convenient due to less frequent dressing changes but is also very costly. It is not the recommended first line therapy.

Although frequently utilized, vitamin C and zinc oral supplements have not been shown to aid in ulcer healing.

Referral for surgical flap and repair may be necessary for refractory pressure ulcers but is usually reserved for patients in whom conservative treatment has failed.

> **KEY POINT**
> - Stage III pressure ulcers, defined by full-thickness tissue loss but without exposure of bone, tendon, or muscle, generally require debridement, proper dressing selection, and treatment of infection, if present.

Bibliography

Reddy M, Gill SS, Kalkar SR, et al. Treatment of pressure ulcers: a systematic review. JAMA. 2008;300(22):2647-2662. [PMID: 19066385]

Item 18   Answer: E
Educational Objective: Diagnose benign prostatic hyperplasia.

The most important diagnostic test to perform next in this patient is urinalysis. Benign prostatic hyperplasia (BPH) is an extremely common cause of lower urinary tract symptoms in men, such as nocturia, urinary frequency and urgency, decreased urinary stream, urinary retention, incomplete bladder emptying, and incontinence. Symptoms may worsen with increasing size of the prostate. The American Urological Association (AUA) recommends screening and following the AUA symptom score to assess need for and effectiveness of treatment. Diagnostic work-up for BPH includes the necessity to rule out underlying infection. Although this patient does not have specific symptoms or clinical findings suggestive of a urinary tract infection, abnormal bladder emptying increases the risk for infection, and even subclinical infection may exacerbate BPH symptoms. Therefore, urinalysis (and if positive, a subsequent urine culture) is indicated in this patient.

Postvoid residual urinary volumes are measured via in-and-out catheterization or by ultrasonography after a patient spontaneously voids. This test is not indicated for routine management of BPH but is useful in evaluation of overflow incontinence or neurogenic bladder. As neither of these conditions is present in this patient, postvoid residual urinary volume measurement is not indicated.

Elevated plasma glucose levels may cause urinary frequency and nocturia due to osmotic diuresis but are unlikely to cause weak stream or urinary hesitancy. Additionally, urinary incontinence due to neurogenic bladder can be seen in late-stage diabetes mellitus with neuropathic complications; however, this patient has no history of diabetes mellitus and is not incontinent.

The U.S. Preventive Services Task Force has concluded that the harms of screening for prostate cancer outweigh the benefits in men of any age regardless of risk factors. Other guidelines, including those of the AUA, recommend offering periodic screening to men older than 50 years who have a life expectancy of at least 10 years. The presence of BPH symptoms does not affect indications for prostate cancer screening.

Transrectal ultrasound of the prostate is most commonly used for evaluation of prostate cancer. Prostate cancer itself rarely causes lower urinary tract symptoms as seen in this patient.

KEY POINT

- Diagnostic work-up for benign prostatic hyperplasia (BPH) includes urinalysis to rule out underlying infection; neither post-void residual urinary volume measurement nor prostate-specific antigen testing is indicated in the routine evaluation of BPH.

Bibliography
McVary KT, Roehrborn CG, Avins AL, et al. Update on AUA guideline on the management of benign prostatic hyperplasia. J Urol. 2011;185(5):1793-1803. [PMID: 21420124]

Item 19   Answer: D
Educational Objective: Treat cancer-related pain.

Sustained-release morphine should be started to better control this patient's cancer-related pain. Long-acting morphine is indicated in cancer patients who develop persistent pain throughout the day or beyond 24 hours of treatment with shorter-acting opioids. The initial dose is usually 30% to 50% of a patient's current 24-hour usage of short-acting opioid. He should also be prescribed short-acting oral morphine for breakthrough pain, and his long-acting morphine should be gradually titrated upward until his pain is well controlled.

A fentanyl patch is convenient and reduces frequency of dosing but will take 24 hours to begin working. Therefore, used alone it would not be the correct choice for this patient who is being discharged today.

Methadone, a long-acting opioid, has an unpredictable half-life that varies from patient to patient making it challenging to dose-adjust. It has also been linked to QT-interval prolongation and other arrhythmias. It should be used with caution, with monitoring of the QT interval. For these reasons, methadone is generally a less ideal choice for long-term pain control in cancer patients.

Short-acting hydromorphone has a rapid onset of action and is dosed every 4 to 6 hours. This would not be optimal in this patient as he requires sustained relief from his pain and would require repeated doses for adequate control, including during hours of sleep. Extended-release hydromorphone preparations are now available, and in conjunction with short-acting hydromorphone for breakthrough pain, these formulations would also be a reasonable treatment option.

KEY POINT

- Long-acting morphine is indicated in cancer patients who develop persistent pain throughout the day or beyond 24 hours of treatment with shorter-acting opioids; the initial dose is usually 30% to 50% of a patient's current 24-hour usage of short-acting opioid.

Bibliography
Swetz KM, Kamal AH. Palliative care. Ann Intern Med. 2012;156(3):ITC2-1-TC2-16. [PMID: 22312158]

Item 20   Answer: C
Educational Objective: Manage unilateral sensorineural hearing loss.

This patient should undergo MRI of the posterior fossa and internal auditory canal. His sensorineural hearing loss is confirmed on physical examination, which demonstrates lateralization of the Weber test to the left ear and demonstration of better hearing with air conduction than bone conduction with the Rinne test. The Rinne test is about 80% sensitive in diagnosing sensorineural hearing loss. In patients with asymmetric sensorineural hearing loss that is not clearly due to Meniere disease, contrast-enhanced MRI of the posterior fossa and internal auditory canal should be considered to exclude acoustic neuroma and meningioma.

Continuous tinnitus most often originates within the auditory system and is usually a consequence of sensorineural hearing loss. A high-pitched continuous tone is most common. Low-pitched tinnitus may be seen in patients with Meniere disease. Other causes are noise exposure, ototoxic medications, presbycusis, otosclerosis, acoustic neuroma, and barotrauma. Treatment of tinnitus should first be directed at the underlying disorder. Behavioral therapies include biofeedback, stress reduction, and cognitive-behavioral therapy directed at improving the patient's ability to cope with tinnitus. Behavioral therapy is not appropriate until other remediable causes of tinnitus are excluded.

Sudden sensorineural hearing loss is defined as hearing loss occurring in 3 days or less. Ninety percent of patients have unilateral hearing loss, and some have tinnitus, ear fullness, and vertigo. It is considered an otologic emergency, and oral corticosteroids are usually given, although randomized trials differ in their conclusions regarding efficacy. This patient's hearing loss has occurred over a period of months, and oral corticosteroids are not indicated.

Benign paroxysmal positional vertigo (BPPV) is the most common cause of vestibular dizziness. BPPV is thought to be caused by otolith debris within the semicircular canal. Otolith repositioning has been shown helpful in resolving symptoms of BPPV, however this patient does not have symptoms compatible with BPPV and therefore this intervention is not warranted.

KEY POINT

- **In patients with asymmetric sensorineural hearing loss that is not clearly due to Meniere disease, contrast-enhanced MRI of the posterior fossa and internal auditory canal should be considered to exclude acoustic neuroma and meningioma.**

Bibliography

McDonald R. Acoustic neuroma: what the evidence says about evaluation and treatment. J Fam Pract. 2011;60(6):E1-4. [PMID: 21647465]

Item 21   Answer: B

Educational Objective: Diagnose the cause of a syncopal episode.

In this elderly woman, given the short prodrome, palpitations, and history of a previous event, a cardiac arrhythmia is the most likely cause of syncope. Arrhythmias are the most common causes of syncope in the elderly population. Patients with an arrhythmogenic cause of syncope usually have had only one or two episodes. A prodrome is usually brief or absent. The patient often experiences palpitations immediately preceding the episode.

Aortic stenosis may cause syncope; however, despite a low-grade systolic murmur, this patient's carotid upstrokes are normal and her episode occurred at rest and not with exertion, making aortic stenosis unlikely.

Myocardial ischemia is a rare cause of syncope, especially in the absence of typical ischemic symptoms. Myocardial ischemia is a consideration in patients with an arrhythmia leading to presyncope or syncope as ischemic myocardium may be arrhythmogenic. However, myocardial ischemia as a cause of hypoperfusion in a patient without symptoms at rest would likely not account for her clinical presentation.

This patient has several risk factors for a possible transient ischemic attack (TIA). However, TIAs typically present with focal neurologic symptoms and findings, and are rarely a cause of syncope.

KEY POINT

- **Arrhythmia is a common cause of syncope in the elderly; arrhythmogenic syncope is characterized by a brief or absent prodrome and palpitations immediately preceding the event.**

Bibliography

Moya A, Sutton R, Ammirati F, et al; Task Force for the Diagnosis and Management of Syncope; European Society of Cardiology (ESC); European Heart Rhythm Association (EHRA); Heart Failure Association (HFA); Heart Rhythm Society (HRS). Guidelines for the diagnosis and management of syncope (version 2009). Eur Heart J. 2009;30(21):2631-2671. [PMID: 19713422]

Item 22   Answer: A

Educational Objective: Treat bilateral symmetric lower extremity edema due to venous stasis.

The most appropriate treatment for this patient is use of compression stockings. This obese woman has dependent symmetric bilateral lower extremity edema caused by venous insufficiency. Her normal cardiovascular and abdominal examinations, along with normal creatinine and albumin levels, urinalysis, and liver chemistry tests, rules out significant heart, lung, kidney, or liver disease as causative. The most effective treatments for edema due to chronic venous stasis are weight reduction, sodium restriction, leg elevation, and compression stockings. External compression decreases accumulation of tissue fluid in the lower extremities that is unable to be removed through the venous system. Compression stockings are particularly effective when used for extended periods when in the upright position to prevent dependent pooling of fluid.

Lower abdominal and pelvic imaging may be useful in assessing for lesions obstructing venous and lymphatic return as a cause of bilateral lower extremity edema. However, this is an uncommon cause of swelling in an otherwise healthy individual with a typical clinical picture of venous insufficiency.

According to expert opinion, diuretics should be avoided in patients with chronic venous insufficiency because they do not predictably lead to mobilization of fluid from the interstitial to the vascular space. Instead, diuretics may lead to decreased intravascular volume followed by orthostatic hypotension and prerenal azotemia.

Lower extremity venous duplex ultrasonography is useful in evaluating for the presence of venous thrombosis. In this patient there is no suspicion of deep vein thrombosis, and imaging is not necessary for a diagnosis of venous insufficiency without additional concerning signs or symptoms.

KEY POINT

- **The most effective treatments for edema due to chronic venous stasis are sodium restriction, leg elevation, weight reduction, and compression stockings; diuretics should be avoided.**

Bibliography

O'Brien JG, Chennubhotla SA, Chennubhotla RV. Treatment of edema. Am Fam Physician. 2005;71(11):2111-2117. [PMID: 15952439]

Item 23   Answer: A

Educational Objective: Manage a suspected rotator cuff tear.

This patient should undergo MRI of the left shoulder. He most likely has a complete left supraspinatus rotator cuff tear. The diagnosis is suggested by his difficulty with abducting the left arm and the positive drop-arm test. The drop-arm test can be performed by the examiner passively abducting the patient's arm and then having the patient slowly lower the arm to the waist. When a complete supraspinatus tear is present, the patient's arm often drops to the waist. Although imaging is not necessary in most patients with uncomplicated shoulder pain, because of the high likelihood of a complete supraspinatus tear by history and examination, it is appropriate to obtain an MRI to confirm the diagnosis. MRI has a high sensitivity (>90%) and specificity in the diagnosis of rotator cuff tears. Not all rotator cuff tears require surgical intervention and many respond to conservative therapy; however, establishing the diagnosis and obtaining more detailed anatomic information are necessary in making the decision about whether surgery would be indicated.

Medication with an NSAID may form a component of the initial treatment plan but a confirmed diagnosis is necessary to make definitive treatment decisions.

Although referral to physical therapy is appropriate for suspected or confirmed incomplete tears, it would not be the appropriate first step in this patient with a suspected complete tear who is young and has no medical comorbidities.

Performing a subacromial corticosteroid injection would not be the most appropriate option in this patient who is suspected of having a complete supraspinatus tear. Subacromial corticosteroid injections have been shown to provide pain relief that lasts up to 9 months in patients with rotator cuff tendinitis or an impingement syndrome, but a significant tear may require surgical intervention, and this should be determined as an initial step in management.

> **KEY POINT**
> - **MRI has a high sensitivity and specificity for diagnosing a rotator cuff tear.**

Bibliography

Seida JC, LeBlanc C, Schouten JR, et al. Systematic review: nonoperative and operative treatments for rotator cuff tears. Ann Intern Med. 2010;153(4):246-255. [PMID: 20621893]

Item 24   Answer: D

Educational Objective: Prevent pressure ulcers in an elderly patient.

The most appropriate intervention for preventing pressure ulcers in this patient is use of a pressure-distributing mattress. He was admitted to the hospital with peritonitis and has a very high risk for pressure ulcer given his limited mobility, ascites, and low serum albumin level. The blanching erythematous patches on his lower back and buttocks must be watched carefully because they are at-risk areas for ulceration. A nonblanching erythematous patch is a stage I pressure ulcer. There is evidence that pressure reduction, accomplished through frequent patient repositioning and use of pressure-distributing support surfaces, is effective in reducing the risk of ulcers. The strongest evidence of benefit exists for higher-specification foam mattresses compared with standard hospital mattresses; beds or mattresses that actively alternate pressure by shifting air or water are of unclear benefit, but may be useful in clinical situations in which prolonged bedrest is required. Medical-grade sheepskin overlays also have some evidence of benefit compared with standard hospital mattresses. Bed overlays made of foam, gel, or water or air-filled pockets are commonly used, although their efficacy in preventing ulcer development has not been established and there is some evidence that they may contribute to additional skin irritation.

Air-filled vinyl boots, water-filled gloves, regular sheepskin, and doughnut-type devices are likely to be harmful and should not be used for prevention of pressure ulcers.

Indwelling urinary catheters increase the risk of urinary tract infection if left in place. Although they are frequently placed specifically to avoid urine contact with skin areas at high risk of ulceration, other mechanisms to avoid moisture contact with the area at risk for breakdown are preferred.

> **KEY POINT**
> - **Pressure-distributing mattresses and medical-grade sheepskin overlays reduce the incidence of pressure ulcers in high-risk patients.**

Bibliography

McInnes E, Jammali-Blasi A, Bell-Syer SE, Dumville JC, Cullum N. Support surfaces for pressure ulcer prevention. Cochrane Database Syst Rev. 2011;(4):CD001735. [PMID: 21491384]

Item 25   Answer: D

Educational Objective: Treat menopausal vaginal symptoms.

The most appropriate management of this patient is vaginal estradiol. The clinical history and physical examination are most helpful for making the diagnosis of vaginal atrophy; pale vaginal walls, decreased rugae, and petechiae are characteristic findings. Approximately 10% to 40% of menopausal women experience symptoms related to vaginal atrophy, which include vulvar itching, vaginal dryness, and dyspareunia. In contrast to menopausal vasomotor symptoms, which may last for a few years and resolve spontaneously, vaginal atrophy is frequently progressive and often requires treatment. Mild to moderate symptoms can be treated with vaginal moisturizers and lubricants, but more severe symptoms, as experienced by this patient, are best treated with vaginal estrogen. Low-dose vaginal estradiol tablets (10-25 micrograms) and the estradiol vaginal ring (8-9 micrograms) are preferred over vaginal estrogen creams, as they result in minimal systemic estrogen absorption.

Although oral estrogen therapy is effective for relieving vaginal atrophy symptoms, it has been associated with several adverse outcomes, including increased rates of coronary heart disease, stroke, venous thromboembolism, and invasive breast cancer. For that reason, current guidelines recommend the use of low-dose local, rather than systemic, estrogen therapy for the treatment of patients who only have vaginal symptoms.

Bacterial vaginosis is characterized by a vaginal discharge, an increased vaginal pH, and clue cells on normal saline preparation and a positive "whiff" test; the absence of these findings in this patient argues against this diagnosis. Treatment for bacterial vaginosis with metronidazole would therefore not be indicated.

Yeast infections are often accompanied by a thick white discharge that is potassium hydroxide–positive. This patient does not have discharge and no hyphae are seen on potassium hydroxide preparation; therefore, she is unlikely to respond to vaginal clotrimazole therapy.

KEY POINT

- **Vaginal estrogen is the recommended therapy for severe symptoms of vaginal atrophy that have not responded to vaginal moisturizers and lubricants.**

Bibliography

North American Menopause Society. The role of local vaginal estrogen for treatment of vaginal atrophy in postmenopausal women: 2007 position statement of The North American Menopause Society. Menopause. 2007;14(3 Pt 1):355-369. [PMID: 17438512]

Item 26   Answer: A

Educational Objective: Diagnosis acromioclavicular joint degeneration.

This patient's pain is originating from his acromioclavicular joint. Given his age, his pain is most likely due to osteoarthritis. Acromioclavicular joint degeneration typically results from trauma (in younger patients) or osteoarthritis (in older patients). Bilateral involvement should raise concern for rheumatoid arthritis. On examination, there is typically pain to palpation of the acromioclavicular joint. Pain on palpation is a very sensitive but not specific sign of acromioclavicular joint disease; absent pain on palpation makes acromioclavicular joint disease unlikely. Palpable osteophytes may be present. Pain

characteristically occurs with shoulder adduction and abduction above 120 degrees.

Adhesive capsulitis is caused by thickening of the capsule surrounding the glenohumeral joint. Pain is characteristically slow in onset and is located near the insertion of the deltoid muscle, and patients often avoid lying on the affected side. On examination, there is loss of both active and passive range of motion. Although this patient's symptoms have been insidious in onset, which could be consistent with adhesive capsulitis, he does not have limited range of motion in all or most planes of motion, which argues against adhesive capsulitis.

Examination findings of a rotator cuff tear include supraspinatus weakness, weakness with external rotation, evidence of impingement, and a positive drop-arm test (inability to slowly and steadily lower the arm completely; the arm drops to the side). The patient has a negative drop-arm sign, which argues against rotator cuff tear.

The patient does not have pain between 60 to 120 degrees of abduction, has normal internal/external rotation, and has a negative Neer and Hawkins sign, all of which argue against the diagnosis of rotator cuff tendinitis.

KEY POINT

- **Acromioclavicular joint degeneration is characterized by pain to palpation of the acromioclavicular joint and pain that occurs with shoulder adduction and abduction above 120 degrees.**

Bibliography

House J, Mooradian A. Evaluation and management of shoulder pain in primary care clinics. South Med J. 2010;103(11):1129-1135. [PMID: 20890250]

Item 27   Answer: A

Educational Objective: Counsel a patient regarding smoking cessation.

Current recommendations are that all clinicians assess tobacco use at every visit, encourage every patient to make a quit attempt, and counsel patients appropriately. Patients who exhibit medical illnesses related to smoking present an opportunity for clinicians to increase the patient's awareness of the connection between the unhealthy behavior and its negative consequences. Even if time does not allow for an in-depth counseling session, all patients should be asked about their smoking at every visit, and a brief, clear message about quitting should be provided to all patients. A recommended strategy for counseling is to follow the "five A's": Ask every patient at every visit about their smoking; Advise all smokers to quit; Assess their current interest in quitting; Assist by offering resources and/or medications, and Arrange for follow-up.

It is not clear yet whether this patient is truly interested in quitting. Thus it would be inappropriate to prescribe either smoking cessation aids or counseling until the physician has determined that the patient is indeed ready to quit.

KEY POINT

- Tobacco use should be assessed at every visit, and patients who smoke should be encouraged to make a quit attempt and counseled appropriately.

Bibliography

2008 PHS Guideline Update Panel, Liasons, and Staff. Treating tobacco use and dependence: 2008 update U.S. Public Health Service Clinical Practice Guideline executive summary. Respir Care. 2008;53(9):1217-1222. [PMID: 18807274]

Item 28   Answer: A

Educational Objective: Manage postoperative venous thromboembolism prophylaxis in a high-risk patient.

The most appropriate treatment for this patient is venous thromboembolism (VTE) prophylactic therapy for up to 5 weeks with a low-molecular-weight heparin (LMWH), such as enoxaparin. VTE is a major preventable postoperative complication, and nearly all surgical patients should receive some VTE prophylaxis postoperatively. Patients at high risk for VTE, including patients with previous VTE, patients who have undergone orthopedic surgery, and patients with some cancers (especially gynecologic malignancy) should receive extended (up to 5 weeks) prophylaxis with LMWH.

Nonpharmacologic prophylaxis against VTE, such as early ambulation, should be encouraged in all postsurgical patients. Other nonpharmacologic treatments include elastic compression stockings and pneumatic compression devices. However, these treatments are only suitable as the sole modality when either the risk of VTE is very low (outpatient surgery) or the morbidity from excess bleeding is unacceptably high (such as in patients undergoing neurosurgery). This patient's surgery for a gynecologic malignancy places her in a high-risk category, and pharmacologic prophylaxis is indicated.

Inferior vena cava (IVC) filters are sometimes used perioperatively, especially in patients with known VTE or patients with a high risk for VTE who cannot receive prophylaxis because of bleeding risk. This patient does not have an excessive bleeding risk, and IVC placement is not indicated. Although newer IVC filters are thought to be extractable following a procedure, the retrieval rate is not typically 100%, and a filter that cannot be removed postoperatively may complicate ongoing care.

Unfractionated subcutaneous heparin is an accepted medication to prevent VTE. However, in this high-risk patient, extended prophylaxis is indicated; therefore, providing prophylaxis only until the patient is discharged is incorrect.

Warfarin, in both fixed doses and adjusted doses, has been studied for VTE prophylaxis, primarily in the orthopedic setting, and been found to be effective in preventing venous thromboembolism in the perioperative period. However, 3 months of prophylaxis would not be indicated

and would substantially increase the risk of bleeding once the perioperative thromboembolism risk has resolved.

KEY POINT

- Surgical patients at high risk for venous thromboembolism, including those with previous venous thromboembolism, patients who have undergone orthopedic surgery, and patients with some cancers (especially gynecologic malignancy), should receive extended (up to 5 weeks) prophylaxis.

Bibliography

Gould MK, Garcia DA, Wren SM, et al; American College of Chest Physicians; Prevention of VTE in nonorthopedic surgical patients: Antithrombotic Therapy and Prevention of Thrombosis, 9th ed: American College of Chest Physicians Evidence-Based Clinical Practice Guidelines. Chest. 2012;141(2 suppl):e227S-e77S.

Item 29   Answer: D

Educational Objective: Diagnose acute retinal detachment.

This patient presents with symptoms consistent with a retinal detachment. Retinal detachment occurs predominantly in myopic patients and is a separation of the retina from underlying retinal epithelium and choroid as fluid from the vitreous cavity enters a tear in the retina and dissects underneath the retina. As with this patient, patients may experience floaters, squiggly lines, flashes of light, and then a sudden peripheral visual defect, appearing as a black curtain that progresses across the visual field. Funduscopic examination usually visualizes the tear and folding of the retina. Treatment is surgical. Prognosis depends upon the extent of the tear and time to surgery, so early recognition and emergent referral are crucial.

Central retinal artery occlusion is marked by painless loss of vision and occurs most frequently in the elderly. It is usually caused by emboli or thrombosis. Examination demonstrates a pale fundus with a cherry-red fovea (accentuated by the pale background).

Central retinal vein occlusion is characterized by abrupt monocular visual loss, and may present with transient episodes of monocular blindness, which can last 2 to 4 hours, longer than is typical for transient arterial retinal ischemia. Patients may report cloudiness of vision rather than frank visual loss. Examination of the retina will show congested, tortuous veins; retinal hemorrhages; and cotton wool spots in the area of the vein occlusion.

Ocular migraine, with or without headache, can cause floaters and squiggly lines but would not cause a visual field defect or a retinal tear and folding seen on funduscopic examination.

The most common presenting symptom in patients with temporal arteritis is a new headache, which this patient does not have. Although visual loss can be sudden and irreversible in the setting of temporal arteritis, it is not preceded by floaters, squiggly lines, or peripheral field defects.

- Patients with a retinal detachment may experience floaters, squiggly lines, flashes of light, and then a sudden peripheral visual defect, appearing as a black curtain that progresses across the visual field.

Bibliography

Magauran B. Conditions requiring emergency ophthalmologic consultation. Emerg Med Clin North Am. 2008;26(1):233-238. [PMID: 18249265]

Item 30   Answer: D

Educational Objective: Implement the Plan-Do-Study-Act (PDSA) cycle in quality improvement.

A specific plan to improve communication of medication allergies from outpatient to inpatient medical records should be developed to attempt to avoid subsequent occurrences. The Plan-Do-Study-Act (PDSA) cycle is a quality improvement approach in which a specific change is planned and implemented on a limited scale, the results are observed, and action is taken based on what is learned. The first step in a PDSA cycle in this case would be to plan an intervention that would remedy the communication deficit between the internist's office records and the hospital's electronic order system and drug allergy alert system. The next steps are to institute the planned intervention in a limited fashion and then to study the outcome of the intervention. The "act" step involves refining the intervention to achieve the ideal outcome based upon what is learned by evaluating the limited intervention. This approach to quality improvement works well in a small-scale health care environment, such as a small office, as well as in a large-scale environment, such as a hospital or health care system.

Most physicians are aware of the importance of patient engagement in their care, but greater involvement by patients may not be adequate in overcoming issues regarding consistent and reliable communication of key medical information across different caregivers in different settings.

Although it is important for patients to know, understand, and communicate their important medical information to other caregivers, not all patients are able to do so in a reliable manner, and this intervention will not address larger systemic issues related to improving quality of care and patient safety.

Electronic health records may be of immeasurable help in improving communication of medical information. However, implementing such systems in institutions and communities is costly, complex, and not easily accomplished, and is not the next step in this case. Clear interventions to avoid known patient safety issues should occur as possible within existing systems, with overall system change to optimize quality of care being the long-term goal.

- The Plan-Do-Study-Act (PDSA) cycle is a quality improvement approach in which a specific change is planned and implemented on a limited scale, the results are observed, and action is taken based on what is learned.

Bibliography

Institute of Medicine of the National Academies. Crossing the Quality Chasm: A New Health System for the 21st Century. www.iom.edu/Reports/2001/Crossing-the-Quality-Chasm-A-New-Health-System-for-the-21st-Century.aspx. Published March 1, 2001. Accessed July 12, 2012.

Item 31   Answer: D

Educational Objective: Evaluate a patient with recurrent syncope.

The most appropriate next step in the evaluation of this patient is tilt-table testing. Tilt-table testing is useful in evaluating recurrent syncope in the absence of heart disease, to discriminate neurocardiogenic from orthostatic syncope, and to evaluate frequent syncope in patients with psychiatric disease. This patient continues to have recurrent syncopal episodes despite normal cardiac and metabolic evaluations without definitive evidence of orthostasis or other explanation for her symptoms.

Electroencephalography may be useful in patients in whom a seizure is suspected as a cause of syncope. However, this patient has no risk factors for seizure and her episodes are without a prodromal aura, evidence of seizure activity, or postictal symptoms suggestive of seizure activity.

Exercise cardiac stress testing has a low yield for syncope in patients at low risk for ischemic heart disease. In this patient with a normal electrocardiogram and echocardiogram, cardiac stress testing would not be expected to contribute significant diagnostic information.

Signal-averaged electrocardiography is a technique designed to detect altered depolarization through the myocardium that could lead to reentrant arrhythmias that may not be evident on surface electrocardiography. It has been studied primarily in patients following myocardial infarction to assess for risk of developing sustained tachyarrhythmias. Its use in evaluating syncope has not been established, however, and its routine use is not recommended.

- Tilt-table testing is useful in evaluating recurrent syncope in the absence of heart disease, to discriminate neurocardiogenic from orthostatic syncope, and to evaluate frequent syncope in patients with psychiatric disease.

Bibliography

Moya A, Sutton R, Ammirati F, et al; Task Force for the Diagnosis and Management of Syncope; European Society of Cardiology (ESC);

European Heart Rhythm Association (EHRA); Heart Failure Association (HFA); Heart Rhythm Society (HRS). Guidelines for the diagnosis and management of syncope (version 2009). Eur Heart J. 2009;30(21):2631-2671. [PMID: 19713422]

Item 32   Answer: C

Educational Objective: Manage medications in a woman who may become pregnant.

The most appropriate treatment for this woman is metformin to treat her type 2 diabetes mellitus. Each visit with a reproductive-age woman represents an opportunity for preconception counseling, as adequate preconception care can reduce the risks for preterm birth and birth anomalies, particularly in a woman actively contemplating pregnancy. If this patient were to become pregnant, her poorly controlled diabetes and hypertension increase her risk for adverse maternal and fetal outcomes. This patient should be counseled about her risk factors for potential medical complications of pregnancy, and she should be referred to a high-risk obstetrician for co-management of her medical and gynecologic issues should she become pregnant. It is essential to avoid prescribing teratogenic medications to reproductive-age women who may become pregnant. Metformin is an FDA pregnancy class B medication and is a reasonable option for controlling this patient's hyperglycemia before pregnancy. If she were to become pregnant, consideration may be given to discontinuing the metformin and starting insulin therapy, which is the preferred treatment of diabetes in pregnancy.

The risk of premature fetal loss is increased in women with systemic lupus erythematosus, particularly in those with the antiphospholipid antibody syndrome. Low-dose aspirin has been used in these patients to attempt to lower this risk, although the effectiveness of this intervention is not clear. As aspirin may interfere with implantation when used near the time of conception and this patient has no clear indication for aspirin therapy at present, it should not be prescribed.

Lisinopril and simvastatin, and all ACE inhibitors and statins, are teratogenic medications and can cause serious fetal anomalies. They are FDA pregnancy class X medications and should not be prescribed to this patient who is anticipating pregnancy. Additionally, although this patient might benefit from treatment with an angiotensin receptor blocker because of her diabetes and proteinuria, this class of medication is also contraindicated in pregnancy owing to its potential teratogenic effects. Labetalol or methyldopa is safely used for the treatment of hypertension in pregnant women, and may be considered for this patient. Bile acid resins, such as colestipol, are not orally absorbed and are FDA pregnancy class B medications. They may be a useful adjunct to diet and lifestyle therapy for managing this patient's dyslipidemia.

KEY POINT

- Avoidance of potentially teratogenic medications is important when treating medical conditions in reproductive-age women contemplating pregnancy.

Bibliography

Berghella V, Buchanan E, Pereira L, Baxter JK. Preconception care. Obstet Gynecol Surv. 2010;65(2):119-131. [PMID: 20100361]

Item 33   Answer: D

Educational Objective: Treat functional urinary incontinence.

This patient would be best managed by establishing a prompted voiding protocol. Urinary incontinence affects more than 50% of nursing home patients and is associated with significant morbidity and cost. Most of these patients have limited mobility or significant cognitive impairment, leading to a high prevalence of functional incontinence, defined as simply not getting to the toilet quickly enough. In a systematic review of 14 randomized controlled studies involving 1161 nursing home patients, the use of prompted voiding (periodically asking the patient about incontinence, reminding the patient to go to the toilet, and providing praise for maintaining continence and using the toilet) was associated with modest short-term improvement in urinary incontinence.

History, focused examination, and urinalysis are often adequate to classify urinary incontinence. Postvoid residual urine volume determination is most useful if overflow incontinence due to outlet obstruction or a flaccid neurogenic bladder is suspected. Detailed urologic evaluations, such as cystoscopy and urodynamic testing, are unnecessary in uncomplicated urinary incontinence.

An indwelling Foley catheter is not advised as a first-line measure to manage urinary incontinence owing to an increased risk of urinary tract infection, resultant antibiotic treatment, and the development of antibiotic complications and resistance.

Pelvic floor muscle training is effective for stress incontinence, which may be coexistent in this patient, but successful implementation requires a cooperative and cognitively intact patient who can understand and participate in the exercise program.

Tolterodine, a selective anticholinergic antimuscarinic medication, is primarily indicated for urge incontinence and is of no benefit in functional incontinence. In addition, adverse side effects, such as dry mouth and worsening cognitive function, render its use in this patient ill advised.

KEY POINT

- Prompted voiding is an effective management strategy for patients with functional urinary incontinence.

Bibliography

Fink HA, Taylor BC, Tacklind JW, Rutks IR, Wilt TJ. Treatment interventions in nursing home residents with urinary incontinence: a systematic review of randomized trials. Mayo Clin Proc. 2008;83(12):1332-1343. [PMID: 19046552]

Item 34   Answer: B

Educational Objective: Screen for cervical cancer.

The patient should have a Pap smear in 2 years. Because she has had multiple normal consecutive satisfactory Pap smears, the most appropriate interval for cervical cancer screening is every 3 years (this patient had a Pap smear 1 year ago and should undergo repeat screening in 2 years). Although the U.S. Preventive Services Task Force (USPSTF), the American College of Obstetrics and Gynecology (ACOG), and the American Cancer Society (ACS) each differ slightly in their specific recommendations, each agrees that the screening interval can be extended beyond 1 year for this patient. The USPSTF recommends screening at least once every 3 years following the initiation of screening. In contrast, the ACOG recommends that screening occur every 2 years between the ages of 21 and 29 years and every 3 years beginning at the age of 30 years if the patient has had three normal consecutive satisfactory Pap smears and has no history of in utero diethylstilbestrol exposure, is not immunocompromised, is not HIV-positive, and does not have a history of cervical intraepithelial neoplasia grade 2 or 3. The ACS recommends that screening should be performed every 3 years between the ages of 21 and 29 years. Between the ages of 30 and 65 years, the preferred method of screening is the combination of a Pap smear and human papillomavirus (HPV) DNA testing every 5 years. Alternatively, a Pap smear alone can be performed every 3 years.

Although medical providers can consider using HPV DNA testing along with cervical cytology in women aged 30 years and older to help guide the appropriate screening interval, it should not be used alone owing to poor specificity.

Discontinuation of screening for cervical cancer at the age of 31 years would not be appropriate despite the patient's having multiple previous normal satisfactory Pap smears. It is generally agreed that screening should be continued into the seventh decade, although controversy exists regarding the exact age to stop screening.

KEY POINT

- **In women older than 30 years with no risk factors for cervical cancer or history of abnormal Pap smears, the cervical cancer screening interval can be extended to 3 years with cytology or 5 years with cytology and human papillomavirus DNA testing.**

Bibliography

Moyer VA. Screening for cervical cancer: U.S. Preventive Services Task Force recommendation statement. Ann Intern Med. 2012;156(12):880-891. [PMID: 22711081]

Item 35   Answer: B

Educational Objective: Diagnose mild cognitive impairment.

This patient most likely has mild cognitive impairment (MCI). Memory is the only cognitive domain that is impaired. Impairment of other domains that might suggest dementia would include impairment of language, apraxia (for example, problems with dressing not related to motor dysfunction), and impaired executive functioning, none of which are abnormal in this patient. Patients with MCI have a single or few areas of cognitive impairment, and this patient's deficit is limited to forgetfulness and recalling names. His age is typical for MCI and about one-fifth of patients older than age 70 years have this condition. His Mini–Mental State Examination (MMSE) score is within the expected range of 24-25 for MCI and may even be falsely elevated because of his high intellectual level.

Alzheimer disease is less likely in this patient because there are no impairments in other domains, such as activities of daily living and instrumental activities of daily living; other language difficulties; or personality changes. MMSE scores of 19 to 24 suggest mild dementia, and scores of 10 to 19 suggest moderate dementia. His MMSE score of 25 suggests MCI rather than dementia.

Pseudodementia is a condition in which the cognitive impairment is secondary to depression. Treatment of the depression leads to improvement in cognition. Whereas this patient is frustrated with his condition, he is not depressed.

Although he has risk factors for cerebrovascular disease, vascular dementia would be less likely with his MMSE score of 25 and normal neurologic examination. In addition, vascular dementia would not affect memory in isolation and would likely affect additional cognitive domains and neurologic functioning.

KEY POINT

- **Patients with mild cognitive impairment have a single or few areas of cognitive impairment, and the Mini–Mental State Examination score is typically 24 or 25.**

Bibliography

Plassman BL, Langa KM, Fisher GG, et al. Prevalence of cognitive impairment without dementia in the United States. Ann Intern Med. 2008;148(6):427-434. [PMID: 18347351]

Item 36   Answer: B

Educational Objective: Manage palliative care discussion.

Palliative care discussions with this patient should begin now. It is important to stress to patients that a palliative care discussion is not a discussion of withholding or withdrawal of treatment or patient abandonment. The primary focus of palliative care is to relieve patient suffering and to improve the quality of patients' lives and those of their caregivers.

Palliative care is often thought of as end-of-life care only, but palliative care addresses pain, suffering, and quality of life across all stages of treatment and does not exclude life-prolonging treatment and rehabilitation. Palliative care may be offered along with curative or life-prolonging therapies for patients with complex, life-threatening disorders. Recent literature suggests that early referral for palliative care improves quality of life and decreases depressive symptoms as compared with patients who only receive standard oncologic care. In a study of 151 patients with metastatic non–small cell lung cancer, patients referred for early palliative care had longer median survival than those referred for oncologic care only.

Waiting until the patient develops symptoms, refuses active treatment, or is admitted to hospice care does not take full advantage of the benefits of early and appropriately administered palliative care.

KEY POINT

- Early referral for palliative care in addition to oncologic care improves quality of life and decreases depressive symptoms as compared with standard oncologic care only.

Bibliography

Temel JS, Greer JA, Muzikansky A, et al. Early palliative care for patients with metastatic non-small-cell lung cancer. N Engl J Med. 2010;363(8):733-742. [PMID: 20818875]

Item 37   Answer: A

Educational Objective: Manage acute cervical radiculopathy.

This patient should be treated with analgesics and avoidance of provocative activities. The initial approach to patients with cervical spine radiculopathy, typically due to nerve root compression, is assessment for weakness and possible involvement of the spinal cord (myelopathy). Weakness due to nerve root compression will be seen in the muscles in the area of distribution of the affected nerve(s); myelopathy is seen as additional neurologic symptoms at and below the affected level of the spinal cord. In patients with acute cervical radiculopathy without appreciable motor deficits, imaging and nerve conduction studies are not initially necessary, even if there are mild focal sensory findings. Management should focus on relief of symptoms, as many patients experience complete resolution without intervention.

A variety of nonsurgical treatments are used for management of cervical radiculopathy in addition to nonnarcotic analgesics, including a short course of systemic corticosteroids, hard and soft cervical collars, and cervical pillows, although evidence that these interventions are effective relative to analgesics and rest alone is of poor quality. Cervical traction has also not been documented to be effective and is not recommended as initial treatment for acute cervical radiculopathy.

Imaging studies should be directed based on suspicions raised during history and physical examination. Except in cases of acute trauma, mechanical neck pain rarely requires imaging. Patients with weakness, hyporeflexia, or symptoms or signs of spinal cord involvement should be evaluated with MRI or CT myelography. An electromyelogram and nerve conduction studies are most helpful in patients with radiculopathy that is poorly defined or in those for whom surgery is being considered to localize the specific area of nerve compression. These studies are not indicated in the initial management of cervical spine radiculopathy.

KEY POINT

- **Conservative treatment of acute cervical radiculopathy without imaging or further testing is appropriate in patients without trauma or evidence of weakness or myelopathy.**

Bibliography

Carette S, Fehlings MG. Clinical practice. Cervical radiculopathy. N Engl J Med. 2005;353:392-399. [PMID: 16049211]

Item 38   Answer: B

Educational Objective: Treat chronic cough due to gastroesophageal reflux disease.

Omeprazole should be continued in this patient. He presents with chronic cough (>8 weeks) most likely due to gastroesophageal reflux disease (GERD). Although typical heartburn symptoms are absent in more than one-third of patients with GERD-related cough, this patient's clinical profile and symptoms of heartburn and cough exacerbated by the recumbent position are classic for GERD. The treatment of chronic cough due to GERD is challenging. If lifestyle modification (weight loss, elevation of the head of the bed, avoidance of tobacco and alcohol) is unsuccessful, targeted and prolonged treatment with histamine blockers or proton pump inhibitors (PPIs) is recommended. In a recent Cochrane review, patients who were treated with PPIs experienced a significant improvement in cough scores. There was no significant difference in total resolution of cough, however (odds ratio [OR] 0.46, 95% CI 0.19-1.15, intention to treat analysis). The duration of therapy was 2 to 3 months. As this patient has been on therapy for only 2 weeks and his clinical picture is without any interim change, continuation for 8 to 12 weeks would be recommended.

The American College of Chest Physicians recommends a symptom-guided, systematic, algorithmic approach to chronic cough. There is no evidence of infection, and therefore, antibiotics are not indicated. The patient does not present with symptoms or signs of upper airway cough syndrome (postnasal drainage, frequent throat clearing, nasal discharge, cobblestone appearance of the oropharyngeal mucosa, or mucus dripping down the oropharynx). The use of antihistamines and decongestants, such as loratadine with pseudoephedrine, should be reserved until the empiric trial of treatment for GERD is completed and found to be ineffective.

Cough-variant asthma (cough is the predominant symptom) occurs in up to 57% of patients with asthma. Cough-variant asthma is suggested by the presence of airway hyperresponsiveness and confirmed when cough resolves with asthma medications. The treatment of cough-variant asthma is the same as asthma in general, but the maximum symptomatic benefit may not occur for 6 to 8 weeks in cough-variant asthma. This patient does not have asthma and has a reasonable alternative explanation for his chronic cough; therefore treatment with an inhaled bronchodilator such as albuterol is not indicated at this time.

KEY POINT

- **The duration of empiric proton pump inhibitor therapy for a patient with gastroesophageal reflux disease–related cough is 8 to 12 weeks.**

Bibliography

Chang AB, Lasserson TJ, Gaffney J, Connor FL, Garske LA. Gastro-oesophageal reflux treatment for prolonged non-specific cough in children and adults. Cochrane Database Syst Rev. 2011;(1): CD004823. [PMID: 21249664]

Item 39 Answer: B

Educational Objective: Diagnose acute pericarditis.

This patient most likely has acute pericarditis. Characteristic findings in acute pericarditis include sharp, pleuritic retrosternal chest pain that is more prominent in the recumbent position, a pericardial friction rub, widespread ST-segment elevation or PR-segment depression on electrocardiogram (ECG), and new or worsening pericardial effusion. This patient has pleuritic chest pain that worsens with recumbency and improves with sitting forward and widespread concave-upward ST-segment elevation, making acute pericarditis the likely diagnosis. The presence of a friction rub is helpful if present but its absence does not exclude the diagnosis. Etiologies of acute pericarditis include infection (especially viral infection, as is likely in this patient), autoimmune disease, neoplasia, uremia, and trauma.

The patient has no risk factors for ischemic heart disease and her description of her chest pain is atypical for that of coronary artery disease. The widespread concave-upward ST-segment ECG changes are more consistent with acute pericarditis rather than ischemia, in which changes localized to leads associated with the specific regions of the involved myocardium would be expected.

Like pericarditis, the pain of acute pleuritis worsens with inspiration, may be positional, and can be accompanied by dyspnea. However, pleuritic chest pain is not confined to the retrosternal area, as it is in pericarditis, and ECG changes would not be expected with pleuritis.

Although the chest pain that accompanies a pulmonary embolism is typically pleuritic, pulmonary embolism is not associated with widespread ST-segment elevation or PR-segment depression on ECG.

KEY POINT

- **The chest pain of acute pericarditis is typically sharp, pleuritic, retrosternal, worsened by recumbency, and improved by sitting forward.**

Bibliography

Khandaker MH, Espinosa RE, Nishimura RA, et al. Pericardial disease: diagnosis and management. Mayo Clin Proc. 2010;85(6):572-593. [PMID: 20511488]

Item 40 Answer: A

Educational Objective: Manage androgen deficiency.

This patient's hydrocodone should be discontinued. Low testosterone levels can lead to decreased energy and libido, fatigue, and erectile dysfunction. Once discovered, low testosterone levels should be investigated further. Many drugs, including opioids, high-dose corticosteroids, and hormonal therapies, can lower testosterone levels, and a review of medications is an important initial step in the evaluation of men with low testosterone levels. It is also important to test morning levels of testosterone as opposed to random levels, as secretion is cyclical. In this patient, hydrocodone may be decreasing testosterone levels and should be discontinued, and the testosterone level should subsequently be retested before any testosterone replacement therapy is given.

Whereas metoprolol and other β-blockers may cause erectile dysfunction and fatigue, they do not generally lower testosterone levels.

While repeat morning testing of testosterone levels is recommended to confirm low values, it would be more appropriate to first discontinue the potential offending agent before retesting the testosterone level.

As testosterone replacement therapy is usually a long-term treatment intervention, it should only be initiated after definitive confirmation of testosterone deficiency in the absence of testosterone-lowering therapies and after weighing the risks and benefits and discussing the multiple potential delivery options for the hormone with the patient.

KEY POINT

- **In men with low testosterone levels, a review of medications should be undertaken; many drugs, including opioids, high-dose corticosteroids, and hormonal therapies, can lower testosterone levels.**

Bibliography

Bhasin S, Cunningham GR, Hayes FJ, et al; Task Force, Endocrine Society. Testosterone therapy in men with androgen deficiency syndromes: an Endocrine Society clinical practice guideline. J Clin Endocrinol Metab. 2010;95(6):2536-2559. [PMID: 20525905]

Item 41   Answer: C
Educational Objective: Treat isolated hypertriglyceridemia.

Among the options listed, fenofibrate is the best treatment option for this patient. His serum triglyceride level is classified as "very high" (≥500 mg/dL [5.65 mmol/L]) according to the National Cholesterol Education Program Adult Treatment Panel III (ATP III) guidelines. He also has a significantly low HDL cholesterol level. The non-HDL cholesterol level (calculated as total cholesterol − HDL cholesterol) correlates closely with elevated LDL and VLDL concentrations, and is considered a secondary target of therapy when triglycerides are elevated. In patients with an LDL cholesterol goal of 130 mg/dL (3.37 mmol/L) or less, as with this patient, the non-HDL cholesterol goal is 160 mg/dL (4.14 mmol/L [30 points higher than the LDL cholesterol goal]). This patient's calculated non-HDL cholesterol level is 165 mg/dL (4.27 mmol/L), and so medical therapy should be initiated. Fenofibrate is very effective for reducing serum triglyceride levels, with observed decreases of 20% to 50%. Additionally, several trials have demonstrated the benefit of fibrate therapy in the primary and secondary prevention of cardiovascular outcomes.

Colesevelam, a bile acid resin, would not be indicated for treatment in this patient with hypertriglyceridemia. Bile acid resins are effective alone or in combination with statins for lowering LDL cholesterol level but may raise serum triglycerides, especially in patients with serum triglyceride levels greater than 400 mg/dL (4.52 mmol/L). These agents should be avoided as monotherapy in patients with triglyceride levels above 200 mg/dL (2.26 mmol/L).

Nicotinic acid will reduce serum triglyceride level by 20% to 50%, decrease LDL cholesterol level by 5% to 25%, and increase the HDL cholesterol level by 15% to 35%. Treatment with nicotinic acid has been shown to reduce cardiovascular outcomes in both primary and secondary prevention trials. However, treatment with nicotinic acid can precipitate gouty attacks, and so should be avoided in patients, such as this one, with a known history of gout.

Omega-3 fatty acids reduce hepatic secretion of triglyceride-rich lipoproteins and thereby lower serum triglyceride levels. However, their effectiveness in reducing cardiovascular risk in high-risk patients has not been established, and these agents thus should be considered alternative therapies for treatment of patients with hypertriglyceridemia who cannot tolerate fibric acids or nicotinic acid.

KEY POINT
- For patients with hypertriglyceridemia, fibric acid derivatives, such as fenofibrate, reduce triglyceride levels and provide benefit in primary and secondary cardiovascular prevention.

Bibliography
McCullough PA, Ahmed AB, Zughaib MT, Glanz ED, Di Loreto MJ. Treatment of hypertriglyceridemia with fibric acid derivatives: impact on lipid subfractions and translation into a reduction in cardiovascular events. Rev Cardiovasc Med. 2011;12(4):173-185. [PMID: 22249508]

Item 42   Answer: B
Educational Objective: Diagnose epididymitis.

This patient most likely has epididymitis. Infection or inflammation of the epididymis often causes pain localized to the superior and posterior aspect of the testicle. The onset may be acute, subacute, or chronic, and pain may occur more gradually compared with torsion. Pain may be accompanied by lower urinary tract symptoms of dysuria, urgency, or frequency. Patients with acute epididymitis may be quite sick, with high fevers and leukocytosis. Risk factors for epididymitis include recent sexual activity, heavy exertion, and bicycle riding. Distribution is bimodal, with occurrences highest in those younger than 35 years and older than 55 years. In younger patients, sexually transmitted infections such as chlamydial infection and gonorrhea are the most likely causes. Older men and men who engage in receptive anal intercourse are more susceptible to *Escherichia coli*, Enterobacteriaceae, and pseudomonal infection.

Acute prostatitis usually presents with pelvic pain and lower urinary tract symptoms, such as dysuria, urgency, and frequency. It may cause fever and leukocytosis, but on examination, the prostate gland is usually exquisitely tender, which is not the case with this patient.

An indirect hernia may lead to discomfort and fullness in the scrotum unilaterally, and also cause palpable changes along the course of the inguinal canal on the affected side. An indirect hernia is unlikely in this patient given lack of a scrotal mass or other physical findings consistent with a hernia; in addition, hernias do not cause fever or leukocytosis.

Orchitis, or inflammation of the testicle, can present as a febrile illness with testicular pain but pain would be expected with direct palpation of the testicle and potentially testicular enlargement.

Testicular torsion, which occurs when the testicle twists on the spermatic cord, usually occurs quite acutely. It leads to decreased blood flow and ischemia and is a surgical emergency. Physical findings usually include severe pain, often accompanied by nausea and vomiting, and a high-riding testicle. This patient's presentation is not consistent with testicular torsion.

KEY POINT
- Epididymitis is characterized by pain localized to the superior and posterior aspect of the testicle; patients may be quite sick, with high fevers and leukocytosis.

Bibliography
Wampler SM, Llanes M. Common scrotal and testicular problems. Prim Care. 2010;37(3):613-626, x. [PMID: 20705202]

Item 43   Answer: B

Educational Objective: Manage life-sustaining care in a critically ill patient.

It is unclear from the clinical scenario whether or not the patient will need dialysis for an extended period of time. However, with the information given, the best course of action is to dialyze temporarily with the hope that the patient will either regain kidney function or improve sufficiently to participate in decision making about long-term dialysis. Although it may be more difficult and resource intensive to initiate dialysis now and stop later if the patient fails to improve, it is the course of action that is most likely to meet both his short-term goal of seeing his great-grandson graduate and his long-term goal of not being dependent on machines. It is important to recognize that from an ethical and legal perspective, stopping a life-sustaining therapy is no different from not starting it, although evidentiary standards among states and cultural and religious beliefs regarding withdrawing or withholding treatment may vary. Interventions should not be withheld for fear they cannot be withdrawn if necessary.

Placing a long-term dialysis catheter may reflect a reasonable assessment of this patient's likelihood of regaining normal kidney function, but implies disregard for his wish not to be dependent on a machine for a long period of time.

Withdrawing all treatment would be in conflict with the wishes of both the patient and his wife so this is not an appropriate choice at this time. However, it would be important to meet with the wife and family to set realistic expectations given the patient's wishes, age, comorbidities, and the severity of illness. They need to be informed that his survival to discharge even with maximal medical support and dialysis is highly unlikely.

Withholding dialysis now would honor his wish not to be dependent on machines, but he would be unlikely to survive. Because it is unclear how long he will need dialysis, it is difficult to tell if it will conflict with his desire not to be on machines for "a long period of time." Although dialysis will not help his poor prognosis from his cancer, it may help him meet his short-term goal of surviving until his great-grandson's graduation, so it is not futile.

KEY POINT

- **From an ethical and legal perspective, stopping a life-sustaining therapy is no different from not starting it; interventions should not be withheld for fear they cannot be withdrawn if necessary.**

Bibliography

Snyder L; American College of Physicians Ethics, Professionalism, and Human Rights Committee. American College of Physicians Ethics Manual: sixth edition. Ann Intern Med. 2012;156(1 Pt 2):73-104. [PMID: 22213573]

Item 44   Answer: B

Educational Objective: Diagnose primary Sjögren syndrome.

This patient has primary Sjögren syndrome. Sjögren syndrome is characterized by keratoconjunctivitis sicca, which causes xerophthalmia (dry eyes), and xerostomia (dry mouth). The absence of oral mucosal moisture often causes difficulty with mastication and swallowing and increases the risk for dental caries and periodontal disease. Vaginal dryness and parotid gland enlargement are frequently present, and fatigue and arthralgia are common. Some patients with Sjögren syndrome also may develop an inflammatory polyarthritis. Additional systemic features of Sjögren syndrome include cutaneous vasculitis, peripheral neuropathy, vasculitis that may be associated with mononeuritis multiplex, and interstitial nephritis with associated distal renal tubular acidosis. Pulmonary involvement may develop in patients with Sjögren syndrome and most commonly manifests with interstitial lung disease; however, bronchial and bronchiolar disease also may occur. Abnormal findings on the Schirmer test, which measures moisture under the lower eyelids, are consistent with Sjögren syndrome. Approximately 50% of patients with this syndrome are antinuclear antibody positive and 60% to 75% of patients with primary Sjögren syndrome are anti-Ro/SSA antibody positive, and approximately 40% of these patients are anti-La/SSB antibody positive. A total of 60% to 80% of patients with this condition are rheumatoid factor positive. The presence of xerophthalmia and xerostomia accompanied by anti-Ro/SSA and anti-La/SSB antibody positivity and abnormal findings on the Schirmer test have a 94% sensitivity and specificity for primary Sjögren syndrome.

Meibomianitis is caused by dysfunction of the meibomian glands responsible for production of the lipid portion of the tear film. Given that this patient also has dry mouth and positive anti-Ro/SSA and anti-La/SSB serology, meibomianitis is unlikely.

Both rheumatoid arthritis and systemic lupus erythematosus can be associated with Sjögren syndrome, in which case, multiple systemic symptoms and findings such as joint involvement, pleuritis, cerebritis, lung dysfunction, and skin changes may all occur. Despite this patient's positive antinuclear antibody and rheumatoid factor test results, her lack of systemic symptoms and a normal physical examination (except for xerophthalmia and xerostomia) argue against rheumatoid arthritis or systemic lupus erythematosus as a cause of secondary Sjögren syndrome.

KEY POINT

- **The presence of xerophthalmia and xerostomia accompanied by anti-Ro/SSA and anti-La/SSB antibody positivity and abnormal findings on the Schirmer test have a 94% sensitivity and specificity for primary Sjögren syndrome.**

Bibliography

Latkany R. Dry eyes: etiology and management. Curr Opin Ophthalmol. 2008;19(4):287-291. [PMID: 185450008]

Item 45   Answer: D

Educational Objective: Evaluate a breast mass in a young woman.

This patient should undergo ultrasonography. A slightly tender, discrete, round, soft, and mobile breast mass, with no nipple discharge and no overlying skin changes, is consistent with a fibroadenoma or benign cyst and not breast cancer. However, no single clinical factor by history or physical examination has sufficient accuracy to rule in or rule out underlying malignancy, and diagnostic imaging should be performed. Ultrasonography serves to distinguish cystic from solid masses. A cystic mass should be aspirated and the fluid sent for cytologic evaluation if bloody or recurrent. A solid mass requires biopsy by fine-needle aspiration, core needle, or excision. A benign biopsy in a woman with a normal mammogram still requires close follow-up, as documented by a study in which breast cancer developed in 707 of 9087 women with previous benign breast biopsies followed for a median of 15 years.

In general, imaging should precede core needle biopsy. A core needle biopsy will not be necessary if the mass is definitively cystic by ultrasonography.

The increased density of breast tissue in women 30 to 35 years of age and younger may limit the utility of mammography, making ultrasonography a better first choice. Ultrasonography can readily distinguish cystic from solid lesions and guide further evaluation, such as aspiration, if needed.

Clinical observation and follow-up in 6 months is not appropriate for a palpable breast mass, which should be evaluated until diagnosis or resolution.

KEY POINT

- **A palpable breast mass should be evaluated until diagnosis or resolution.**

Bibliography

Rungruang B, Kelley JL 3rd. Benign breast diseases: epidemiology, evaluation, and management. Clin Obstet Gynecol. 2011;54(1):110-124. [PMID: 21278510]

Item 46   Answer: B

Educational Objective: Recognize a medication-related adverse effect in an elderly patient.

The patient's clinical presentation is likely the result of overmedication in an elderly patient who has significant medical comorbidities and is taking numerous medications. She was recently hospitalized and had medication adjustments made in the setting of chronic kidney disease, including an increase in her diuretic dose, that have led to volume depletion, which, in turn, may have led to changes in her kidneys' ability to metabolize drugs that are renally cleared.

Polypharmacy is becoming more common as the population ages. Twelve percent of patients in the United States older than 65 years take 10 or more medications each week, and adverse drug reactions in the elderly account for 10% of emergency department visits and up to 17% of acute hospitalizations. Numerous medications on this patient's list could cause adverse reactions. For example, gabapentin can cause dizziness and weakness and needs to be dose-adjusted in the setting of kidney disease. A review of every patient's medications, particularly in the elderly, should be a part of routine care to avoid polypharmacy and potential medication-related adverse events.

Although this patient has an apparent decline in her kidney function as estimated by her serum creatinine level, there is no clear evidence of acute kidney injury being the primary cause of her altered mental status.

Infection should always be a primary consideration in elderly patients presenting with mental status changes and failure to thrive. However, in this patient there is no evidence of infection as a cause of her symptoms.

The patient has atrial fibrillation and is not receiving anticoagulation therapy. She does, therefore, have an increased risk for thromboembolic disease. However, her neurologic examination is nonfocal, which would be less consistent with stroke as the underlying cause of her presentation.

KEY POINT

- **Polypharmacy, particularly in elderly patients with multiple comorbid medical conditions, is a frequent cause of adverse events; ongoing review of the need and appropriate dosing of medications should be a part of routine care.**

Bibliography

Hayes BD, Klein-Schwartz W, Barrueto F Jr. Polypharmacy and the geriatric patient. Clin Geriatr Med. 2007;23(2):371-390. [PMID: 17462523]

Item 47   Answer: C

Educational Objective: Manage preoperative care of a patient with COPD scheduled for an intermediate-risk procedure.

This patient with COPD undergoing hip surgery should begin performing incentive spirometry preoperatively to reduce his risk of perioperative pulmonary complications (PPCs). Risk factors for PPCs including chronic lung disease, older age, use of spinal or general anesthesia, and surgery around the diaphragm. Patients with COPD are two to five times more likely to experience PPCs. The only therapy proved effective for reducing the risk of PPCs in the immediate postoperative period is pre- and postoperative lung volume expansion, either via deep breathing or incentive spirometry.

Positive airway pressure can be used postoperatively to minimize atelectasis in patients unable to adequately perform incentive spirometry (such as those with musculoskeletal or neuromuscular limitations to full lung expansion). However, there is no clear role for perioperative positive airway pressure in those who are able to perform incentive spirometry. Additionally, continuous positive airway pressure (CPAP) is not indicated during the day, nocturnally, or both, in the preoperative management of patients with COPD unless they already have an indication for treatment or are unable to use an incentive spirometer.

Chest radiographs are often ordered preoperatively. Only 1% to 3% show a clinically significant abnormality, however, of which only approximately 0.1% affect clinical care. Furthermore, most clinically significant chest radiograph abnormalities can be predicted by history and physical examination. Given this patient's unchanged clinical symptoms and stable pulmonary examination, imaging would not be expected to lead to an improved clinical outcome associated with surgery.

Results of pulmonary function testing do not predict the risk of PPCs, and these tests have no role in routine preoperative evaluation. Pulmonary function testing should be reserved for the evaluation of dyspnea when the cause is not known.

KEY POINT

- The only therapy proved effective for reducing the risk of postoperative pulmonary complications in the immediate perioperative period is pre- and postoperative lung volume expansion, either via deep breathing or incentive spirometry.

Bibliography

Qaseem A, Snow V, Fitterman N, et al; Clinical Efficacy Assessment Subcommittee of the American College of Physicians. Risk assessment for and strategies to reduce perioperative pulmonary complications for patients undergoing noncardiothoracic surgery: a guideline from the American College of Physicians. Ann Intern Med. 2006;144(8):575-580. [PMID: 16618955]

Item 48   Answer: B
Educational Objective: Manage rectal bleeding.

In this average-risk patient, the most appropriate next step would be to proceed to endoscopic evaluation, such as colonoscopy, to rule out colonic neoplasia as a source of bleeding. Typically, patients with hemorrhoidal bleeding report streaks of bright red blood on the toilet paper or on the outside of a firm stool. There is usually pain associated with defecation. However, the hemorrhoids themselves are not painful because there is no innervation to the colonic mucosa proximal to the dentate line. Hemorrhoids are unlikely to cause serious bleeding. Although hemorrhoids are a common cause of bright red blood from the rectum, rectal bleeding should not be considered hemorrhoidal without additional investigation in older patients. Most authorities

agree that the nature of the evaluation is governed by the patient's risk for colon cancer. In young patients (age <40 years) with typical symptoms of hemorrhoid bleeding and low risk for colon cancer, additional evaluation of the colon is unnecessary. Because of the increasing incidence of colon cancer with age, patients 40 to 50 years old with typical hemorrhoidal symptoms but at low risk for colon cancer should probably have at least sigmoidoscopy. Patients aged 50 years and older should undergo colonoscopy to evaluate the source of bleeding provided that routine screening has not been recently performed.

If colon cancer is excluded by colonoscopy, his hemorrhoids can be treated conservatively. Banding and other invasive procedures are reserved for patients whose hemorrhoids do not respond to conservative therapy.

Fiber supplementation is an appropriate treatment for this patient with hard stools but as the only management for his hematochezia is inappropriate, as this option potentially puts him at risk for a missed diagnosis of colon cancer.

Home fecal occult blood testing would likely be positive, but whether positive or negative, the recommendation for this 46-year-old patient remains the same; colonoscopy or sigmoidoscopy based upon the report of bright red rectal bleeding.

KEY POINT

- Patients older than 40 years with hematochezia should undergo colon cancer evaluation with colonoscopy or sigmoidoscopy.

Bibliography

Schubert MC, Sridhar S, Schade RR, Wexner SD. What every gastroenterologist needs to know about common anorectal disorders. World J Gastroenterol. 2009;15(26):3201-3209. [PMID: 19598294]

Item 49   Answer: A
Educational Objective: Manage prostate cancer screening.

The most appropriate management is to have an informed discussion with the patient regarding the risks and benefits of prostate cancer screening. The European Randomized Study of Screening for Prostate Cancer included 162,243 men aged 55 to 69 years. During a median of 9 years, the rate of diagnosis of prostate cancer was higher in the prostate-specific antigen (PSA)–screened group (8.2%) compared with the control (non-screened) group (4.8%) and there was an absolute, albeit small, mortality benefit (1410 men would need to be screened and an additional 48 men would need to be treated for prostate cancer to prevent one death from prostate cancer). In contrast, the Prostate, Lung, Colorectal, and Prostate Cancer Screening Trial found no benefit for annual concurrent PSA and digital rectal examination (DRE) after 7 to 10 years of follow up. Given the conflicting evidence regarding the benefit of prostate cancer screening, the decision of whether or not to screen an individual patient should begin with the clinician having an informed discussion with the patient regarding the risks and benefits of screening and the limitations of the methods used to screen. Based on the conflicting results of these trials, it is not surprising that there is little consensus in terms of screening recommendations. The American Cancer Society supports the need for men to be involved in the decision of whether or not to be screened. In 2012, the U.S. Preventive Services Task Force (USPSTF) published a formal recommendation statement based on a review of existing evidence advising against PSA testing for prostate cancer screening in all men.

Performing a DRE alone is not recommended for screening owing to the poor test characteristics (positive likelihood ratio, 0.53-1.33; negative likelihood ratio, 0.65-14.9).

Although obtaining a PSA level alone and performing a DRE in combination with obtaining a PSA level are frequently employed in screening for prostate cancer, neither approach should be performed without first having an informed discussion with the patient.

> **KEY POINT**
>
> - The decision of whether or not to screen for prostate cancer in an individual man should begin with an informed discussion regarding the risks and benefits of screening and the limitations of the methods used to screen.

Bibliography

Chou R, Croswell JM, Dana T, et al. Screening for prostate cancer: a review of the evidence for the U.S. Preventive Services Task Force. Ann Intern Med. 2011;155(11):762-771. Epub 2011 Oct 7. [PMID: 21984740]

Item 50   Answer: B

Educational Objective: Diagnose central vertigo.

This patient demonstrates vertigo of central origin, a medical emergency. He should undergo MRI with angiography of the brain. Acute vertigo accompanied by vertical nystagmus and nystagmus that is immediate, prolonged (>1 min), and nonfatigable on the Dix-Hallpike maneuver is characteristic of a central origin. Central vertigo may be caused by ischemia or infarct in the brainstem or cerebellum. The patient's inability to stand without support and the absence of diplopia or dysarthria likely puts his lesion in the cerebellum. Up to one quarter of patients with traditional risk factors for stroke who present with severe vertigo and nystagmus and who are unable to stand without support have ischemia or infarction of the cerebellum.

Diffusion-weighted MRI is recommended over CT scanning as the first-line evaluation for stroke within 12 hours of symptom onset owing to its superior sensitivity. Although CT scanning without contrast has excellent sensitivity for intracranial hemorrhage, is widely available, and,

in most cases, can be performed more quickly and with less cost, it is less sensitive than MRI for acute ischemic stroke and does not provide adequate imaging of the vasculature of the posterior circulation.

Otolith repositioning, commonly known as the Epley maneuver, has been shown helpful in resolving symptoms of benign paroxysmal positional vertigo (BPPV). BPPV is the most common cause of vestibular (peripheral) dizziness. Patients with BPPV describe vertigo lasting minutes in duration, with multiple episodes occurring over weeks to months. Tinnitus, ear pain, and hearing loss are absent, and nausea that is sufficiently severe or prolonged to cause vomiting is rare. The patient's findings are not consistent with BPPV.

Symptomatic treatment with vestibular suppressants is generally reserved for peripheral causes. The patient's recent upper respiratory tract infection is a risk factor for vestibular neuritis. However, his history and bedside examination are inconsistent with peripheral vertigo. On the Dix-Hallpike maneuver, vertigo of peripheral origin is usually severe, lasts less than 1 minute, has a latency of 2 to 40 seconds, and fatigues with time. The direction of peripheral nystagmus is not vertical but is horizontal with a rotational component.

> **KEY POINT**
>
> - Acute vertigo accompanied by vertical nystagmus and nystagmus that is immediate, prolonged, and nonfatigable on the Dix-Hallpike maneuver is characteristic of central vertigo.

Bibliography

Post RE, Dickerson LM. Dizziness: a diagnostic approach. Am Fam Physician. 2010;82(4):361-368, 369. [PMID: 20704166]

Item 51   Answer: D

Educational Objective: Counsel an obese patient regarding weight reduction.

This patient should reduce her current caloric intake by 500 to 1000 kcal/d. Consistent reduction in daily dietary caloric intake is the most successful long-term and safest weight loss strategy in obese and overweight patients. Patients who follow a diet that reduces their caloric intake by 500 to 1000 kcal/d as compared with their intake that is currently maintaining weight will lose an average of 0.45 to 0.91 kg (1-2 lb) per week. The initial goal should be a loss of 10% of total body weight. If this patient adheres to this recommendation, she should lose 9.1 kg (20 lb) in 4 to 5 months. This degree of weight loss has been shown to decrease the health-related consequences of obesity, including diabetes mellitus. Because she already has prediabetes, weight loss is important to her long-term health.

Exercise is an important part of a comprehensive weight loss program that focuses on lifestyle modification.

However, without attention to eating habits and caloric restriction, exercise alone is not adequate for weight loss.

Current National Institutes of Health and Veterans Affairs guidelines recommend consideration of bariatric interventions, such as laparoscopic band surgery, in patients with a BMI greater than 40 or patients with a BMI of 35 to 40 with obesity-related comorbidities, such as diabetes mellitus, obstructive sleep apnea, or severe joint disease. This patient does not meet these recommendations.

Orlistat is a lipase inhibitor that leads to fat malabsorption. It is FDA approved when used in conjunction with a reduced calorie diet. It is moderately effective in weight loss (2.9 kg [6.4 lb] at 12 months) but gastrointestinal side effects are common. More serious adverse effects, such as severe liver injury and malabsorption of fat-soluble vitamins, have been reported. Lifestyle management with diet and exercise should be the first step in any weight loss program. Medications can be used in conjunction with, but not as a substitute for, diet and exercise.

KEY POINT

- **Consistent reduction in daily dietary caloric intake is the most successful long-term and safest weight loss strategy in obese and overweight patients.**

Bibliography
Management of Overweight and Obesity Working Group. VA/DoD clinical practice guideline for screening and management of overweight and obesity. Washington (DC): Department of Veterans Affairs, Department of Defense; 2006.

Item 52   Answer: B

Educational Objective: Treat elevated LDL cholesterol level.

Pravastatin is the safest choice for lowering LDL cholesterol level in this patient. She has recently diagnosed peripheral arterial disease, which is associated with atherosclerosis; her goal LDL cholesterol level is, therefore, less than 100 mg/dL (2.59 mmol/L). Pravastatin is one of the preferred statins in patients who are being treated with multiple medications.

Statins should be considered first-line therapy for lowering LDL cholesterol levels in this patient, as studies have shown that older patients (ages 65-80 years) derive similar benefit as younger patients for secondary prevention of cardiovascular disease. However, advanced age is also a risk factor for statin-related myopathy, and therapy should be chosen carefully to minimize this risk. Female sex, small body frame, hypothyroidism, statin dosage, and treatment with multiple medications also influence the likelihood of developing statin-related myopathy. Pravastatin is metabolized by the kidneys; therefore, its concentration will be unaffected by cytochrome isoenzymes that affect the metabolism of other statins or warfarin.

In contrast, atorvastatin, lovastatin, and simvastatin are primarily metabolized through the cytochrome P-450 3A4 isoenzyme, and treatment with these medications in combination with diltiazem can increase serum statin levels, placing the patient at higher risk for statin myopathy. These statins should not be combined with diltiazem in a patient who is at already high risk for statin-induced myopathy based on her age, small body frame, hypothyroidism, and multiple medications.

Rosuvastatin and fluvastatin are metabolized through the cytochrome P-450 CYP2C9 isoenzyme, and would effectively lower this patient's LDL cholesterol level. However, rosuvastatin may affect the metabolism of warfarin, leading to an increased INR. Caution is therefore necessary when combining these medications, and this is not the safest choice for this patient.

KEY POINT

- **In patients who require lipid-lowering therapy and who are taking multiple medications, a statin that is renally metabolized, such as pravastatin, has a lower risk of drug-drug interactions.**

Bibliography
Joy TR, Hegele RA. Narrative review: statin-related myopathy. Ann Intern Med. 2009;150(12):858-868. [PMID: 19528564]

Item 53   Answer: C

Educational Objective: Treat heavy menstrual bleeding.

The most appropriate next management step is oral medroxyprogesterone acetate. In patients who present with menorrhagia (heavy menstrual bleeding) with a known etiology, several therapeutic agents can decrease bleeding. For moderate bleeding that can be managed on an outpatient basis, a progestational agent such as medroxyprogesterone acetate can be given for 10 to 21 days. The progesterone will typically act to stabilize the endometrium and stop uterine blood flow.

Estrogen/progesterone-containing oral contraceptives may be useful in decreasing menstrual blood loss, although the doses of both agents in most typical formulations would likely be inadequate to control the degree of bleeding in this patient, particularly with a multiphasic preparation. If a specific progestational agent is not available, a monophasic oral contraceptive may be dosed four times daily for 5 to 7 days, and subsequently reduced to daily dosing until definitive treatment is undertaken.

If the patient were orthostatic or dizzy from blood loss, intravenous estrogen would be appropriate. Parenteral conjugated estrogens are approximately 70% effective in stopping the bleeding entirely. Pulmonary embolism and venous thrombosis are complications of intravenous estrogen therapy.

Monitoring the patient for an additional week of observation is not appropriate given her significant, ongoing blood loss.

KEY POINT

- Medroxyprogesterone acetate for 10 to 21 days is effective treatment for moderate menstrual bleeding.

Bibliography

Fazio SB, Ship AN. Abnormal uterine bleeding. South Med J. 2007;100(4):376-382; quiz 383, 402. [PMID: 17458397]

Item 54   Answer: B

Educational Objective: Diagnose patellofemoral pain syndrome.

This patient most likely has patellofemoral pain syndrome, the most common cause of knee pain in patients younger than 45 years. Patellofemoral pain syndrome is a clinical diagnosis and further diagnostic testing such as radiographs is not necessary. Patellofemoral pain syndrome is more common in women than in men and is characterized by anterior knee pain that is made worse with prolonged sitting and with going up and down stairs. The pain is reproduced by applying pressure to the patella with the knee in extension and moving the patella both medially and laterally (patellofemoral compression test).

According to the American College of Rheumatology's clinical criteria, osteoarthritis of the knee can be diagnosed if knee pain is accompanied by at least three of the following features: age greater than 50 years, stiffness lasting less than 30 minutes, crepitus, bony tenderness, bony enlargement, and no palpable warmth. These criteria are 95% sensitive and 69% specific but have not been validated for clinical practice. Crepitus of the knee is common in patients with osteoarthritis between the patella and the femur. Passive range of motion of the knee often elicits pain at the extremes of flexion and extension. Palpation of the knee discloses only mild tenderness. This patient has no clinical evidence of knee osteoarthritis.

Pes anserine bursitis characteristically produces pain that is located near the anteromedial aspect of the proximal tibia. On examination, tenderness is elicited at the level of the tibial tuberosity (approximately 3.8 cm [1.5 in] below the level of the medial joint line). Swelling may be present at the insertion of the medial hamstring muscles. This patient's presentation is not consistent with pes anserine bursitis.

Prepatellar bursitis is often caused by recurrent trauma, such as repeated kneeling ("housemaid's knee") but can also be caused by infection or gout. Although the pain is located anteriorly, examination reveals swelling, tenderness to palpation (usually localized near the lower pole of the patella), and erythema, all of which are lacking in this patient.

KEY POINT

- Patellofemoral pain syndrome is more common in women than in men and is characterized by anterior knee pain that is made worse with prolonged sitting and with going up and down stairs.

Bibliography

Collado H, Fredericson M. Patellofemoral pain syndrome. Clin Sports Med. 2010;29(3):379-398. [PMID: 20610028]

Item 55   Answer: A

Educational Objective: Manage chronic dizziness in an elderly patient.

This elderly woman with chronic dizziness should receive physical therapy with gait evaluation. Chronic dizziness is a common problem in the elderly. Although not associated with excess mortality, chronic dizziness is associated with falls, syncope, and self-rated health decline. It is often multifactorial and exhaustive work-ups are costly and often unrewarding, particularly in the absence of suggestive or supporting findings on history or physical examination. Common contributing factors, including medications, sensory impairments, neuropathy, muscle weakness, deconditioning, anxiety, depression, and postural hypotension, should be identified and addressed. This patient specifically presents with dysequilibrium, a nonvertiginous feeling of imbalance or unsteadiness while standing or walking. She has impairments in vision and hearing. She is at high risk for falls. In addition to evaluation for visual and hearing aids, referral to physical therapy for balance and gait training is an appropriate first step. In a recent systematic review and meta-analysis of community- and residential care–dwelling older adults, programs that included exercise and that focused on exercises that challenge balance had the greatest relative effects on fall rates (RR = 0.58, 95% CI = 0.48-0.69).

Administration of topical ophthalmic medication carries some risk of systemic absorption. This patient is being treated with latanoprost, a prostaglandin analogue that typically has minimal systemic effects. β-Blocker ophthalmic drops, such as timolol, are associated with systemic absorption, which may worsen her symptoms.

Although medication side effects and polypharmacy can contribute to dizziness, this patient is not orthostatic, and changing from an ACE inhibitor to an angiotensin receptor blocker would not likely relieve her symptoms.

Vestibular rehabilitation therapy is most useful for patients with benign paroxysmal positional vertigo. This patient presents with nonspecific dizziness and not true vertigo.

KEY POINT

- Physical therapy is an effective intervention to decrease fall risk in elderly patients with dysequilibrium.

Bibliography

Sherrington C, Whitney JC, Lord SR, Herbert RD, Cumming RG, Close JC. Effective exercise for the prevention of falls: a systematic review and meta-analysis. J Am Geriatr Soc. 2008;56(12):2234-2243. [PMID: 19093923]

Item 56   Answer: C
Educational Objective: Treat depression.

The most appropriate next treatment step for this patient is to discontinue bupropion and begin a different antidepressant, such as sertraline. She has moderate depression that is refractory to initial single-agent treatment. The goal of treatment is to achieve complete remission within 6 to 12 weeks and continue treatment for 4 to 9 months thereafter. Patients should be assessed 2 and 4 weeks after starting therapy for adherence, adverse drug reactions, and suicide risk, and again at 6 to 8 weeks for response to therapy. Using a formal tool for severity assessment (such as the PHQ-9) helps quantify the nature of the response; patients are considered to have at least a partial response if a 50% or greater decrease in symptom score has occurred. Using the PHQ-9, patients can be classified as complete responders, partial responders, or nonresponders. Complete responders should continue the same therapy modality for an additional 4 to 9 months. Treatment options for partial responders and nonresponders include using a higher dose of the same agent (ineffective in this patient), adding a second agent, switching to a new drug, or adding psychotherapy (patient not interested). Any change in therapy requires periodic follow-up as outlined above.

Buspirone is an anxiolytic. Given the patient's lack of anxiety symptoms and her total lack of response to bupropion, adding this medication is not appropriate.

This patient remains unresponsive to treatment with bupropion following a dose escalated to the maximal dose. Waiting an additional 8 weeks is unlikely to change management and will slow this patient's recovery. Switching to a new drug, either of the same class (unavailable in this case) or different class, is indicated. Selective serotonin reuptake inhibitors (SSRIs), such as sertraline, are the most commonly prescribed class of antidepressants. In general, SSRIs are well tolerated with low toxicity; however, sexual side effects are common.

Electroconvulsive therapy is indicated in severely depressed patients, such as those with profound suicidal ideation or psychotic features in whom a rapid response to therapy is particularly desirable. This patient has no indication for electroconvulsive therapy.

> **KEY POINT**
>
> - **Patients refractory to a single antidepressant may respond to a change in therapy, which may include replacement with another antidepressant, either from the same or a different class; addition of a second antidepressant; or a psychotherapeutic intervention.**

Bibliography

Fancher TL, Kravitz RL. In the clinic. Depression. Ann Intern Med. 2010;152(9):ITC51-15; quiz ITC5-16. [PMID: 20439571]

Item 57   Answer: D
Educational Objective: Prevent type 2 diabetes mellitus in an overweight patient.

The most appropriate therapies to prevent type 2 diabetes mellitus in this patient are weight loss and exercise. This patient has a strong family history of type 2 diabetes mellitus and impaired fasting glucose, defined as a fasting plasma glucose level of 100 to 125 mg/dL (5.6 to 7.0 mmol/L). Based on multiple clinical trials, lifestyle modification has been shown to be the most effective intervention to prevent type 2 diabetes and its associated cardiovascular consequences. The Finnish Diabetes Prevention Study and the U.S. Diabetes Prevention Program (USDPP) both demonstrated a 58% relative risk reduction in the progression to diabetes with these methods in generally obese, middle-aged persons with impaired glucose tolerance. The American Diabetes Association recommends that lifestyle modifications continue to be the standard approach in diabetes prevention, with the goal being to increase regular physical activity by approximately 30 minutes on most days of the week and to reduce calories (to reduce weight) by 7%.

The USDPP reported a 31% risk reduction in the development of diabetes in patients treated with metformin. Acarbose reduced the risk of diabetes by 25% in the Study to Prevent Non–Insulin-Dependent Diabetes Mellitus (STOP-NIDDM) trial but had a high drop-out rate owing to gastrointestinal adverse effects. Other studies have shown a 62% reduction in progression to diabetes with rosiglitazone in patients with impaired glucose tolerance or impaired fasting glucose and an 82% reduction in the progression to diabetes with pioglitazone. However, the thiazolidinediones are associated with significant potential adverse effects, and the harm of these drugs may outweigh the benefit of their use in this patient population. Despite these findings, currently no drugs are FDA-approved for the prevention of diabetes. In patients with impaired fasting glucose and other risk factors (BMI ≥35, a strong family history, elevated triglyceride level, reduced HDL cholesterol level, hypertension, hemoglobin A_{1c} >6.0%), some clinicians will use metformin if lifestyle modifications have not been successful.

> **KEY POINT**
>
> - **The most appropriate therapies to prevent type 2 diabetes mellitus are weight loss and exercise.**

Bibliography

Knowler WC, Fowler SE, Hamman RF, et al; Diabetes Prevention Program Research Group. 10-year follow-up of diabetes incidence and weight loss in the Diabetes Prevention Program Outcomes Study. Lancet. 2009;374(9702):1677-1686. [PMID: 19878986]

Item 58   Answer: D

Educational Objective: Evaluate relative versus absolute risk.

The number needed to treat (NNT) with drug Z compared with drug C to prevent one additional case of deep venous thrombosis (DVT) is 100.

Absolute risk (AR) is the risk of a specific disease based on its actual occurrence, or its event rate (ER), in a group of patients being studied, and is expressed as:

$$AR = \frac{\text{patients with event in group}}{\text{total patients in group}}$$

As seen in the table, in this study, the AR for DVT in the group treated with drug Z is 25/2500, or 1%, and the AR for the group treated with drug C is 50/2500, or 2%.

Often, the event rate of a disease in an experimental group (EER) is compared with the event rate in a control group (CER). When the risk between groups is reduced, this difference is termed the absolute risk reduction (ARR), or if the outcome is of benefit, the difference is called the absolute benefit index (ABI). In this case, patients treated with drug Z (EER) appear to benefit from treatment with a lower risk of DVT than patients in the group treated with drug C (CER). This is expressed as:

$$ABI = |\,EER - CER\,|$$
$$ABI = |1\% - 2\%| = 1\% \text{ or } 0.01$$

This means that treatment with drug Z benefits patients compared with drug C by lowering the risk of DVT from 2% to 1%, or an absolute difference of 1%.

Assessing treatment studies using absolute measures also allows determination of "numbers needed," which are estimates of the clinical magnitude of the differences between treatments. In this case, the NNT indicates the number of patients needed to be treated with drug Z, compared with drug C, to obtain one additional beneficial outcome. The NNT is calculated as:

$$NNT = 1/ABI$$
$$NNT = 1 \div 0.01 = 100$$

This means that 100 patients would need to be treated with drug Z compared with drug C in order to prevent one additional case of DVT.

Treatment study results may also be reported as relative measures; these measures compare the ratio of two outcomes without regard to the actual frequency of the outcome in a given study population. In this case, treatment with drug Z leads to a 50% reduction in risk of DVT compared with treatment with drug C (25 compared with 50 events), even though the actual frequency of DVT in the study populations does not exceed 2%. Therefore, outcomes expressed in relative terms usually appear of greater magnitude than when expressed in absolute terms; they also do not allow calculations of number needed to estimate clinical impact.

KEY POINT

- Treatment study outcomes reported in absolute terms reflect the frequency of a disease in the study population and allow estimation of "numbers needed"; outcomes reported in relative terms tend to appear to be of greater magnitude.

Bibliography

Guyatt GH, Sackett DL, Cook DJ. Users' guides to the medical literature. II. How to use an article about therapy or prevention. B. What were the results and will they help me in caring for my patients? Evidence-Based Medicine Working Group. JAMA. 1994;271(1):59-63. [PMID: 8258890]

Item 59   Answer: D

Educational Objective: Manage ankle sprain.

The most appropriate management of this patient's ankle sprain is splinting. This patient most likely has a grade II ankle sprain. Correct grading of ankle sprains is important both in terms of predicting prognosis and for helping to ensure appropriate treatment. Grade II ankle sprains involve partial tears of one or more ankle ligaments and manifest clinically with moderate pain and some difficulty with bearing weight, which is occurring in this patient. Mild ankle instability and limited range of motion may also be present. In addition to conservative therapy (rest, ice, compression, elevation) and NSAIDs, joint stabilization is indicated and may be achieved with an elastic bandage and ankle splint. Adequate splinting will also support early ambulation and help protect against repeat injury. The optimal duration of splinting is unclear, although several weeks is reasonable with improvement of symptoms. Formal rehabilitation, including proprioceptive training, may be helpful in preventing chronic instability in grade II sprains.

Corticosteroid injections do not have a role in acute ankle injuries and should not be performed.

Although MRI may provide more detailed information than plain radiographs, they offer no advantage if acute imaging is indicated. MRIs are reserved primarily for evaluation of ankle sprains that fail to respond to a course of standard therapy or complex ankle injuries.

An inability to bear weight, although common with severe sprains, should raise concern for the possibility of a fracture. Fractures of the base of the fifth metatarsal are associated with tenderness to palpation of this area on examination. Lateral malleolar fractures are associated with tenderness to palpation of the lateral malleolus. According to the Ottawa ankle rules, ankle radiographs should be obtained only in patients with ankle pain who are unable to bear weight or who have bony tenderness to palpation at the posterior edge of either the lateral or medial malleoli. One systematic review found this set of criteria to be almost 100% sensitive in diagnosing fractures. Thus, it would not be appropriate to obtain ankle radiographs in this patient.

Urgent surgical referral would be appropriate for a patient with a grade III ankle sprain, which is characterized by complete rupture of one or more ligaments and presents with severe swelling, ecchymosis, instability, and the inability to bear weight. Urgent surgical referral is not needed in a patient with a grade II ankle sprain.

KEY POINT

- Ankle radiographs should only be obtained in patients with acute ankle pain who are unable to bear weight or who have bony tenderness to palpation at the posterior edge of either the lateral or medial malleoli.

Bibliography

Seah R, Mani-Babu S. Managing ankle sprains in primary care: what is best practice? A systematic review of the last 10 years of evidence. Br Med Bull. 2011;97:105-135. [PMID: 20710025]

Item 60　　Answer:　E

Educational Objective: Treat menopausal vasomotor symptoms.

This 61-year-old woman with cardiovascular risk factors and a history of deep venous thrombosis should be started on a nonhormonal therapy for her hot flushes. Certain antidepressants, including serotonin-norepinephrine reuptake inhibitors such as venlafaxine, are effective nonhormonal medications for reducing menopausal vasomotor symptoms.

Approximately 10% of menopausal women experience hot flushes for 7 to 10 years after the cessation of menses. This patient is continuing to experience frequent and severe hot flushes which have been refractory to conservative therapy and are decreasing her quality of life; thus, pharmacologic therapy is warranted. Systemic estrogen therapy is the most effective treatment for the relief of menopausal hot flushes and must be coadministered with progesterone in women with an intact uterus. However, combined estrogen and progesterone therapy has been shown to increase the risk of several adverse outcomes, including coronary heart disease, stroke, invasive breast cancer, and venous thromboembolism. The North American Menopause Society guideline notes that women older than 60 years who experienced natural menopause at the median age and have never used hormone therapy will have elevated baseline risks of cardiovascular disease, venous thromboembolism, and breast cancer; hormone therapy, therefore, should not be initiated in this population without a compelling indication and only after appropriate counseling and attention to cardiovascular risk factors. Moreover, this patient has a history of deep venous thrombosis, which is an absolute contraindication to initiating hormone therapy.

Several nonhormonal medications have been found to be effective for the treatment of menopausal hot flushes. Notably, there is a significant placebo effect: in most studies, approximately one-third of women will experience relief of hot flushes, even if they do not receive active treatment. In numerous studies, venlafaxine, administered at doses of 37.5 mg/d to 150 mg/d, decreases hot flush severity and frequency in approximately 60% of patients (as compared with 30% who experienced benefit with placebo treatment). Paroxetine is similarly beneficial; in contrast, few studies have shown efficacy with fluoxetine or citalopram. Gabapentin and clonidine are two additional nonhormonal treatments that reduce hot flushes, but attendant side effects may limit their use in some patients.

Vaginal estrogen therapy is typically used for the isolated treatment of vaginal dryness, pruritus, and dyspareunia. Treatment with vaginal estrogen tablets will improve local vaginal symptoms, but will not improve menopausal vasomotor symptoms.

KEY POINT

- Owing to cardiovascular and thromboembolic risks, systemic hormone therapy is not recommended for treatment of menopausal vasomotor symptoms in women older than 60 years who experienced menopause at the median age.

Bibliography

Nelson HD, Vesco KK, Haney E, et al. Nonhormonal therapies for menopausal hot flashes: systematic review and meta-analysis. JAMA. 2006;295(17):2057-2071. [PMID: 16670414]

Item 61　　Answer:　C

Educational Objective: Diagnose central retinal vein occlusion.

This patient most likely has central retinal vein occlusion (CRVO). Patients with CRVO experience acute onset of painless blurry vision due to reduced venous outflow and vascular edema in the eye. CRVO is characterized by optic disc swelling, dilated and tortuous veins, flame-shaped retinal hemorrhages, and cotton-wool spots ("blood and thunder"). Because the nerve supply to the eye remains intact but vision is decreased, an afferent pupillary defect in the affected eye may be present. CRVO is most commonly encountered in older patients with hypertension and atherosclerotic vascular disease. Cases have also been associated with acute carotid artery dissection and conditions associated with increased blood viscosity, such as polycythemia vera, sickle cell disease, and leukemia. Prognosis depends on the degree of visual impairment at the onset of symptoms. There is no generally accepted acute management, but a thorough investigation into possible etiologies should be undertaken.

Acute angle closure glaucoma is characterized by narrowing or closure of the anterior chamber angle, which impedes the trabecular drainage system in the anterior chamber, resulting in elevated intraocular pressure and damage to the optic nerve. Typical signs and symptoms include significant pain, diminished visual acuity, seeing halos around lights, a red eye, headache, and a dilated pupil.

The globe may feel firm owing to increased intraocular pressure (often to 30 mm Hg or higher). Retinal examination may be normal or demonstrate optic cupping if chronic narrow-angle glaucoma is present.

Central retinal artery occlusion (CRAO) classically presents in a 50- to 70-year-old patient as a painless, abrupt blurring or loss of vision that occurs in the early morning hours—usually between midnight and 6 AM. It results from an embolic or thrombotic event in the ophthalmic artery. It is typically unilateral. On examination, visual acuity is markedly diminished in the affected eye to either finger counting or light perception. There is an afferent pupillary defect. On funduscopic examination, the retina appears pale, either segmentally or completely. The fovea may appear as a cherry red spot. Interruption of the venous blood columns may be recognized with the appearance of "box-carring"—rows of slowly moving corpuscles separated by clear intervals. These findings are not present in this patient.

Symptoms of retinal detachment include diminished vision, photopsia (flashes of light), abrupt onset of multiple floaters in the vision, and metamorphopsia (wavy vision). Retinal detachment may result from trauma or occur spontaneously, particularly in persons with myopia. It is typically unilateral. On funduscopic examination, retinal detachment is characterized by distortion, folding, and tearing of the retina, which were not seen in this patient.

KEY POINT

- Central retinal vein occlusion is characterized by acute onset of painless blurry vision and optic disc swelling, dilated and tortuous veins, flame-shaped retinal hemorrhages, and cotton-wool spots ("blood and thunder").

Bibliography

Ahmed R, Foroozan R. Transient monocular visual loss. Neurol Clin. 2010;28(3):619-629. [PMID: 20637992]

Item 62 Answer: C

Educational Objective: Manage a perioperative patient with cirrhosis.

This patient has cirrhotic liver disease, placing him at a high risk of perioperative complications, and nonoperative management of his hip osteoarthritis should be recommended. Patients with cirrhosis have an increased risk of perioperative morbidity and mortality. Surgery and anesthesia in these patients are risk factors for fulminant hepatic failure, and cirrhosis itself can predispose to bleeding, infection, adverse reactions to drugs, and poor wound healing. The risk of perioperative complications can be quantified using a number of scales, including Child-Turcotte-Pugh (CTP) classification. The CTP score is based on the presence of ascites and encephalopathy, as well as serum bilirubin, albumin, and INR values. Patients with CTP class A (0-6 points), class B (7-9 points), and class C (≥10 points) scores have postoperative mortality rates of approximately 10%, 30%, and 80%, respectively. Patients with a CTP class C score are usually advised to avoid elective surgery.

Patients with acute alcoholic hepatitis may present with leukocytosis, jaundice, hepatomegaly, and right upper quadrant pain. In addition to abstinence from alcohol and nutritional therapy, pharmacologic therapy with corticosteroids may be beneficial in patients with severe alcoholic hepatitis. However, this patient's cirrhosis is a result of long-term chronic alcohol use, and there is no indication for corticosteroid therapy.

Patients with cirrhosis are predisposed to bleeding because of quantitative and qualitative platelet dysfunction as well as a deficiency of hepatically produced clotting factors. The INR elevation in these patients is usually not caused by vitamin K deficiency. Although patients with coagulopathy are sometimes treated with oral vitamin K to reverse any nutritional deficiencies, administration of vitamin K would only minimally change the inherent risks of surgery in this patient.

KEY POINT

- Patients with a Child-Turcotte-Pugh class C score are usually advised to avoid elective surgery.

Bibliography

O'Leary JG, Yachimski PS, Friedman LS. Surgery in the patient with liver disease. Clin Liver Dis. 2009;13(2):211-231. [PMID: 19442915]

Item 63 Answer: B

Educational Objective: Counsel a patient using motivational interviewing.

It would be appropriate to determine which lifestyle change this patient believes is most important to implement. Key features of motivational interviewing are that the patient chooses the agenda, the provider is not in "control" and does not tell the patient what he or she should do, and the provider assesses the patient's sense of the importance of issues for them and their level of confidence in making these changes, which should be small and incremental. Physicians can support the patient's choice and provide advice on how to overcome barriers to implementation.

The patient has indicated a willingness to make important lifestyle changes; he now needs to be empowered to identify those changes he wishes to make and identify barriers and facilitators to those changes. He does not need to be told to lose weight; the patient has already acknowledged the need to make lifestyle changes. After the patient identifies the changes that are important to him, it would be appropriate to ascertain his confidence in making those changes, but to do so prior to this step would be premature. Having the patient control the agenda and select the changes he believes are most important and identify the associated barriers and facilitators is more likely to be effective than the physician providing advice on smoking or other lifestyle changes that the patient may deem as less important.

- Key features of motivational interviewing are that the patient chooses the agenda, the provider is not in "control" and does not tell the patient what he or she should do, and the provider assesses the patient's sense of the importance of issues and level of confidence in making changes.

Bibliography

Rollnick S, Butler CC, Kinnersley P, Gregory J, Mash B. Motivational interviewing. BMJ. 2010;340:1242-1245. [PMID: 20423957]

Item 64   Answer: C

Educational Objective: Diagnose metabolic syndrome.

Given this patient's hypertension, lipid profile, and abdominal obesity, she meets the criteria for metabolic syndrome. The diagnosis of metabolic syndrome (Adult Treatment Panel III criteria) is made by the presence of three or more of the following five criteria: (1) waist circumference >40 in (102 cm) in men and >35 in (88 cm) in women; (2) systolic blood pressure ≥130 mm Hg or diastolic blood pressure ≥85 mm Hg; (3) HDL cholesterol level <40 mg/dL (1.04 mmol/L) in men and <50 mg/dL (1.30 mmol/L) in women; (4) triglyceride level ≥150 mg/dL (1.70 mmol/L); and (5) fasting plasma glucose level ≥110 mg/dL (6.1 mmol/L).

The clinical importance of identifying the metabolic syndrome is the increased risk for cardiovascular disease and type 2 diabetes mellitus in those with this diagnosis. Persons with the metabolic syndrome should receive aggressive intervention focused on lifestyle modification to decrease weight, increase physical activity, and implement a nonatherogenic diet, in addition to treating the significant metabolic abnormalities that define the syndrome. The metabolic syndrome is frequently identified in patients with polycystic ovary syndrome, and has also been associated with the development of other disorders, including fatty liver disease, obstructive sleep apnea, hyperuricemia, and gout.

The patient does not meet the criteria for hypertriglyceridemia, although American Heart Association guidelines recommend an optimal triglyceride level of below 100 mg/dL (1.13 mmol/L), and this would be an appropriate goal for this patient for lifestyle modifications.

Impaired fasting glucose (prediabetes) is defined as a fasting blood glucose level of 100 to 125 mg/dL (5.6-6.9 mmol/L). She does not have this diagnosis, and the diagnosis of the metabolic syndrome does not strictly require abnormalities in glucose metabolism.

- Metabolic syndrome is diagnosed by the presence of three or more of five abnormalities: increased waist circumference, elevated systolic or diastolic blood pressure, decreased HDL cholesterol level, elevated triglyceride level, and elevated fasting plasma glucose level.

Bibliography

Tota-Maharaj R, Defilippis AP, Blumenthal RS, Blaha MJ. A practical approach to the metabolic syndrome: review of current concepts and management. Curr Opin Cardiol. 2010;25(5):502-512. [PMID: 20644468]

Item 65   Answer: B

Educational Objective: Manage advanced cancer pain.

The next step in the treatment protocol for this patient would be a NSAID, such as ibuprofen. The World Health Organization analgesic ladder represents a useful framework for pharmacologic treatment of pain. Nonnarcotic treatments, such as aspirin, acetaminophen, or NSAIDs, are used for mild pain (score of 1-3 on the 0-10 pain intensity scale). Moderate pain (pain score 4-6) is treated with a combination of opioids and nonnarcotic pain relievers. If these agents are combined in a single pill (such as oxycodone and acetaminophen) to reduce polypharmacy, care must be taken to avoid inadvertent overdosing of the nonnarcotic component when the need for the opioid ingredient increases. The daily cumulative acetaminophen dose (<4 g) limits the dosing of the opioid in combination medications. Severe pain (pain score 7-10) is mainly treated with opioids. Adjunctive therapies (antidepressants, anticonvulsants, corticosteroids, muscle relaxants) can be used at all levels of the analgesic ladder. NSAIDs can be especially effective in patients with bone pain, particularly if there is an inflammatory component.

The use of gabapentin, an anticonvulsant, is a useful adjuvant pain medication and may be particularly helpful in patients with neuropathic pain but would be a poor choice for this patient with bone pain.

Meperidine is rarely appropriate for oral use owing to variable oral bioavailability and the accumulation of active metabolites with prolonged use at high doses or in kidney failure. Such accumulation lowers the seizure threshold and causes central nervous system symptoms, such as tremors, twitching, and nervousness.

Oral administration is the preferred route for opioid analgesics because of its convenience, low cost, and ability to produce stable opioid blood levels. Intramuscular injections are not recommended because of the associated pain, unreliable absorption, and relatively long interval to peak drug concentrations. This patient should be tried on a NSAID prior to an opioid medication.

KEY POINT

- Nonopioid agents are the first step in the management of mild cancer pain and should be initiated before progressing to an opioid agent.

Bibliography

Swetz KM, Kamal AH. Palliative care. Ann Intern Med. 2012;156(3):ITC21. [PMID: 22312158]

Item 66   Answer: D

Educational Objective: Treat dyslipidemia.

This patient should be started on statin therapy. He has a very high LDL cholesterol level despite a healthy diet and regular vigorous exercise. According to the National Cholesterol Education Program (NCEP) Adult Treatment Panel III guidelines, persons with two or more cardiovascular risk factors, such as this patient, should have an LDL cholesterol goal of below 130 mg/dL (3.37 mmol/L), and drug therapy should be considered in those with LDL cholesterol levels of 160 mg/dL (4.14 mmol/L) or above.

The non-HDL cholesterol level is calculated by subtracting the measured HDL cholesterol from the total cholesterol level. In patients with elevated triglycerides, the non-HDL level correlates with high concentrations of atherogenic lipoproteins, including VLDL remnants. The NCEP guidelines designate the non-HDL cholesterol level as a secondary target for therapy, after goal LDL cholesterol levels have been achieved. Calculation of the non-HDL cholesterol level will not alter this patient's current management strategy.

The U.S. Preventive Services Task Force (USPSTF) has recently reviewed the utility of adding several novel cardiac risk markers to traditional methods of cardiac risk stratification. According to their guidelines, there is insufficient evidence to recommend for or against the use of high-sensitivity C-reactive protein levels for assessing cardiovascular risk. Measurement of the high-sensitivity C-reactive protein level in this patient is not likely to affect management.

Fibric acid derivatives are effective at lowering triglyceride levels, but have a lesser effect on LDL cholesterol level. Although this patient has borderline-high triglyceride levels, lowering his LDL cholesterol level would significantly reduce his cardiovascular risk, and some reduction in his triglyceride levels would be expected with statin therapy.

KEY POINT

- In moderate-risk patients with LDL cholesterol levels of 160 mg/dL (4.14 mmol/L) or above, therapeutic lifestyle changes and pharmacologic lipid-lowering therapy are warranted.

Bibliography

U.S. Preventive Services Task Force. Using nontraditional risk factors in coronary heart disease risk assessment: U.S. Preventive Services Task Force recommendation statement. Ann Intern Med. 2009;151(7):474-482. [PMID: 19805770]

Item 67   Answer: A

Educational Objective: Manage fall risk in an elderly patient.

This patient appears to have had a fall without any indication of gait abnormality, visual deficit, or weakness. Her bumping into a wall at night may have caused the fall. It would be important to know if she has night lights in each room, because lack of proper lighting would contribute to her risk for falls. Installing night lights in each room is a simple and inexpensive fall prevention strategy. Additionally, an evaluation for home safety is always an appropriate consideration for patients who have fallen, because hazards can be found in two-thirds of homes. Other causes for falls, such as the presence of rugs and thresholds between rooms, have been ruled out. If the patient was already using night lights, then a home safety evaluation for other hazards, including general clutter, uneven lighting, and unsafe or absent hand rails, would be important.

In the Timed "Up & Go" (TUG) test, the patient is asked to arise from a chair, walk 10 feet, turn around, and sit in the same chair. Those completing the task in more than 14 seconds are considered high risk for subsequent falling. This patient's gait and TUG test are normal. An individualized exercise program is probably unnecessary in this patient with normal gait and motor examination. Additionally, meta-analyses have shown some harm with exercise programs in the elderly, especially in frail patients.

This patient's normal gross visual acuity on office testing suggests against an ophthalmologic contribution to her fall. Her normal gait and timed Up & Go test indicate that she does not require a walker.

KEY POINT

- An evaluation for home safety is important for patients who have fallen and may include the presence of rugs and thresholds between rooms, use of night lights, general clutter, uneven lighting, and unsafe or absent hand rails.

Bibliography

Wyman JF, Croghan CF, Nachreiner NM, et al. Effectiveness of education and individualized counseling in reducing environmental hazards in the homes of community-dwelling older women. J Am Geriatr Soc. 2007;55(10):1548-1556. [PMID: 17908058]

Item 68   Answer: D

Educational Objective: Diagnose schizophrenia.

This patient's negative symptoms of social withdrawal and flat affect and positive symptoms of paranoia and hearing voices are consistent with schizophrenia. Signs and symptoms should be present for at least 1 month and some for at least 6 months, as in this patient. Her family history of schizophrenia in a first-degree relative puts this patient's lifetime risk for developing this disorder between 6% and

17%. Positive symptoms of schizophrenia include paranoid delusions, hearing voices, and hallucinations; negative symptoms include flat affect, social withdrawal, and lack of interest or enjoyment in life. Thought tends to be disorganized, with confused speech and rapid shifts in topic. No symptom or sign is pathognomonic for schizophrenia. Women tend to present later in life than males, who tend to present in their teenage years or early twenties.

Both bipolar disorder and major depressive disorder should be included in the differential diagnosis at this time. Up to 22% of patients diagnosed with schizophrenia will have their diagnosis changed during subsequent hospitalizations, so it is important to keep other medical and psychiatric causes of paranoia, auditory hallucinations, and social withdrawal in the differential diagnosis. This patient requires urgent psychiatric evaluation and possibly admission to the hospital for further evaluation.

Although this patient has been using marijuana, there is little evidence that *Cannabis* dependence or abuse leads to psychosis to the degree she is experiencing.

> **KEY POINT**
> - To make a diagnosis of schizophrenia, signs and symptoms should be present for at least 1 month and some for at least 6 months.

Bibliography

Schultz SH, North SW, Shields CG. Schizophrenia: a review. Am Fam Physician. 2007;75(12):1821-1829. [PMID: 17619525]

Item 69   Answer: B
Educational Objective: Recommend contraception options for a young woman.

Given this patient's demographic profile and behavior pattern, her risks of unintended pregnancy and sexually transmitted infection (STI) are very high, and a combination of barrier and hormonal methods is recommended. Condom use with a repository form of progesterone would both help prevent STIs and minimize the risk of contraceptive failure due to medication noncompliance.

Although condom use with combination estrogen-progesterone pills would be an effective regimen for both prevention of STIs and contraception, it would require daily medication adherence.

Although long-acting progesterone compounds such as depot medroxyprogesterone acetate are recommended in adolescents and young adults in whom user compliance may be unreliable, they do not offer protection from STIs.

A contraceptive vaginal ring containing estrogen and progesterone is a method of non–coitally based contraception that many users find more convenient than daily pills. It is an effective means of contraception, although it does require that the user be able to properly place the ring. It does not, however, confer protection against STIs, and therefore would not be a method of choice in this patient.

> **KEY POINT**
> - Contraception with a combination of a barrier method and a hormonal method is recommended in patients in whom the risks of unintended pregnancy and STIs are high.

Bibliography

Workowski KA, Berman S; Centers for Disease Control and Prevention (CDC). Sexually transmitted diseases treatment guidelines, 2010. MMWR Recomm Rep. 2010;59(RR-12):1-110. [PMID: 21160459]

Item 70   Answer: A
Educational Objective: Treat benign prostatic hyperplasia.

This patient has classic findings of symptomatic benign prostatic hyperplasia (BPH), and combination therapy with both an α-blocker and a 5α-reductase inhibitor is indicated. The American Urological Association (AUA) guideline on treatment of BPH recommends that patients with an AUA symptom score greater than 7 (questionnaire available at www2.niddk.nih.gov/NR/rdonlyres/8E99FCF4-8A92-43EE-8E47-5B70D634938A/0/AUABPH.pdf) or who are bothered by their symptoms receive treatment for BPH. 5α-Reductase inhibitors (5-ARIs), such as finasteride and dutasteride, may be suitable in patients who have failed to respond to or do not tolerate α-antagonists and those with severe symptoms. The Medical Therapy of Prostate Symptoms Study demonstrated that in the long term, among men with larger prostates, combination therapy is superior to either α-blocker or 5-ARI therapy in preventing progression and improving symptoms. Similarly, the ComBAT trial demonstrated that combination therapy resulted in significantly greater improvements than single-agent therapy. Combination therapy was associated with a higher incidence of adverse effects than monotherapy.

5-ARIs decrease the production of dihydrotestosterone, thereby arresting prostatic hyperplasia. Because shrinkage is slow, symptoms often do not improve until after 6 months of therapy. Therefore, these agents are not typically used as initial monotherapy for BPH, and switching this patient from an α-antagonist to a 5-ARI would not be indicated. Side effects include erectile and ejaculatory dysfunction, reduced libido, gynecomastia, and breast tenderness.

α-Antagonists (terazosin, doxazosin, alfuzosin, tamsulosin, silodosin) relax the prostatic smooth muscle in the bladder outflow tract, act rapidly (usually within 48 hours), and are considered first-line treatment, producing a clinical response in 70% of men. All drugs in this class have similar efficacy and tend to improve symptoms by 30% to 40%. Although some agents are more selective for prostate-specific α-receptors and therefore have less effect on systemic blood pressure, there is not a significant difference in effectiveness in treating BPH. Therefore, there is no benefit in switching between α-antagonists in this patient, as he has tolerated his current treatment well. Abnormal ejaculation is a side effect and appears similar for all α-antagonists. Elderly patients are less likely to discontinue treatment because of ejaculatory dysfunction than because of cardiovascular side effects, such as postural hypotension, dizziness, and headaches.

A 4-week course of a fluoroquinolone antibiotic would be appropriate therapy for chronic bacterial prostatitis. However, this patient has no symptoms or signs of prostatitis on examination and a normal urinalysis, making this diagnosis unlikely.

KEY POINT

- In patients with symptomatic benign prostatic hyperplasia, the combination of an α-blocker and a 5α-reductase inhibitor is associated with greater improvement in symptoms and more side effects than treatment with either agent alone.

Bibliography
Juliao AA, Plata M, Kazzazi A, Bostanci Y, Djavan B. American Urological Association and European Association of Urology guidelines in the management of benign prostatic hypertrophy: revisited. Curr Opin Urol. 2012;22(1):34-39. [PMID: 22123290]

Item 71   Answer: C
Educational Objective: Manage influenza vaccination in a healthy woman.

This healthy 30-year-old woman should receive a seasonal influenza vaccination. The Centers for Disease Control and Prevention currently recommends that all adults be vaccinated annually against influenza, regardless of risk factors. Vaccination usually takes place between September and March in the Northern hemisphere. Healthy adults can be vaccinated with either an inactivated vaccine injected intramuscularly or a live attenuated intranasal vaccine.

The hepatitis B vaccine is indicated for all children and adolescents through age 18 years, persons with HIV or other recent sexually transmitted infections, persons who are sexually active but not monogamous, workers with occupational exposure to blood, clients and staff of institutions for the developmentally disabled, correctional facility inmates, illicit drug users, persons with diabetes mellitus who are younger than 60 years, and persons with advanced chronic kidney disease who are approaching hemodialysis. Hepatitis B vaccination is also indicated for those planning travel to an endemic area and those with an increased risk for morbidity related to the disease, as well as for persons who request vaccination. This patient has no indication for hepatitis B vaccination.

The human papillomavirus vaccine is licensed for males and females aged 9 through 26 years and is recommended for females between the ages of 11 and 26 years and males

between the ages of 11 and 21 years. The vaccine is not indicated for this 30-year-old woman.

Current recommendations are that a tetanus and diphtheria (Td) vaccine be routinely administered every 10 years. Owing to an increased incidence of pertussis, thought in part to be related to waning immunity from childhood vaccination, all adults are recommended to receive a single tetanus, diphtheria, and acellular pertussis (Tdap) vaccination regardless of the interval since their last Td booster (although it may be given in place of a decennial Td booster if scheduled); this is a particularly important recommendation for persons aged 65 years or older because of the high burden of associated disease in this patient population. In addition, all postpartum women, health care workers, and adults who have close contact with infants younger than 12 months should receive a one-time Tdap booster if not already given. This patient is not due for a routine repeat Td booster for another 5 years and has no indications to receive either a Td or Tdap vaccination at this time.

KEY POINT

- Annual seasonal influenza vaccination is recommended for all adults, regardless of risk factors.

Bibliography
National Center for Immunization and Respiratory Diseases. General recommendations on immunization —- recommendations of the Advisory Committee on Immunization Practices (ACIP). MMWR Recomm Rep. 2011;60(2):1-64. [PMID: 21293327]

Item 72   Answer: C
Educational Objective: Manage chronic fatigue syndrome.

The most appropriate management for this patient is to begin a graded exercise program. Chronic fatigue syndrome (CFS) is defined as medically unexplained fatigue that persists for 6 months or more and is accompanied by at least four of the following symptoms: subjective memory impairment, sore throat, tender lymph nodes, muscle or joint pain, headache, unrefreshing sleep, and postexertional malaise lasting longer than 24 hours. Management of CFS is challenging and is geared toward managing symptoms and maintaining function, rather than seeking cure. A comprehensive, individually tailored approach is required, typically based on nonpharmacologic therapy, such as lifestyle modification and sleep hygiene. Specific treatment options that have been demonstrated to improve symptoms include graded exercise programs and cognitive-behavioral therapy (CBT). CBT in this setting is targeted in part at breaking the cycle of effort avoidance, decline in physical conditioning, and increase in fatigue, and can work well in combination with graded exercise in this regard. CBT reduces fatigue and improves functional status.

Although Epstein-Barr virus and a host of other infectious agents have been considered in the pathogenesis of

CFS, none have been borne out by careful study; therefore, antiviral therapy, including acyclovir, has no role in the treatment of CFS. A variety of other medications have been tried, including corticosteroids, mineralocorticoids, growth hormone, and melatonin, but with no clear evidence of benefit, and are not indicated for this patient.

Current evidence is not sufficiently robust to recommend dietary supplements, herbal preparations (evening primrose oil), homeopathy, or even pharmacotherapy. Patients with concomitant depression should be treated with antidepressants. Although no specific class of antidepressant is recommended in this setting, tricyclic antidepressants are often utilized in patients with CFS and depression owing to their adjunct effectiveness in treating muscle pain.

KEY POINT

- **Effective treatment options for chronic fatigue syndrome include graded exercise programs and cognitive-behavioral therapy.**

Bibliography

Reid S, Chalder T, Cleare A, Hotopf M, Wessely S. Chronic fatigue syndrome. Clin Evid (Online). 2011;05:(1101)1-52. [PMID: 21615974]

Item 73   Answer: A

Educational Objective: Manage a difficult clinical encounter.

In this case of a patient with persistent symptoms not attributable to a specific cause and who is angry and demanding, an appropriate response is to provide empathetic supportive care at relatively frequent intervals. This would be best accomplished by initiating an ongoing discussion with the patient to better understand the potential causes and significance of her pain symptoms.

Multiple studies indicate that physicians classify about 15% of clinical encounters as difficult. Difficult encounters often involve patients who have a depressive or anxiety disorder, poorer functional status, unmet expectations, reduced satisfaction, and greater use of health care services. Physicians often report the most difficulty with patients by whom they feel manipulated or frustrated, patients who are time consuming and have unrealistic demands, patients who express anger, patients who do not follow the physician's recommendations, and those who interrupt physician routine and make extra work. Patients who have somatization disorder, chronic pain, substance abuse, or have an undiagnosable medical problem are often labeled as difficult. Patients with identifiable personality disorders such as borderline, dependent, histrionic, obsessive, or antisocial personality disorders also are frequently labeled as difficult.

It would be inappropriate to treat this patient's nonspecific pain with opioid medications based only on a patient's request without a better understanding of its etiology. Although this is an expedient way of dealing with a difficult situation, it would not address the potentially complex causes of her symptoms or allow identification of more appropriate therapeutic interventions.

Patients with physical complaints that are inconsistent or without evidence of underlying pathology are particularly difficult to manage, especially in the context of a busy medical practice. These persons are often evaluated by multiple subspecialist physicians and undergo extensive testing, both as an attempt to achieve a diagnosis and because of time considerations. In this patient, while not inappropriate, gastroenterology evaluation would likely not be of high yield given her nonspecific clinical symptoms and examination findings, and would likely not address the issues underlying her complaints.

Transferring the care of the patient to another physician would not be desirable. One of the most important aspects of dealing with patients seen as difficult is to recognize the potential psychosocial and emotional factors that may be contributing to a patient's symptoms, even if they are not recognized as such by the individual. Equally important is for physicians to understand their own, potentially negative, emotions about the patient. Having some insight into these factors will hopefully allow the patient and physician to work together collaboratively to develop an appropriate diagnostic and treatment plan.

KEY POINT

- **When involved in a difficult clinical encounter, an understanding of the patient's psychosocial and emotional factors potentially contributing to his or her symptoms as well as the physician's own feelings about the patient is essential in establishing and maintaining an effective therapeutic relationship.**

Bibliography

Kroenke K. Unburdening the difficult clinical encounter. Arch Intern Med. 2009;169(4):333-334. [PMID: 19237715]

Item 74   Answer: D

Educational Objective: Appropriately administer the pneumococcal vaccine in a patient who has been previously vaccinated.

This man should receive a single pneumococcal polysaccharide vaccination at age 65 years. Adults 65 years and older should be immunized against pneumococcal pneumonia. The vaccine contains 23 antigen types of *Streptococcus pneumoniae* and protects against 60% of bacteremic disease. The vaccine is also recommended in some populations of younger patients, including Alaskan natives and certain American Indian populations; residents of long-term care facilities; patients who are undergoing radiation therapy or are on immunosuppressive medication; patients who smoke; and patients with chronic pulmonary disorders (including asthma), diabetes mellitus, cardiovascular disease, chronic liver or kidney disease, cochlear implants, asplenia, immune disorders, or malignancies. There is no information on vaccine safety during pregnancy. The vaccine is reasonably effective, with high levels of antibody typically found for at least 5 years. Currently, immunocompetent persons vaccinated after age 65 years are not recommended to receive a booster. Immunocompetent persons vaccinated before age 65 years, such as this patient, should receive a single booster vaccination at age 65 years, or 5 years after their first vaccination if they were vaccinated between the ages of 60 and 64 years.

Immunocompromised patients (including those with HIV infection and kidney disease) as well as patients with asplenia should receive a single pneumococcal vaccine booster 5 years after their first vaccine. This strategy would be inappropriate for this patient.

Current recommendations do not support more than a single booster after initial pneumococcal vaccination for any persons. Hence, a strategy of vaccination every 5 years would be inappropriate.

All patients vaccinated before age 65 years need a booster at some point. Hence, withholding further pneumococcal vaccination is inappropriate.

KEY POINT

- Immunocompetent persons who received the pneumococcal polysaccharide vaccine before age 65 years should receive a single booster vaccination at age 65 years, or 5 years after their first vaccination if they were vaccinated between the ages of 60 and 64 years.

Bibliography

Targonski PV, Poland GA. Pneumococcal vaccination in adults: recommendations, trends, and prospects. Cleve Clin J Med. 2007;74(6):401-406, 408-410, 413-414. [PMID: 17569198]

Item 75   Answer: A

Educational Objective: Treat hyperlipidemia in a woman who desires pregnancy.

This patient should be started on colesevelam. She has several risk factors for cardiovascular disease, including poorly controlled diabetes mellitus, hypertension, dyslipidemia, and a family history of premature myocardial infarction. Her goal LDL cholesterol level is below 100 mg/dL (2.59 mmol/L). Therapeutic lifestyle changes, which include a low-saturated fat diet and at least 120 minutes of aerobic exercise weekly, will reduce LDL cholesterol levels by 7% to 15%. Thus, this patient needs additional therapy to achieve her LDL cholesterol goal.

Ezetimibe is a cholesterol absorption inhibitor that can reduce LDL cholesterol levels by up to 19%. Treatment with ezetimibe has not been shown to have beneficial effects on cardiovascular morbidity or mortality. Moreover, ezetimibe is FDA pregnancy class X, and should be avoided in women who may become pregnant.

Gemfibrozil is a fibric acid that is typically used for the treatment of hypertriglyceridemia. It reduces LDL cholesterol levels by 10% or less; in addition, gemfibrozil monotherapy in patients with hypertriglyceridemia can actually raise LDL cholesterol levels. Gemfibrozil is not contraindicated in pregnancy (FDA pregnancy class C) but would not be effective for achieving this patient's LDL cholesterol goal.

Although statins (such as simvastatin) are typically the first-line treatment for lowering LDL cholesterol levels, statins are teratogenic (FDA pregnancy class X) and should be avoided in women who may be or wish to become pregnant. Colesevelam, which is a bile acid sequestrant that lowers LDL cholesterol levels by up to 18%, is the best initial treatment option for this patient. Colesevelam is FDA pregnancy class B and so is safe to use in premenopausal women who are sexually active. Bile acid sequestrants have been shown to reduce the risk of coronary heart disease in primary prevention trials. The most common side effects associated with bile acid sequestrants include constipation, abdominal pain and bloating, and flatulence. Bile acid sequestrants can bind to and reduce the absorption of other drugs; this effect can be minimized by administering the other drugs 1 hour before or 4 hours after taking a bile acid sequestrant.

KEY POINT

- Bile acid sequestrants are an option for reducing LDL cholesterol levels in women with hyperlipidemia who wish to become pregnant.

Bibliography

Pande RL. Approach to lipid therapy in the patient with atherosclerotic vascular disease. Curr Treat Options Cardiovasc Med. 2012;14(2)177-183. [PMID: 22270374]

Item 76   Answer: D

Educational Objective: Initiate nonhospice palliative care in a patient with newly diagnosed cancer.

In this patient with a newly diagnosed advanced malignancy, palliative care consultation is an important component of her care. Palliative care focuses on improving and maintaining the quality of life in individuals with any severe illness. Palliative care is a multidisciplinary, boarded specialty that focuses on preventing and relieving suffering and establishing goals of treatment that are consistent with the patient's wishes. This often involves efforts at pain and symptom control and encouraging and enabling patients to be actively involved in the decisions regarding their care. Nonhospice palliative care does not exclude testing, treatment, or hospitalization, but seeks to ensure that these interventions are consistent with what the patient wants and the expected goals and outcomes of care. Whereas care in a hospice setting may be palliative in nature, not all palliative care takes place in patients with terminal illness. Palliative care input may be particularly valuable in assisting this patient, who has a new diagnosis of severe

H
CONT.

disease, with understanding her illness and making decisions regarding her care. Although studies are limited, palliative care has been shown to improve overall quality of life in the setting of various diseases relative to usual care for severely ill individuals.

Although depression may be seen in some patients with severe illness, starting therapy for depression without clear evidence the patient is having significant depressive symptoms or that pharmacologic treatment is indicated would be inappropriate.

It is not clear that this patient is either medically or emotionally ready for hospice care. Although her newly diagnosed malignancy may carry a poor prognosis, her currently stable condition and expressed desire to explore possible treatment options would make a decision to pursue hospice care premature without further characterization of her disease and discussion of her long-term treatment goals.

Opioid therapy is commonly used in cancers and particularly malignancies involving the respiratory tract to reduce both pain and dyspnea. However, this patient does not have significant pain and has only mild shortness of breath, which should improve as her pulmonary embolism resolves. Therefore, initiation of ongoing opioid therapy is not indicated.

KEY POINT

- Palliative care focuses on improving and maintaining the quality of life in any patient with severe illness; it is not limited to those with terminal illness or inpatient settings.

Bibliography

Bakitas M, Lyons KD, Hegel MT, et al. Effects of a palliative care intervention on clinical outcomes in patients with advanced cancer: the Project ENABLE II randomized control trial. JAMA. 2009;302(7):741-749. [PMID: 19690306]

Item 77   Answer: D

Educational Objective: Diagnose nonasthmatic eosinophilic bronchitis.

This patient's presentation is consistent with nonasthmatic eosinophilic bronchitis (NAEB), and the next diagnostic step would be sputum testing for eosinophils. NAEB is an increasingly recognized cause of chronic cough, particularly in patients such as this one who lack risk factors or findings for the more common causes of chronic cough (smoking, cough-variant asthma, gastroesophageal reflux disease, upper airways disease). Patients with NAEB do not exhibit symptoms of or pulmonary function testing evidence of airflow obstruction or hyperresponsiveness, with or without provocation with methacholine, which differentiates this entity from asthma. The diagnosis is supported by airway eosinophilia in an induced sputum sample (greater than 3%), bronchial washings, or biopsy. Although bronchial mucosal biopsies are required to definitively diagnose eosinophilic bronchitis, most experts recommend a therapeutic trial of

inhaled corticosteroid therapy as initial therapy, as most patients with NAEB will respond to this intervention.

Targeted and optimized empiric treatment of common causes of chronic cough is generally recommended prior to more invasive or costly testing. Treatment with antihistamines or decongestants should begin first, without need for sinus radiographs to evaluate for sinus disease in patients with suspected upper airway cough syndrome. Similarly, diet and lifestyle modification plus proton pump inhibitors for 1 to 3 months should be prescribed prior to considering 24-hour esophageal pH manometry to evaluate for acid reflux disease.

KEY POINT

- A diagnosis of nonasthmatic eosinophilic bronchitis should be considered in patients with chronic, nonproductive cough without an apparent cause, including asthma; sputum examination for eosinophils is useful in establishing the diagnosis.

Bibliography

Desai D, Brightling C. Cough due to asthma, cough-variant asthma and non-asthmatic eosinophilic bronchitis. Otolaryngol Clin North Am. 2010;43(1):123-130, x. [PMID: 20172262]

Item 78   Answer: A

Educational Objective: Evaluate an elderly patient with a recent fall.

This patient who has recently fallen should be assessed for gait and mobility. The Timed "Up & Go" (TUG) is a validated test for mobility that can be easily performed in the clinic and may be useful in predicting the likelihood of future falls. The test is performed by asking the patient to arise from a chair, walk 10 feet, turn around, and sit back down in the same chair. A time of more than 14 seconds indicates an increased risk for future falls. The sensitivity and specificity for one or more falls during the 6 months after the TUG test are 96% and 32%, respectively. In patients who have fallen, it is important to get a detailed history of the circumstances of the fall and whether the patient has fallen before or has problems with balance. A complete list of medications, particularly psychotropic medications, should be obtained. This patient had what sounds like a mechanical fall, without any evidence of syncope, lightheadedness, or dizziness. She remembers the entire event and was not confused after the fall, making a seizure unlikely.

Discontinuing lisinopril is not likely to reduce this patient's risk for falls because her blood pressure is not low, she has no orthostatic blood pressure changes, and she has no symptoms of lightheadedness or dizziness. Discontinuing antihypertensive medication would be indicated if it were deemed likely that hypotension or orthostatic hypotension were present and a possible cause for her fall.

Prescribing an exercise program would be indicated if physical examination revealed weakness or poor balance.

Some studies have shown that there may be harms associated with exercise programs in the frail older adult, so all such programs should be supervised.

Whereas providing an assistive device such as a walker would be indicated for patients with weakness, poor balance, or gait disturbance, assessment of gait and mobility should be performed first. If the TUG were abnormal, further assessment by a physical therapist could be performed to determine if an assistive device is indicated and which assistive device might be most helpful.

KEY POINT

- The Timed "Up & Go" (TUG) test for evaluating gait and mobility is performed by asking the patient to arise from a chair, walk 10 feet, turn around and sit back down in the same chair; a time of more than 14 seconds indicates an increased risk for future falls.

Bibliography

Nordin E, Lindelöf N, Rosendahl E, Jensen J, Lundin-Olsson L. Prognostic validity of the Timed Up-and-Go test, a modified Get-Up-and-Go test, staff's global judgement and fall history in evaluating fall risk in residential care facilities. Age Ageing. 2008;37(4):442-448. [PMID: 18515291]

Item 79   Answer: C

Educational Objective: Diagnose pes anserine bursitis.

This patient most likely has pes anserine bursitis. Although pes anserine bursitis most commonly occurs in patients with medial compartment osteoarthritis, it also occurs in the setting of overuse, as is the case with this patient. The pain is typically located along the anteromedial aspect of proximal tibia distal to the joint line of the knee. Pain is worse with climbing steps and frequently worsens at night.

Iliotibial band syndrome is a common cause of knife-like lateral knee pain that occurs with vigorous flexion-extension activities of the knee, such as running. It is treated conservatively with rest and stretching exercises. This patient's presentation is not consistent with iliotibial band syndrome as the patient's pain is located medially. Also, the pain with iliotibial band syndrome is characteristically worsened with walking both up and down steps, which this patient does not report.

The most common cause of knee pain in persons younger than 45 years, especially in women, is the patellofemoral syndrome. The pain is peripatellar and exacerbated by overuse (such as running), descending stairs, or prolonged sitting. On examination, pain and apprehension can often be elicited by applying pressure on the patella (the patellofemoral compression test).

Prepatellar bursitis presents with pain in the anterior aspect of the knee. On examination, swelling and tenderness to palpation are frequently present near the lower pole of the patella.

KEY POINT

- The pain of pes anserine bursitis is typically located along the anteromedial aspect of the proximal tibia distal to the joint line of the knee and characteristically worsens with step climbing and at night.

Bibliography

Schraeder TL, Terek RM, Smith CC. Clinical evaluation of the knee. New Engl J Med. 2010;363(4):e5. [PMID: 20660399]

Item 80   Answer: B

Educational Objective: Treat vulvovaginal candidiasis in a pregnant patient.

The most appropriate treatment for this pregnant woman is a topical imidazole, such as clotrimazole. She has classic symptoms and signs of vulvovaginal candidiasis (VVC), including itching, discomfort, and a thick, white vaginal discharge with evidence of vulvar edema and erythema on examination. The vaginal pH is normal, and potassium hydroxide preparation shows evidence of hyphae and yeast, supporting this diagnosis. Uncomplicated VVC is diagnosed when an otherwise healthy, nonpregnant patient has mild to moderate symptoms and suspected *Candida albicans* infection. Complicated VVC is diagnosed in women with severe symptoms (extensive vulvar erythema, edema, excoriation, and fissure formation), immunosuppression, multiple recurrences, or diabetes mellitus; and in women who are pregnant. As compared with treatment of uncomplicated VVC, patients with complicated VVC, such as this pregnant woman, typically require longer and more aggressive therapy. Regimens for treatment of complicated *C. albicans* vulvovaginitis include topical imidazole therapy for up to 14 days or two 150-mg doses of oral fluconazole given in two sequential doses 72 hours apart (compared with single-dose therapy). Topical imidazole therapy should be used preferentially in pregnant women, and a variety of regimens are available for treatment. Seven days of topical clotrimazole cream is an appropriate option in this patient.

Oral fluconazole is an appropriate treatment for uncomplicated VVC, and is associated with high treatment success rates. However, it should not be given in pregnancy as the effect on the fetus is unknown (FDA pregnancy category C medication), and topical therapy is equally efficacious.

Although 30% of women will experience two or more episodes of VVC, recurrent VVC is diagnosed if a patient experiences more than four symptomatic episodes per year. Frequently, recurrent VVC is associated with non-*albicans Candida* infection. Initial treatment of culture-proven non-*albicans* VVC includes 7 to 14 days of an oral or topical non-imidazole therapy, such as voriconazole, a second-generation triazole antifungal agent; recurrent VVC may be treated with intravaginal boric acid for 2 weeks. Because this patient has had only one previous episode of symptomatic VVC, which responded well to treatment, she can be empirically treated for *Candida albicans* infection again.

> **KEY POINT**
>
> - Treatment of *Candida albicans* vulvovaginal candidiasis in pregnant women typically requires longer and more aggressive therapy; topical imidazole therapy for 7 days is the preferred treatment.

Bibliography

ACOG Committee on Practice Bulletins—Gynecology. ACOG Practice Bulletin. Clinical management guidelines for obstetrician-gynecologists, Number 72, May 2006: Vaginitis. Obstet Gynecol. 2006;107(5):1195-1206. [PMID: 16648432]

Item 81   Answer: B

Educational Objective: Treat cough in a patient taking an ACE inhibitor.

In this patient with a nonproductive cough, the best option is to discontinue lisinopril. Clinical evaluation of chronic cough (>8 weeks in duration) includes a careful history and physical examination focusing on the common causes of chronic cough. All patients should undergo chest radiography. Smoking cessation and discontinuation of ACE inhibitors should be recommended for 4 weeks before additional workup. Cough is a common side effect of ACE inhibitors. Approximately 15% of patients who are prescribed these medications will develop a nonproductive cough. Reported causative factors include bradykinin and substance P, which are metabolized by angiotensin-converting enzyme and prostaglandins. The onset may be delayed, as in this patient, and may take up to 4 weeks to resolve upon discontinuation of the drug (rarely, up to 3 months). Although the cough is frequently mild, in some patients it is significant enough to interfere with quality of life, and alternate therapy needs to be considered. Substitution of an angiotensin receptor blocker, such as losartan, is a good alternative in this patient; these medications generally do not cause cough (incidence is similar to that of placebo) and evidence supports their renal protective benefits in patients with diabetes mellitus.

Because this patient's cough has been present for 8 weeks, other causes of chronic cough should be considered. As the clinical picture is most consistent with ACE inhibitor–induced cough and there is no symptom predominance to support bronchospasm (history of asthma, wheezing and cough with exertion, exposure to allergens or cold air), upper airway cough syndrome (postnasal drip with frequent nasal discharge, a sensation of liquid dripping into the back of the throat, and frequent throat clearing), or gastroesophageal reflux disease (heartburn or regurgitation), initial empiric treatment with albuterol, an antihistamine, intranasal corticosteroids, or omeprazole is not indicated at this time. ACE inhibitor–induced cough generally abates within 4 weeks

after the drug is discontinued. If this patient's cough persists beyond this time, a systemic approach to treatment of chronic cough should ensue.

> **KEY POINT**
>
> - In patients with chronic cough and a normal chest radiograph, smoking cessation and discontinuation of ACE inhibitors should be recommended for 4 weeks before additional evaluation for the cough.

Bibliography

Dicpinigaitis PV. Angiotensin-converting enzyme inhibitor-induced cough: ACCP evidence-based clinical practice guidelines. Chest. 2006;129(1 suppl):169S-173S. [PMID: 16428706]

Item 82   Answer: A

Educational Objective: Manage medications perioperatively.

This patient should continue all of his current medications. Antiplatelet therapy (including aspirin and clopidogrel), antihypertensive medications, and anticonvulsant drugs can be continued during low-risk surgeries, such as cataract surgery, if the benefit outweighs the risk. In a preoperative evaluation each medication should be assessed for its individual risk and benefit. Those for which risk outweighs benefit should be temporarily discontinued perioperatively.

Dual antiplatelet therapy with clopidogrel and aspirin should be continued for at least 1 year in patients who have received a drug-eluting stent. This patient's drug-eluting stent was inserted only 6 months ago; therefore, the patient remains at increased risk for in-stent thrombosis if clopidogrel is discontinued and at no increased risk of bleeding related to the cataract surgery if clopidogrel is continued.

The use of β-blockers in the perioperative period is controversial, with well-designed randomized controlled trials showing both benefit and harm. Current recommendations are that patients currently on a β-blocker should continue taking it. Thus, metoprolol should not be discontinued.

Any medication that can produce withdrawal symptoms, such as benzodiazepines, long-acting narcotics, and antiseizure drugs, are typically continued the morning of surgery.

> **KEY POINT**
>
> - In a preoperative evaluation, each medication should be assessed for its individual risk and benefit, and those for which risk outweighs benefit should be temporarily discontinued perioperatively.

Bibliography

Whinney C. Perioperative medication management: general principles and practical applications. Cleve Clin J Med. 2009;76(suppl 4):S126-32. [PMID: 19880829]

Item 83   Answer: A

Educational Objective: Manage a request for physician-assisted suicide.

When approached with a request for assistance in dying, it is best to respond to the request with empathy and compassion, and assess whether or not the patient is receiving adequate palliative interventions. Optimizing care interventions focused on maintaining or improving the quality of life may not always occur in the context of treating the underlying disease process; thus, reviewing the patient's overall care to address comfort and functional issues in severe illness is essential to appropriate management. Involving physicians trained specifically in palliative care medicine may also be helpful in such situations.

Physician-assisted suicide is a controversial area of ethics. Most ethicists agree that it is acceptable to consider interventions that may hasten the death of a terminally ill patient if the primary intent is therapeutic (the principle of "double effect"). However, physician-assisted suicide using prescriptions or interventions with the specific intent to kill the patient is illegal in most states. The American Medical Association and the American College of Physicians have both taken positions against the practice.

Seeking legal counsel may be advisable if one intends to provide the patient assistance in dying, as states in which it is legal have specific protocols that must be followed. However, this step would not be appropriate until alternatives such as improved palliative care were assessed.

Categorically refusing to discuss a request for physician-assisted suicide can close the door to a discussion of why the patient is making the request and may jeopardize the therapeutic relationship with the patient.

Writing a prescription for medication to assist a patient in dying without a detailed assessment of the patient's situation and motives would be irresponsible.

KEY POINT

- **When approached with a request for assistance in dying, it is best to respond to the request with empathy and compassion, and assess whether or not the patient is receiving adequate palliative care.**

Bibliography

Snyder L, Sulmasy DP; Ethics and Human Rights Committee, American College of Physicians-American Society of Internal Medicine. Physician-assisted suicide. Ann Intern Med. 2001;135(3):209-216. [PMID: 11487490]

Item 84   Answer: C

Educational Objective: Diagnose Morton neuroma.

This patient most likely has Morton neuroma, which is thought to be caused by inflammation, edema, and scarring of the small interdigital nerves. It commonly occurs in overuse syndromes (such as running) and with wearing tight shoes. It classically presents with burning pain on the plantar surface in the space between the third and fourth toes but may also occur between the second and third toes. Women are more commonly affected than men, and the wearing of high heels is a recognized risk factor. Treatment is typically conservative, with the goal of reducing pressure across the metatarsal heads through the use of padding, orthotics, and the removal of likely inciting footwear or activities. If conservative measures fail, a local corticosteroid injection is usually successful.

A hammer toe is characterized by a flexion deformity of the proximal interphalangeal joints with normal distal interphalangeal joints and metatarsophalangeal joints. Presenting symptoms include pain and difficulty wearing shoes because of the resulting toe structure. A corn may also develop on the dorsal surface of the proximal interphalangeal joint.

In metatarsal stress fractures, the examination is notable for tenderness to palpation of the fracture site. It would not be expected to cause pain between toes, as is the case in this patient.

Tarsal tunnel syndrome is entrapment of the posterior tibial nerve or one of its branches as it travels behind the medial malleolus. Although this may cause pain and a burning sensation, symptoms tend to occur on the medial plantar aspect of the foot, occasionally mimicking plantar fasciitis.

KEY POINT

- **Morton neuroma is characterized by burning pain on the plantar surface in the space between the third and fourth toes.**

Bibliography

Wu KK. Morton neuroma and metatarsalgia. Curr Opin Rheumatol. 2000;12:131-142. [PMID: 10751016]

Item 85   Answer: A

Educational Objective: Manage body dysmorphic disorder.

Cognitive-behavioral therapy (CBT) would be appropriate in the management of this patient. This patient's presentation is consistent with body dysmorphic disorder, a somatoform disorder in which a patient is focused on a single real or imagined symptom. In order to qualify as a psychiatric disorder, somatoform symptoms need to be medically unexplained or out of proportion to medically expected findings, should persist over time, and cause impairment in a patient's ability to function. Although no therapy has been shown to be consistently helpful in treating somatoform disorders, multiple trials have found benefit in patients who undergo CBT.

Benzodiazepines such as diazepam have not been shown to be of benefit for somatoform disorders, and would likely be a poor choice because of their ability to induce tolerance and long-term dependence.

It is unlikely that this patient would have any additional abnormal findings on further abdominal imaging. As patients with somatoform disorders have a true psychiatric disease, additional normal diagnostic tests are ineffective in alleviating symptoms.

Psychosis encompasses delusions, hallucinations, disorganized speech, and disorganized or catatonic behavior. Psychotic features may occur in depression as well as other psychiatric or organic disorders, but schizophrenia is a disorder in which psychosis is a defining feature. The diagnosis requires at least 6 months of symptoms, including 1 month or more of at least two active-phase symptoms, such as hallucinations, delusions, disorganized speech, grossly disorganized or catatonic behavior; and negative symptoms, such as flattened affect. This patient is not psychotic and treatment with an antipsychotic medication such as olanzapine is not indicted.

KEY POINT

- **Although no therapy has been shown to be consistently helpful in treating somatoform disorders, multiple trials have found benefit in patients who undergo cognitive-behavioral therapy.**

Bibliography

Kroenke K. Efficacy of treatment for somatoform disorders: a review of randomized controlled trials. Psychosom Med. 2007;69(9):881-888. [PMID: 18040099]

Item 86   Answer: E

Educational Objective: Evaluate vasovagal syncope.

No further testing is required for this patient. Her symptoms are consistent with the most common form of syncope, vasovagal neurocardiogenic syncope, the common "faint." Suggestive features of vasovagal syncope include any of the "3 P's": Posture (occurrence during prolonged standing, or similar previous episodes that have been aborted by lying down); Provoking factors (e.g., pain, a medical procedure); and Prodromal symptoms (sweating, feeling warm before loss of consciousness). Persons with an uncomplicated faint, situational syncope, or orthostatic hypotension should undergo electrocardiography but do not otherwise require immediate further investigation or specialist referral.

Admission to the hospital for telemetry should be considered in patients with undiagnosed syncope but with known structural heart disease and at high risk for arrhythmia. Even in this selected group, however, the diagnostic yield is low (approximately 16%), and there is no benefit for patients with symptoms compatible with vasovagal syncope in the absence of known heart disease.

Neuroimaging, such as CT scanning, is of limited use in evaluating syncope. It has the highest yield in patients who are older than 65 years and have neurologic symptoms, such as headache, neurologic examination abnormalities, head trauma, or are on anticoagulants. This patient has no features to suggest a neurologic cause of syncope and a head CT scan is not indicated.

If structural heart disease is suspected, further assessment should include cardiac imaging, usually by echocardiography, as the first diagnostic test. There is nothing in the patient's history or physical examination that suggests structural heart disease, and echocardiography is not indicated.

Tilt-table testing is reserved for patients with suspected neurocardiogenic syncope not confirmed by history and physical examination, those with recurrent episodes, and those with a suspected cardiac cause. As this patient's history and physical examination are consistent with vasovagal syncope and there is no history of recurrent episodes, tilt-table testing is not indicated.

KEY POINT

- **Persons with uncomplicated faint, situational syncope, or orthostatic hypotension do not require further investigation if the initial physical examination and electrocardiogram are normal.**

Bibliography

Cooper PN, Westby M, Pitcher DW, Bullock I. Synopsis of the National Institute for Health and Clinical Excellence Guideline for management of transient loss of consciousness. Ann Intern Med. 2011;155(8):543-549. [PMID: 21930835]

Item 87   Answer: B

Educational Objective: Manage a fall in an elderly patient.

In this patient with generalized weakness as well as leg muscle weakness, slow gait, and a recent fall, it is appropriate to prescribe vitamin D. Vitamin D deficiency increases the risk for falls in the elderly and vitamin D supplementation reduces this risk. According to U.S. Preventive Services Task Force recommendations, vitamin D supplementation can be prescribed without first obtaining a serum vitamin D level for patients with an increased risk of falling. The proposed mechanism of action of vitamin D is its beneficial effect on muscle strength and function and on gait. Although calcium supplementation may have a beneficial effect on bone loss, there is no clear benefit to adding calcium in reducing falls.

Discontinuing lisinopril is not appropriate because she does not demonstrate orthostatic blood pressure changes that would account for her fall, and discontinuing antihypertensive medication would likely result in elevated blood pressure.

Zolpidem is a nonbenzodiazepine sedative hypnotic with a short half-life that can be prescribed for a limited time period for insomnia. Caution must be exercised, however, because of adverse effects, including an increased risk for falls, especially among older adults. Reviewing sleep hygiene would be a better first step in managing her insomnia.

Although this patient demonstrates a mild near-vision deficit, it is not likely that this deficit contributed significantly to her fall. Furthermore, bifocal lenses are associated with an increased risk for falling. If needed, reading glasses could be obtained.

KEY POINT

- **Vitamin D supplementation reduces the risk for falls in elderly patients, and can be prescribed without obtaining a serum vitamin D level in patients with an increased risk of falling.**

Bibliography

Kalyani RR, Stein B, Valiyil R, et al. Vitamin D treatment for the prevention of falls in older adults: systematic review and meta-analysis. J Am Geriatr Soc. 2010;58(7):1299-1310. [PMID: 20579169]

Item 88   Answer: A

Educational Objective: Treat stress urinary incontinence.

This patient has stress urinary incontinence and should receive pelvic floor muscle training (PFMT). Stress urinary incontinence, defined as loss of urine with physical activity, cough, or sneeze, is caused by sphincter incompetence. Findings on physical examination include weakened anterior or posterior vaginal wall support (cystocele or rectocele, respectively). PFMT is considered first-line therapy for urinary stress incontinence. In PFMT, women learn repetitive exercises (Kegel exercises) to strengthen the voluntary urethral sphincter and levator ani muscles. For PFMT to be effective, it is important that the patient learn to correctly contract her muscles without straining, which increases abdominal pressure. Each contraction is held for approximately 10 seconds, followed by an equal relaxation period. The number of repetitions should be increased weekly until the patient is performing 8 to 12 repetitions three times daily, every day or at least 3 to 4 days per week. In a systematic review of nonsurgical therapy, PFMT improved stress urinary incontinence episodes. Outcomes were even better when PFMT was combined with biofeedback and when skilled therapists directed the treatment.

Prompted voiding is indicated in and is effective in patients with significant mobility or cognitive impairments that may hinder the patient's ability to reach the toilet in time, neither of which this patient has.

Sling procedures are effective for moderate to severe stress incontinence, but surgery is usually reserved for patients who do not benefit from more conservative approaches, including behavioral or appropriate pharmacologic therapy.

Tolterodine, a selective antimuscarinic anticholinergic medication, is most effective for patients with urge, rather than stress, incontinence. This patient does not experience the classic sense of urinary urgency with her incontinence episodes, and, therefore, tolterodine would not be an appropriate first choice.

KEY POINT

- **Pelvic floor muscle training is first-line treatment for stress urinary incontinence.**

Bibliography

Shamliyna TA, Kane RL, Wyman J, Wilt TJ. Systematic review: randomized, controlled trials of nonsurgical treatments for urinary incontinence in women. Ann Intern Med. 2008;148(6):459-473. [PMID: 18268288]

Item 89   Answer: D

Educational Objective: Initiate a discussion about palliative care with the family of a cancer patient.

The cornerstone of establishing goals of care in the end-of-life setting is to communicate in a patient-centered, open-ended format. This is true regardless of whether a patient or patient's family is angry or is requesting inappropriately aggressive care. The first step in this process in this case is to ask the family to tell you what they understand about the patient's condition. Active, empathic listening allows the caregiver to establish what the patient and family understand about the diagnosis and prognosis. It also shows respect for the myriad ways in which loved ones process information about medical conditions and helps to establish trust. The family should be allowed to vent their frustration and to articulate what they believe the patient's condition and chance of meaningful recovery to be. Given the feelings of distress about the patient's condition, it is entirely possible that one meeting may not be enough to establish clearly defined goals of care. Asking open-ended questions and being comfortable with silences are important in building a trusting relationship with the patient and family.

The upcoming dialogue with the family is likely to be emotionally charged, and a series of visits may be needed to cover all appropriate areas. It would not be appropriate to initiate the discussion with the patient and family about advanced directives until it is learned what the family knows about the diagnosis and prognosis.

It would not be helpful to begin a meeting with a distraught family or patient by stating curative therapy would be futile. This approach is likely to further alienate a family struggling with a distressing diagnosis.

Although explaining the diagnosis and prognosis may be an important goal for a family meeting, it is usually more effective to begin the meeting with an open-ended question that allows the physician to better understand the family's perspective. Explanations can then be better tailored to what the family knows and understands about the patient's condition.

KEY POINT

- The cornerstone of establishing goals of care in the end-of-life setting is to communicate in a patient-centered, open-ended format.

Bibliography

Swetz KM, Kamal AH. Palliative care. Ann Intern Med. 2012;156(3):ITC21. [PMID: 22312158]

Item 90   Answer: C

Educational Objective: Evaluate a breast mass in a postmenopausal woman.

This patient should undergo core needle biopsy of the mass. She presents with a normal mammogram but with suspicious findings on physical examination for breast cancer. The palpable mass is nonpainful, persistent, and firm. Although her normal mammogram could be interpreted as reassuring, approximately 10% to 20% of palpable breast cancers can be missed by either ultrasonography or screening mammography. She requires further evaluation to definitively rule in or rule out malignancy. Core needle biopsy, with or without ultrasonographic or stereotactic guidance, provides excellent tissue sampling for pathology and receptor status. It is the test of choice for most solid lesions.

Breast MRI would likely better define the breast lesion radiographically that was not visualized on mammography, but would not replace the need for a tissue diagnosis in this patient.

Breast ultrasonography is particularly useful in defining possible cystic lesions identified on examination or mammography. However, given the highly suspicious nature of this patient's breast mass, ultrasonography would not be indicated.

Reassurance is inappropriate as definitive diagnosis of the mass via tissue sampling is imperative in this postmenopausal woman.

KEY POINT

- Core needle biopsy is the test of choice for most solid breast masses.

Bibliography

Barlow WE, Lehman CD, Zheng Y, et al. Performance of diagnostic mammography for women with signs or symptoms of breast cancer. J Natl Cancer Inst. 2002;94(15):1151-1159. [PMID: 12165640]

Item 91   Answer: A

Educational Objective: Manage acute low back pain.

In this patient presenting with uncomplicated low back pain and examination findings suggesting radiculopathy,

initial treatment with nonopioid analgesics and mobilization as tolerated is most appropriate. The overall prognosis for acute musculoskeletal low back pain is excellent; most patients without sciatica show substantial improvement within 2 weeks, and three quarters of those with sciatica are substantially better after 3 months; therefore, therapeutic interventions should focus on mitigating symptoms and maintaining function while the patient recovers.

Complete blood count and erythrocyte sedimentation rate are helpful in assessing for infection, inflammatory spondylitis, and malignancy. This patient has no signs or symptoms suggestive of systemic illness, and specific laboratory testing is therefore not indicated at this time.

Epidural corticosteroid injection is sometimes considered in patients with chronic radiculopathy, although the literature is mixed regarding its value. This patient has an excellent prognosis without intervention, so invasive treatments would be inappropriate as initial therapy.

Lumbar spine imaging is not indicated for most patients with acute lumbosacral back pain with radiculopathy as it does not add clinically significant information. Situations in which imaging is necessary include patients with rapidly progressing neurologic symptoms, evidence of cord compression, cauda equina syndrome, or if infection or malignancy is a possible cause of the patient's symptoms and examination findings.

Lumbar spine radiography is helpful to assess for possible malignancy or compression fracture. In this younger patient without evidence of systemic illness, radiography is not indicated. An MRI would likely demonstrate the disk herniation and nerve root compression that are already evident on physical examination, but the management plan would still be analgesics and gentle mobilization.

KEY POINT

- Therapeutic interventions for most patients with acute low back pain should focus on mitigating symptoms and maintaining function while the patient recovers.

Bibliography

Chou R, Qaseem A, Snow V, et al; Clinical Efficacy Assessment Subcommittee of the American College of Physicians; American College of Physicians; American Pain Society Low Back Pain Guidelines Panel. Diagnosis and treatment of low back pain: a joint clinical practice guideline from the American College of Physicians and the American Pain Society. Ann Intern Med. 2007;147(7):478-491. [PMID: 17909209]

Item 92   Answer: A

Educational Objective: Recognize threats to validity in a medical study.

The main reason that it is difficult to determine the effectiveness of this drug based on the published study is that there is no comparison, or control, group. When evaluating the medical literature, it is important to consider the quality of the study design. Studies assessing treatment effectiveness should always have a control group, which can receive either an alternative treatment or a placebo. A control group is critical because it tells the investigators what would have happened if the intervention had not been done. Depending on the study type, patients can be assigned to a control group (in an experimental study), or be part of a "natural" control (observational study). The primary threat to validity of this study is the absence of a control group; that is, there is no group with which the patients taking "drug X" can be compared.

In general, it is always best for outcomes in any study to be assessed by an independent evaluator who is unaware of treatment assignment ("blinded"). In the case of unambiguous outcomes such as death, however, an unblinded outcomes assessment is permissible.

In experimental study designs, investigators often randomly assign patients to a therapy in order to equalize the group for measured and unmeasured confounding variables. This trial has no comparison group, so randomization would not be possible.

Increased numbers of patients in studies generally yield greater precision in measurement. In this trial, however, the key threat to validity is not trial size but absence of a control group.

KEY POINT

- **The primary threat to validity in a case series is the absence of a control group.**

Bibliography

Ho PM, Peterson PN, Masoudi FA. Evaluating the evidence: is there a rigid hierarchy? Circulation. 2008;118(16):1675-1684. [PMID: 18852378]

Item 93   Answer: E

Educational Objective: Manage attention-deficit/hyperactivity disorder in an adult.

The most appropriate management for this patient with attention-deficit/hyperactivity disorder (ADHD) is to stop his ADHD medication and reassess his need for treatment. ADHD is characterized by difficulty paying attention, impulsivity, and motor restlessness or hyperactivity, with onset before the age of 7 years. There must also be some impairment in social, occupational, or academic functioning, and the symptoms must be manifest in at least two different environments, such as school and home. There are three subtypes: predominantly inattentive, predominantly hyperactive, and a combined type. The presence of symptoms in childhood is crucial to the diagnosis of ADHD, and this patient gives a history that is compatible with ADHD. However, he also has new-onset hypertension and a heart rate at the higher end of normal, which could be related to sympathomimetic drug use. He has had relatively few symptoms related to ADHD for the past 2 years. Periodic "drug holidays" for adult patients with ADHD may be useful to assess

need for ongoing medications; this would be an opportune moment for a drug holiday in this patient.

Atomoxetine is a selective norepinephrine reuptake inhibitor that is specifically approved for treatment of ADHD in adults. It is not associated with hypertension and would be a reasonable option after his drug holiday if there is a need for ongoing medications; however, first it should be ascertained whether he still needs pharmacologic treatment for his ADHD. Atomoxetine carries a black box warning of increased suicidal ideation in the pediatric population and has been associated with rare but serious hepatotoxicity.

Fluoxetine and other selective serotonin reuptake inhibitors have not been shown to be useful for the treatment of ADHD. Bupropion and tricyclic antidepressants may be helpful for ADHD, although this is an off-label use of these drugs.

Methylphenidate has sympathomimetic properties, and could contribute to his hypertension. Therefore, switching to this agent would not be beneficial.

KEY POINT

- **In adult patients with attention-deficit/hyperactivity disorder (ADHD), it is important to reassess the need for ADHD medications periodically.**

Bibliography

Okie S. ADHD in Adults. N Engl J Med. 2006;354:2637-2641. [PMID: 16790695]

Item 94   Answer: D

Educational Objective: Manage a transition of care in an elderly patient undergoing hospital discharge.

The patient should be evaluated for placement in a skilled nursing facility. Although discharge home is preferable if a patient is safe and medically stable for care in that setting, this patient is not able to return home to a setting in which she was not doing well prior to admission. Her complicated hospitalization has left her significantly debilitated. Skilled nursing facilities provide nursing level services, such as intravenous medications and medication management, wound care, and other medical services in addition to low-level rehabilitation services. With further recovery, her long-term care options may be reassessed and the most appropriate type pursued.

Inpatient rehabilitation is focused on intensive physical and occupational therapy and other forms of rehabilitative treatment as needed. Although patients with active medical issues may be candidates for inpatient rehabilitation, these issues need to be stable, and patients are generally required to participate in therapy for a minimum of 3 hours daily.

Long-term acute care hospitals (LTACHs) provide care similar to that in an acute hospital setting but for patients who are considered stable with the need for hospital-based

H **CONT.**

testing or interventions and with few anticipated changes in the care plan. This setting is overseen by physicians and is appropriate for patients who require significant medical monitoring but are expected to have a more prolonged (more than 25 days) time to recovery. This patient's medical needs are minimal and could be appropriately provided in a skilled nursing setting.

Although this patient may have been declining for several years, she does not have a diagnosis or condition indicative of a prognosis of less than 6 months. To qualify for hospice care, her physician must feel that her expected prognosis is less than 6 months of life remaining.

Establishing appropriate discharge care plans involves close coordination with the physician, patient and family, and the care coordination staff. Understanding the patient's medical needs is critical in determining the appropriate options available, and this process should be started as early as possible in the course of hospitalization.

KEY POINT

- **Understanding a patient's medical needs in conjunction with the wishes and resources available to the patient and family is critical in determining appropriate posthospital care, and this process should be started as early as possible in the course of hospitalization.**

Bibliography

Kane RL. Finding the right level of posthospital care: "We didn't realize there was any other option for him". JAMA. 2011;305(3):284-293. [PMID: 21245184]

Item 95   Answer: A

Educational Objective: Diagnose acute angle-closure glaucoma.

This patient most likely has acute angle-closure glaucoma. Angle-closure glaucoma is characterized by narrowing or closure of the anterior chamber angle, which impedes the trabecular drainage system in the anterior chamber, resulting in elevated intraocular pressure and damage to the optic nerve. Acute angle-closure glaucoma is an ophthalmologic emergency. Symptoms depend upon the rapidity of the elevation of intraocular pressure. Typical history of acute angle-closure glaucoma may include seeing halos around lights, severe unilateral eye pain, headache, and nausea and vomiting. Occasionally, patients may present with only nausea and vomiting and be mistaken as having cardiac or abdominal pathology. Physical examination may show conjunctival erythema; a sluggish or nonreactive, mid-range dilated pupil; corneal cloudiness; and, on funduscopic examination, cupping of the optic nerve. Treatment in this case would be immediate referral to an ophthalmologist or emergency department for initiation of topical β-adrenergic antagonists and pilocarpine and carbonic anhydrase inhibitors.

Central retinal artery occlusion (CRAO) classically presents in a 50- to 70-year-old patient as a painless, abrupt

loss of vision that occurs in the early morning hours—usually between midnight and 6 AM and, second most commonly, between 6 AM and noon. It results from an embolic or thrombotic event in the ophthalmic artery. Although this patient is at risk for CRAO owing to her atrial fibrillation, CRAO would not cause red eye, a firm globe, ocular pain, nausea, or vomiting.

Ocular migraine, also known as retinal migraine, typically occurs in persons with a family history or personal history of migraine, which this patient does not have. Symptoms include flashing lights, scintillating scotomas, visual blurring, and even total unilateral vision loss. Patients with ocular migraine tend to be younger than 40 years, making this diagnosis highly unlikely in this 76-year-old patient.

Temporal arteritis should be considered in patients older than 50 years presenting with a severe new headache. Visual loss in temporal arteritis is painless, however, and would not cause a red eye, nausea, or vomiting.

KEY POINT

- **Acute angle-closure glaucoma is characterized by severe unilateral eye pain, headache, nausea and vomiting, and seeing halos around lights; physical examination findings include conjunctival erythema; a sluggish or nonreactive, mid-range dilated pupil; corneal cloudiness; and cupping of the optic nerve.**

Bibliography

Magauran B. Conditions requiring emergency ophthalmologic consultation. Emerg Med Clin North Am. 2008;26(1):233-238. [PMID: 18249265]

Item 96   Answer: B

Educational Objective: Diagnose de Quervain tenosynovitis.

This patient's presentation is most consistent with de Quervain tenosynovitis, which refers to swelling or stenosis of the abductor pollicis longus and extensor pollicis brevis tendon sheaths at the level of the wrist. It is most commonly caused by repetitive motion of the thumb but can also be associated with underlying conditions including pregnancy and rheumatoid arthritis. This condition commonly presents with pain and swelling located over the radial styloid. The pain occurs with use of the thumb. On examination, there is localized tenderness of the distal radial styloid. Pain is elicited with both resisted thumb abduction and extension. The Finkelstein test is frequently positive (as with this patient).

Carpometacarpal arthritis presents with pain at the base of the thumb that occurs with thumb gripping and pinching. This pain may radiate into the distal forearm. On examination, there is tenderness to palpation on both the dorsal and palmar surfaces of the joint. Compressing the joint by applying a longitudinal load frequently produces pain. In advanced cases, joint stiffness and loss of range of motion may be present. The absence of these findings, as well as the patient's young age, argues against carpometacarpal arthritis as the cause of his pain.

A ganglion is a cyst that forms on the tendon sheath and results from inflammation, often following trauma. The anatomic location of the patient's pain and the absence of a palpable cystic structure do not support this diagnosis.

Patients with a scaphoid fracture usually have a history of an injury that involves wrist dorsiflexion. Pain is located in the anatomic snuffbox (the radial side of the wrist between the abductor and long thumb extensor tendons just distal to the radial styloid). On examination, there is significant tenderness to palpation of the anatomic snuffbox.

KEY POINT

- de Quervain tenosynovitis is pain that occurs with thumb use, characterized by pain and swelling over the radial styloid that is is elicited with both resisted thumb abduction and extension.

Bibliography

Moore JS. De Quervain's tenosynovitis. Stenosing tenosynovitis of the first dorsal compartment. J Occup Environ Med. 1997;39(10):990-1002. [PMID: 9343764]

Item 97   Answer: D

Educational Objective: Manage temporomandibular joint disorder.

This patient likely has a temporomandibular disorder. Initial treatment of temporomandibular disorders focuses on noninterventional, nonpharmacologic strategies. Jaw relaxation, heat, and therapeutic exercises may be helpful. Temporomandibular disorders are more common in women and typically present in the third or fourth decade of life. Patients typically report unilateral jaw discomfort in the masticatory muscles, often with radiation to the ear or posterior neck; chewing almost always makes the pain worse. Some patients report a history of clicking with jaw movement.

There is insufficient evidence for or against the effectiveness of simple analgesics such as ibuprofen or the use of tricyclic drugs to treat temporomandibular disorders. Evidence for the effectiveness for selective serotonin reuptake inhibitors such as fluoxetine is lacking. Furthermore, fluoxetine and paroxetine should be avoided as they can sometimes cause bruxism and exacerbate the problem.

The diagnosis of temporomandibular disorders is primarily clinical. Radiography is usually not helpful but may be considered when dental disease is suspected based on visual inspection or tooth percussion or if the patient does not respond to conservative therapy. If structural (nondental) changes of the jaw are suspected and the patient has not responded to conservative therapy or jaw locking is present, jaw MRI is the imaging procedure of choice but is not indicated in most patients.

For patients with chronic temporomandibular disorders, cognitive-behavioral therapy has been shown to reduce pain, depression, and interference with activities. Biofeedback may also be of value. Jaw appliances and occlusal splints have been a prominent part of temporomandibular disorder therapy for years despite questionable evidence of benefit.

KEY POINT

- Initial treatment of temporomandibular disorders focuses on noninterventional, nonpharmacologic strategies.

Bibliography

Mujakperuo HR, Watson M, Morrison R, Macfarlane TV. Pharmacological interventions for pain in patients with temporomandibular disorders. Cochrane Database Syst Rev. 2010;(10):CD004715. [PMID: 20927737]

Item 98   Answer: D

Educational Objective: Manage peripheral vertigo.

This patient should be referred for vestibular rehabilitation, which involves balance exercises and physical therapy. She presents with persistent symptoms of benign paroxysmal positional vertigo (BPPV), the most common cause of vertigo. Patients with BPPV classically report recurrent episodes of vertigo with rapid change in head position. The Dix-Hallpike maneuver is performed by having the examiner support the patient's head in 20 degrees of extension while sitting, then assisting the patient rapidly to the supine position with the head turned to one side and hanging over the edge of the examining table; the test is repeated with the head turned to the other side. A positive test results in horizontal nystagmus with latency 2 to 40 seconds and duration less than 1 minute with reproduction of symptoms that will fatigue and habituate.

BPPV is thought to be caused by movement of debris in the semicircular canals and resultant perturbation of sensory receptors. The Epley maneuver is a particle repositioning procedure intended to move the debris within the semicircular canal; it can successfully relieve symptoms in more than 60% of patients. In this patient, however, the maneuver was unsuccessful, and, based on her symptoms, further treatment is warranted. Vestibular rehabilitation, especially if initiated early, is effective in treating peripheral vertigo. Studies have shown improvement in symptoms, balance, and activities of daily living. Referral to a therapist trained in vestibular rehabilitation is recommended.

With a classic presentation for BPPV and no focal neurologic findings, brain imaging is not indicated in this patient. The severity of vertiginous symptoms is highly concerning for many patients, who seek reassurance that their condition is benign by undergoing imaging. However, such testing is typically of very low yield and does not alter the course of clinical management.

Meniere disease is characterized by the symptomatic triad of vertigo, tinnitus, and hearing loss, although it can present with vertigo alone. The vertigo is usually episodic and may not be positional. It can be accompanied by a sensation of aural fullness. Diuretic therapy (hydrochlorothiazide) is advocated for patients with this disease by some experts, but robust efficacy data are lacking. This patient's presentation is most consistent with BPPV, and therapeutic interventions should be targeted toward this diagnosis.

In general, medications are ineffective for the treatment of BPPV. Benzodiazepines and centrally acting anticholinergic antihistamines (meclizine) may modify the intensity of symptoms for some patients, particularly those with vestibular neuritis. When medications are used, they should be prescribed for less than 24 to 48 hours, since longer use may prolong symptoms by suppressing vestibular feedback and central compensation mechanisms.

KEY POINT

- **Vestibular rehabilitation is effective in treating peripheral vertigo.**

Bibliography

Bhattacharyya N, Baugh RF, Orvidas L, et al. Clinical practice guideline: benign paroxysmal positional vertigo. Otolaryngol Head Neck Surg. 2008;139(5)(suppl 4):S47-S81. [PMID: 18973840]

Item 99   Answer: C

Educational Objective: Diagnose depression in an older adult.

This patient should be assessed for depression. Elderly patients with depression may present with somatic and vegetative symptoms rather than dysphoria. The PHQ-9 is a validated depression assessment tool with a sensitivity of 80% and specificity of 92% for major depression using a score 10 or above as a cut off value. Administering the PHQ-9 in this patient is appropriate because depression in older adults is often underdiagnosed as changes in mood or behavior are often perceived as a consequence of underlying chronic illnesses. This patient's risk factors for depression include living in an institutional facility, chronic illness, and the recent death of his wife. The PHQ-9 assesses anhedonia, depressed mood, sleeping difficulties, decreased energy, changes in appetite, feelings of guilt or worthlessness, concentration impairment, psychomotor changes, and suicidal ideation. Alternatively, the Geriatric Depression Scale, consisting of 15 questions, could be administered. Its sensitivity of 80% to 90% and specificity of 70% to 85% are similar to the sensitivity and specificity of the PHQ-9.

The Dix-Hallpike maneuver is often performed in patients with dizziness to assess for benign paroxysmal positional vertigo. To perform the maneuver, the patient is directed to assume the supine position with the head allowed to lie below the horizontal and turned to one side. The maneuver is repeated with the head turned to the other side. The examiner observes for nystagmus and vertigo. Dizziness is not a symptom in this patient.

The Mini–Mental State Examination (MMSE) is a validated instrument to test cognition. Although the MMSE is an appropriate screening test in older adults, this patient's normal orientation and lack of symptoms regarding cognition would make this test less of a priority at this time. Furthermore, false-positive MMSE results can be seen in patients with untreated depression.

In the Timed "Up & Go" (TUG) test, the patient is asked to arise from a chair, walk 10 feet, turn around, and return to sit in the same chair. Those completing the task in more than 14 seconds are considered to be at high risk for subsequent falling. Although the TUG test is appropriate for assessing fall risk, it would not address the causes of his diminished activity or his somatic symptoms.

KEY POINT

- **Elderly patients with depression may present with somatic and vegetative symptoms rather than dysphoria.**

Bibliography

Kroenke K, Spitzer RL, Williams JB. The PHQ-9: validity of a brief depression severity measure. J Gen Intern Med. 2001;16(9):606-613. [PMID: 11556941]

Item 100   Answer: D

Educational Objective: Diagnose posttraumatic stress disorder.

This patient most likely has posttraumatic stress disorder (PTSD). PTSD occurs in response to exposure to a traumatic event that involves serious threat to oneself or others. PTSD is characterized by at least 1 month of symptoms that include intrusive thoughts about the trauma, nightmares or flashbacks, avoidance of reminders of the event, and hypervigilance with sleep disturbance. To meet DSM-IV criteria, the symptoms must be in each of three areas: re-experiencing the event, avoiding reminders of the event, and heightened arousal. Comorbid psychiatric conditions are common, so screening for depression, anxiety, and substance abuse is essential. PTSD symptoms often require multimodal treatments, and early intervention may prevent chronicity of symptoms. Trauma-focused cognitive-behavioral therapy focuses on cognitively reframing distorted thinking patterns while gradually re-exposing the patient to the traumatic experience. Simple stress management interventions can also be helpful in alleviating some symptoms. The most effective pharmacotherapy is selective serotonin reuptake inhibitors. However, no advantage has been identified for either psychotherapy or pharmacotherapy.

Generalized anxiety disorder is characterized by excessive anxiety and worry about a variety of events or activities on most days for at least 6 months, with difficulty controlling worrying. Physical symptoms of headache, nausea, and tremulousness may occur. In generalized anxiety disorder there is usually not a link to a particular inciting incident, and interfering nightmares are not a hallmark.

A major depressive episode is diagnosed according to the DSM-IV by the presence of five or more of the nine cardinal symptoms of depression during the same 2-week period, at least one of which is either depressed mood or loss of interest or pleasure. Symptoms should represent a change from previous functioning and cause clinically significant distress or impairment in functioning. This patient does not have significant mood disturbance or anhedonia.

Patients with obsessive-compulsive disorder report recurrent obsessions or compulsions sufficiently severe to occupy 1 hour daily or result in marked distress or impaired social function. Obsessions are persistent ideas, thoughts, impulses, or images experienced as intrusive and are associated with significant anxiety or distress. Examples include fears of having left doors unlocked and fears of germ contamination. Compulsions are repetitive behaviors, such as handwashing, checking, ordering, or counting, that are repeated to decrease the anxiety related to the obsessions. This patient's presentation is not consistent with obsessive-compulsive disorder.

KEY POINT

- **Posttraumatic stress disorder is characterized by at least 1 month of symptoms that include intrusive thoughts about the trauma, nightmares or flashbacks, avoidance of reminders of the event, and hypervigilance with sleep disturbance; symptoms must be in each of three areas: re-experiencing the event, avoiding reminders of the event, and heightened arousal.**

Bibliography
Ravindran LN, Stein MB. Pharmacotherapy of PTSD: premises, principles, and priorities. Brain Res. 2009;1293:24-39. [PMID: 19332035]

Item 101   Answer: B

Educational Objective: Manage chest pain due to an acute coronary syndrome.

This patient should be admitted to the coronary care unit for further treatment. Because chest pain is a common clinical symptom and may have noncardiac causes, assessment of the probability that chest pain has a cardiac etiology is critical to pursuing appropriate diagnosis and treatment. This is done through an understanding of existing cardiac risk factors, the nature of the presenting symptoms, findings on physical examination, and the results of specific initial diagnostic studies, such as chest radiography and electrocardiography. Her cardiac risk factors include her age, hypertension, and hyperlipidemia, and the substernal nature of her chest pain places her in an intermediate risk

category for cardiac-related pain. Coupled with her electrocardiogram (ECG) showing anterolateral ST-segment depression, her clinical picture is consistent with coronary ischemia as the cause of her chest pain. She therefore requires emergent treatment for coronary ischemia and admission to a coronary care unit.

Low-risk patients without evidence of myocardial infarction can be evaluated with an exercise or pharmacologic stress test. However, a stress test in a patient with probable acute coronary syndrome could provoke an extension of her myocardial infarction or a life-threatening arrhythmia.

CT pulmonary angiography would be helpful if there were a high probability of acute pulmonary embolism. Because this patient has symptoms and ECG findings of acute coronary syndrome and the probability of pulmonary embolism is low (she has no risk factors or physical examination findings to support the diagnosis of venous thromboembolism and her symptoms can be explained by an alternative diagnosis), a CT pulmonary angiogram is not indicated.

NSAIDs are indicated for the treatment of acute pericarditis or musculoskeletal chest wall pain. The pain of pericarditis is characteristically pleuritic in nature. In addition, the characteristic ECG finding in pericarditis is ST-segment elevation throughout the precordial and limb leads rather than regional ST-segment depression, as in this patient. ECG changes are not present in musculoskeletal chest pain.

KEY POINT

- **Assessment of chest pain is based on preexisting risks for cardiac or other diseases, elements of the history and physical examination, and appropriate, directed testing based on the likely cause of chest symptoms.**

Bibliography
Panju AA, Hemmelgarn BR, Guyatt GH, Simel DL. The rational clinical examination. Is this patient having a myocardial infarction? JAMA. 1998;280(14):1256-1263. [PMID: 9786377]

Item 102   Answer: B

Educational Objective: Screen for essential hypertension.

It is recommended that this patient be screened again for hypertension in 2 years. Although there are not strong data on outcomes with different screening intervals, the Seventh Report of the Joint National Committee on Prevention, Detection, Evaluation, and Treatment of High Blood Pressure (JNC 7) recommends that persons with blood pressure below 120/80 mm Hg should be screened every 2 years. The mean of two or more seated clinic measurements should be used to evaluate for possible hypertension.

The JNC 7 recommends that yearly screening should be reserved for patients with systolic blood pressures of 120 mm Hg to 139 mm Hg and diastolic blood pressures of 80 mm Hg to 89 mm Hg.

Benefits of screening for hypertension at intervals longer than 2 years have not been established.

KEY POINT

- All adults aged 18 years and older should be screened for hypertension; screening every 2 years is appropriate for those with blood pressure below 120/80 mm Hg.

Bibliography

Chobanian AV, Bakris GL, Black HR, et al; Joint National Committee on Prevention, Detection, Evaluation, and Treatment of High Blood Pressure; National Heart, Lung, and Blood Institute; National High Blood Pressure Education Program Coordinating Committee. Seventh report of the Joint National Committee on Prevention, Detection, Evaluation, and Treatment of High Blood Pressure. Hypertension. 2003;42(6):1206-1252. [PMID: 14656957]

Item 103   Answer: B

Educational Objective: Manage mild cognitive impairment.

This patient has mild cognitive impairment (MCI) as evidenced by reported memory loss, some impaired functioning, and no involvement of other cognitive domains. Her Mini–Mental State Examination (MMSE) score of 26 is typical for MCI. She does not demonstrate involvement of other domains of mental impairment that might suggest dementia, including problems with executive functioning, language difficulties, or activities of daily living. Patient concern about memory loss is more likely with MCI than it is with dementia, in which concerns are usually raised by family members. Although there is no widely accepted treatment for MCI, cognitive rehabilitation has been shown to have some effectiveness in improving functioning in some patients. Cognitive rehabilitation is performed by neuropsychologists and occupational therapists and involves using external memory aids as well as teaching patients organizational and attention skills.

In patients with Alzheimer disease, anticholinesterase inhibitors, such as donepezil, galantamine, and rivastigmine, may be tried because their use may result in modest improvement of cognition, performance of activities of daily living, and functioning, as determined by global assessment. However, the use of anticholinesterase inhibitors has not been shown to delay the progression from MCI to dementia.

Although PET scanning can detect pathologic levels of amyloid in patients with MCI and dementia, and possibly differentiate between the two, its use at this time is still investigational.

Reassurance that the patient will not progress to dementia is not appropriate because persons with MCI appear to be at increased risk for further declines in

cognition relative to those with normal cognitive function. The annual incidence rate of dementia in the general elderly population is 1% to 3%, whereas the annual incidence rate of dementia in patients with a diagnosis of MCI is approximately 12%, suggesting a significant increased risk of progression to dementia from their baseline level of cognitive impairment.

KEY POINT

- Although there is no widely accepted treatment for mild cognitive impairment, cognitive rehabilitation has been shown to have some effectiveness in improving functioning in some patients.

Bibliography

Kinsella GJ, Mullaly E, Rand E, et al. Early intervention for mild cognitive impairment: a randomised controlled trial. J Neurol Neurosurg Psychiatry. 2009;80(7):730-736. [PMID: 19332424]

Item 104   Answer: B

Educational Objective: Evaluate a patient with pleuritic chest pain.

This patient should undergo radiography of the chest. He has severe COPD and findings consistent with spontaneous secondary pneumothorax. These findings include sudden, sharp, nonradiating pleuritic chest pain and shortness of breath with hyperresonance, decreased breath sounds, and decreased chest wall expansion on the side of the pneumothorax in a patient with underlying lung disease. Pneumothorax should be considered in any patient with sudden onset of pleuritic chest pain and dyspnea. The diagnostic test of choice if pneumothorax is suspected is an upright chest radiograph. Findings on chest radiograph include separation of the parietal and visceral pleura by a collection of gas and the absence of vessels in this space. The diagnosis of pneumothorax may be difficult in patients with COPD because the pleural line may be difficult to visualize in hyperlucent lung tissue, and a pneumothorax may be difficult to distinguish from a large bulla.

Chest CT also can be used to diagnose a pneumothorax. Chest CTs may be more sensitive in delineating smaller collections of gas in the pleural space and in providing more information about the pulmonary parenchyma and pleura. Plain film radiography remains the initial test of choice for most patients, however, and CT of the chest should be reserved for patients in whom the chest radiograph does not provide information to guide further treatment or evaluation.

The patient's history and physical examination are classic for pneumothorax and his pain descriptors do not strongly suggest ischemia or other primary cardiovascular disease. An electrocardiogram or echocardiogram, tests of choice to evaluate ischemic heart disease, valvular heart disease or cardiomyopathy, would not be the first diagnostic test of choice for suspected pneumothorax.

- Pneumothorax should be considered in any patient with sudden onset of pleuritic chest pain and dyspnea, and the diagnostic test of choice if pneumothorax is suspected is an upright chest radiograph.

Bibliography

Noppen M. Spontaneous pneumothorax: epidemiology, pathophysiology and cause. Eur Respir Rev. 2010;19(117):217-219. [PMID: 20956196]

Item 105   Answer: D

Educational Objective: Diagnose somatization disorder.

This patient most likely has somatization disorder. Although medically unexplained symptoms are common, as are patient concerns and anxiety regarding the possible presence of disease for which they seek evaluation, somatization disorder is a relatively rare psychiatric disease related to an extreme focus on medical symptoms and their evaluation. DSM-IV criteria for somatization disorder include a constellation of symptoms, including two gastrointestinal symptoms, four pain symptoms, one pseudoneurologic symptom, and one sexual symptom. The symptoms must start before age 30 years, persist (although they often wax and wane), and cause significant impairment for the patient. In addition, each symptom must be medically unexplained after evaluation. Somatization disorder should always be distinguished from depression with somatic features; the latter will meet diagnostic criteria for depression. This patient meets DSM-IV criteria for somatization disorder.

Celiac disease may be difficult to diagnose and may cause diffuse symptoms, including nausea, but would most likely cause weight loss and other gastrointestinal symptoms. In addition, celiac disease would not fully explain the focal neurologic and other symptoms experienced by the patient.

Patients who are malingering consciously fabricate symptoms for some secondary gain, whereas patients with somatoform disorders are unaware that their symptoms are a manifestation of psychiatric disease. This patient's history gives no suggestion of secondary gain.

Patients with multiple sclerosis can have nausea. However, this patient's neurologic symptoms affect the right face and body and thus do not follow neuroanatomy. Furthermore, multiple sclerosis is an unlikely cause of the patient's multiple somatic symptoms, and the patient's recent neuroimaging study did not show evidence of demyelination.

- Criteria for somatization disorder include a constellation of medically unexplained, persistent symptoms, including gastrointestinal, pain, pseudoneurologic, and sexual, that begin before age 30 years and cause significant impairment for the patient.

Bibliography

Oyama O, Paltoo C, Greengold J. Somatoform disorders. Am Fam Physician. 2007;76(9):1333-1338. [PMID: 18019877]

Item 106   Answer: B

Educational Objective: Treat chronic bacterial prostatitis.

The most appropriate treatment for this patient is a 1-month course of a fluoroquinolone antibiotic. This patient has chronic bacterial prostatitis (National Institutes of Health category II), which presents with pain and urinary symptoms with recurrent bacterial infection. The prostate in patients with chronic bacterial prostatitis may be less inflamed than with acute prostatitis. The recommendation for treatment of category II prostatitis is a prolonged (1 month) course of a fluoroquinolone antibiotic such as ciprofloxacin, which covers common bacterial infections of the prostate with good penetration of the prostate.

A 1-week course of trimethoprim-sulfamethoxazole would be appropriate for acute bacterial prostatitis (category I prostatitis) or urinary tract infection; however, this patient has had short-course antibiotics for three prior infections, placing him in category II and warranting a longer course of antibiotics.

Category III prostatitis (chronic abacterial prostatitis/chronic pelvic pain syndrome) is noninfectious and therefore does not respond to antibiotics. This patient's urinary findings of bacteria and leukocytes support an infectious cause of his symptoms, and not this form of prostatitis. There is some evidence that cognitive-behavioral therapy may provide some benefit to patients with chronic pelvic pain syndrome, although there is not a role for this intervention in bacterial prostatitis. Symptoms of category III chronic pelvic pain syndrome are often refractory, and empathetic supportive care is often required.

Finasteride is a 5-α-reductase inhibitor that decreases prostate volume and is used primarily in the treatment of benign prostatic hyperplasia. It does not have an established use in either acute or chronic bacterial prostatitis.

- The recommended treatment for chronic bacterial prostatitis is a prolonged course of a fluoroquinolone antibiotic.

Bibliography

Touma NJ, Nickel JC. Prostatitis and chronic pelvic pain syndrome in men. Med Clin North Am. 2011;95:75-86. [PMID: 21095412]

Item 107   Answer: B

Educational Objective: Manage acute sinusitis.

This patient with clinical findings typical of acute sinusitis should be observed and given symptomatic treatment, such as chlorpheniramine. Most cases of acute sinusitis are caused by viruses and typically resolve in 7 to 10 days without directed therapy. The clinical presentation is not helpful in determining whether the cause of symptoms is viral or bacterial. However, because most cases of viral or bacterial sinusitis resolve spontaneously within 10 days, observation and treatment of the associated symptoms with analgesics and decongestants is appropriate.

Antibiotics are generally reserved for sinusitis accompanied by high or continued fever or worsening symptoms, and even in this setting, their efficacy is not well documented. When used, an antibiotic focused on common respiratory organisms is reasonable.

Nasal cultures have not been shown to be helpful in diagnosing a bacterial etiology for sinusitis or in guiding antibiotic therapy.

Sinus imaging is not part of the initial management of acute sinusitis because imaging results are frequently abnormal in symptomatic patients with either a viral or bacterial sinusitis, and also in a high percentage of asymptomatic patients. Imaging is generally indicated in patients with a complicated presentation, such as those with visual changes or severe headache.

Inhaled nasal corticosteroids are frequently prescribed for acute symptom relief for sinusitis and have some efficacy in this setting; however, the role of systemic corticosteroids in acute sinusitis is not clear, and they are not recommended.

KEY POINT

- **Most cases of viral or bacterial sinusitis resolve spontaneously within 10 days, and observation and treatment of the associated symptoms with analgesics and decongestants is appropriate.**

Bibliography

Chow AW, Benninger MS, Brook I, et al. IDSA clinical practice guideline for acute bacterial rhinosinusitis in children and adults. Clin Infect Dis. 2012;54(8):e72-e112. [PMID: 22438350]

Item 108   Answer: D

Educational Objective: Manage sudden sensorineural hearing loss.

This woman with sudden-onset unilateral sensorineural hearing loss requires urgent audiometry and otorhinolaryngology referral because early diagnosis and treatment may be associated with improved outcomes. Based on the initial examination, this patient does not have conductive hearing loss because she hears better when sound is transmitted via air (through the external ear canal and middle ear) than when it is transmitted via bone vibration. Sudden sensorineural hearing loss (SSNHL) is an alarming problem that is defined as sensorineural hearing loss occurring in 3 days or less. Patients often report immediate or rapid hearing loss or loss of hearing upon awakening. Ninety percent have unilateral hearing loss, and some have tinnitus, ear fullness, and vertigo. SSNHL constitutes a considerable diagnostic challenge because it may be caused by many conditions, including infection, neoplasm, trauma, autoimmune disease, vascular events, and ototoxic drugs. Immediate otorhinolaryngologic referral is required. Improvement occurs in about two thirds of patients. Oral or intratympanic corticosteroids are usually given, although randomized trials differ in their conclusions regarding efficacy.

Otic herpes zoster (Ramsay Hunt syndrome) is characterized by herpetic lesions in the external canal and ipsilateral facial palsy neither of which is seen in this patient. Acyclovir may be considered in a clear case of Ramsay Hunt syndrome but has been shown to be unhelpful in idiopathic SSNHL.

Neomycin, polymyxin B, and hydrocortisone ear drops are a possible treatment for acute otitis externa. This patient is unlikely to have otitis externa because she does not have otalgia, otorrhea, itching, or pain intensified by jaw motion. She does not have internal tenderness when the tragus or pinna is pushed or pulled. Her ear canal erythema is most likely secondary to the trauma of recent cerumen removal than otitis externa.

Triethanolamine ear drops may help to treat or prevent cerumen impaction, but cerumen impaction causes conductive hearing loss, not sudden sensorineural hearing loss. After her cerumen was successfully removed, the patient's conductive hearing was intact, making this an unlikely cause of her sudden hearing loss in her left ear. Cerumen impaction is also unlikely to cause tinnitus.

KEY POINT

- **Patients with sudden sensorineural hearing loss should be urgently evaluated by audiometry and considered for oral or intratympanic corticosteroid treatment by an otorhinolaryngologist.**

Bibliography

Stachler RJ, Chandrasekhar SS, Archer SM, et al; American Academy of Otolaryngology-Head and Neck Surgery. Clinical practice guideline: sudden hearing loss. Otolaryngol Head Neck Surg. 2012;146(3 suppl):S1-S35. [PMID: 22383545]

Item 109   Answer: D

Educational Objective: Employ the principle of substituted judgment in managing care of a patient without decisional capacity.

Although the patient is unconscious and unable to make his own decisions, the ethical obligation of both the practitioner and the surrogate decision maker (his wife) is to continue to make decisions that are consistent with his previously expressed wishes and values. The principle, called "substituted judgment," essentially asks, "What would the patient want if he or she could decide?"

In patients who present to the emergency department unable to make decisions, lifesaving therapy is both ethical and necessary under the principle of implied consent. However, once a patient's wishes are known, it is unethical to specifically defy those wishes simply because the patient has lost decisional capacity; therefore, it would be unethical to transfuse the patient knowing that he specifically did not want transfusion.

Obtaining a court-appointed guardian is not indicated in this case because the patient clearly stated his views, and subsequent care decisions will be made by his duly appointed surrogate based on his wishes.

Seeking the permission of the patient's wife to allow transfusion or attempting to convince her that transfusion would be in her husband's best interest is ethically unacceptable; all available evidence suggests that he was consistent in his wishes to avoid transfusion, and it would be inappropriate to place her in a difficult ethical position, especially in this stressful situation.

KEY POINT

- When a patient is unable to make his or her own decisions, the ethical principle of substituted judgment obliges surrogate decision makers to make decisions that are consistent with the patient's previously expressed wishes and values.

Bibliography
Snyder L; American College of Physicians Ethics, Professionalism, and Human Rights Committee. American College of Physicians Ethics Manual: sixth edition. Ann Intern Med. 2012;156(1 Pt 2):73-104. [PMID: 22213573]

Item 110   Answer: D

Educational Objective: Diagnose testicular torsion.

This patient has testicular torsion, which occurs when the testicle twists on the spermatic cord, leading to decreased blood flow and ischemia. It is more common in children and in men younger than 30 years. Pain is usually sudden in onset and examination often reveals a high-riding testicle with the longitudinal axis abnormally oriented transversely. Absence of the cremasteric reflex on the affected side is nearly 99% sensitive for torsion. Treatment of torsion includes rapid surgical decompression to resume blood flow. In the absence of rapid access to surgery, manual decompression may be attempted.

Men with epididymitis typically present with subacute onset of scrotal pain, dysuria, urinary frequency, and fever. Inflammation and infection of the epididymis cause pain localizing to the posterior and superior aspect of the testicle. The scrotum may be edematous and erythematous. It does not result in malpositioning of the testicle or an absent cremasteric reflex.

Clinical presentations of inguinal hernias can vary from an asymptomatic bulge to a feeling of groin or abdominal pressure to severe pain when incarceration or strangulation occurs. A strangulated hernia may present as a painful mass in the scrotum or as a tender bulge in the inguinal area; signs of bowel obstruction may also be present. This patient does not have findings consistent with a strangulated inguinal hernia.

Orchitis, an inflammation of the testicle, is usually caused by viral infection (mumps) or extension of a bacterial infection from epididymitis or urinary tract infection; in mumps, parotiditis begins about 5 days prior to orchitis. The testicle is diffusely tender and may be swollen; the position of the testicle in the scrotum is normal and the cremasteric reflex is present.

KEY POINT

- Testicular torsion is characterized by severe pain and an elevated high-riding testicle with the longitudinal axis abnormally oriented transversely and an absent cremasteric reflex.

Bibliography
Wampler SM, Llanes M. Common scrotal and testicular problems. Prim Care. 2010;37(3):613-626, x. [PMID: 20705202]

Item 111   Answer: C

Educational Objective: Treat bacterial vaginosis.

The most appropriate treatment for this patient is a 7-day oral regimen of metronidazole (500 mg twice daily). She has bacterial vaginosis (BV), a polymicrobial infection characterized by an overgrowth of multiple anaerobic bacteria. Although BV is not a sexually transmitted infection, risk factors include lack of condom use and multiple or new sexual partners. BV can be diagnosed clinically using Amsel criteria, which include the following symptoms or signs: (1) homogeneous thin discharge that coats the vaginal walls; (2) clue cells (epithelial cells with borders obscured by small bacteria) on saline microscopy; (3) pH of vaginal fluid >4.5; and (4) fishy odor of vaginal discharge before or after the addition of 10% potassium hydroxide to the secretions (the "whiff" test). The presence of at least three of these clinical findings has a high sensitivity and specificity for diagnosing BV when compared with Gram stain of collected secretions, which is the gold standard. Because this woman is symptomatic, treatment should be offered with either oral metronidazole, vaginal metronidazole gel, or vaginal clindamycin cream; patient preference should dictate treatment choice. Topical clindamycin should be avoided during pregnancy as it may increase the risk of adverse outcomes. Women treated with oral metronidazole should be cautioned to avoid alcohol, which can cause a disulfiram-like reaction.

This patient's abnormal vaginal pH and lack of yeast and hyphae on potassium hydroxide preparation make vulvovaginal candidiasis an unlikely explanation for her symptoms. Treatment with oral fluconazole or topical clotrimazole cream, effective therapies for vulvovaginal candidiasis, is not warranted.

This patient has multiple sexual partners, increasing her risk for trichomoniasis. Characteristic symptoms and signs include a malodorous discharge with vulvar itching, burning, and postcoital bleeding. Although the vaginal pH will be elevated and the whiff test may be positive (as noted with this patient), clue cells are not a characteristic finding on saline microscopy, making trichomoniasis an unlikely diagnosis in this patient.

Oral metronidazole is also used for the treatment of trichomoniasis, but it is typically given as a single 2-g dose, which would not be appropriate for treatment of BV.

KEY POINT

- **Bacterial vaginosis is the likely diagnosis in women with at least three of the following features: (1) homogeneous thin discharge that coats the vaginal walls; (2) clue cells on saline microscopy; (3) pH of vaginal fluid >4.5; and (4) fishy odor of vaginal discharge (positive "whiff" test).**

Bibliography

Wilson, JF. In the clinic. Vaginitis and cervicitis. Ann Intern Med. 2009;151(5):ITC3-1-ITC3-15. [PMID: 19721016]

Item 112   Answer: C
Educational Objective: Treat erectile dysfunction.

Since this patient has not yet taken anything for his erectile dysfunction (ED), it would be most appropriate to treat him with sildenafil, a phosphodiesterase type 5 (PDE-5) inhibitor. PDE-5 inhibitors are generally considered first-line pharmacologic therapy for ED and include sildenafil, vardenafil, and tadalafil. These agents increase penile cyclic guanosine monophosphate (cGMP), facilitating smooth muscle relaxation and allowing inflow of blood. All of these drugs have been shown to improve erectile function, as measured by successful sexual intercourse attempts and improved scores on various survey instruments. There are no direct comparisons to support superiority of any one agent, as the populations studied differ in various characteristics.

The PDE-5 inhibitors vary in their duration of action, interaction with food and other medications, and adverse effects. Treatment failure may result from lack of patient education or improper use (timing, taking with food, inadequate sexual stimulation, inadequate dose, inadequate trial), performance anxiety or unrealistic expectations, hypogonadism, or an incorrect diagnosis

(premature ejaculation or hypoactive sexual desire disorder). An adequate trial is generally deemed to constitute patient reeducation and gradual escalation of the dose to maximum dose and at least six attempts on maximum-dose therapy. PDE-5 inhibitors should be avoided in patients receiving any form of nitrate therapy.

Second-line therapies for ED should be reserved for men who fail to improve with lifestyle modifications or with use of PDE-5 inhibitors. These include alprostadil (either intraurethral or intracavernosal), penile pumps, and penile prostheses. Intraurethral alprostadil is more effective than that administered intracavernosally and is associated with fewer side effects.

Testosterone replacement therapy should be limited to patients with clinical symptoms and signs consistent with androgen deficiency and a subnormal serum testosterone level (generally an 8 AM total testosterone level <200 ng/dL [7 nmol/L]).

KEY POINT

- **First-line pharmacologic therapy for erectile dysfunction consists of phosphodiesterase type 5 inhibitors.**

Bibliography

Tsertsvadze A, Fink HA, Yazdi F, et al. Oral phosphodiesterase-5 inhibitors and hormonal treatments for erectile dysfunction: a systematic review and meta-analysis. Ann Intern Med. 2009;151(9):650-661. [PMID: 19884626]

Item 113   Answer: C
Educational Objective: Prevent medication errors from occurring during a transition in care.

The most likely cause for this patient's readmission is a medication error stemming from her medication changes at discharge. It is likely that she either did not receive or did not take the medications at the increased dosages. One in five patients discharged from the hospital will suffer an adverse event related to medical management within 3 weeks of hospital discharge, with 66% of these being adverse events related to medications. Most medication errors result from inadequate communication by hospital caregivers with patients and their primary care clinicians. Medication reconciliation is the process by which medications are reviewed at every step of the care process, with a focus on ensuring that the patient is taking only those medications intended, and that this is clear to the patient and all others involved in that patient's care. Patients should receive a list of medications at the time of discharge, be informed of previous medications that have been discontinued or changed, any new medications that have been added, and the reasons for these changes.

True diuretic resistance is uncommon, although the bioavailability of oral diuretics may be highly variable, particularly in the edematous state. She responded to intravenous diuretics as an inpatient with a return of her weight to a nonedematous level, and her oral diuretic dose was appropriately increased at the time of discharge. Her rapid decompensation from her normal baseline weight on an increased dose of diuretic with the addition of a second agent at the time of discharge makes clinically significant resistance to diuretics unlikely.

Inadequate post-hospital follow-up is a potential cause for readmission, particularly with complex patients who have had extended hospitalizations and multiple changes to their treatment regimen. In general, for most patients admitted for heart failure exacerbation, a follow-up appointment in 1 week should be scheduled at the time of discharge, preferably with direct contact with the primary care physician. This patient was scheduled for a 1-week follow-up, but worsening of her symptoms shortly after discharge suggests an issue with treatment of her initial problem, or development of an additional medical complication.

Spironolactone has been shown to decrease mortality in selected patients with systolic heart failure. Its primary complications are hyperkalemia and other effects of aldosterone blockade. However, it is unlikely to be an independent cause of her acute heart failure decompensation.

KEY POINT

- **Hospitalized patients should receive a list of medications at the time of discharge and be informed of previous medications that have been discontinued or changed.**

Bibliography

Kripalani S, Jackson AT, Schnipper JL, Coleman EA. Promoting effective transitions of care at hospital discharge: a review of key issues for hospitalists. J Hosp Med. 2007;2(5):314-323. [PMID: 17935242]

Item 114   Answer: D

Educational Objective: Manage upper respiratory tract infection with ear pain.

This patient presents with signs and symptoms of a viral upper respiratory tract infection (URI). The recent development of ear pain and the findings of a dull tympanic membrane with a small middle ear effusion are compatible with either otitis media or a viral URI without otitis media. Treatment of otitis media in adults has not been well studied. There are no guidelines for antibiotic use in adults separate from those for children. In children older than 2 years without severe illness, outcomes appear to be similar for observation without antibiotics compared with antibiotic treatment. This strategy to reduce use of antimicrobials has not been evaluated in adults, and it is not known if antibiotics are associated with improved short- or long-term outcomes. However, antibiotic use is associated with adverse effects and higher levels of antibiotic resistance that should be considered in conjunction with the lack of evidence regarding benefit. Considering the patient's equivocal

diagnosis of otitis media and mild symptoms, it would be reasonable to withhold antibiotic therapy.

If an antibiotic was prescribed, amoxicillin is recommended as first-line therapy in adults. Erythromycin could be used in a penicillin-allergic patient, but there is no evidence that it is more efficacious.

An otorhinolaryngology consultation is not indicated at this time because the patient only has a URI.

KEY POINT

- **Do not routinely prescribe antibiotic therapy for adults with otitis media.**

Bibliography

Coco A, Vernacchio L, Horst M, Anderson A. Management of acute otitis media after publication of the 2004 AAP and AAFP clinical practice guideline. Pediatrics. 2010;125(2):214-220. [PMID: 20100746]

Item 115   Answer: D

Educational Objective: Manage secondary insomnia.

This patient's history of daytime fatigue and obesity and large neck size put him at risk for obstructive sleep apnea, which can be diagnosed with an overnight polysomnography study. It would be helpful to obtain corroborating information from his wife regarding symptoms of snoring, gasping, other breathing problems, or abnormal leg movements. Referral for polysomnography is indicated when a primary sleep disorder is suspected (obstructive sleep apnea, restless legs syndrome, periodic limb movement disorder). A sleep study may also include multiple sleep latency testing, in which a patient takes four or five 20-minute naps, and sleep latency (the time from deciding to sleep to actually falling asleep) is measured. Sleep latency of less than 8 minutes is associated with hypersomnia, which occurs with sleep disorders such as narcolepsy, insufficient sleep syndrome, medication adverse effects, sleep apnea syndromes, and periodic limb movements of sleep.

Although alcohol can contribute to insomnia, this patient's pattern of alcohol use does not support its having a role in his symptoms, since he is having daily fatigue symptoms despite only using alcohol on weekends.

Pharmacotherapy would not be appropriate in this patient until a secondary cause of insomnia is ruled out. Prescription drug therapy for insomnia is reserved for patients with primary insomnia who have not benefited from nonpharmacologic and behavioral therapies.

Restless legs syndrome is a clinical diagnosis. Besides an urge to move the legs, other symptoms that patients may exhibit in support of this diagnosis include an uncomfortable or unpleasant sensation in the legs that may begin or worsen during periods of rest or inactivity, is partially or totally relieved by movement as long as activity continues, and is worse in the evening or night or is present only at night. Restless legs syndrome can be divided into primary and secondary forms. The primary form refers to patients without another condition known to be associated with restless legs syndrome. Conditions associated with secondary restless legs syndrome include pregnancy, end-stage kidney disease, and iron deficiency. Since this patient does not have restless legs syndrome, iron studies are not indicated.

> **KEY POINT**
> - Referral for polysomnography is indicated when a primary sleep disorder is suspected (obstructive sleep apnea, restless legs syndrome, periodic limb movement disorder).

Bibliography
Wilson JF: In the clinic: Insomnia. Ann Intern Med. 2008;148(1): ITC13-1-ITC13-16. [PMID: 18166757]

Item 116   Answer: C
Educational Objective: Diagnose osteonecrosis of the hip.

This patient's presentation is most consistent with osteonecrosis of the hip. Osteonecrosis of the hip commonly presents with dull, aching groin pain (most commonly) or thigh or buttock pain that is indolent in onset. Occasionally, as is the case in this patient, severe pain may be reported in the early stages as bone death is occurring. Corticosteroid use and excessive use of alcohol account for more than 90% of hip osteonecrosis cases. On examination, patients have limited range of motion of the hip. During the early stages of this disease, radiographic imaging may be normal. Eventually, patchy areas of sclerosis and lucency may be seen. Hip MRI is the most sensitive imaging test for osteonecrosis and is typically positive early in the course of the disease.

Osteoarthritis of the hip can be established in patients with a history of chronic pain in the groin and medial thigh that worsens with activity and is relieved by rest. Although osteoarthritis of the hip can present with slowly progressive hip pain, severe pain at the onset of symptoms does not usually occur. Radiographs in patients with osteoarthritis may show joint-space narrowing, subchondral sclerosis, and osteophyte formation. Although there is a poor correlation between radiographic evidence of osteoarthritis and symptoms, it would be unusual for a patient with osteoarthritis of the hip to have a normal radiographic series.

L1 radiculopathy is rare. Symptoms include pain, paresthesia, and sensory loss in the groin. On examination, this patient has limited internal and external range of motion and pain with log-rolling of the hip. Each of these findings supports a joint etiology of this patient's hip pain and argues against lumbar disk disease at the L1 level.

Septic arthritis would be expected to present acutely with fever and limited range of motion. This patient's slow onset of symptoms and prolonged course are not consistent with septic arthritis.

> **KEY POINT**
> - Osteonecrosis of the hip commonly presents with dull, aching groin pain that is indolent in onset; risk factors include corticosteroid use and excessive alcohol use.

Bibliography
Amanatullah DF, Strauss EJ, Di Cesare PE. Current management options for osteonecrosis of the femoral head: part 1, diagnosis and nonoperative management. Am J Orthop (Belle Mead NJ). 2011;40(9):E186-92. [PMID: 22022684]

Item 117   Answer: B
Educational Objective: Manage a patient with a chronic pain syndrome.

This patient should be evaluated for possible intimate partner violence. It is essential to perform a comprehensive assessment in the evaluation of patients with chronic pain syndromes. This patient has a chronic pain syndrome, fibromyalgia that had previously been well controlled but has worsened recently, significantly affecting her functional status. In patients with chronic pain conditions, overlying psychosocial stressors, including domestic violence, may exacerbate or destabilize symptoms. Therefore, in addition to questioning the patient more thoroughly about pain onset and relieving and exacerbating factors, the provider should also inquire about threats to the patient's safety as well as other potential psychosocial events or situations that may be contributing to her worsened clinical status.

There is no specific role for diagnostic testing or imaging in the evaluation of patients with most chronic pain syndromes in the absence of objective physical examination findings or laboratory abnormalities suggesting a specific underlying disorder. Although various studies are frequently obtained in patients with chronic pain, they are typically not revealing, and abnormalities that are identified on diagnostic testing may not be the source of the patient's pain. This patient is experiencing worsening of her typical fibromyalgia pain, and obtaining muscle and nerve conduction studies without focal symptoms or clinical findings is unlikely to change management.

NSAIDs are most effective for treating the pain associated with rheumatoid arthritis, inflammatory arthropathies, and musculoskeletal pain. They are generally ineffective in the management of neuropathic and muscular pain syndromes, such as fibromyalgia, and can be associated with significant gastrointestinal and cardiovascular toxicities. Adding high-dose ibuprofen to this patient's pain regimen is unlikely to significantly improve her symptoms.

Opioid therapy should generally be avoided in patients with chronic pain syndromes given the expected chronicity of use, lack of demonstrated efficacy, and the potential for significant side effects and dependency.

- Patients with chronic pain syndromes should be evaluated for concurrent psychosocial stressors, particularly in those in whom symptoms have worsened without explanation.

Bibliography

Bradley LA. Pathophysiology of fibromyalgia. Am J Med. 2009;122(12 suppl):S22-30. [PMID: 19962493]

Item 118　　Answer:　C

Educational Objective: Manage risk for motor vehicle accidents in an older adult driver.

This patient has a number of factors that increase his risk of being involved in a motor vehicle accident and his physician has a responsibility to reduce this risk. This patient's risk factors for a motor vehicle accident include his age, likely visual deficits, decreased motor function (including a history of falling), and decreased cognitive function. The first step in assessing driving ability in older adults is to ask the patient and family members about driving difficulties. This assessment should include questions about whether friends and family members are worried about their driving, getting lost while driving, near misses, and recent accidents. A more complete set of questions to assess driving risk can be found in the "Am I a Safe Driver" self-assessment tool (www.ama-assn.org/ama1/pub/upload/mm/433/am_i _a_safe_driver.pdf). A positive response to any of the questions suggests unsafe driving.

It would be premature to advise this patient to stop driving before assessing driving-related skills, providing the patient with information on safe driving, and suggesting that the patient enroll in a driving course designed to improve skills. Referral to a driver rehabilitation specialist can also assist in assessment and skill improvement.

Advising the patient to drive only locally is not advised because so-called "low-mileage" drivers may be at the greatest risk. Older drivers who are having driving difficulties often self-restrict their driving, but local roads often have more hazards, including more signs and signals and confusing and congested intersections.

Guidelines for reporting patients to the department of transportation vary by state and include immediate threats to driving safety such as new seizures. Even in states that require reporting of immediate threats to driving safety, there is no indication to report this patient before a more complete evaluation is performed.

- The first step in assessing driving ability in older adults is to ask the patient and family members about driving difficulties, including whether friends and family members are worried about their driving, getting lost while driving, near misses, and recent accidents.

Bibliography

Carr DB, Schwartzberg JG, Manning L, Sempek J. Physician's Guide to Assessing and Counseling Older Drivers. 2nd edition. Washington, DC. NHTSA. 2010. Available at www.ama-assn .org/ama/pub/physician-resources/public-health/promoting -healthy-lifestyles/geriatric-health/older-driver-safety/assessing -counseling-older-drivers.page.

Item 119　　Answer:　D

Educational Objective: Manage panic disorder.

The most appropriate management of this patient is to prescribe a selective serotonin reuptake inhibitor. Panic disorder is a syndrome characterized by sudden panic attacks with the acute onset of somatic symptoms, which may include chest pain, palpitations, sweating, nausea, dizziness, dyspnea, and numbness. These symptoms usually last from 5 to 60 minutes. About 50% of patients with panic disorder also have associated agoraphobia, with fears of being in crowds or in places from which escape would be difficult. Diagnosis is based on clinical descriptors and setting, but care should be made to consider underlying medical disorders, such as cardiac disease, thyroid disease, or pheochromocytoma, particularly in patients at increased risk for one of these disorders. However, extensive testing is not necessary in most patients with a characteristic presentation and normal physical examination and basic laboratory studies. Treatment options for panic disorder include medication and psychotherapy. Cognitive-behavioral therapy (CBT) has been shown to be the most effective psychotherapeutic intervention in controlled trials. Selective serotonin reuptake inhibitors and serotonin-norepinephrine reuptake inhibitors have been shown to be effective. Panic disorder that is severe or refractory appears to be most amenable to the combination of CBT and pharmacotherapy compared with either treatment alone.

This patient has classic symptoms of panic disorder and no cardiac risk factors. It would be inappropriate to order further cardiac testing in the setting of a normal electrocardiogram and classic symptoms. This patient's symptoms are also atypical for gastroesophageal reflux disease, rendering empiric proton pump inhibitor therapy an incorrect choice.

- Panic disorder is characterized by sudden panic attacks with the acute onset of somatic symptoms, which may include chest pain, palpitations, sweating, nausea, dizziness, dyspnea, and numbness.

Bibliography

Work Group on Panic Disorder; American Psychiatric Association; Practice guideline for the treatment of patients with panic disorder. Am J Psychiatry. 1998;155(5 suppl):1-34. [PMID: 9585731]

Item 120   Answer: A

Educational Objective: Manage a patient with harmful alcohol use.

This patient is exhibiting harmful use of alcohol and should be counseled appropriately, including connecting her drinking habits with the negative consequences that she has recently experienced. Harmful drinking is drinking that causes physical or psychological harm. This patient's drinking has resulted in serious illness as well as an arrest for driving while intoxicated. Optimal management would include a discussion of appropriate amounts of alcohol, negative consequences, and agreement of goals for reducing alcohol intake. This should be performed in the setting of frequent follow-up and reassessment and should incorporate the patient's ideas about her drinking behaviors and ways to change them, barriers she may face in reducing her alcohol consumption, and previous experiences with attempting to stop or reduce her drinking.

Labeling a patient an alcoholic is neither productive nor a medically useful term. Goals of managing this patient may not require complete abstinence, and abstinence may be difficult for the patient to accomplish immediately.

Adjunct management strategies may include medications or referral to Alcoholics Anonymous or psychiatry, but these measures are more effective when done in combination with primary counseling.

The National Institute on Alcohol Abuse and Alcoholism defines at-risk drinking as more than 14 drinks per week or 4 drinks per occasion in men and more than 7 drinks per week or 3 drinks per occasion in women. However, harmful drinking is defined by consequences and not by the quantity consumed.

KEY POINT

- **Management of harmful drinking patterns includes counseling to help patients connect the negative consequences to their drinking, discussion of appropriate amounts of alcohol, and agreement of goals for reducing alcohol intake, performed in a patient-centered manner in a setting of frequent follow-up and reassessment.**

Bibliography

U.S. Preventive Services Task Force. Screening and behavioral counseling interventions in primary care to reduce alcohol misuse: recommendation statement. Ann Intern Med. 2004;140(7):554-556. [PMID: 15068984]

Item 121   Answer: B

Educational Objective: Manage a patient with suspected obstructive sleep apnea in the postoperative period.

This patient most likely has undiagnosed obstructive sleep apnea (OSA). OSA is a major risk factor for perioperative pulmonary complications, although a large number of patients in the community have unrecognized OSA. Patients with more than a negligible risk for OSA should be screened preoperatively. One instrument that may be used is the STOP-BANG questionnaire, a screen based on eight parameters: Snoring, Tired, Observed stopping breathing during sleep, high blood Pressure, BMI (>35), Age (>50 years), Neck circumference (>40 cm), and Gender (male). Patients with three or more positive responses have a high risk of OSA. Had he been screened, this patient would have scored at least 5 points (tiredness, hypertension, high BMI, age >50 years, male), and would have qualified for evaluation for possible OSA.

Although myocardial ischemia may lead to transient respiratory failure, this patient has a negative cardiac history, no chest pain, and a normal electrocardiogram, making this less likely than OSA.

Extubation following surgery is typically performed after careful assessment of stability following removal of sedating and paralyzing medications, with subsequent monitoring in a postanesthesia care unit. It is likely that he met criteria for extubation following his procedure, but patients with unrecognized OSA can develop acute respiratory failure induced by the sleep apnea combined with the respiratory depression caused by narcotics for postoperative analgesia and the lingering effects of anesthesia.

Sepsis can cause perioperative respiratory failure; however, patients with sepsis are typically febrile, hypotensive, and show evidence of a metabolic acidosis. The absence of any of these findings makes sepsis a less likely cause of his respiratory failure.

KEY POINT

- **Patients with more than a negligible risk for obstructive sleep apnea (OSA) should be screened preoperatively; those with three or more of the following parameters have a high risk of OSA: snoring, tired, observed stopping breathing during sleep, hypertension, BMI >35, age >50 years, neck circumference >40 cm, and male sex.**

Bibliography

Vasu TS, Doghramji K, Cavallazzi R, et al. Obstructive sleep apnea syndrome and postoperative complications: clinical use of the STOP-BANG questionnaire. Arch Otolaryngol Head Neck Surg. 2010;136(10):1020-1024. [PMID: 20956751]

Item 122   Answer: C

Educational Objective: Diagnose rotator cuff tendinitis.

This patient most likely has rotator cuff impingement syndrome from underlying tendinitis. She presented with pain in her shoulder that began after performing the repetitive overhead motion of painting, and her pain is most pronounced with abduction of her arm. On examination, her pain occurs between 60 and 120 degrees of abduction, which supports the diagnosis of rotator cuff tendinitis. She also has a positive Hawkins test, which has a high sensitivity (92%) but poor specificity (25%) for rotator cuff impingement.

Acromioclavicular joint degeneration is typically associated with trauma (in younger patients) or osteoarthritis (in older patients). Palpable osteophytes may be present, and radiographs, if obtained, may demonstrate degenerative changes. It characteristically presents with pain that occurs with shoulder adduction and abduction above 120 degrees. This diagnosis is unlikely in this patient given that she has no history of trauma and that there is no acromioclavicular joint tenderness on examination.

Adhesive capsulitis is caused by thickening of the capsule surrounding the glenohumeral joint. Adhesive capsulitis presents with loss of both passive and active range of motion in multiple planes and patient reports of stiffness, which are not present in this patient. Also, pain is typically slow in onset and is located near the insertion of the deltoid muscle.

Rotator cuff tears are usually accompanied by weakness and loss of function. Examination findings include supraspinatus weakness, weakness with external rotation, and a positive drop-arm test. The absence of weakness along with the negative drop-arm test argues against the presence of a rotator cuff tear in this patient.

KEY POINT

- **Rotator cuff impingement syndrome due to underlying tendinitis is a common cause of nontraumatic shoulder pain; characteristic findings are pain with arm abduction and a positive Hawkins test.**

Bibliography

House J, Mooradian A. Evaluation and management of shoulder pain in primary care clinics. South Med J. 2010;103(11):1129-1135. [PMID: 20890250]

Item 123   Answer: C
Educational Objective: Screen for HIV infection.

According to guidelines published by the Centers for Disease Control and Prevention (CDC), this man should be screened for HIV infection using enzyme immunoassay antibody (EIA) testing. The guidelines recommend that all persons between the ages of 13 and 64 years be screened for HIV infection. This recommendation is based on evidence from several studies that have demonstrated that screening for HIV is effective even in low-prevalence settings. This is particularly true when screening is coupled to the availability of antiretroviral therapy. All positive results using EIA testing should be confirmed by Western blot testing. Western blot testing should not be used as the initial screening test owing to its high rate of false-positive and false-negative results. In contrast to the CDC guidelines, the U.S. Preventive Services Task Force (USPSTF) assigns

a C grade to HIV screening, making no recommendation for or against routine HIV screening.

The National Cholesterol Education Program (NCEP) recommends that screening be initiated at the age of 20 years and then continued at least every 5 years thereafter if normal. This patient's lipid levels were normal 4 years ago; therefore, it would not be appropriate to screen him according to the NCEP guideline. The USPSTF recommends lipid screening for all men 35 years or older and for men 20 to 35 years of age with increased cardiovascular risk. Because this patient is not at increased risk for atherosclerotic heart disease, according to the USPSTF guidelines, screening for hyperlipidemia should begin at the age of 35 years.

The USPSTF recommends diabetes screening for all adults with a sustained blood pressure of 135/80 mm Hg or greater. In contrast, the American Diabetes Association recommends screening all adults who are 45 years and older and all adults who have a BMI of 25 or greater who have one or more additional risk factors (gestational diabetes, hypertension, hyperlipidemia, family history of type 2 diabetes mellitus in a first-degree relative). Screening for diabetes would be inappropriate in this patient owing to his age, absence of hypertension or obesity, and lack of other risk factors.

There is no agreement among major groups related to screening for hypothyroidism. The American Academy of Family Physicians and the American Association of Clinical Endocrinologists recommend screening for hypothyroidism in older women. The American Thyroid Association recommends screening adults by measuring thyroid-stimulating hormone (TSH) beginning at age 35 years, but the USPSTF does not recommend routine screening. This patient is not in a high-risk group defined by either age or sex, and screening for thyroid disease with a TSH level is not appropriate.

KEY POINT

- **The Centers for Disease Control and Prevention recommend that all persons between the ages of 13 and 64 years be screened for HIV infection.**

Bibliography

Qaseem A, Snow V, Shekelle P, Hopkins R Jr, Owens DK; Clinical Efficacy Assessment Subcommittee, American College of Physicians. Screening for HIV in health care settings: a guidance statement from the American College of Physicians and HIV Medicine Association. Ann Intern Med. 2009;150(2):125-131. [PMID: 19047022]

Item 124   Answer: A
Educational Objective: Manage an encounter with an impaired colleague.

In this situation, there is considerable evidence that the colleague's judgment is impaired by both the amount and rate

CONT.

of alcohol consumption and her response to an expression of concern. The ethical obligation is to prevent her from potentially harming a patient, which means contacting the hospital tonight.

Reporting to state authorities on Monday may help this physician and her future patients but would not protect the patient she is admitting tonight.

Taking her aside later is unlikely to be helpful, and puts the unimpaired physician in the position of monitoring whatever action she may take to address the issue.

Members of the medical profession have an obligation to protect the welfare of patients, which includes taking action when a colleague puts patients at risk. Many states have mandatory reporting statutes. Nevertheless, almost 75% of respondents in a 2009 survey did not believe they had a duty to report a known impaired colleague to the relevant authority, raising significant concerns about physicians' understanding of their personal and professional ethical obligations.

> **KEY POINT**
>
> - Members of the medical profession have an obligation to protect the welfare of patients, which includes taking action when a colleague puts patients at risk.

Bibliography

DesRoches CM, Rao SR, Fromson JA, et al. Physicians' perceptions, preparedness for reporting, and experiences related to impaired and incompetent colleagues. JAMA. 2010;304(2):187-193. [PMID: 20628132]

Item 125   Answer: D

Educational Objective: Manage a patient undergoing low-risk surgery.

This patient undergoing endoscopic sinus surgery should proceed to surgery without further testing. Patients undergoing low-risk surgery, which includes endoscopic surgery, cataract surgery, superficial surgery, breast surgery, and ambulatory surgery, do not need perioperative cardiac testing unless they have high-risk ("active") conditions such as an unstable coronary syndrome (myocardial infarction <30 days ago, unstable or severe angina), decompensated heart failure, significant arrhythmia, or severe valvular disease. Although this patient has three clinical risk factors (coronary artery disease, chronic kidney disease, diabetes mellitus requiring insulin) for a major perioperative cardiac complication, he does not require further cardiac testing because the anticipated surgery is low risk.

The use of β-blockers in the perioperative period is controversial, with well-designed randomized controlled trials showing both benefit and harm. Current recommendations are that patients currently on a β-blocker should continue taking it. Thus, metoprolol should not be discontinued.

Cardiac testing is reserved for patients undergoing surgery at the highest risk of a perioperative cardiac event as predicted by their Revised Cardiac Risk Index (clinical risk factors), exercise tolerance, and the nature of the proposed surgery. Patients with a low or unknown exercise tolerance who have three or more clinical risk factors undergoing intermediate- or higher-risk surgery should be considered for preoperative cardiac testing if it will change management; however, in this patient who is undergoing low-risk surgery, no testing is needed.

Percutaneous cardiac interventions have no demonstrated value in the perioperative setting. Thus, perioperative cardiac risk assessment, if needed, should be done through noninvasive stress testing. In general, the overriding theme of perioperative cardiac risk assessment is that testing should only be done if the results will affect management, and prophylactic revascularization is rarely necessary just to get a patient through surgery. This patient has no indications for cardiac catheterization.

> **KEY POINT**
>
> - In patients without active cardiac conditions undergoing low-risk surgery, preoperative cardiovascular testing is not routinely needed.

Bibliography

Fleisher LA, Beckman JA, Brown KA, et al. 2009 ACCF/AHA focused update on perioperative beta blockade incorporated into the ACC/AHA 2007 guidelines on perioperative cardiovascular evaluation and care for noncardiac surgery: a report of the American College of Cardiology Foundation/American Heart Association Task Force on Practice Guidelines. Circulation. 2009;120(21):e169-276. [PMID: 19884473]

Item 126   Answer: C

Educational Objective: Manage a patient who is a victim of intimate partner violence.

The primary responsibility of the provider for a patient who is a victim of intimate partner violence is to assist with health; assess for safety; and provide validation, support, and empathy.

Leaving the abuser is neither necessary nor recommended without a well thought-out plan unless the patient is in imminent danger, in which case immediate intervention is indicated. Advising victims of intimate partner violence to simply leave the situation, to utilize a shelter, contact an intimate partner violence counseling service, or press criminal charges is generally not helpful as the circumstances surrounding intimate partner abuse relationships are complex, and the abused individual may have significant reasons for not pursuing these actions that need to be understood. An appreciation of the individual circumstances in the context of a supportive relationship will help in developing a plan that may ultimately involve the use of these valuable resources.

It is not recommended that the potential abuser be confronted directly or legal action be undertaken as an initial step in most cases as this may potentially put the victim in greater danger.

Psychiatry intervention may be necessary for refractory depression, or when the patient is deemed a risk to harm herself or others. However, this would not be an appropriate next step in management of this patient.

A substantial number of patients remain in adverse relationships yet demonstrate improved health and health outcomes after disclosure of their situation with appropriate support and management.

KEY POINT

- The primary responsibility of the provider for a patient who is a victim of intimate partner violence is to assist with health; assess for safety; and provide validation, support, and empathy.

Bibliography
Zolotor AJ, Denham AC, Weil A. Intimate partner violence. Prim Care. 2009;36(1):167-179. [PMID: 19231608]

Item 127   Answer: A

Educational Objective: Evaluate a randomized controlled trial for generalizability.

This patient with cardiomyopathy is asymptomatic, placing her in the category of New York Heart Association (NYHA) functional class I heart failure. Therefore, her heart failure is too mild for her to take drug H, which was tested on patients with NYHA class III and IV heart failure.

Randomized controlled trials (RCTs) are often considered the "gold standard" for evaluating new therapies because their experimental design allows confounding variables that might obscure the benefit of a therapy to be balanced between groups. Thus, any finding in a well-designed RCT is typically considered valid. In order to maximize the ability of a given study to find a meaningful result, RCTs are typically restricted to relatively homogeneous individuals who meet rigidly defined inclusion and exclusion criteria. The proscribed nature of patient selection and intervention in RCTs therefore make their conclusions narrow. Clinicians must use caution when generalizing these results to other populations. Drug H was shown to be effective for patients with NYHA class III or IV heart failure, and it may not be effective for a patient with more mild heart failure, such as this patient.

Although the mean age of participants in the trial was 63 years, the drug was tested on patients between the ages of 40 and 80 years. Thus, based on her age, the patient would have been eligible for the trial, and age alone is not a reason to withhold the drug from her.

Despite rigid criteria for inclusion and exclusion in a RCT, there will still likely be some variability between individual patients included in a particular study, such as concurrent medications being used. Even with these differences, however, a net benefit of treatment was found in the study population. Although most patients in the study were already on a β-blocker, it cannot be inferred from the

study whether this treatment is required to see the benefit of drug H.

There is no arbitrary level of risk of harm that would impact a decision to use a medication; rather, each medication should be evaluated according to its risk and benefit profile. Furthermore, in this trial, drug H had net benefit despite its rate of serious adverse events.

KEY POINT

- Caution should be used when generalizing the results of randomized controlled trials to populations other than those who would meet the inclusion and exclusion criteria of the study.

Bibliography
Ho PM, Peterson PN, Masoudi FA. Evaluating the evidence: is there a rigid hierarchy? Circulation. 2008;118(16):1675-1684. [PMID: 18852378]

Item 128   Answer: A

Educational Objective: Diagnose an autism spectrum disorder.

The diagnosis is autism spectrum disorder. Autism is characterized by a triad of impaired communication; impaired social interactions; and restrictive, repetitive, and stereotyped behaviors and interests. In addition, classic autism is often associated with some degree of learning disability or mental retardation and is typically diagnosed in early childhood. Less severe variants include high-functioning autism (HFA) and Asperger syndrome, which may not be diagnosed until adolescence or even adulthood. HFA is a category of autistic disorder with less severe clinical features and without cognitive impairment. Asperger syndrome differs from HFA in that early language development is not delayed. Many experts believe that autism, HFA, and Asperger syndrome are variants along a single spectrum.

The hallmark of obsessive-compulsive disorder is the presence of recurrent obsessions or compulsions that are of sufficient severity to occupy at least 1 hour per day or to result in marked distress or functional impairment. The person should recognize that the obsessions or compulsions are excessive or unreasonable. Obsessions are defined as persistent ideas, thoughts, impulses, or images that are experienced as intrusive, inappropriate, and associated with significant anxiety or distress. This patient has compulsions but has additional symptoms not characteristic of obsessive-compulsive disorder.

Schizophrenia is defined by the presence of psychosis. Psychosis encompasses delusions, hallucinations, disorganized speech, and disorganized or catatonic behavior. The diagnosis requires at least 6 months of symptoms, including 1 month or more of at least two active-phase symptoms, such as hallucinations, delusions, disorganized speech, grossly disorganized or catatonic behavior; and negative symptoms, such as flattened affect. There must also be significant impairment in social or occupational function. This patient's symptoms are not consistent with schizophrenia.

The primary feature of social anxiety disorder is a severe and persistent fear of social or performance situations, such as public speaking or taking an examination. Persons with more generalized social anxiety disorder avoid many occupational and social situations because of fears of interacting with other people. This patient's symptoms of emotional outbursts, echolalia, and stereotyped interest in trains do not suggest social anxiety disorder.

KEY POINT

- Autism is characterized by a triad of impaired communication; impaired social interactions; and restrictive, repetitive, and stereotyped behaviors and interests.

Bibliography
Rao S, Salmon G. Autism spectrum disorders. Br J Hosp Med (Lond). 2010;71(12):699-703. [PMID: 21135768]

Item 129   Answer: E
Educational Objective: Select an appropriate vaccination strategy for an HIV-positive patient.

A CD4 cell count should be obtained in this patient before any vaccines are administered. This woman is entering school to become a certified nursing assistant; all health care workers should be vaccinated against or have serologic evidence of immunity to hepatitis B, varicella, measles, mumps, and rubella. In addition, health care workers should receive a one-time tetanus, diphtheria, and acellular pertussis (Tdap) vaccine as well as annual influenza vaccination. In general, vaccines can either be inactivated viral proteins or live attenuated viruses. Inactivated viral proteins are safe to administer in all patients, including those with HIV infection, except those with a documented allergy to the vaccine or its growth media (such as eggs). Live attenuated vaccines, on the other hand, should be withheld in patients with immune deficiency, including HIV-positive patients with a CD4 cell count below 200/microliter. Therefore, before administering any vaccines, however, it is important to determine whether or not she is functionally immunodeficient.

The measles, mumps, and rubella vaccine contains live, attenuated virus, and for this patient, it would be inappropriate to administer it before verifying that she is immunocompetent and also that she needs revaccination (based on negative serologic studies).

Live, attenuated influenza vaccine should be avoided in patients with immunodeficiency. Regardless of her CD4 cell count, the inactivated influenza vaccine would likely be preferred for this patient.

Hepatitis B vaccination is indicated in health care workers and in HIV-positive patients, as well as in patients with unknown hepatitis B status for whom hepatitis B vaccination is needed. As for other vaccines, it would be best to determine this patient's immune status before providing the vaccine.

Persons born after 1980, health care workers, and those born before 1980 who have a high risk for disseminated varicella should receive a two-dose varicella vaccination series unless they have serologic evidence of varicella immunity or physician-documented evidence of either varicella or varicella vaccination. Patient or parent self-report is not considered reliable.

KEY POINT

- In patients who are HIV-positive, CD4 cell counts should be obtained before administering live attenuated vaccines.

Bibliography
Advisory Committee on Immunization Practices; Centers for Disease Control and Prevention (CDC). Immunization of health-care personnel: recommendations of the Advisory Committee on Immunization Practices (ACIP). MMWR Recomm Rep. 2011;60(RR-7):1-45. [PMID: 22108587]

Item 130   Answer: C
Educational Objective: Diagnose costochondritis.

This patient most likely has costochondritis. The etiology of chest pain can be determined in most cases after a careful history and physical examination. Musculoskeletal chest pain has an insidious onset and may last for hours to weeks. It is most recognizable when sharp and localized to a specific area of the chest; however, it can also be poorly localized. The pain may be worsened by turning, deep breathing, or arm movement. Chest pain may or may not be reproducible by chest palpation (pain reproduced by palpation does not exclude ischemic heart disease), and the cardiovascular examination is often normal. Importantly, his findings are not consistent with an alternative cause of chest pain.

The chest pain associated with acute pericarditis is typically pleuritic in nature and is worsened when the patient lies down. A two- or three-component friction rub is often present. This patient does not have any risk factors for pericarditis; specifically, there is no history of recent viral infection, myocardial infarction, trauma, malignancy, medications, connective tissue disease, or uremia. Pericarditis, therefore, is highly unlikely.

Aortic dissection is generally described as a tearing or ripping pain with radiation to the back. It is more commonly seen in patients with a history of hypertension. Although physical examination findings may be missed, asymmetric intensity of peripheral pulses has a positive likelihood ratio of 5.7. This patient's chest pain description, physical examination, and absence of risk factors are inconsistent with aortic dissection.

This patient has no risk factors for cardiac disease. His history is inconsistent with descriptors that increase the probability of ischemic chest pain, including unstable angina. Specifically, there is no radiation to the arms, exertional component, relief with rest, diaphoresis, nausea, vomiting, or pressure description. Considering the patient's age and description of his chest pain, the probability of unstable angina or an acute coronary syndrome is low.

KEY POINT

- **Musculoskeletal chest pain has an insidious onset and may last for hours to weeks; it is most recognizable when sharp and localized to a specific area of the chest; and the pain may be worsened by turning, deep breathing, or arm movement.**

Bibliography

Stochkendahl MJ, Christensen HW. Chest pain in focal musculoskeletal disorders. Med Clin North Am. 2010;94(2):259-273. [PMID: 20380955]

Item 131 Answer: C

Educational Objective: Manage primary dysmenorrhea.

The most appropriate management option for this patient is a trial of NSAID therapy, such as ibuprofen. This patient has dysmenorrhea associated with normal menstrual cycles and no pelvic pathology. Initial treatment options for primary dysmenorrhea include NSAIDs and cyclooxygenase-2 inhibitors, which inhibit the inflammation, vasoconstriction, and uterine ischemia that are thought to cause the symptoms.

If symptoms are not relieved with NSAID therapy or the patient requests contraception or is sexually active, a combination estrogen-progesterone contraceptive would be appropriate. Extended-cycle formulations are particularly useful for this indication.

Depot medroxyprogesterone acetate (DMPA) is a long-acting progesterone compound, administered intramuscularly or subcutaneously every 12 to 14 weeks. Long-acting progesterone therapy is a treatment option for dysmenorrhea, and also provides contraception. For adolescents and young adults, however, long-term use of progesterone therapy decreases bone mineral density owing to prolonged estrogen deficiency. Therefore, such treatment should be used with caution for dysmenorrhea or for contraception in younger women based on the risks and benefits of treatment in a given patient. In general, NSAIDs should be tried before hormonal therapy.

In the absence of worrisome symptoms such as severe pelvic pain or significant bleeding abnormalities, treatment for dysmenorrhea may be initiated without further evaluation, such as pelvic imaging, hormonal testing, or gynecologic referral.

KEY POINT

- **The first-line treatment for primary dysmenorrhea is NSAID therapy.**

Bibliography

Harel Z. Dysmenorrhea in adolescents and young adults: from pathophysiology to pharmacological treatment and management strategies. Expert Opin Pharmacother. 2008;9(15):2661-2672. [PMID: 18803452]

Item 132 Answer: D

Educational Objective: Diagnose ulnar nerve entrapment at the level of the elbow.

This patient's presentation is consistent with ulnar nerve entrapment at the elbow (cubital tunnel syndrome). The cubital tunnel is the path followed by the ulnar nerve as it passes around the elbow toward the hand. In this region, the nerve is near the surface of the skin and therefore susceptible to injury. Injury may occur from mild and often unrecognized trauma, sustained pressure on the nerve as may occur during sleep, or activities that involve sustained flexion of the elbow and stretching of the nerve. Diagnostically, maneuvers that compress or stretch the injured nerve, such as flexing the arm (as seen in this patient), result in elbow pain. Paresthesias are also commonly present in the ulnar nerve distribution in the hand. These paresthesias are characteristically located on both the palmar and dorsal surfaces of the hand, which contrasts with entrapment of the ulnar nerve at the wrist, which only involves the palmar surface.

Patients with lateral epicondylitis (tennis elbow) typically present with pain in the lateral elbow that radiates down the forearm to the dorsal hand. On examination, there is tenderness to palpation at the location of the insertion of extensor muscles on the lateral epicondyle. Pain is reproduced by forced extension of the wrist.

Patients with medial epicondylitis (golfer's elbow) typically present with pain in the medial elbow and proximal forearm. On examination, there is tenderness to palpation from the medial epicondyle to the pronator teres and flexor carpi radialis muscles. Pain can be reproduced with wrist flexion and resisted forearm supination.

Olecranon bursitis is characterized by pain in the posterior elbow and swelling of the bursal sac that overlies the olecranon process. Range of motion of the elbow is not limited.

KEY POINT

- **Ulnar nerve entrapment at the elbow is characterized by pain that occurs with flexion of the arm and paresthesias on both the palmar and dorsal surfaces of the hand, in the distribution of the ulnar nerve.**

Bibliography

Caliendro P, La Torre G, Padua R, Giannini F, Padua L. Treatment for ulnar neuropathy at the elbow. Cochrane Database Syst Rev. 2011;(2):CD006839. [PMID: 21328287]

Item 133 Answer: D

Educational Objective: Understand the principles of informed consent.

The principles of informed consent were not followed in this case. The three key elements of informed consent are: understanding of the proposed treatment, understanding of alternatives to the proposed treatment, and understanding the risks and benefits of both the treatment and the alternatives. In this case, the patient says he was not given either information about risks of antibiotics or alternative options. This calls into question whether he received adequate information to give informed consent.

Informed consent applies to all health care decisions, not only to invasive procedures. It requires an active dialogue around the three key elements.

Many practitioners obtain written informed consent for invasive procedures because this entails documentation of consent, but it does not exempt physicians from having a discussion of risks, benefits, and alternatives for all treatments that have the potential to cause harm.

KEY POINT

- The three key elements of informed consent are: understanding of the proposed treatment, understanding of alternatives to the proposed treatment, and understanding the risks and benefits of both the treatment and the alternatives.

Bibliography

Snyder L; American College of Physicians Ethics, Professionalism, and Human Rights Committee. American College of Physicians Ethics Manual: sixth edition. Ann Intern Med. 2012;156(1 Pt 2):73-104. [PMID: 22213573]

Item 134   Answer: D
Educational Objective: Treat chronic cervical radiculopathy with neurologic deficits.

This patient should be referred for surgical evaluation. He has clinical and imaging evidence of cervical radiculopathy, and progressive weakness in the affected arm that correlates with his disk herniation. Surgical intervention is generally indicated in patients with progressive neurologic symptoms resulting from a defined anatomic abnormality to preserve and avoid permanent loss of function.

In the absence of progressive motor deficits, a conservative approach is indicated as most patients experience improvement in symptoms without more aggressive imaging or intervention. Local corticosteroid injections may provide faster pain relief, although long-term outcomes are similar to conservative therapy. Physical therapy is also a useful intervention in patients with uncomplicated cervical radiculopathy to decrease discomfort and possibly strengthen the neck muscles to prevent recurrent episodes. However, these interventions, including continued analgesics and rest, would not be appropriate in this patient with worsening neurologic function.

KEY POINT

- Surgical referral is indicated for patients with cervical radiculopathy with progressive motor deficits.

Bibliography

Nikolaidis I, Fouyas IP, Sandercock PA, Statham PF. Surgery for cervical radiculopathy or myelopathy. Cochrane Database Syst Rev. 2010;(1):CD001466. [PMID: 20091520]

Item 135   Answer: B
Educational Objective: Diagnose interstitial cystitis as a cause of chronic pelvic pain.

This most likely diagnosis in this patient with chronic pelvic pain is interstitial cystitis. Chronic pelvic pain is defined as noncyclic pain of at least 6 months' duration that localizes to the anatomic pelvis, the anterior abdominal wall at or below the umbilicus, the lumbosacral back, or the buttocks, and is of sufficient severity to impair quality of life. Potential causes of chronic pelvic pain include interstitial cystitis, endometriosis, pelvic adhesions, and irritable bowel syndrome. In this patient, the combination of chronic pelvic pain in association with unexplained urinary symptoms is most consistent with a diagnosis of interstitial cystitis. Interstitial cystitis is a chronic inflammatory condition of the bladder that causes symptoms of urinary urgency, frequency, and pelvic discomfort. The pelvic discomfort may be worsened by sexual intercourse, and patients may urinate numerous times per day. Although urinalysis and urine cultures are almost always negative, most women with interstitial cystitis have been treated empirically several times for urinary tract infections.

Endometriosis is a common cause of chronic pelvic pain, and patients typically report severe dysmenorrhea, cyclic pain, and dyspareunia. The absence of severe dysmenorrhea and the noncyclic nature of this patient's pelvic pain make endometriosis a less likely diagnosis. Similarly, irritable bowel syndrome is unlikely to explain her symptoms in the absence of any associated gastrointestinal symptoms.

Adhesions are diagnosed in 25% to 50% of women with chronic pelvic pain. Pelvic adhesions typically form in the setting of acute or chronic inflammatory processes, such as infection, or surgery. This patient has no history of pelvic infection and has never had pelvic surgery, making this an unlikely cause of her symptoms.

KEY POINT

- Interstitial cystitis is a likely diagnosis in women with chronic pelvic pain associated with unexplained urinary symptoms; most women with interstitial cystitis have been treated empirically several times for urinary tract infections.

Bibliography

Vercellini P, Somigliana E, Viganò P, Abbiati A, Barbara G, Fedele L. Chronic pelvic pain in women: etiology, pathogenesis, and diagnostic approach. Gynecol Endocrinol. 2009;25(3):149-158. [PMID: 19347704]

Item 136   Answer: D

Educational Objective: Treat chronic neuropathic pain with opioid therapy.

Long-acting opioid therapy, such as sustained-release morphine, would be the best treatment option in this patient. Although opioid medications are generally not recommended for use in patients with chronic noncancer pain, they are appropriately considered in patients with moderate to severe neuropathic pain that has not responded to adequate trials of multiple nonopioid therapies. As with all patients being considered for long-term opioid treatment, he should have a thorough understanding of its risks and benefits and should work together with the physician to develop an opioid management plan, or pain contract, that outlines agreed-upon goals and rules of treatment.

Long-acting opioids provide more consistent serum drug levels and are generally preferred to intermittent dosing of shorter-acting agents that may lead to significant fluctuations in pain level. Although this patient's pain is reasonably well controlled on his current regimen of oxycodone-acetaminophen, it is also a short-acting preparation and is less desirable for long-term use. When used chronically, the overall daily dose of acetaminophen needs to be taken into account; daily doses should be below 4 g and less in patients with liver disease, significant alcohol use, or those being treated with other potentially hepatotoxic medications.

Tramadol is a weak opioid agonist and may be effective for mild, episodic neuropathic pain, although it may require a relatively high daily dose with an increased risk of associated side effects, such as gastrointestinal symptoms. It also has a short period of action and requires multiple daily dosing, which would not be preferable in this patient.

Methadone is a long-acting opioid that can be very effective for pain control but can be associated with significant adverse cardiovascular outcomes, such as QT-interval prolongation, hypotension, and cardiac arrhythmias. It should be avoided in this patient with a history of ischemic cardiomyopathy and conduction defects noted on the electrocardiogram.

> **KEY POINT**
> • Long-acting opioid therapy should be considered in a patient with moderate to severe neuropathic pain that has not responded to nonopioid therapies.

Bibliography

Bril V, England J, Franklin GM, et al; American Academy of Neurology; American Association of Neuromuscular and Electrodiagnostic Medicine; American Academy of Physical Medicine and Rehabilitation. Evidence-based guideline: Treatment of painful diabetic neuropathy: report of the American Academy of Neurology, the American Association of Neuromuscular and Electrodiagnostic Medicine, and the American Academy of Physical Medicine and Rehabilitation. Neurology. 2011;76:1758-1765. [PMID: 21482920]

Item 137   Answer: B

Educational Objective: Diagnose complicated grief.

This patient is likely suffering from complicated grief stemming from his wife's death 9 months ago. Complicated grief, also referred to as complicated bereavement, is an abnormal response to bereavement persisting more than 6 months, at least 6 months after a death. Its chief symptom is yearning for a loved one so intensely that all other desires are incapacitated. Although interventions have been attempted to prevent this severe grief reaction, none have proved beneficial. It is important for health care providers to be watchful for this disorder in bereaved survivors.

Drugs with the potential for anticholinergic adverse effects, such as diphenhydramine, are generally not a good choice in the elderly. Although the anticholinergic properties of diphenhydramine could be responsible for acute confusion and hallucinations, this patient's persistent symptoms, such as anhedonia and early morning wakening, would not be explained by such a short-acting agent.

Generalized anxiety disorder is characterized by excessive anxiety and worry about a variety of events or activities over at least a 6-month period; difficulty exercising control over worrying; several symptoms associated with the anxiety, such as fatigue, irritability, restlessness, sleep disturbance, and difficulty concentrating; and functional impairment. Although an anxiety disorder should also be considered in the differential diagnosis of this patient given his sleep disturbance, his lack of excessive anxiety and worry make it less likely.

Although this patient could also have major depression, his intense feelings that his wife is beside him are more indicative of complicated grief marked by an unwillingness to accept her death. His sense that his wife is beside him when he wakes up in the middle of the night and his visions of his wife's face when he closes his eyes are not consistent with hallucinations because the patient is aware that they are not real. Patients with true psychosis are convinced their hallucinations and delusions are real.

> **KEY POINT**
> • Complicated grief is grief persisting more than 6 months, at least 6 months after a death; its chief symptom is yearning for a loved one so intensely that all other desires are incapacitated.

Bibliography

Wittouck C, Van Autreve S, De Jaegere E, Portzky G, van Heeringen K. The prevention and treatment of complicated grief: a meta-analysis. Clin Psychol Rev. 2011;31(1):69-78. [PMID: 21130937]

Item 138   Answer: D

Educational Objective: Diagnose rhinitis medicamentosa.

This patient most likely has rhinitis medicamentosa. The key clue in this patient's presentation is ongoing use of a topical nasal vasoconstrictor (oxymetazoline). In some patients, this produces a syndrome of tolerance (rhinitis medicamentosa) in which continued use of the vasoconstrictor produces diminishing returns, but withdrawal of it causes severe nasal congestion. Withdrawal of the offending agent is the only reliable way to treat this condition. Sometimes, use of nasal corticosteroids or nasal saline rinses can mitigate symptoms of decongestant withdrawal.

A 2011 trial randomized 60 patients with perennial allergic rhinitis to fluticasone, oxymetazoline, a combination of both agents, and placebo. After 4 weeks of treatment, no evidence of rhinitis medicamentosa was seen in either of the oxymetazoline-treated groups, raising the possibility that rhinitis medicamentosa is much less common than previously thought.

Chronic rhinosinusitis is characterized by mucopurulent drainage or facial pain or pressure typical of sinusitis. In the absence of these findings and the presence of ongoing oxymetazoline use, rhinitis medicamentosa is the more likely diagnosis.

Chronic nonallergic (vasomotor) rhinitis is a syndrome characterized by the presence of at least one typical symptom of rhinitis (sneezing, rhinorrhea, nasal congestion, postnasal drainage) in the absence of a specific etiology. Chronic nonallergic rhinitis is a possibility in this patient, but the diagnosis cannot be made until the oxymetazoline is stopped.

Granulomatosis with polyangiitis (Wegener granulomatosis) is a necrotizing vasculitis that typically affects the respiratory tract and the kidneys. More than 70% of patients present with upper airway symptoms, particularly sinusitis. Up to 90% of patients have pulmonary manifestations that can include cough, hemoptysis, or pleurisy. The patient's findings are not consistent with granulomatosis with polyangiitis.

KEY POINT

- Ongoing use of a topical nasal vasoconstrictor may cause rhinitis medicamentosa, in which continued use of the vasoconstrictor produces diminishing returns, but withdrawal of it causes severe nasal congestion.

Bibliography

Doshi J. Rhinitis medicamentosa: what an otorhinolaryngologist needs to know. Eur Arch Otorhinolaryngol. 2009;266(5):623-625. [PMID: 19096862]

Item 139   Answer: C
Educational Objective: Manage cyclical mastalgia.

This patient has cyclical mastalgia, which affects up to 40% of premenopausal women. It is most prominent during the luteal phase of the menstrual cycle and is typically described as a bilateral, throbbing discomfort. Education, reassurance, and the use of a well-fitting bra are recommended for all women with cyclical mastalgia, and 20% of patients will experience resolution of their pain without any intervention. This patient has recently increased her level of physical activity, and lack of a supportive sports bra may have exacerbated her discomfort.

Medical treatment is typically reserved for women who have severe and persistent pain that interferes with their quality of life. Danazol is the only treatment that has been approved by the FDA for cyclical mastalgia, although it would not be appropriate in this patient without a trial of nonmedical therapy.

A thorough history and physical examination are typically sufficient to rule out more serious causes of breast discomfort. A patient can be diagnosed with benign mastalgia if there is no evidence of extramammary causes of breast discomfort, such as pneumonia, pleuritis, myocardial ischemia, infection, or costochondritis. In the absence of a palpable breast mass or skin changes suggestive of malignancy, there is no role for diagnostic mammography in the management of cyclical mastalgia.

Tamoxifen has been used off-label for treatment of benign mastalgia, and rarely can be associated with hot flushes and menstrual irregularities. It could be considered for this patient, but only if she does not benefit from conservative measures, including use of a well-fitting bra.

KEY POINT

- Conservative measures, including education, reassurance, and the use of a well-fitting support bra, are recommended for all women with cyclical mastalgia and should be tried before initiating medical treatment.

Bibliography

Miltenburg DM, Speights VO Jr. Benign breast disease. Obstet Gynecol Clin North Am. 2008;35(2):285-300, ix. [PMID: 18486842]

Item 140   Answer: B
Educational Objective: Treat a depressive episode of bipolar disorder.

The most appropriate treatment for this patient is lamotrigine. He most likely is having a depressive episode of bipolar disorder. Careful questioning of patients who present with depressive symptoms to elucidate a history of hypomanic or manic episodes is important in order to identify bipolar disorder. The Mood Disorders Questionnaire (MDQ) is a relatively brief, validated questionnaire to screen for bipolar disorder. A cut-off of seven or more positive responses out of the thirteen items on question 1 yields a sensitivity of 73% and specificity of 90%. Pharmacotherapy for bipolar disorder is more complicated than for unipolar depression, and a psychiatrist should be involved in the care of most patients with the disorder. Lithium has long been a mainstay of bipolar disorder therapy; however, it has a narrow therapeutic window and is teratogenic, nephrotoxic, and can cause hypothyroidism. Alternative first-line therapies include mood stabilizing agents, such as lamotrigine, valproic acid, or carbamazepine. In addition, atypical antipsychotic agents, such as aripiprazole or quetiapine, can be used for frank mania. Simply prescribing antidepressants alone places the patient at risk for experiencing a frank manic episode.

Duloxetine, a serotonin-norepinephrine reuptake inhibitor, is an appropriate therapy for the treatment of depressive disorders. Most classes of antidepressants have equal efficacy (about 70% in most studies) and should be chosen on the basis of previous patient response, side-effect profile, and cost. This patient has bipolar disorder, and an antidepressant alone would not be the appropriate treatment.

Benzodiazepines, such as lorazepam, are ineffective single agents for depression or bipolar disorder, but may be used as an adjunct therapy in patients with mania or hypomania. This patient is having a depressive episode, and there is no role for lorazepam in treating his condition.

Selective serotonin reuptake inhibitors (SSRIs), such as sertraline, may trigger a manic episode in patients with bipolar disease and should not be used in this population. For this reason, in any patient being considered for initiation of SSRIs for depression, it is important that the history be assessed for manic symptoms.

KEY POINT

- **In patients with depressive symptoms, it is important to elucidate a history of hypomanic or manic episodes in order to identify bipolar disorder, which is treated with mood stabilizers rather than antidepressants.**

Bibliography

Belmaker RH. Treatment of bipolar depression. N Engl J Med. 2007;356(17):1771-1773. [PMID: 17392296]

Item 141   Answer: D

Educational Objective: Diagnose secondary causes of dyslipidemia.

This patient's serum thyroid-stimulating hormone level should be measured. Her total cholesterol and LDL cholesterol levels are markedly elevated despite adherence to treatment with simvastatin. Secondary causes of dyslipidemia should be considered, as statin therapy may be ineffective in the setting of untreated hypothyroidism, diabetes mellitus, obstructive liver disease, or nephrotic syndrome. There are several clinical clues that suggest the diagnosis of hypothyroidism in this patient, including symptoms of fatigue and constipation and dry skin noted on physical examination. Undiagnosed thyroid disease is likely contributing to this patient's apparent treatment-refractory dyslipidemia.

Gemfibrozil is a fibric acid derivative that is typically used for the treatment of hypertriglyceridemia. Adding gemfibrozil to this patient's regimen will likely reduce her triglyceride levels by up to 50%, but will not substantially decrease her LDL cholesterol (typical reductions of 5%-20%). Moreover, gemfibrozil raises the serum concentration of statins by two-fold, thereby increasing the risk for statin-induced myopathy. The risks adding gemfibrozil to her statin therapy, therefore, outweigh the benefits for this patient.

A review of data from several large clinical trials found that the risk of myopathy with the 80-mg dose of simvastatin was significantly higher than the risk observed with other statin therapies. In patients who have not achieved goal LDL cholesterol levels with a 40-mg dose of simvastatin, the FDA has now recommended that therapy be switched to atorvastatin or rosuvastatin. These statins are more potent and can achieve LDL cholesterol goals at lower doses, thereby decreasing the risk for statin-induced myopathy. Increasing the simvastatin dose to 80 mg/d, therefore, is inappropriate for this patient's management.

Undiagnosed diabetes mellitus should be considered in patients with unresponsive hyperlipidemia and may be diagnosed by a hemoglobin A_{1c} level of 6.5% or greater. In this patient, her fasting glucose and triglyceride levels are normal, making a diagnosis of diabetes less likely; therefore, obtaining a hemoglobin A_{1c} level would not be an appropriate next step in management.

KEY POINT

- **In patients with hyperlipidemia that is refractory to medical therapy, secondary causes, including hypothyroidism, diabetes mellitus, nephrotic syndrome, and obstructive liver disease, should be considered.**

Bibliography

Alwaili K, Alrasadi K, Awan Z, Genest J. Approach to the diagnosis and management of lipoprotein disorders. Curr Opin Endocrinol Diabetes Obes. 2009;16(2):132-140. [PMID: 19306526]

Item 142   Answer: D

Educational Objective: Manage warfarin perioperatively in a high-risk patient.

For this patient with a high risk for a perioperative thromboembolic event, the most appropriate treatment is to discontinue warfarin 5 days before surgery and provide bridging anticoagulation with a low-molecular-weight heparin (LMWH), such as enoxaparin, until the morning of surgery. In general, patients using warfarin have three possible preoperative treatment options: stop warfarin, receive bridging therapy with a parenteral anticoagulant, or continue the warfarin. This patient has atrial fibrillation with a high $CHADS_2$ score (1 point each for diabetes mellitus, heart failure, and hypertension, and 2 points for previous stroke or transient ischemic attack [TIA] = 5) and her TIA is recent, placing her at a high risk for thrombosis; such patients should not have anticoagulation withheld for a prolonged period of time. Thus, warfarin should be changed to an agent with a shorter and more predictable half-life, usually LMWH. This agent is then withheld just before surgery and restarted after surgery, thus minimizing the amount of time the patient is not therapeutically anticoagulated.

The effect of dose adjustment of warfarin on INR is hard to predict. Thus, it would be inappropriate to recommend a fixed half dose of warfarin. This may result in an inappropriately high INR level for surgery (as would continuing the current dose of warfarin up to surgery) or a prolonged period of time with an inadequate INR, putting the patient at risk for thromboembolism.

In patients taking warfarin who have a low risk of thromboembolism, including those with a history of venous thromboembolism more than 12 months ago and those with atrial fibrillation with a CHADS$_2$ score of 2 or less, stopping warfarin without providing bridging anticoagulation is acceptable. However, this patient's CHADS$_2$ score is 5, and withholding anticoagulation for 5 days preoperatively is not recommended.

KEY POINT

• Patients taking warfarin who are at high risk of postoperative venous thromboembolism and are undergoing intermediate- or high-risk surgery should have warfarin discontinued 5 days before surgery and receive bridging anticoagulation, usually with low-molecular-weight heparin.

Bibliography

Douketis JD, Spyropoulos AC, Spencer FA, et al; American College of Chest Physicians. Perioperative management of antithrombotic therapy: Antithrombotic Therapy and Prevention of Thrombosis, 9th ed: American College of Chest Physicians Evidence-Based Clinical Practice Guidelines. Chest. 2012;141(2 suppl):e326S-e50S. [PMID: 22315266]

Item 143   Answer: C
Educational Objective: Treat anorexia nervosa.

The most appropriate treatment for this patient with anorexia nervosa is cognitive-behavioral therapy (CBT). Anorexia nervosa is characterized by an abnormally low body weight (<85% of expected) in association with a fear of gaining weight, an excessive emphasis of body weight on self-perception, and amenorrhea for at least three menstrual cycles. Overall recovery rates range from 35% to 85%, and many patients relapse. The goals of treatment are to restore healthy weight, treat physical and metabolic complications, address abnormal attitudes and feelings related to eating, and treat associated psychiatric conditions. Behavioral interventions include CBT, cognitive analytic therapy, and family therapy; among these, CBT appears to be the most effective for reducing relapse after weight restoration has been initiated.

Antidepressants, when used as monotherapy for anorexia nervosa, have not been shown to increase weight gain or improve the underlying attitudes or behaviors associated with anorexia nervosa. In particular, amitriptyline and bupropion should be avoided in patients with anorexia nervosa because of the high risk of adverse effects of these agents when given in the setting of metabolic derangements, which are common in this patient population.

Megestrol acetate is an appetite stimulant that is approved for palliative treatment of patients with cancer and AIDS complicated by anorexia and significant weight loss. It is not approved for patients with anorexia nervosa and has not been studied in this population.

Amenorrhea is a diagnostic criterion for anorexia nervosa, and oral contraceptive pills will restore menses. However, there are no convincing data to support this practice, and restoration of menses through hormonal manipulation may decrease a patient's motivation for weight gain.

KEY POINT

• In patients with anorexia nervosa, cognitive-behavioral therapy can be effective for reducing relapse after weight restoration has been initiated.

Bibliography

Bulik CM, Berkman ND, Brownley KA, Sedway JA, Lohr KN. Anorexia nervosa treatment: a systematic review of randomized controlled trials. Int J Eat Disord. 2007;40(4):310-320. [PMID: 17370290]

Item 144   Answer: A
Educational Objective: Treat chronic pain in an elderly patient.

Acetaminophen is the best medication for the initial treatment of this patient's chronic pain secondary to spinal stenosis, and is recommended as first-line therapy for chronic noncancer pain by the American Geriatrics Society. It is effective for the relief of mechanical/compressive pain and has an excellent safety profile. This patient has no underlying liver disease and does not drink alcohol, so he has no contraindications to this medication. He should not exceed a dose of 4 g in 24 hours; the FDA has recently limited the dose of prescription acetaminophen to 325 mg to decrease the risk of toxicity.

Several medications are effective for treating mechanical/compressive pain, including tricyclic antidepressants, NSAIDs, acetaminophen, and duloxetine. However, older patients are more likely to experience medication-related side effects, and comorbid conditions may predispose to impaired drug metabolism. Careful selection of pain medications is therefore essential. Tricyclic antidepressants, such as amitriptyline, should be avoided in the elderly owing to their potential for adverse effects, including cardiac conduction abnormalities, orthostasis, and anticholinergic effects.

Muscle relaxants, such as cyclobenzaprine, have demonstrated limited effectiveness in the treatment of mechanical/compressive pain.

Although NSAIDs can be very effective for the relief of pain, their associated risks for gastrointestinal, cardiovascular, and renal toxicities limit their use in older patients with comorbidities. This patient has a history of peptic ulcer disease, and the addition of ibuprofen to his medication regimen may increase his risk for gastrointestinal bleeding.

KEY POINT

- First-line therapy for chronic pain in the elderly is acetaminophen.

Bibliography

American Geriatrics Society Panel on the Pharmacologic Management of Persistent Pain in Older Persons. Pharmacologic management of persistent pain in older persons. J Am Geriatr Soc. 2009;57(8):1331-1346. [PMID: 19573219]

Item 145   Answer: B
Educational Objective: Screen for depression.

This woman should be screened for depression. The U.S. Preventive Services Task Force (USPSTF) recommends screening all adults for depression provided that adequate resources are available to ensure adequate treatment and follow up. Little evidence supports using one screening method over another. However, asking two questions, "During the past 2 weeks, have you felt down, depressed, or hopeless?" and "During the past 2 weeks, have you felt little interest or pleasure in doing things?" appears to have similar effectiveness compared with longer instruments.

One-time abdominal ultrasonography to screen for abdominal aortic aneurysm (AAA) is recommended only for men between the ages of 65 to 75 years who have previously smoked. The USPSTF recommends against screening women for AAA regardless of age or whether or not they have ever smoked.

The USPSTF strongly recommends screening for hepatitis B virus infection in all pregnant women at their first prenatal visit. Owing to the low prevalence of hepatitis B in the general population in the United States, however, routine screening is not cost effective and is not recommended.

The USPSTF recommends screening for osteoporosis in all women age 65 years or older and also in younger women with an elevated fracture risk. Screening this patient for osteoporosis would not be appropriate as she is younger than 65 years and does not have a fracture risk that is equal to or greater than that of a 65-year-old woman without additional risk factors, such as alcoholism, corticosteroid use for more than 3 months, low body mass, current tobacco use, dementia, or use of anticonvulsants.

KEY POINT

- Screening for depression is recommended for all adults as long as appropriate supports are in place to ensure adequate treatment and follow up.

Bibliography

O'Connor EA, Whitlock EP, Beil TL, Gaynes BN. Screening for depression in adult patients in primary care settings: a systematic evidence review. Ann Intern Med. 2009;151(11):793-803. [PMID: 19949145]

Item 146   Answer: C
Educational Objective: Diagnose generalized anxiety disorder.

This patient most likely has generalized anxiety disorder (GAD). Anxiety disorders are among the most common psychiatric disorders in the general population; of these, GAD is the most common, occurring in approximately 4% of the population. GAD is characterized by excessive anxiety and worry about a variety of events or activities on most days for at least 6 months, with difficulty controlling worrying. Associated symptoms include fatigue, irritability, restlessness, insomnia, and difficulty concentrating. Patients with GAD often have comorbid anxiety disorders, depression, or substance abuse. Patients with GAD often have somatoform symptoms, which can make them high utilizers of health care resources.

Attention-deficit/hyperactivity disorder first manifests in childhood and is characterized by inattention, hyperactivity, and impulsivity accompanied by functional impairment in at least two settings (home, work, school). This patient's presentation is not consistent with attention-deficit/hyperactivity disorder.

Bipolar disorder is characterized by manic or hypomanic mood episodes and depressive episodes. A manic episode is marked by a persistent period of elevated mood, irritability, lack of need for sleep, racing thoughts, high energy levels, increased talkativeness, spending sprees, hypersexuality, and increased self confidence, with possible delusions of grandeur or psychosis.

A major depressive episode is diagnosed by the presence of five or more of the following symptoms occurring nearly every day during the same 2-week period, at least one of which is either depressed mood or loss of interest or pleasure: depressed mood most of the day, loss of interest or pleasure in most activities, significant unintentional weight or appetite gain or loss, insomnia or hypersomnia, psychomotor agitation or retardation, fatigue or loss of energy, feelings of worthlessness or guilt, diminished concentration, or recurrent thoughts of death or suicide without a specific plan or prior attempt. This patient's symptom complex does not fit with a diagnosis of depression.

KEY POINT

- Generalized anxiety disorder is characterized by excessive anxiety and worry about a variety of events or activities on most days for at least 6 months, with difficulty controlling worrying.

Bibliography

Kroenke K, Spitzer RL, Williams JB, Monahan PO, Löwe B. Anxiety disorders in primary care: prevalence, impairment, comorbidity, and detection. Ann Intern Med. 2007;146(5):317-325. [PMID: 17339617]

Item 147   Answer: A

Educational Objective: Manage hypoactive sexual desire disorder.

This woman has hypoactive sexual desire disorder (HSDD), which is diagnosed if a patient reports personal distress associated with a persistent lack of sexual thoughts, desire for, or receptiveness to sexual activity. HSDD is the most common female sexual disorder, with prevalence ranging from 12% to 19%. In studies of menopausal women, predictors of sexual function included feelings for partner, change in partner status, and previous level of sexual function. As this patient's current feelings about the relationship with her partner may be causing distress, individual or couples sex therapy, which provides information about the normal female sexual response and facilitates communication about sexual issues, may be beneficial. There is no FDA-approved medication for the treatment of female HSDD.

Sildenafil is an effective treatment for male erectile dysfunction but generally is not indicated for the treatment of sexual disorders in women. It was found to be no better than placebo for increasing the frequency of enjoyable sexual encounters or improving any aspect of sexual function in women. It may be used to improve sexual arousal and orgasm in women experiencing sexual dysfunction related to selective serotonin reuptake inhibitor therapy but does not impact sexual desire.

Systemic estrogen and progesterone therapy improves many symptoms associated with menopause, including hot flushes and vaginal atrophy (unresponsive to topical therapy). This patient has no signs or symptoms of vaginal atrophy and does not report vasomotor symptoms, so this treatment is not indicated.

Several studies have shown that systemic testosterone therapy, either as monotherapy or in combination with estrogen therapy, increases sexual function scores and number of satisfying sexual episodes in menopausal women but has significant adverse effects. Treated women experienced unwanted hair growth, vaginal bleeding, and had a trend toward an increased incidence of breast cancer. The FDA has not approved any testosterone therapy for the treatment of sexual dysfunction.

KEY POINT

- For women with hypoactive sexual desire disorder, individual or couples sex therapy may be beneficial.

Bibliography

Nappi RE, Martini E, Terreno E, et al. Management of hypoactive sexual desire disorder in women: current and emerging therapies. Int J Womens Health. 2010;2:167-175. [PMID: 21072309]

Item 148   Answer: A

Educational Objective: Diagnose macular degeneration.

This patient has age-related macular degeneration (AMD). In the early stages, AMD is often asymptomatic. Common symptoms, when present, include distortion of vision or a notable loss of central vision. Those with advanced AMD and profound visual loss may experience visual hallucinations (Charles Bonnet syndrome). In both dry and wet AMD, drusen are common findings. Drusen are amorphous deposits behind the retina that lead to visual loss through direct (space occupying) and indirect (inflammatory response) means. A few small, hard drusen are common as people age, but numerous large, soft drusen are a harbinger of severe AMD. Wet AMD, which is less common than dry AMD and typically more aggressive, is characterized by neovascularization with subsequent vessel leakage and hemorrhage. Smoking is a risk factor for AMD.

Cataract, or any opacification of the otherwise optically clear lens behind the pupil and iris, is the most common cause of blindness and low vision worldwide. Vision loss is slowly progressive and is usually worse in bright light or at night, with glaring headlights while driving. This patient's clear lens is not consistent with cataract.

Primary open angle glaucoma (POAG) is a progressive optic neuropathy associated with increased intraocular pressure. POAG is characterized by painless, gradual loss of peripheral vision in both eyes that may go unnoticed by the patient. In later stages, the central vision may also be affected. This patient's vision distortion and central vision loss and the funduscopic findings are not consistent with POAG.

Retinal detachment is a separation of the neurosensory layer of the retina from the choroid beneath. It may result from trauma or occur spontaneously, particularly in persons with myopia. Symptoms include diminished vision, photopsia (flashes of light), abrupt onset of multiple floaters in the vision, or metamorphopsia (wavy vision). Funduscopic examination reveals the folds of the retinal tear and detachment, which are not present in this patient.

KEY POINT

- Age-related macular degeneration causes painless progressive vision loss, characterized by distortion of vision and loss of central vision.

Bibliography

Jager RD, Mieler WF, Miller JW. Age-related macular degeneration. N Engl J Med. 2008;358(24):2606-2617. [PMID: 18550876]

Item 149   Answer: D

Educational Objective: Assess cardiac risk in a patient scheduled for intermediate-risk surgery.

This patient needs no further testing before surgery. Current recommendations are to reserve preoperative cardiac evaluation for patients at highest risk for perioperative cardiac events undergoing intermediate- or high-risk surgeries when testing would influence patient management. These are typically patients with both a low exercise tolerance and multiple risk factors. (Adequate exercise tolerance is defined as the ability to perform physical exertion of ≥4 metabolic equivalents [METs] without symptoms.) The Revised Cardiac Risk Index (RCRI) is a validated risk assessment tool that assigns one point each for a history of ischemic heart disease, compensated or prior chronic heart failure, diabetes mellitus requiring insulin, chronic kidney disease, or history of cerebrovascular disease. Although this patient has poor exercise tolerance and is undergoing an intermediate-risk procedure (orthopedic surgery), he has no RCRI risk factors. The American Heart Association/American College of Cardiology guidelines on perioperative cardiac evaluation recommend that patients with no RCRI risk factors undergoing an intermediate-risk procedure proceed to surgery without further cardiac evaluation. Cardiac complications occur in less than 1% of patients with zero or one RCRI risk factors. Thus, despite this patient's age and comorbidities, the current recommendations are for no preoperative cardiac testing.

Cardiac catheterization is not recommended as an initial preoperative cardiac evaluation, because of the good test performance characteristics of stress tests and the invasive nature a cardiac catheterization.

CT coronary angiography is a noninvasive means of defining cardiac anatomy. It has not been studied for perioperative cardiac risk assessment.

Noninvasive pharmacologic stress testing, either dobutamine stress echocardiography or nuclear perfusion stress tests, are recommended for patients in whom preoperative cardiac testing is indicated. However, this patient's cardiovascular risk is estimated to be low enough to not warrant stress testing.

KEY POINT

- **Low-risk patients who are not undergoing higher-risk surgery can proceed to surgery without preoperative cardiac testing.**

Bibliography

Fleisher LA, Beckman JA, Brown KA, et al. 2009 ACCF/AHA focused update on perioperative beta blockade incorporated into the ACC/AHA 2007 guidelines on perioperative cardiovascular evaluation and care for noncardiac surgery: a report of the American College of Cardiology Foundation/American Heart Association Task Force on Practice Guidelines. Circulation. 2009;120(21):e169-276. [PMID: 19884473]

Item 150   Answer: A

Educational Objective: Manage obesity with bariatric surgery.

This patient should be referred for bariatric surgery. For patients with class III obesity (BMI ≥40) or class II obesity (BMI 35.0-39.9) with obesity-related complications, the National Institutes of Health Consensus Development Conference recommends consideration of bariatric surgery if diet, exercise, and/or medication are ineffective. Patients should be motivated and well informed about this option and undergo multidisciplinary evaluation by a medical, surgical, psychiatric, and nutritionist team. The most common procedure is gastric bypass surgery, but laparoscopic banding is becoming common, as well. Bariatric surgery results in more dramatic and sustained weight loss than nonsurgical interventions and leads to improvement in obesity-related complications (diabetes mellitus, obstructive sleep apnea, hypertension, and hyperlipidemia). This patient has not attained his goal weight loss after a 6-month trial of diet and medication and has obesity-related complications that likely will improve with weight loss.

Phentermine is a sympathomimetic drug that is FDA-approved for short-term use (up to 12 weeks) as an adjunctive treatment of obesity. This patient's weight loss goal is 45.4 kg (100 lb), which will take much longer than 12 weeks. In addition, most persons regain any weight that is lost with this medication upon its discontinuation.

Restricting caloric intake to below 800 kcal/d (a very-low-calorie diet) is no more effective for long-term weight loss than a moderate strategy of restricting intake to 500-1000 kcal/d below what is estimated to maintain current body weight. In addition, long-term compliance with a very-low-calorie diet is nearly impossible.

Exercise is an important part of a comprehensive weight loss program that focuses on lifestyle modification. However, the patient has already not benefited from an exercise program. It is unlikely that exercise alone will meet his weight loss goals.

KEY POINT

- **Bariatric surgery should be considered for patients with BMI of 40 or greater or BMI of 35.0 to 39.9 with obesity-related complications in whom diet, exercise, and/or medication are ineffective.**

Bibliography

Colquitt JL, Picot J, Loveman E, Clegg AJ. Surgery for obesity. Cochrane Database Syst Rev. 2009;(2):CD003641. [PMID: 19370590]

Item 151   Answer: A

Educational Objective: Screen for abdominal aortic aneurysm.

This patient should undergo one-time abdominal ultrasonography to screen for an abdominal aortic aneurysm

(AAA) because he is a man between the ages of 65 to 75 years who has ever smoked (defined as 100 lifetime cigarettes). In the Multicentre Aneurysm Screening Study, a population-based sample of 67,770 men between the ages of 65 and 74 years were offered either screening for AAAs with an abdominal ultrasound or no screening. After 10 years of follow up, it was determined that screening offered a 14% absolute risk reduction in mortality from AAAs and a reduction in all-cause mortality that was of borderline significance.

Coronary artery calcium (CAC) determination by electron beam CT has high sensitivity for detecting stenoses of greater than 50% but low specificity. Because of this low specificity, a 2007 American College of Cardiology Foundation/American Heart Association consensus document states that determination of CAC by electron beam CT is not recommended in asymptomatic persons. Therefore, it would not be appropriate to order this screening test in this patient.

Although this patient is a former smoker, the U.S. Preventive Services Task Force (USPSTF) concludes that there is insufficient evidence to recommend for or against screening for lung cancer with either chest radiography, low-dose CT, sputum cytology, or a combination of these tests.

The USPSTF recommends screening for lipid disorders in men aged 35 years and older and in men or women aged 20 years and older who are at increased risk for cardiovascular disease. The Adult Treatment Panel of the National Cholesterol Education Program (ATP III) guidelines recommend that patients with 0 to 1 risk factor and a normal fasting lipid profile or normal nonfasting total cholesterol and HDL cholesterol levels do not have to be screened again for 5 years; the USPSTF acknowledges that the optimal screening interval is uncertain but that every 5 years is reasonable for low-risk persons. The patient's only risk factor is hypertension and his lipid levels were normal 1 year ago; therefore, there is no reason to repeat the test annually.

KEY POINT

- One-time abdominal ultrasonography to screen for an abdominal aortic aneurysm is recommended in men between the ages of 65 to 75 years who have ever smoked (defined as 100 lifetime cigarettes).

Bibliography

Thompson SG, Ashthon HA, Gao L, Scott RA; Multicentre Aneurysm Screening Study Group. Screening men for abdominal aortic aneurysm: 10 year mortality and cost effectiveness results from the randomised Multicentre Aneurysm Screening Study. BMJ. 2009;338:b2307. [PMID: 19553269]

Item 152   Answer: C

Educational Objective: Avoid adverse outcomes associated with opioid treatment for chronic pain.

This patient should be evaluated for opioid dependency. He has received definitive surgical treatment for chronic lower back pain secondary to spinal stenosis, and has continued to experience pain out of proportion to usual postoperative pain without evidence of ongoing spinal or nerve compression. Additionally, his not participating in further treatment, including physical therapy and home exercise, is concerning. He is currently on opioid therapy, which he has not tapered downward, and has risk factors that have been associated with aberrant drug-taking behaviors, including age younger than 45 years, cigarette smoking, a history of depression, and a family history of alcohol abuse. The possibility of opioid dependency should be discussed directly with the patient and a plan for managing his opioid use developed and mutually agreed upon, possibly including development of a pain management contract.

Amitriptyline can be a useful adjunctive therapy in the management of chronic pain, and might be a useful adjunctive treatment in this patient, although it would be inappropriate to start this therapy before addressing his opioid use.

It is generally preferable to avoid long-term opioid use for chronic pain. In situations in which they must be used, long-acting opioids, such as sustained-release morphine sulfate, are preferable to short-acting agents as they avoid the serum peaks and troughs that occur with short-acting opioids and provide more stable pain control.

Although this patient is post–spinal surgery, his surgical course has been uneventful and he has no focal findings suggestive of an operative complication or intervening issue, such as infection. Therefore, further imaging is not indicated.

KEY POINT

- Opioid dependency should be suspected in patients with risk factors for aberrant drug use and an inability to stop opioid medications after being treated with these agents for legitimate indications.

Bibliography

Dunn KM, Saunders KW, Rutter CM, et al. Opioid prescriptions for chronic pain and overdose, a cohort study. Ann Intern Med. 2010;152(2):85-92. [PMID: 20083827]

Item 153   Answer: C

Educational Objective: Manage chronic primary insomnia.

This patient should be counseled regarding sleep hygiene, which refers to behavioral and environmental factors that affect sleep. This patient is experiencing a primary sleep disturbance likely related to environmental factors in his new apartment. Although sleep hygiene alone is often ineffective in completely relieving insomnia, it provides a foundation of good sleep habits to which other therapies may be added. In the case described, resolution may be as simple as adjusting the temperature in the bedroom; other environmental factors that may be contributing include noise level, bed comfort, and the patient's psychosocial adjustment in the new apartment.

Although alcohol can contribute to insomnia or be used inappropriately to treat insomnia, this patient's pattern of alcohol use does not suggest either of these. He is not using alcohol to help him fall asleep, and he is having nightly insomnia despite only using alcohol on weekends.

When nonpharmacologic approaches such as improving sleep hygiene are unsuccessful in treating insomnia, pharmacotherapy may be indicated. Although many patients take over-the-counter antihistamines as sleep aids, they are not recommended owing to their potential anticholinergic side effects and next-day drowsiness. If this patient requires medication, the nonbenzodiazepine hypnotics zolpidem or zaleplon are considered first line because they do not alter sleep architecture and have a favorable side-effect profile. Benzodiazepines, such as diazepam, may be used as second-line agents, preferably for short-term use only.

> **KEY POINT**
> • The first-line treatment of insomnia is counseling regarding sleep hygiene.

Bibliography
Wilson JF. In the clinic: Insomnia. Ann Intern Med. 2008;148(1):ITC13-1-ITC13-16. [PMID: 18166757]

Item 154   Answer: C

Educational Objective: Diagnose bulimia nervosa.

This patient most likely has bulimia nervosa, which is an eating disorder characterized by recurrent episodes of binge eating with subsequent compensatory behavior aimed at preventing weight gain. The compensatory behaviors may include self-induced vomiting and misuse of medications, such as laxatives (purging subtype), or fasting and excessive exercise. The purging subtype of bulimia nervosa may be suspected by metabolic abnormalities, including hypokalemia, hypomagnesemia, and metabolic alkalosis, as seen in this patient. Diagnostic behavior includes engaging in bingeing and compensatory behaviors at least twice a week for 3 months, and having one's self-perception be excessively influenced by body weight and shape. Most patients with bulimia nervosa have a normal weight; the presence of dental caries, enlarged salivary glands, and scarring on the dorsum of the hand are highly suggestive of purging behaviors.

Anorexia nervosa is characterized by an abnormally low body weight (<85% of expected) in association with an intense fear of gaining weight, an overemphasis of body weight on self-evaluation, and amenorrhea for three consecutive menstrual cycles. The restricting subtype of anorexia nervosa is associated with regular caloric restriction; the binge-eating/purging subtype is characterized by

binge-eating, which may or may not be associated with self-induced vomiting or the misuse of medications. This patient's normal body weight and regular menses are more suggestive of bulimia nervosa rather than anorexia nervosa. Notably, 30% of patients with the restricting subtype of anorexia nervosa go on to develop bulimia nervosa, as seen with this patient.

Binge-eating disorder is more common than either anorexia nervosa or bulimia nervosa, affecting 2% to 3% of the general population. It is differentiated from bulimia nervosa in that there is no associated compensatory behavior after the binge.

Night-eating syndrome is characterized by excessive eating at night, difficulty sleeping, and morning anorexia. It is a prevalent disorder in obese patients and those seeking bariatric surgery.

> **KEY POINT**
> • Bulimia nervosa is an eating disorder characterized by recurrent episodes of binge eating with subsequent compensatory behavior aimed at preventing weight gain.

Bibliography
Sim LA, McAlpine DE, Grothe KB, Himes SM, Cockerill RG, Clark MM. Identification and treatment of eating disorders in the primary care setting. Mayo Clin Proc. 2010;85(8):746-751. [PMID: 20605951]

Item 155   Answer: D

Educational Objective: Diagnose meralgia paresthetica.

This patient most likely has meralgia paresthetica, or entrapment of the lateral femoral cutaneous nerve beneath the inguinal ligament. Meralgia paresthetica is characterized by paresthesia (burning/numbness) located over the anterolateral thigh. There are no motor symptoms because the lateral femoral cutaneous nerve is a purely sensory nerve. Risk factors for developing meralgia paresthetica include diabetes mellitus, obesity, and the wearing of tight-fitting pants or belts. On examination, dysesthesia or hypoesthesia is present in the distribution of the lateral femoral cutaneous nerve. The remainder of the examination is typically normal.

Patients with greater trochanteric bursitis report pain in the region of the greater trochanter that is made worse with lying on the affected side. On examination, there is tenderness to palpation approximately 2.5 cm (1 in) posterior and superior to the greater trochanter.

Iliotibial band syndrome typically presents with pain in the anterolateral knee that is worse with running downhill or cycling. The pain is typically absent during rest. On examination, patients frequently have pain to palpation of the lateral femoral epicondyle.

Lumbar disk herniation at L5 typically presents with back pain that radiates down the lateral thigh to the foot. There is weakness in foot dorsiflexion, toe extension, foot inversion, and foot eversion. The straight leg raising test is more than 90% sensitive for lumbar radiculopathy and its absence is strong evidence against lumbar disk disease. Deep tendon reflexes are typically normal in L5 radiculopathy. This patient's findings are not compatible with L5 radiculopathy.

KEY POINT

- **Meralgia paresthetica is a nerve entrapment syndrome of the lateral femoral cutaneous nerve of the anterior thigh typified by pain and burning.**

Bibliography

Plante M, Wallace R, Busconi BD. Clinical diagnosis of hip pain. Clin Sports Med. 2011;30(2):225-238. [PMID: 21419954]

Item 156   Answer: C

Educational Objective: Manage syncope in an elderly patient.

Cardiac arrhythmia is the most likely cause of syncope in this patient, given his prodrome, time course, and complete recovery immediately following the event. Cardiac causes of syncope carry a high mortality, and patients with suspected cardiac causes warrant further evaluation in the hospital regardless of age. High-risk patients requiring immediate in-hospital telemetry are those with exertional or supine syncope, palpitations prior to the event, a family history of sudden death, nonsustained ventricular tachycardia, and abnormal electrocardiographic findings. Thus, monitoring by telemetry in the hospital is appropriate for this high-risk patient.

Neurologic abnormalities are uncommon causes of syncope. Therefore, studies to assess for an intracranial or carotid process are very low yield in patients without new neurologic findings; thus, neither carotid Doppler ultrasonography nor head CT scan is indicated. Brain imaging may be appropriate to assess head trauma associated with his syncopal event, but not as a routine component of syncope evaluation.

Echocardiography for evaluation of syncope is also low yield except in patients suspected of having structural heart disease or with significant findings on cardiovascular examination, neither of which is the case in this patient.

KEY POINT

- **Cardiac causes of syncope carry a high mortality, and patients with suspected cardiac causes warrant further evaluation in the hospital.**

Bibliography

Mendu ML, McAvay G, Lampert R, Stoehr J, Tinetti ME. Yield of diagnostic tests in evaluating syncopal episodes in older patients. Arch Intern Med. 2009;169(14):1299-1305. [PMID: 19636031]

Item 157   Answer: B

Educational Objective: Diagnose Lemierre syndrome.

This patient should undergo CT of the neck with contrast. She has fever, leukocytosis, sore throat, unilateral neck tenderness, and multiple densities on her chest radiograph, suggestive of septic emboli. The combination of these factors points strongly toward Lemierre syndrome, which is septic thrombosis of the internal jugular vein. The diagnosis should be suspected in anyone with pharyngitis, persistent fever, neck pain, and septic pulmonary emboli. CT of the affected vessel with contrast would confirm the diagnosis. Treatment should include intravenous antibiotics that cover streptococci, anaerobes, and β-lactamase–producing organisms. Penicillins with β-lactamase inhibitors and carbapenems are both reasonable choices (such as ampicillin-sulbactam, piperacillin-tazobactam, and ticarcillin-clavulanate).

Chest CT would better characterize the pulmonary infiltrates, but such information would not provide specific diagnostic information that would guide therapy.

Soft tissue radiography of the neck is incapable of detecting jugular vein filling defects or thromboses, which are diagnostic of septic thrombophlebitis.

Echocardiography would be helpful to rule out right-sided endocarditis as a cause of septic emboli; however, there is nothing in the history or on the cardiac examination to suggest a cardiac source of septic emboli.

KEY POINT

- **The diagnosis of septic thrombosis of the jugular vein (Lemierre syndrome) should be suspected in anyone with pharyngitis, persistent fever, neck pain and septic pulmonary emboli.**

Bibliography

Centor RM, Samlowski R. Avoiding sore throat morbidity and mortality: when is it not "just a sore throat?". Am Fam Physician. 2011;83(1):26, 28. [PMID: 21888123]

Item 158   Answer: D

Educational Objective: Manage elevated liver chemistry test results in a patient on statin therapy.

No change in management of this patient's lipid levels is indicated, including repeat liver chemistry testing or change in statin medication. Statins work by inhibiting the hepatic HMG-CoA reductase enzyme, and can be associated with an elevation of aminotransferase levels, and rarely hepatotoxicity and acute liver failure. Aminotransferase elevations less than three times the upper limit of normal may occur in up to 3% of statin-treated patients. Conversely, statin-related hepatotoxicity (defined as alanine aminotransferase level more than three times the upper limit of normal and total bilirubin level more than twice the upper limit of normal) and acute liver failure are very rare. Acknowledging this, the FDA has recently recommended that baseline liver chemistry tests be measured prior to initiating statin therapy and then only as clinically indicated thereafter.

This patient has minor elevations of aminotransferase levels that were discovered incidentally. Statin-related minor elevation of aminotransferase levels is usually asymptomatic, occurs within the first 12 weeks of therapy, and resolves spontaneously without discontinuation of therapy. It is thought to represent a "leak" of liver enzymes related to increased hepatocyte permeability; there are no associated histopathologic changes. This phenomenon has been observed with all of the statins but is more common with higher doses.

Simvastatin should only be discontinued if there is clinical evidence of drug-related hepatotoxicity. This occurs most commonly in the setting of underlying liver conditions or as a result of drug interactions (such as acetaminophen).

In the setting of possible hepatotoxicity on treatment, persistent elevations of liver chemistry test results after discontinuation of the statin warrant further evaluation. Common causes of liver disease should be sought, including hepatitis C virus infection, nonalcoholic fatty liver disease, and autoimmune hepatitis. Serum antibody studies and liver ultrasonography may be helpful in this situation, and statin therapy should be withheld until investigations are complete.

KEY POINT

- **Baseline liver chemistry tests should be obtained in patients prior to starting statin therapy; however, routine follow-up of liver chemistry testing is not needed and is indicated only if there is clinical evidence of liver dysfunction.**

Bibliography

FDA Drug Safety Communication: Important safety label changes to cholesterol-lowering statin drugs. Additional Information for Healthcare Professionals. Available at: www.fda.gov/Drugs/DrugSafety/ucm293101.htm#hcp. Accessed June 7, 2012.

Item 159   Answer: D

Educational Objective: **Appropriately administer the pneumococcal vaccine in a young adult.**

This young man with asthma should receive the pneumococcal polysaccharide vaccine. Pneumococcal vaccination is currently indicated for adults aged 65 years and older and for adults younger than 65 years who have risk factors for acquisition of pneumococcal disease or morbidity from it. This includes persons with chronic cardiovascular disease (including hypertension), chronic pulmonary disease (including asthma), chronic liver disease, diabetes mellitus, alcoholism, and persons who smoke. Vaccination is generally considered safe in patients with mild to moderate illness and should not be routinely withheld in hospitalized patients. In fact, pneumococcal vaccination is routinely administered to inpatients and is part of the Joint Commission's Core Measures for patients with pneumonia.

Hepatitis B vaccination is reserved for persons at highest risk for either hepatitis B acquisition or its sequelae, as well as persons who request the vaccine. This includes travelers to endemic regions as well as persons with an increased risk of sexual, percutaneous, and mucosal transmission, such as those with multiple sex partners or men who have sex with men, injection drug users, and health care workers. This patient has none of these risk factors and should not be routinely vaccinated.

Human papillomavirus (HPV) vaccination is recommended for males between the ages of 11 and 21 years, and is permitted in men ages 22 to 26 years. The rationale for vaccinating men is the prevention of genital warts, anal carcinoma (in men who have sex with men), and transmission of HPV to women. This patient is 30 years old and the vaccination is not indicated.

Meningococcal vaccination is reserved for adolescents and for adults living in college dormitories or military barracks or who are asplenic. It is not indicated in this patient.

KEY POINT

- **The pneumococcal polysaccharide vaccine is indicated for adults with asthma; it is considered safe in patients with mild to moderate illness and should not be routinely withheld in hospitalized patients.**

Bibliography

Advisory Committee on Immunization Practices. Recommended adult immunization schedule: United States, 2012. Ann Intern Med. 2012;156(3):211-217. [PMID: 22298576]

Item 160   Answer: B

Educational Objective: **Manage a patient with type 2 diabetes mellitus postoperatively.**

This patient with type 2 diabetes mellitus should be given long- and short-acting insulin postoperatively to control her glucose level. Both the stress of surgery and anesthesia independently contribute to intra- and postoperative hyperglycemia. Therefore, many patients, even those who have previously been well controlled with diet or oral medications, may need insulin during the perioperative period.

Oral agents are challenging to use perioperatively owing to variability in the patient's ability to eat as well as the long-acting nature of these agents; in general, these medications should be avoided during the perioperative period.

Sliding scale insulin, the administration of short-acting insulin in a dose based on periodic blood glucose measurements (usually every 4-6 hours), has been a traditional method of treating patients with diabetes in acute care and perioperative settings. However, because basal hypoglycemic treatment is not provided and the dosing of insulin is "retrospective" based on current glucose levels, control with this approach is typically poor,

CONT.

with the potential for significant fluctuations in glucose levels. Providing a basal level of long-acting insulin with as-needed short-acting insulin is the preferred method of glucose control in acute care settings.

The optimal plasma glucose level postoperatively is controversial. Overt hyperglycemia likely contributes to postoperative dehydration as well as poor wound healing, although there is no reduction in mortality when intensive insulin therapies are used to lower plasma glucose level to a target of 80 to 180 mg/dL (4.4 to 10.0 mmol/L) among patients in the postoperative period. Therefore, most experts advocate using insulin to keep random glucose level below 180 mg/dL. As this patient's plasma glucose level is 250 mg/dL (13.9 mmol/L), she should be treated to reduce her glucose level.

KEY POINT

- Owing to the stresses of surgery and the potential adverse effects of oral diabetic agents, many patients with type 2 diabetes mellitus require insulin during the perioperative period even if their diabetes was well controlled with diet or oral medications previously.

Bibliography

Lipshutz AK, Gropper MA. Perioperative glycemic control: an evidence-based review. Anesthesiology. 2009;110(2):408-421. [PMID: 19194167]

Item 161   Answer: B
Educational Objective: Manage acute pharyngitis.

This patient should be given a rapid streptococcal antigen test before beginning antibiotic therapy. The patient's primary symptoms (fever, cough, and sore throat) are compatible with either a viral upper respiratory tract infection or streptococcal pharyngitis. The Centor criteria (presence of fever >38.1 °C [100.5 °F], tonsillar exudates, tender cervical lymphadenopathy; absence of cough) predict the likelihood of streptococcal pharyngitis and is a reasonable way to triage patients with pharyngitis to empiric treatment with antibiotics, symptomatic treatment only, or testing with treatment if the test is positive. Patients with all four criteria have a 40% or greater chance of having group A β-hemolytic streptococcal (GABHS) pharyngitis; patients with zero or one criterion have a low (<3%) probability of GABHS pharyngitis. Patients with two criteria, such as this patient, or three criteria have an intermediate probability of GABHS pharyngitis; for these patients, some guidelines recommend throat culture and others recommend the rapid antigen detection test (RADT) with confirmation of negative results. The advantage of RADT is the immediate availability of the results. RADT has comparable sensitivity and specificity to throat culture. The throat swab for either culture or RADT should be obtained from both tonsils or tonsillar fossae and the posterior pharyngeal wall. In high-risk patients, a negative antigen test should be confirmed by throat culture.

No guidelines recommend antibiotic treatment without further testing. Some recommend treating patients with three or four Centor criteria while test results are pending, although guidelines differ on this point.

KEY POINT

- Use of the four-point Centor criteria is a reasonable way to triage patients with pharyngitis to empiric treatment with antibiotics, symptomatic treatment only, or testing with treatment if the test is positive.

Bibliography

Wessels MR. Clinical practice. Streptococcal pharyngitis. N Engl J Med. 2011;364(7):648-655. [PMID: 21323542]

Item 162   Answer: A
Educational Objective: Manage vaccination in a patient in whom a multidose vaccination series has been interrupted.

This patient who received only the first of a three-dose series of hepatitis B vaccine 3 years ago should finish the series. Many vaccines require multiple doses to achieve an optimal immune response. However, the interval between doses is a minimum interval, not a maximum, and a longer than desired interval is not thought to reduce the overall antibody concentration following completion of the series. Thus, in patients with a prolonged interval since the previous dose of vaccine, the series does not need to be restarted but should be resumed with the next injection as soon as possible after the missed prescribed interval and completed as recommended.

An adequate response to immunization against hepatitis B virus is suggested by the presence of greater than 10 milliunits/mL of anti-HBs antibody in the blood. However, because the seroconversion rate in a general patient population is approximately 95%, antibody titer testing to confirm an adequate response following completion of a vaccination series is not routinely indicated except in certain high-risk patient populations (such as health care workers at high risk for exposure to bodily fluids, hemodialysis patients, and those who may be repeatedly exposed to hepatitis B virus). As this patient has not yet completed the vaccination series, antibody titer testing is not currently indicated and would not affect the recommendation to complete his remaining injections. He would require post-vaccination antibody testing only if he is in a known high-risk group or if there are concerns regarding his ability to generate an immune response owing to his existing liver disease.

Hepatitis B vaccine is currently indicated for adults at increased risk of seroconversion or increased risk of complications for hepatitis, such as patients with chronic liver disease. The patient has chronic liver disease and thus should complete a vaccination series against hepatitis B.

KEY POINT

- In patients with a prolonged interval since the previous dose of a multiple-dose vaccine, the series should be resumed rather than restarted.

Bibliography

Poland GA, Jacobson RM. Clinical practice: prevention of hepatitis B with the hepatitis B vaccine. N Engl J Med. 2004;351(27):2832-2838. [Erratum in: N Engl J Med. 2005;352(22):2362 and N Engl J Med. 2005;352(7):740]. [PMID: 15625334]

Item 163   Answer: A

Educational Objective: Diagnose acute otitis externa.

This patient most likely has uncomplicated acute otitis externa. Her swimming puts her at risk for otitis externa owing to moist conditions created by daily water immersion. Symptoms include otalgia, itching or fullness with or without hearing loss, and pain intensified by jaw motion. Signs include internal tenderness when the tragus or pinna is pushed or pulled and diffuse ear canal edema, purulent debris, and erythema, with or without otorrhea. Otitis externa can cause erythema of the tympanic membrane and mimic otitis media. In otitis externa, however, pneumatic otoscopy shows good tympanic membrane mobility. Management consists of clearing the canal of as much debris as possible to optimize penetration of ototopical agents as well as to visualize the tympanic membrane to ensure it is intact before initiating treatment. Topical agents have been the mainstay of therapy for uncomplicated otitis, although there is a paucity of data regarding the effectiveness of one topical treatment compared with another. An ototopical agent containing neomycin, polymyxin B, and hydrocortisone is frequently used and is effective when given for 7 to 10 days. Mild otitis externa can be treated with a dilute acetic acid solution.

Whereas an allergic reaction to plastic ear plugs should be considered, the purulent discharge and the much higher likelihood of this being bacterial acute otitis externa make a delayed type (type IV) hypersensitivity reaction unlikely. Delayed hypersensitivity reactions (contact dermatitis) are typically characterized by erythema and edema with vesicles or bullae that often rupture, leaving a crust. Allergic reactions to the plastic in hearing aids, metal in earrings, or even to otic suspension drops used to treat otitis externa should always be considered in the differential diagnosis of an inflamed external auditory canal.

Malignant otitis externa is a much more serious entity in which the infection in the ear canal spreads to the cartilage and bones nearby. It is frequently accompanied by fever, significant pain, and otorrhea, and patients usually appear much more ill than this healthy-appearing woman with localized ear discomfort. On physical examination, granulation tissue is often visible along the inferior margin of the external canal.

Pain with tugging on the pinna and movement of the tragus and an inflamed external auditory canal make otitis media highly unlikely as a diagnostic possibility. In addition, acute otitis media is associated with signs of middle ear effusion and middle ear inflammation (erythema of the tympanic membrane), which are not present in this patient.

KEY POINT

- Symptoms of otitis externa include otalgia, itching or fullness, and pain intensified by jaw motion; signs include internal tenderness when the tragus or pinna is pushed or pulled and diffuse ear canal edema, purulent debris, and erythema.

Bibliography

Osguthorpe JD, Nielsen DR. Otitis externa: Review and clinical update. Am Fam Physician. 2006;74(9):1510-1516. [PMID: 17111889]

Item 164   Answer: C

Educational Objective: Recommend contraception options for a woman who smokes.

The best hormonal contraception option for this 38-year-old woman who smokes is a progesterone-only preparation. Women older than 35 years who smoke more than 15 cigarettes daily should not be prescribed estrogen-containing preparations because of the increased risk of thromboembolic disease. A family history of stroke itself is not a contraindication to the use of estrogen-containing preparations, although a personal history of stroke or thromboembolic disease is; progesterone-only contraceptives are considered safe in these women. Progesterone-only options for women with contraindications to estrogen include the "mini-pill," long-acting progesterone compounds (such as depot medroxyprogesterone acetate), subcutaneous progesterone implants, and progesterone-containing intrauterine devices.

Estrogen-only patches are never appropriate for contraception; they may be used as hormone replacement therapy in postmenopausal women without an intact uterus.

Combined estrogen-progesterone preparations are available in the form of patches and vaginal rings, which avoid first-pass hepatic metabolism and may limit estrogen's effects on the liver and on lipids. These products do not negate the thrombogenic effects of estrogen, however, and so they are still contraindicated in women who smoke.

KEY POINT

- Estrogen-containing contraceptives are contraindicated in women older than 35 years who smoke more than 15 cigarettes daily because of the increased risk of thromboembolic disease.

Bibliography

ACOG Committee on Practice Bulletins-Gynecology. ACOG practice bulletin. No. 73: Use of hormonal contraception in women with coexisting medical conditions. Obstet Gynecol. 2006;107(6):1453-1472. [PMID: 16738183]

Item 165   Answer: E

Educational Objective: Recognize the adverse effects of glaucoma treatment options.

This patient's timolol drops should be discontinued. Glaucoma is a frequent cause of blindness in the elderly and is characterized by increased intraocular pressure causing damage to the optic nerve. Many classes of drugs, local and systemic, have been used to reduce intraocular pressure, by either decreasing inflow or increasing outflow of the aqueous humor. Timolol decreases the inflow of aqueous humor and is generally well tolerated, but even locally applied drugs can have systemic side effects. Most adverse reactions of timolol are manifestations of its therapeutic effect and may include heart block, sinus bradycardia, and hypotension; most reactions are not serious and can be alleviated by eliminating the drug or decreasing the dosage. Other associated adverse effects of topical β-blocker therapy include bronchospasm, decreased libido, central nervous system depression, and mood swings.

Amlodipine, a systemic antihypertensive agent, has the main side effects of hypotension, peripheral edema, dizziness, and headache. Fewer than 1% of patients taking amlodipine experience bradycardia, but a cause and effect relationship has not been established.

Carbonic anhydrase inhibitors, which may be administered orally or topically, reduce intraocular pressure by decreasing aqueous humor inflow. Dorzolamide, a topical carbonic anhydrase inhibitor, has fewer side effects than systemic carbonic anhydrase inhibitors, such as acetazolamide, which can cause acidosis, malaise, hirsutism, diarrhea, and blood dyscrasias.

Latanoprost, a topical prostaglandin analogue, increases outflow of the aqueous humor. It can cause flu-like symptoms and muscle aches.

ACE inhibitors, such as lisinopril, have adverse effects of cough, hyperkalemia, and kidney failure but not bradycardia.

KEY POINT

- **Timolol, a topically applied β-blocker for treatment of glaucoma, may have systemic adverse effects, including bradycardia and heart block.**

Bibliography
Fogagnolo P, Rossetti L. Medical treatment of glaucoma: present and future. Expert Opin Investig Drugs. 2011;20(7):947-959. Epub 2011 May 3. [PMID: 21534887]

Item 166   Answer: A

Educational Objective: Manage erectile dysfunction in a patient with coronary artery disease.

The most appropriate treatment for this man with erectile dysfunction is initiation of a phosphodiesterase type 5 (PDE-5) inhibitor, such as sildenafil. Cardiovascular disease is common in men with erectile dysfunction (ED), and ED is a warning sign of future cardiovascular events similar in magnitude to smoking or a family history of myocardial infarction. It is essential to accurately assess cardiovascular risk prior to treating ED. According to the Second Princeton Consensus Conference risk classification for sexual activity, this patient would be classified as having low cardiovascular risk as he is asymptomatic and has fewer than three of the following major cardiovascular risk factors: age, hypertension, diabetes mellitus, smoking, dyslipidemia, sedentary lifestyle, and family history of premature coronary artery disease. Although he underwent prior coronary revascularization, this intervention was successful, it was performed more than 8 weeks ago, and he is currently asymptomatic. As a result of his low cardiovascular risk classification, it is appropriate to initiate therapy for his ED without performing further cardiac evaluation. Because he is not on a nitrate drug, first-line therapy with a PDE-5 inhibitor would be most appropriate.

Testosterone replacement therapy should only be initiated in patients with ED who have symptoms and signs of hypogonadism and whose testosterone level is measured and found to be low.

Although stopping his metoprolol may improve his ED, the cardiovascular mortality benefit of this medication makes it unwise to stop.

KEY POINT

- **Patients with coronary artery disease who have successfully undergone previous coronary revascularization, are without cardiovascular symptoms, and have fewer than three major cardiovascular risk factors are considered to be at low risk and can safely engage in sexual activity without cardiac evaluation.**

Bibliography
Schwartz BG, Kloner RA. Clinical cardiology: physician update: erectile dysfunction and cardiovascular disease. Circulation. 2011;123(1):98-101. [PMID: 21200016]

Item 167   Answer: A

Educational Objective: Treat plantar fasciitis.

The most appropriate next step in the management of this patient is arch supports. Plantar fasciitis is the most common cause of heel pain in adults. Initial therapy for plantar fasciitis should focus on nonpharmacologic measures with acetaminophen or NSAIDs for pain control. Although this patient has been doing heel stretches and has been using acetaminophen, her pes planus has not yet been addressed. Pes planus, the loss of the arch of the foot, leads to decreased cushioning with standing and walking and allows the redistribution of forces across the foot and ankle, commonly resulting in pain and exacerbation of other foot issues. Arch supports to correct her pes planus should therefore be tried. The patient should also be educated that the expected period of time until recovery is long and is often measured in months.

Although corticosteroid injections (15 to 30 mg of methylprednisolone injected into the origin of the plantar fascia) appear to provide short-term improvement in symptoms, one meta-analysis found that there was no improvement in long-term outcomes. Given the lack of proven benefit in long-term outcomes, corticosteroid injection is best reserved for patients who do not respond to a conservative management plan that has included addressing pes planus, if present.

Multiple studies have investigated the role of extracorporeal shock wave therapy in the treatment of plantar fasciitis with conflicting results. In a meta-analysis that only included studies considered to be of high quality, there was no statistically significant benefit observed. Consequently, although extracorporeal shock wave therapy is well tolerated (the only significant side effect is a temporary increase in pain), it should not be routinely recommended owing to a lack of evidence supporting its use.

Plantar fascia release surgery should be reserved for patients with refractory plantar fasciitis.

KEY POINT

- Initial therapy for plantar fasciitis should focus on nonpharmacologic measures with acetaminophen or NSAIDs for pain control.

Bibliography
Young C. In the clinic. Plantar fasciitis. Ann Intern Med. 2012;156(1 pt 1):ITC1-1-16. [PMID: 22213510]

Item 168   Answer: D
Educational Objective: Manage perioperative risk in a patient undergoing intermediate-risk surgery.

This patient can proceed to surgery without further testing. The American College of Cardiology/American Heart Association recommendations for perioperative cardiac risk assessment suggest that preoperative stress testing be reserved for patients at greatest likelihood of a perioperative cardiac event. Risk is based on the nature of the planned surgery as well as the patient's clinical risk for a perioperative cardiac event, usually derived from the number of Revised Cardiac Risk Index (RCRI) risk factors present and exercise tolerance. Stress testing is reserved for patients undergoing non–low risk surgeries who have three or more RCRI risk factors and are unable to achieve four metabolic equivalents (METs) of exercise without symptoms suggestive of angina, and in whom testing will result in changes in management. Although this patient will be undergoing an intermediate-risk procedure, she has two RCRI risk factors (diabetes mellitus, chronic kidney disease with serum creatinine level >2.0 mg/dL [177 µmol/L]) and a good self-reported level of exercise. Therefore, no further testing is required.

Electrocardiographic stress testing, and pharmacologic stress testing for those unable to physically exercise, can be used for perioperative risk stratification. However, based on this patient's good functional capacity, as seen by her ability to exercise to a reasonable rate without significant difficulty, no further cardiovascular testing is needed.

Preoperative percutaneous coronary interventions have not been shown to improve postoperative outcomes and are not routinely indicated preoperatively even in high-risk patients. In patients for whom testing is required, stress testing is preferred. In addition, coronary angiography would put this patient at risk for worsening kidney injury and should be avoided unless absolutely necessary.

KEY POINT

- In patients undergoing non–low risk surgeries, preoperative stress testing is reserved for those who have three or more clinical cardiac risk factors and are unable to achieve four metabolic equivalents (METs) of exercise without symptoms suggestive of angina.

Bibliography
Fleisher LA, Beckman JA, Brown KA, et al. 2009 ACCF/AHA focused update on perioperative beta blockade incorporated into the ACC/AHA 2007 guidelines on perioperative cardiovascular evaluation and care for noncardiac surgery: a report of the American College of Cardiology Foundation/American Heart Association Task Force on Practice Guidelines. Circulation. 2009;120(21):e169-276. [PMID: 19884473]

Index

Note: Page numbers followed by f and t denote figures and tables, respectively. Test questions are indicated by Q.

Abdominal aortic aneurysms
    screening for, 7t, 8, Q151
    surgical repair of, 128
Abortifacients, 86
Abscesses, anorectal, 108
Absolute risk (AR), 3, 3t, Q58
Absolute risk reduction (ARR), 3, 3t, 4
Accountable care organizations (ACOs), 6t
ACE inhibitors, cough and, 37, Q81
Acetaminophen
    for plantar fasciitis, Q167
    use in liver disease, 35
    use in older patients, 35, Q144
Achilles tendon
    rupture of, 62
    tendinopathy of, 61–62
Acromioclavicular joint, degeneration of, 56, Q26
Activities of daily living (ADLs), 116–117, 117t
Acupuncture, 35
Acute coronary syndrome (ACS)
    chest pain in, 48, 49, Q101
    hospitalization for, 49
Adhesive capsulitis, 55–56
Adolescents
    medical confidentiality for, 26
    sexually active, 18
Adrenal insufficiency, perioperative management of, 132–133
Advance directives, 24
Alcohol dependence, 17
Alcohol use/abuse
    insomnia in, 44, Q153
    interventions for, 18, Q120
    in physicians, 27, 27t
    screening for, 7t, 8, 9, 17–18
Alcohol Use Disorders Identification Test (AUDIT), 17
α-blockers, for benign prostatic hyperplasia, 78, 78t, Q70
Alzheimer's disease, 118
Amenorrhea, anorexia nervosa and, 113
American Academy of Family Physicians, cancer screening guidelines from, 10
American Academy of Ophthalmology, 119
American Cancer Society
    cancer screening guidelines from, 10
    cervical cancer screening guidelines from, 10t
    mammography recommendations from, 9–10
    osteoporosis screening guidelines from, 9
American College of Cardiology/American Heart Association, 125, 127, Q151, Q168
American College of Chest Physicians, 36
American College of Obstetricians and Gynecologists
    mammography recommendation from, 9
    pelvic pain treatment recommendation from, 92
American College of Physicians
    cancer screening guidelines from, 10
    clinical practice guidelines from, 4, 7
    evidence-based medicine resources from, 4
    High-Value Cost-Conscious Care initiative of, 23
    low back pain diagnostic testing recommendation from, 51
    position on physician-assisted suicide, 25, Q83
American Diabetes Association, diabetes screening recommendation from, 70
American Geriatrics Society, 35, 117
American Heart Association
    optimal triglyceride levels guidelines from, 63
    stroke prevention guidelines from, 69
American Medical Association
    alcohol abuse screening recommendation from, 8
    mammography recommendation from, 9
    older driver evaluation recommendation from, 120
    position on physician-assisted suicide, 25, Q83

American Society of Addictive Medicine, alcohol abuse screening recommendation from, 8
American Urological Society, 78
Aminotransferases, statin-related increase in, 65, 66t, 67, Q158
Anal cancer, screening for, 10
Anal fissures, 108
Analgesic ladder, 29–30, 29f, 35, Q65
Analgesics. See also Opioid analgesics
    perioperative use of, 126t
Anchoring heuristic, 21t, Q12
Androgen deficiency, 77, 77t, Q40
Anemia, perioperative management of, 131
Angiotensin-converting enzyme inhibitors. See ACE inhibitors
Ankle, sprains of, 61, Q59
Anorectal abscesses, 108
Anorectal disorders, 107–108
Anorectal pain, chronic, 108
Anorexia, 32
Anorexia nervosa, 113–114, Q143
Anterior cruciate ligament
    examination of, 59, 59f
    injuries to, 59
Anterior drawer test, 59, 59f
Anticoagulant therapy, perioperative management of, 126t, 129–130, 131t, 132, Q142
Antidepressants, 109, 110t, Q56
    for insomnia, 44
Antiemetics, 32
Antihistamines, for insomnia, 44, 45
Anti-La/SSB antibodies, Q44
Antiplatelet medications, perioperative management of, 126t, 130–131, 132
Anti-Ro/SSA antibodies, Q44
Antiseizure medications, perioperative management of, 126t
Anxiety, in anorexia nervosa, 114
Anxiety disorders, 110–112, Q146
Aortic dissection, chest pain in, 49, 50
Apley scratch test, 54, 54t
Apolipoprotein A-1, 64
Apolipoprotein B, 64
Apprehension test, 54, 54t, 55f
Arrhythmias, as syncope cause, 46, Q156
Arteritis, temporal, 99, Q95
Arthritis, septic, of the knee, 58
Aspergillosis, in immunocompromised patients, 39
Aspirin
    as adjunct to dyslipidemia management, 69, 69t
    gastrointestinal bleeding and, 69, 69t
    for metabolic syndrome, 68, 68t
    perioperative management of, 130, 132
Asthma
    cough-variant, 37, 38f, 39
    as indication for pneumococcal vaccination, 14, 16, Q159
Atherosclerosis, 68
Atorvastatin, 64–65
Attention-deficit/hyperactivity disorder, 115, Q93
Autism spectrum disorders, 115–116, Q128

Bacteriuria, screening for, 7t, 9
Baker (popliteal) cyst, 61
Bariatric surgery, 73–74, 73f, 74t, Q150
Bayes theorem, 4
β-blockers, perioperative use of, 126t, 127, 128, Q125
Behavioral counseling, 16
Behavioral health. See Mental and behavioral health
Behavioral therapy. See also Cognitive-behavioral therapy
    for obesity, 72
    for urinary incontinence, 121–122
Benign paroxysmal positional vertigo, 41, 42f, 43, Q14, Q20
Benign prostatic hyperplasia, 78, 78t, Q18, Q70

Benzodiazepines
    contraindication for cancer pain, 30
    for insomnia, 44, 45, 45t, Q153
Bereavement, 32, 109
Bias, in study design, 1
    lead-time, 7
    length, 7
Bile acid sequestrants, 65, 65t, Q75
Binge-eating disorder, 114, Q154
Bipolar disorder, 109, 112, Q140
Bladder, overactive, in benign prostatic hypertrophy, 78
Bladder cancer, 10
Bladder outlet obstruction (BOO), 78
Blepharitis, 95
Body dysmorphic disorder, 113, Q85
Body mass index (BMI), 69, 70, 70t, Q150
BRCA1/BRCA2 gene mutations, 9
Breast, cystic, 83
Breast cancer, 84
    hormone therapy and, 88–89
    screening for, 7t, 9–10, 11
Breast masses, palpable, evaluation of, 82–84, 83t, Q45, Q90
Breast pain, 84
Brief advice, 16
Brief interventions, 16
Brief Pain Inventory (BPI), 33
Bronchitis, nonasthmatic eosinophilic, 37, 38f, 39, Q77
Bulimia nervosa, 114, Q154
Bupropion, 17
Burning mouth syndrome, 106
Bursitis
    olecranon, 56, Q132
    pes anserine, 60, Q79
    prepatellar, 60
    trochanteric, 58

CAGE questionnaire, for alcohol abuse diagnosis, 17
Caloric restriction, for weight loss, 72, Q51
Canadian Task Force on Preventive Health Care, 8
Canadian Task Force on the Periodic Health Examination, 119
Cancer. See also specific types of cancer
    clinical course of, 28, 28f
    constipation in, 30
    dyspnea in, 32
    fatigue in, 30
    low back pain in, 51t
    screening for, 7t, 9–10
Cancer pain, 29–30, 31t, Q19, Q65
Candidiasis, vulvovaginal, 92, 93, Q80
Capsulitis, adhesive, 55–56
Cardiac risk assessment, perioperative, 125, 128t, Q149, Q168
Cardiac Risk Index (RCRI), Revised, 125, 128t, Q168
Cardiovascular disease
    chest pain in, 48–50, 48t, Q101
    clinical course of, 28f
    dyslipidemia as risk factor for, 62–64, 63t
    risk stratification for, Q66
    syncope in, 46, 47
Cardiovascular medications, perioperative management of, 126t
Cardiovascular perioperative medicine, 125, 127–128, 127f, 128t, Q125
Cardiovascular testing, preoperative, 125, Q125
Carpal tunnel syndrome, 57, Q2
Case-control studies, 2, 2t
Case series, 2
Cataracts, 97
Cauda equina syndrome, 50, 51t
Celecoxib, 35
Cellulitis, orbital, 99
Centers for Disease Control and Prevention (CDC), 9
    Advisory Committee on Immunization Practices, 12
Centor criteria, for pharyngitis triage, 104, Q161
Central adiposity, 70
Central retinal artery occlusion, 99, 99f, Q95
Central retinal vein occlusion, 99, Q61
Cerumen, impaction of, 103
Cervical cancer, screening for, 7t, 10, 10t, 11, Q34
Cervical neurogenic pain, 53
Charter on Medical Professionalism, 23, 23t
Chemical injuries, ocular, 99
Chest pain, 47–50
    cardiovascular causes of, 48–50, 48t, Q101
    differential diagnosis of, 47–49

    gastrointestinal causes of, 49
    hospitalization for, 49–50
    misdiagnosis of, 47
    musculoskeletal causes of, 49, Q130
    pleuritic, 49, 50, Q104
    pulmonary causes of, 49
Child abuse, 18
    mandated reporting of, 26
Children, medical confidentiality for, 26
Chlamydial infection, 18
    bacterial vaginosis as risk factor for, 92
    screening for, 7t, 9, 11
Chronic diseases, screening for, 7t, 8–9
Chronic fatigue, 39–40
Chronic fatigue syndrome, 39–40, Q7, Q72
Chronic obstructive pulmonary disease (COPD)
    as perioperative pulmonary complications cause, 128, 128t
    preoperative care in, 128, Q47
Chronic pain
    in elderly patients, Q144
    noncancer, 33–36, 34t, Q117
    pelvic
        in men, 80–81
        in women, 91–92, 91t, Q135
Chronic Prostatitis Symptom Index, 80
Cirrhosis, perioperative management of, 133–134, Q62
Clinical decision support, 22
Clinical practice guidelines, 4, 7
Clopidogrel, perioperative management of, 130, 132
Clue cells, 92, 92f
"Clunk" sign, 54t
Cluster-randomized trials, 1, 2t
Coagulopathies, preoperative evaluation of, 131
Cochrane collection, 4
Codeine, 31t
Cognitive-behavioral therapy
    for anxiety disorders, 111
    for chronic fatigue, 40
    for chronic pain, 34–35
    for depression, 109
    for eating disorders, 114
    for insomnia, 44
    for obsessive-compulsive disorder, 112, Q3
    for social anxiety disorder, 111
Cohort studies, 2, 2t
Colon cancer, 107
    screening for, 7t, 11, Q48
Colonoscopy, 107, Q48
Common symptoms, 32–50
    chest pain, 47–50
    chronic fatigue, 39–40
    chronic noncancer pain, 33–36
    cough, 36–39
    dizziness, 40–43
    edema, 50
    insomnia, 43–45
    syncope, 45–47
Comparative effectiveness research (CER), 3
Compression stockings, 50, Q22
Computerized physician order entry (CPOE), 22
Concierge medicine, 6t
Condoms, 85t, 86
Confidence interval (CI), 1
Confidentiality, 25–26
Conflicts of interest, 26, 27t
Confounding, 1
Conjunctivitis, 93–94, 95
    bacterial, 94, 94f
    viral, 93, 94f, Q11
Constipation, in cancer patients, 30
Contraception
    emergency, 85t, 86
    for men, 85t, 86
    for women, 84–86, Q69, Q164
    for women smokers, 84, 86, Q164
Control groups, Q92
Conversion disorder, 112–113
Core measure sets, 20
Cornea
    abrasions to, 94–95
    edema of, 97
    ulcers of, 95

Coronary artery bypass grafting, 125, 130
Coronary artery disease (CAD)
    chest pain in, 48, 48t
    erectile dysfunction management in, Q166
    screening for, 8–9
Coronary heart disease (CHD)
    dyslipidemia management in, 63, 63t
    hormone therapy and, 88
Coronary revascularization, 125
Corticosteroids, 30, 32
    perioperative management of, 126t, 132–133
Costochondritis, Q130
Cough, 36–39
    ACE inhibitors and, Q81
    acute, 37
    chronic, 37–39, 38f, Q38
    in gastroesophageal reflux disease, 37, 38f, 39, Q38
    in immunocompromised patients, 39
    in nonasthmatic eosinophilic bronchitis, 37, Q77
    subacute, 37–39
C-reactive protein, 64, Q66
Creatine kinase, 65, 67
Cross-arm test, 54t
Crossed straight-leg raise test, 51
Cross-sectional studies, 2
Cubital tunnel syndrome, 56, Q132
Cyclooxygenase-2 (COX-2) inhibitors, 35
Cystitis, interstitial, 91, 91t, Q135
Cysts
    Baker (popliteal), 61
    breast, 83
    epididymal, 79
    ganglion, 57
Cytochrome P-450 3A4 isoenzyme inhibitors, 64–65

Decisional capacity, 24–25, 26, Q109
Delirium, in terminally ill patients, 32
Dementia, 118
    clinical course of, 28f
Dental disease/infection, 105, 106
Depression, 108–110
    in anorexia nervosa, 114
    in bipolar disorder, 109, 112, Q140
    in chronic fatigue, 40
    in elderly patients, 119, Q99
    in low back pain, 50
    management of, 109, 110t, Q56
    in pain, 35
    postpartum, 109
    screening for, 7t, 8, Q145
    in terminally ill patients, 32
Depressive disorders, diagnosis of, 108–109
De Quervain tenosynovitis, 57, Q96
Dexamethasone, 32
Diabetes mellitus
    dyslipidemia management in, 63
    metabolic syndrome and, 67
    obesity and, 70, Q51, Q57
    perioperative management of, 132, Q160
    prevention of, 72
    screening for, 7t, 8, 70
Diabetes Recognition Program (DRP), 6t
Diagnostic errors, 20, 21t, Q12
Diagnostic tests
    interpretation of, 3–4, 5t
    preoperative, 124, Q8
    properties of, 4, 5t
Diet
    for dyslipidemia management, 64
    for weight loss, 72, Q51
Dietary behavioral counseling, 16
Difficult patient encounters, 116
Diphenhydramine, for insomnia, 44, 45
Diphtheria vaccine, 12t, 13
DIRE score, 35–36
Discharge, from hospital, 21, Q94
Discharge summaries, 21, 22t
Diuretics, for edema, 50, Q22
Dix-Hallpike maneuver, 41, 41t, Q14, Q50
Dizziness, 40–43, Q55
    nonspecific, 43
Domestic violence, 18–19, Q117, Q126

Drivers, older, 120, Q118
Drop-arm test, 54t
Drug abuse, 18
    of opioids, 36
    in physicians, 27, 27t
Drug Abuse Screening Test (DAST-10), 18
Dry eye, 97–98, Q44
Durable power of attorney for healthcare, 24
Dysequilibrium, 43
Dyslipidemia
    in elderly patients, 68–69
    evaluation of, 62–64, 63t, Q141
    management of, 64–67, 65t, 66t, 68t, Q66
    in pregnancy, Q75
    screening for, 62
Dysmenorrhea, 90–91, Q131
Dyspareunia, 82, 88, 89, Q5
Dyspnea, at end of life, 32, Q6

Ear, nose, mouth and throat disorders, 100–107
    cerumen impaction, 103
    epistaxis, 105
    hearing loss, 100–101, 101t
    oral health, 105–106
    otitis externa, 102–103
    otitis media, 102
    temporomandibular disorders, 106–107
    tinnitus, 101–102
    upper respiratory tract infections, 103–105
Eating disorder not otherwise specified (EDNOS), 114
Eating disorders, 113–114, Q143, Q154
    domestic violence and, 19
    in men, 77
Ecologic fallacy, 2–3
Edema, 50
    corneal, 97
    of the knee, 58–59
    venous stasis–related, 50, Q22
Edmonton Symptom Assessment Scale, 29
Effect size, 4
Eicosapentaenoic acid, 66–67
Elbow, golfer's, 56, Q132
Elbow pain, 56
Elder abuse, 18
Elderly patients. See Geriatric medicine
Electrocardiography (ECG), for syncope evaluation, 46, 47
Electronic Health Record (EHR) Incentive program, 6t
Electronic health records (EHRs), 22
Electronic prescribing, 6t
Embolism, pulmonary, chest pain in, 49
Endocrine diseases, perioperative management of, 132–133
End-of-life care, 25, 28-29, 28f. See also Palliative care
Endolymphatic hydrops, 41
Endometriosis, 91, 91t, 92
Endophthalmitis, 97, 99
Epicondylitis, 56, Q132
Epidemiologic studies, 2–3
Epididymitis, 78, 79, Q42
Epiphora, 98
Episcleritis, 95, 95f
Epistaxis, 105, Q4
Epley maneuver, 41, 42f
Erectile dysfunction, 74–76, 75t, 76t, Q112
    in cardiovascular disease patients, 75, 76t, Q166
    management of, 75, 76t, Q112, Q166
Errors, medical. See Medical errors
Estrogen therapy
    for hypoactive sexual desire disorder, 82, Q147
    for menopause symptoms, 88–89, 89t, Q25
    perioperative, 126t
Ethics, 22–27, 23t
Euthanasia, 25
Evidence, sources of, 4
Evidence-based medicine, 4
Exercise, for weight control, 72, Q51
Experimental studies, 1, 2t
External validity, 1
Eye disorders, 93–100
    blepharitis, 95
    cataracts, 97
    conjunctivitis, 93–94, 94f, 95, Q11
    corneal conditions, 94–95, 97

Eye disorders (*continued*)
  dry eye, 97–98, Q44
  episcleritis, 95, 95f
  excessive tearing, 98
  eye emergencies, 99–100, 99t
  glaucoma, 96–97, 97t, 119, Q95, Q165
  macular degeneration, 96, 96f, 119, Q148
  retinal detachment, 98, 98f, Q29
  retinal vascular occlusion, 99, 99f
  scleritis, 95
  subconjunctival hematoma, 94, 94f
  uveitis, 95
Eye examinations, in elderly patients, 119
Ezetimibe, 65, 65t, 66

FABER test, 58, 58f
Falls, in elderly patients
  management of, Q87
  patient assessment after, 117–118, Q78
  prevention of, 117–118, 119, Q67
Family history, 11
Fatigue
  chronic, 39–40, Q7, Q72
  end-stage illness–related, 30
Feeding tubes, 32
Fenofibrate, 66, Q41
Fentanyl transdermal patches, 30, 31t, Q19
Fibrates, 64–65, 65t, 66, 67, 68, Q41, Q66
Fibroadenomas, 83
Fish oil supplementation, cardioprotective effects of, 66–67
5α-reductase inhibitors, for benign prostatic hyperplasia, 78, 78t, Q70
Fluvastatin, 65
Folic acid supplementation, 87
Follicle-stimulating hormone (FSH), 87–88
Foot pain
  forefoot, 62
  hindfoot, 61–62
  midfoot, 62
Forefoot pain, 62
Fractures
  compression, as low back pain cause, 51t
  of wrist and hand, 57
Frail elderly. *See also* Geriatric medicine
  clinical course in, 28f
  outcome measures for, 5
  urinary incontinence screening in, 121
FRAMES model, of brief interventions, 16
Functional assessment, of elderly patients, 116–120

Gabapentin, 35, Q65
Gait analysis, in elderly patients, 117
Gastric bypass surgery, 73, 73f, 74t, Q15
Gastroesophageal reflux disease (GERD)
  chest pain in, 49
  cough in, 37, 38f, 39, Q38
Gastrointestinal medications, perioperative management of, 126t
Generalizability, of study results, Q127
Generalized anxiety disorder (GAD), 110–111, Q146
Genetic counseling, referral for, 11–12, Q1, Q16
Genetic testing, 11, Q1, Q16
Genital herpes, bacterial vaginosis as risk factor for, 92
Geographic tongue, 106
Geriatric medicine, 116–124
  acetaminophen use, 35, Q144
  chronic pain management, Q144
  depression, 119, Q99
  dizziness, 40, Q55
  driving, 120, Q118
  dyslipidemia management, 68–69
  falls, 117–118, 119, Q67, Q78, Q87
  frail elderly, 5, 28f, 121
  functional assessment, 116–120
  levels of care in, 120
  polypharmacy, 120–121, Q46
  pressure ulcers, 123–124, 124t, Q17, Q24
  syncope management, Q156
  urinary incontinence, 121–123, 122f
Glaucoma, 119
  acute angle closure, 97, Q95
  adverse effects of treatment for, 96, 97t, Q165
  primary open angle, 96–97, 97t
Globe, traumatic injury to, 99
Glossitis, atrophic, 106
Golfer's elbow, 56, Q132
Gonorrhea
  bacterial vaginosis and, 92
  screening for, 7t, 9, 11
Granulomatosis
  with polyangiitis, 104, Q138
  Wegener, 104, Q138
Grief, 32, 109, Q137
Groin pain, 58
Group A streptococcal pharyngitis, 104

Halitosis, 106
Hallux valgus, 62
Hamate bone, fractures of, 57
Hand, innervation of, 56f
Hand pain, 57
Hawkins test, 54, 54t, 55f
Hazard ratio, 3
Healthcare Effectiveness Data and Information Set (HEDIS), 6, 6t
Healthcare industry, conflicts of interest with, 26, 27t
Healthcare services, unsafe and low-value, 23, 24
Health care workers, vaccinations for, 15, 16
Health examinations, periodic, 8
Health information technology (HIT), 22
Hearing loss
  cerumen impaction and, 103
  common causes of, 100, 101t
  evaluation of, 100
  in older adults, 119
  otitis media and, 102
  screening for, 119
  sudden sensorineural, 100, Q20, Q108
  unilateral sensorineural, 100, Q20
Heart failure, preoperative, 127
Hematochezia, 107, Q48
Hematologic perioperative medicine, 129–132
Hematoma, subconjunctival, 94, 94f
Hemoptysis, 39
Hemorrhage
  abnormal uterine, 90, Q53
  rectal, 107, Q48
Hemorrhoids, 107, Q48
Heparin therapy, perioperative, 129–130
Hepatitis, perioperative management of, 133
Hepatitis A vaccine, 12t, 15
Hepatitis B, 18
  screening for, 7t, 9, 11
Hepatitis B vaccine, 12t, 15, 15t, 16, Q162
Hepatitis C, 18
  screening for, 7t, 9, 11
Hepatotoxicity, statin-related, 65, Q158
Herbal supplements
  for menopausal symptoms, 89
  for pain, 35
  preoperative discontinuation of, 126t
Hernia, inguinal, 81
Herpes simplex virus, 18
Herpes zoster ophthalmicus, 99–100
Herpes zoster virus, chest pain and, 47
Herpes zoster virus vaccine, 12t, 14
Heuristics, 21t, Q12
High-density lipoprotein (HDL) cholesterol, 62, 63t, 64, 65t, 66
  low-carbohydrate diet and, 72
  smoking cessation and, 67
Hindfoot pain, 61–62
Hip, osteonecrosis of, 58, Q116
Hip pain, 58, 58f
Home safety, for elderly patients, 118
Hormone therapy. *See also* Estrogen therapy; Testosterone therapy
  for menopause symptoms, 88–89, 89t, Q25, Q60
Hospice care, 28-29. *See also* Palliative care
Hot flushes, 88
"Housemaid's knee," 60
Human immunodeficiency virus (HIV) infection
  bacterial vaginosis as risk factor for, 92
  screening for, 7t, 9, 11, Q123
  sexual transmission of, 18

Human immunodeficiency virus–positive patients, vaccination of, 13, Q129
Human papillomavirus, 10, 18
Human papillomavirus vaccine, 12t, 14–15
Hutchinson sign, 99–100
Hydrocele, 79
Hydrocodone, 31t
Hydromorphone, 30, 31t, Q19
Hyperlipidemia. *See* Dyslipidemia
Hyperplasia
    benign prostatic, 78, 78t, Q18, Q70
    gingival, 105
Hypertension
    pulmonary, as chest pain cause, 49
    screening for, 7t, 8, Q102
Hypertriglyceridemia, 63–64
    management of, 65t, 66–67, Q41
Hypoactive sexual desire disorder, 81–82, Q5, Q147
Hypochondriasis, 113
Hypoglycemic agents, perioperative management of, 126t
Hypotension, orthostatic, 46, 47, Q86

Iliotibial band syndrome, 60
Immunization. *See also specific vaccines*
    for adults, 12–16, 12t
    multiple-dose, 15, Q162
    preconception administration of, 87
Immunocompromised patients. *See also* Human immunodeficiency virus (HIV)
        infection
    cough in, 39
    pneumococcal immunization in, 14, 14t
Immunomodulators, perioperative management of, 126t
Infection, low back pain and, 51t
Infectious diseases
    reporting of, 26
    screening for, 7t, 9
Inferior vena cava filters, 129
Influenza vaccine, 12t, 13, 15, 87, Q71
Informed consent, 24, Q133
Insomnia, 43–45
    anxiety disorders and, 110
    evaluation of, 44, Q115
    management of, 44–45, 45t, Q115, Q153
Institute for Clinical Systems Improvement, 33
Institute of Medicine (IOM)
    To Err is Human: Building a Safer Health System, 19
    fall prevention recommendations of, 117
    obesity definition of, 69
    vitamin D supplementation recommendation of, 118
Instructive directives, 24
Instrumental activities of daily living (IADLs), 116–117, 117t
Insulin resistance, 68
Insulin therapy, perioperative, 132, Q160
Intermittent explosive disorder, 112
Internal validity, in study design, 1
International Index of Erectile Dysfunction-5 (IIEF-5), 75
Intimate partner violence, 18–19, Q117, Q126
Intraocular pressure (IOP), 96–97
Irritable bowel syndrome, 91, 92

Joint Commission (formerly JCAHO), 20, 22
Joint National Committee on Prevention, Detection, Evaluation, and
    Treatment of High Blood Pressure, 8, Q102

Kegel exercises, 121, Q33, Q88
Keratoconjunctivitis sicca, 97–98, Q44
Kidney disease, perioperative management of, 133
Knee
    ligamentous injuries to, 59
    osteoarthritis of, 58, 59
Knee pain, 58–61
    diagnosis and evaluation of, 58–59, 59f, 60f

Lachman test, 59, 59f
Lacrimation, 98
Lateral femoral cutaneous nerve, entrapment syndrome of, 58, Q155
Laxatives, 30
Lemierre syndrome, 104, Q157
Libido, decreased
    in men, 77
    in women, 81–82, Q5, Q147

Lifestyle risk factors, interventions for, 16–19
Life-sustaining treatment, withholding or withdrawing of, 25, Q43
Likelihood ratio (LR), 4, 5t
Liver chemistry tests, in statin use, 65, Q158
Liver disease, perioperative management of, 133–134
Living wills, 24
Long-term care, 120
Lorcaserin, 73
Lovastatin, 64–65
Low back pain, acute, 50–52, 51t, Q91
Low-density lipoprotein (LDL) cholesterol
    evaluation of, 62–63
    goal level of, 62, 63, 63t
    management of, 63t, 64–66, 65t, 67, 68t, 69, Q52, Q75
    metabolic syndrome and, 68, 68t
    pregnancy and, 65t, Q75
    stroke and, 69
Lower respiratory tract infections, as cough cause, 37
Lower urinary tract symptoms (LUTS), in men, 78
Lp(a) lipoprotein, 64
Lumbar disk disease, 58
Lung volume expansion, perioperative, 128, 129, Q47

Macular degeneration, 96, 96f, 119, Q148
Malcolm Baldrige Model for Performance Excellence, 19
Mammography
    for palpable breast mass evaluation, 83
    screening, 7t, 9–10, 11
Mastalgia, 84, Q139
McMurray test, 59, 59f
Measles, mumps, rubella vaccine, 12t, 15, 16
Medial collateral ligament injuries, 59
Medial-lateral grind test, 59, 61
Median nerve, 56f
Medical errors, 19–22, 21t, Q12
    disclosure of, 26
    medication-related, 20, Q113
    sources of, 20
    "Swiss cheese" model of, 19, 19f
Medical literature, interpretation of, 1–4
    statistical analysis, 3–4
    study design, 1–3, 2t
    terminology, 3t
Medically unexplained symptoms (MUSs), 112
Medicare, 28
Medication errors, 20, Q113
Medications. *See also specific medications*
    erectile dysfunction and, 74–75, 75t
    perioperative management of, 125, 126t, Q82
    teratogenic, 86, 87t, Q32
    weight gain and, 70t
Melatonin, for insomnia, 44–45
Melatonin-receptor agonists, for insomnia, 44–45, 45t
Meniere disease, 41, Q14, Q20
Meningococcal vaccine, 12t, 15
Menisci
    examination of, 59, 59f, 61
    injuries to, 59
Menometrorrhagia, 90
Menopause
    urogenital symptom management in, 89, Q25
    vasomotor symptom management in, 88–89, 89t, Q60
Menorrhagia, 90
Men's health, 74–81
    acute testicular and scrotal pain, 78–79
    androgen deficiency, 77, 77t, Q40
    benign prostatic hyperplasia, 78, 78t, Q18, Q70
    epididymal cysts, 79–80
    hernia, 81
    hydrocele, 79
    pelvic pain, 80–81
    prostatitis, 80–81, 80t
    sexual dysfunction, 74–77, 75t, 76t
    varicocele, 79–80
Mental and behavioral health, 108–116
    anxiety disorders, 110–112, Q146
    attention-deficit/hyperactivity disorder, 115, Q93
    autism spectrum disorders, 115–116
    bipolar disorder, 109, 112, Q140

Mental and behavioral health *(continued)*
    depression, 108–110
        anorexia nervosa and, 114
        bipolar disorder and, 109, 112, Q140
        chronic fatigue and, 40
        in elderly patients, 119, Q99
        low back pain and, 50
        management of, 109, 110t, Q56
        pain and, 35
        postpartum, 109
        screening for, 7t, 8, Q145
        in terminally ill patients, 32
    difficult patient encounters, 116, Q73
    eating disorders, 19, 77, 113–114, Q143, Q154
    intermittent explosive disorder, 112
    schizophrenia, 77, 114–115, Q68
    somatoform disorders, 112–113, Q105
Meralgia paresthetica, 58, Q155
Meta-analyses, 3
Metabolic equivalents (METs), 125, 127f, Q168
Metabolic syndrome, 67–68, 67t, Q64
    "ABCDE" approach to management of, 67–68, 68t
Methadone, 30, 36, Q136
Metrorrhagia, 90
Midfoot pain, 62
Migraine, ocular/retinal, Q95
Mild cognitive impairment, 118–119, 120, Q35, Q103
Mini-Mental State Examination (MMSE), 118
Morphine, 30, 31t, Q19
Motivational interviewing, 16, 72, Q63
Motor vehicle accidents, in older drivers, 120, Q118
Mucosal lesions, oral, 105, 106
Multiple sclerosis, perioperative management of, 134
Mumps vaccine, 12t, 15, 16
Muscle relaxants
    for low back pain, 52
    for neck pain, 53
Musculoskeletal pain, 50–62
    acute low back, 50–52, 51t, Q91
    ankle and foot, 61–62, 61f, Q59
    elbow, 56, 56f
    hip, 58, 58f
    knee, 58–61, 59f, 60f
    neck, 52–53, Q37, Q134
    shoulder, 53–56, 54f, 54t, 55f
    wrist and hand, 57
Myocardial infarction
    chest pain in, 50
    perioperative, 125
Myopathy, statins and, 64, 66t

National Cholesterol Education Program Adult Treatment Panel III (ATP III), 8, 62, 63, 63t, 64, 65, 69, Q151
National Committee for Quality Assurance (NCQA), 6
National Comprehensive Cancer Network, 9
National Institutes of Health (NIH)
    Chronic Prostatitis Symptom Index, 80
    obesity screening guidelines from, 70
National Quality Forum, 26
Nausea, chronic, 32
Neck pain, 52–53, Q37, Q134
Neer test, 54f, 54, 54t
Negative likelihood ratio (LR–), 5t
Negative predictive value (NPV), 4, 5t
Neural tube defects, 87
Neuritis, optic, 99, 100
Neurologic disease, perioperative management of, 134
Neuroma, Morton, 62, Q84
Neuronitis, vestibular, 41, 43, Q14
Neuropathic pain, 34t, 35, Q136
Niacin, 66
Nicotinic acid, 65t, 66, 67
Noble test, 60
Nonsteroidal anti-inflammatory drugs (NSAIDs), 29, 29f, 35
    for abnormal uterine bleeding, 90
    for acromioclavicular joint degeneration, 56
    for adhesive capsulitis, 56
    for ankle pain, 61
    for cancer pain, 29, Q65
    for chronic pain, Q117
    for dysmenorrhea, 91, Q131

    for elbow pain, 56
    for foot pain, 62
    for knee pain, 60
    for low back pain, 52
    for neck pain, 53
    nephrotoxicity of, 133
    for pelvic pain, 80, 81, 91
    for rotator cuff disorders, 55
    use in elderly patients, 35
    for wrist and hand pain, 57
Nosebleed, 105
Number needed to harm (NNH), 3t, 4
Number needed to treat (NNT), 3–4, 3t, Q58

Obesity, 69–74
    adverse health effects of, 70, 74, Q57
    definition of, 69–70, 70t
    epidemiology of, 69
    erectile dysfunction in, 74
    evaluation of, 70
    screening for, 7t, 8, 70
    treatment of, 71–74, 71f, 73f, 74t, Q51, Q150
Observational studies, 1–3, 2t
Obsessive-compulsive disorder, 111–112, 113, Q3
Obstructive sleep apnea (OSA), perioperative management of, 128–129, 129t, Q121
Odds ratio, 3
Older patients. *See* Geriatric medicine
Olecranon bursitis, 56, Q132
Omega-3 fatty acids, 65t
Opioid analgesics, 29–30, 29f, 31t, 34t, 35–36
    abuse of, 30, 35, 36, Q152
    for cancer pain, 29–30, 31t, Q19, Q65
    for chronic neuropathic pain, 34t, 35, Q136
    for chronic noncancer pain, 34t, 35–36
    constipation and, 30
    for low back pain, 52
    for neck pain, 53
Oral cancer, 10, 105
    screening for, 106
Oral contraceptives, 84, 85t
    for abnormal uterine bleeding, 90
    for dysmenorrhea, 90–91
Oral health, 105–106
Oral infections, 106
Oral ulcers, 106
Orchitis, 78–79
Orgasmic disorder, 82
Orlistat, 72–73
ORYX initiative, 20
Osteoarthritis
    of the hand, 57
    of the hip, 58
    of the knee, 58, 59
Osteonecrosis, of the hip, 58, Q116
Osteoporosis, screening for, 7t, 8, 9
Otitis externa, 102–103, Q163
Otitis media, 102
Ottawa ankle and foot rules, 61, 61f
Outcome measures, of healthcare, 5–6
Ovarian cancer, 10
Overdiagnosis, 7
Overuse syndrome, of the knee, 59–60
Overweight, 70t
Oxycodone, 30, 31t

Pain
    cancer, 29–30, 31t, Q19, Q65
    chest, 47–50
        cardiovascular causes of, 48–50, 48t, Q101
        differential diagnosis of, 47–49
        gastrointestinal causes of, 49
        hospitalization for, 49–50
        misdiagnosis of, 47
        musculoskeletal causes of, 49, Q130
        pleuritic, 49, 50, Q104
        pulmonary causes of, 49
    chronic
        in elderly patients, Q144
        noncancer, 33–36, 34t, Q117
    groin, 58

musculoskeletal, 50–62
    acute low back, 50–52, 51t, Q91
    ankle and foot, 61–62, 61f, Q59
    elbow, 56, 56f
    hip, 58, 58f
    knee, 58–61, 59f, 60f
    neck, 52–53, Q37, Q134
    shoulder, 53–56, 54f, 54t, 55f
    wrist and hand, 57
neuropathic, 34t, 35, Q136
palliative care management of, 29–30, 29f, 31t
pelvic pain, chronic
    in men, 80–81
    in women, 91–92, 91t, Q135
scrotal, 78–79
testicular, 78–79
Pain contracts, 36
Palliative care, 27–32
    assessment and communication in, 29, Q36, Q89
    hospice, 28–29
    nonhospice, 28, 29, Q76
    symptom management in, 29–32
Pancreatic cancer, 10
Panic disorder, 110, 111, Q119
Parkinson disease, perioperative management of, 134
Patellofemoral pain syndrome, 59–60, Q54
Patient-centered medical home (PCMH), 6t
Patient Health Questionnaire (PHQ-9), 109, 119
Patient identification, 22
Patient refusal, of treatment, 25
Patients, difficult encounters with, 116, Q73
Patient safety, 19–22
    health information technology and, 22
    national goals for, 22
Pay for performance (P4P), 6t
Pelvic adhesions, 91, 91t
Pelvic floor muscle training, 121, Q33, Q88
Pelvic pain, chronic
    in men, 80–81
    in women, 91–92, 91t, Q135
Pelvic varices, 91, 91t
Percutaneous coronary intervention (PCI), 125, 127
Performance measures, 5–6, 6t
Pericarditis, acute, chest pain in, 49, Q39
Periodontal disease, 105, 106
Perioperative medicine, 124–134
    cardiovascular, 125, 127–128, 127f, 128t
    endocrine, 132–133
    general recommendations for, 124–125
    hematologic, 129–132
    kidney disease, 133
    liver disease, 133–134
    neurologic disease, 134
    pulmonary, 128–129, 128t
Pertussis, 37
Pertussis vaccine, 12t, 13, 87
Pes anserine bursitis, 60, Q79
Pharyngitis, 104, Q161
Phosphodiesterase inhibitors, 75–76, 78, Q166
Physical activity. *See also* Exercise
    promotion of, 16
Physician-assisted suicide, 25, Q83
Physician health programs, 27
Physician Quality Reporting System (PQRS), 6t
Physicians, impaired, 27, 27t, Q124
Piriformis syndrome, 58
Pivot test, 59f
Plan-Do-Study-Act (PDSA) model, for quality improvement, 19, 20f, Q30
Plantar fasciitis, 61, Q167
Platelet deficiencies, perioperative management of, 131
Pleuritis, as chest pain cause, 49, 50
Pneumococcal polysaccharide vaccine, 12t, 14, 14t, 16, Q74, Q159
Pneumonia
    Pneumocystis jirovecii, 39
    as shoulder pain cause, 53
Pneumothorax, as chest pain cause, 49, Q104
Polymenorrhagia, 90
Polypharmacy, 120–121, Q46
Positive likelihood ratio (LR+), 5t
Positive predictive value (PPV), 4, 5t
Postconcussion syndrome, 111
Posterior drawer test, 59

Posterior vitreous detachment, 98
Posttest odds, 5t
Posttest probability, 5t
Posttraumatic stress disorder (PTSD), 111, Q100
Pravastatin, 65, Q52
Preconception counseling, 86–87, 87t
Predictive value, of diagnostic tests, 4
Pregabalin, 35
Pregnancy
    alcohol abuse screening during, 17
    hyperlipidemia management and, Q75
    medication management during, 86, 87t, Q32
    preconception counseling for, 86–87, 87t
    vaccination during, 13
    vulvovaginal candidiasis during, 93, Q80
Premature ejaculation, 76
Premenstrual dysphoric disorder, 109
Preoperative risk assessment, 124
Preoperative testing, 124, Q8
Prepatellar bursitis, 60
Pressure ulcers, 123–124, 124t, Q17, Q24
Presyncope, 43
Pretest odds, 5t
Pretest probability, 5t
Prevalence, 5t
Professionalism, 22–27, 23t
Prostate cancer, screening for, 10, Q49
Prostate-specific antigen (PSA), 10, 77
Prostatitis, 80–81, 80t, Q106
Proxy directives, 24
Pruritus ani, 108
Psychiatric medications, perioperative management of, 126t
PubMed, 4
Pulmonary medications, perioperative management of, 126t
Pulmonary perioperative medicine, 128–129, 128t, 129t
P value, 4

Quality improvement, 6
    measurement of, 20
Quality improvement models, 19–20, 20f
Quasi-experimental study design, 1, 2t

Radial nerve, 56f
Radiculopathy
    cervical, 134, Q37
    low back pain in, 51, 51t, 52
Raloxifene, 10
Randomized controlled trials (RCTs), 1, 2t, Q127
Rectum, bleeding from, 107, Q48
Relative risk, 3
Relative risk reduction (RRR), 3, 3t
Relative risk (RR), 3, 3t, Q58
Relocation test, 54t
Respiratory depression, morphine and, 30
Retinal detachment, 98, 98f, Q29
Retinal vascular occlusion, 99, 99f
Revised Cardiac Risk Index (RCRI), 125, 128t, Q168
Rhabdomyolysis, statins and, 66t
Rheumatoid arthritis, of the knee, 58
Rhinitis
    allergic, 103–104
    nonallergic, 104, Q138
Rhinitis medicamentosa, 104, Q138
Rhinorrhea, 103
Rhinosinusitis, 37, Q13
Rinne test, 100, Q20
Romberg test, 51
Rosuvastatin, 65
Rotator cuff disorders, 54–55, 56, Q23, Q122
Routine care, of healthy patients, 4–19
    family history, 11
    genetic testing and counseling, 11–12
    immunization, 12–16, 12t
    lifestyle risk factors management, 16–19
    screening tests, 6–11
Roux-en-Y gastric bypass surgery, 73, 73f, 74t, Q15
Rubella vaccine, 12t, 15, 16, 87

Sacroiliitis, 58
Scaphoid bone, fractures of, 57
Schirmer test, Q44
Schizophrenia, 114–115, Q68

Sciatica, 51–52, 51t
Scleritis, 95
SCOFF questionnaire, for eating disorders screening, 113, 113t, 114
Screening, 6–11
    for abdominal aortic aneurysms, 7t, 8, Q151
    for alcohol abuse, 7t, 8, 9, 17–18
    for breast cancer, 7t, 9–10, 11
    for cancer, 7t, 9–10
    for cervical cancer, 7t, 10, 10t, 11, Q34
    for colon cancer, 7t, 11, Q48
    for coronary artery disease, 8–9
    for depression, 7t, 8, Q145
    for diabetes mellitus, 7t, 8, 70
    for drug abuse, 18
    for dyslipidemia, 62
    for eating disorders, 113, 113t, 114
    for hearing loss, 119
    for hepatitis B, 7t, 9, 11
    for hepatitis C, 7t, 9, 11
    during history and physical examination, 8
    for human immunodeficiency virus (HIV) infection, 7t, 9, 11, Q123
    for infectious diseases, 7t, 9
    for obesity, 7t, 8, 70
    for oral cancer, 106
    for osteoporosis, 7t, 8, 9
    for prostate cancer, 10, Q49
    for sexually transmitted diseases, 7t, 9, 11, 18
    for urinary incontinence, 121, 122f
Seasonal affective disorder, 109
Sedative-hypnotics, for insomnia, 44, 45t
Seizure disorders, perioperative management of, 134
Selective serotonin reuptake inhibitors (SSRIs), 109, 110t, 111, 114, 119
Sensitivity, of diagnostic tests, 4, 5t
Sexual arousal disorder, 82
Sexual aversion disorder, 81–82, Q5
Sexual behavior
    risky, 18, 19
    sexual contact between physician and patient, 26
Sexual behavior counseling, 18
Sexual desire disorders, 81–82, Q5, Q147
Sexual dysfunction
    in men, 74–77, 75t, 76t, Q112, Q166
    in women, 81–82, 81t, 88, 89, Q5, Q147
Sexually transmitted diseases
    in adolescents, 18
    screening for, 7t, 9, 11, 18
    in victims of intimate partner violence, 18–19
Sexual pain disorders, 82
Shoulder, "frozen," 55–56
Shoulder pain, 53–56, 54f, 54t, 55f
Sigmoidoscopy, 107, Q48
Simvastatin, 64–65, 66, Q158
Sinusitis, 103, Q107
Six Sigma model, for quality improvement, 19–20
Sjögren syndrome, 98, Q44
Skin cancer, 10
Sleep hygiene, 44, Q153
Smoking, 17
    abdominal aortic aneurysm and, 7t, Q151
    cough and, 37
    erectile dysfunction and, 74
    implication for female contraception, 84, 86, Q164
    sinusitis and, 103
Smoking cessation
    chronic cough and, 37
    counseling in, 17, 18, Q10, Q27
    high-density lipoprotein cholesterol levels and, 67
    pharmacotherapy in, 17, 18
Social anxiety disorder, 111
Somatization, 50, 112, Q105
Somatoform disorders, 112–113, Q105
Specificity, of diagnostic tests, 4, 5t
Speed maneuver, 54t
Spinal cord compression, 53, Q37
Spinal stenosis, low back pain and, 51, 51t, 52
Spirometry, preoperative, 128, 129
Spondyloarthropathies, 50
Spurling test, 54t
"Squeeze" test, 61
Statins, 64–65, 65t, 68, Q52
    adverse effects of, 64–65, 66t, Q158

Statistical analysis, 3–4
Sterilization
    female, 85t, 86
    male, 85t
STOP-BANG questionnaire, for sleep apnea, 128–129, 129t
Straight-leg raise test, 51
Stress testing, preoperative, 125, Q168
Stroke
    perioperative, 134
    prevention of, 69
Study design, 1–3, 2t
    experimental studies, 1, 2t
    observational studies, 1–3, 2t
    validity, 1
Substance use disorders, 17-18. See also Alcohol use/abuse; Drug abuse
    domestic violence and, 19
    in physicians, 27, 27t
Substituted judgment, 24–25, Q109
Suicide
    bipolar disorder and, 112
    physician-assisted, 25, Q83
    tramadol and, 35
Sulcus sign, 54t
Surrogate decision-making, 24–25
Sympathomimetic drugs, for weight loss, 72
Syncope, 45–47
    cardiac causes of, 46, 47, Q21, Q156
    diagnostic evaluation of, 46–47, Q31
    in elderly patients, 46, 47, Q21, Q156
    management of, 47
    neurocardiogenic, 45–46, 47
    orthostatic, 46, 47, Q86
    risk stratification of, 47
    vasovagal, Q86
Syphilis, screening for, 7t, 11
Systematic reviews, 3

Tamoxifen, 10
Tarsal tunnel syndrome, 62
Tearing, excessive, 98
Temporomandibular disorders, 106–107, Q97
Tendinitis, rotator cuff, 54, 55, Q122
Tendinopathy, Achilles, 61–62
Tennis elbow, 56, Q132
Tenosynovitis, de Quervain, 57, Q96
Teratogens, 86, 87t, Q32
Terminally ill patients
    end-of-life care for, 25, 28–29, 28f
    palliative care for, 27–32
Testicular torsion, 78, 79, Q110
Testosterone deficiency, 77, 77t, Q40
Testosterone therapy, 77, Q166
Tests. See Diagnostic tests
Tetanus, diphtheria, pertussis vaccine, 12t, 13, 15, 16, 87
3 Incontinence Questions (3IQ), 121, 122f
Thromboembolic disease, estrogen-containing contraceptives and, 84, 86, Q164
Thrombosis, perioperative deep venous, 129–130, 130t, 131t, Q28
Thrombotic thrombocytopenic purpura, 131
Thyroid diseases, perioperative management of, 132
Thyroid medications, perioperative management of, 126t
Tilt-table testing, for syncope, 47, Q31
Timed "Up and Go" (TUG) test, 117, Q78
Tinel sign, 62
Tinnitus, 101–102
    pulsatile, 101, Q9
To Err is Human: Building a Safer Health System (Institute of Medicine), 19
Tongue syndromes, 106
Toxic shock syndrome, 105
Tramadol
    for low back pain, 52
    for noncancer chronic pain, 35, Q136
Transitions in care, 20–21, 22t, Q94, Q113
Transjugular intrahepatic portosystemic shunt (TIPS), 134
Transurethral resection of the prostate (TURP), 78
Traumatic brain injury, 111
Trichomoniasis, 92–93
Tricyclic antidepressants
    for pain, 35
    perioperative management of, 126t
Triglycerides, 63–64

Trochanteric bursitis, 58
Tubal ligation, 85t, 86
Tuberculosis, in immunocompromised patients, 39
TWEAK test, 17

Ulcers
    corneal, 95
    oral, 106
    pressure, 123–124, 124t, Q17, Q24
Ulnar nerve, 56f
    entrapment of, 56, Q132
Ultrasonography, for abdominal aortic aneurysm screening, 8, Q151
Underweight, 70t
United States Preventive Services Task Force (USPSTF)
    obesity management recommendations from, 72
    screening recommendations from, 7, 7t, 8, 9, 10t, 11, 62, 64, 70, 106, 119, Q151
Upper airway cough syndrome (UACS), 37, 38f
Upper respiratory tract infections, 103–105
    cough in, 37
    ear pain in, Q114
Urinary incontinence, 121–123, 122f, Q33, Q88
Uterine bleeding, abnormal, 90, Q53
Uveitis, 95

Vaginal estrogen therapy, 89, Q25
Vaginal symptoms, postmenopausal, 89, Q25
Vaginismus, 82, Q5
Vaginosis, bacterial, 92, 92f, Q111
Valgus stress test, 59f, 60f
Validity, threats to, 1, Q92
Value, in healthcare, 5
Varenicline, 17
Varicella vaccine, 12t, 13–14, 15, 16, 87
Varicocele, 79–80
Varus stress test, 59, 59f, 60f
Vasectomy, 85t
Vasomotor symptoms, of menopause, 88–89, 89t, Q60
Venous stasis, as edema cause, 50, Q22
Vertigo, 40–43
    benign paroxysmal positional, 41, 42f, 43, Q14, Q20, Q98
    central, 41t, 43, Q14, Q50
    peripheral, 41, 41t, 42f, 43, Q14, Q98

Very-low-density lipoprotein (VLDL) cholesterol, 63
Visual acuity test, 119
Visual impairment, in older adults, 119
Vitamin B_{12} deficiency
    atrophic glossitis and, 106
    in bariatric surgery patients, 74, 74t, Q15
Vitamin D supplementation, for older adults, 118, Q87

Warfarin, perioperative management of, 126t, 129–130, 131t, 132, Q142
Weber test, 100
Wegener granulomatosis, 104, Q138
Weight gain, medication-related, 70t
Weight loss, for obesity control, 71, Q51
Whooping cough. See Pertussis
Withholding/withdrawing, of treatment, 25, Q43
Women's health, 81–93
    abnormal uterine bleeding, 90, Q53
    breast cancer, 84
    breast masses, 82–84, 83t
    breast pain, 84
    chronic pelvic pain, 91–92, 91t
    contraception, 84–86
    dysmenorrhea, 90–91
    menopause, 87–89, 89t
    postpartum depression, 109
    preconception counseling, 86–87, 87t
    premenstrual dysphoric disorder, 109
    sexual dysfunction, 81–82, 81t, 88, 89, Q5, Q147
    vaginitis, 92–93
Women's Health Initiative, 88
World Health Organization, analgesic ladder of, 29–30, 29f, 35
Wrist pain, 57

Xerophthalmia, 97–98, Q44
Xerostomia, 105, 106

Yergason test, 54, 54t, 55f

Zaleplon, for insomnia, 44, 45t, Q153
Zolpidem, for insomnia, 44, 45t, Q153

A

NAME AND ADDRESS (Please complete.)

_____
Last Name   First Name   Middle Initial

_____
Address

_____
Address cont.

_____
City   State   ZIP Code

_____
Country

_____
Email address

B

Order Number

(Use the Order Number on your MKSAP materials packing slip.)

C

ACP ID Number

(Refer to packing slip in your MKSAP materials
for your ACP ID Number.)

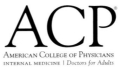

ACP
AMERICAN COLLEGE OF PHYSICIANS
INTERNAL MEDICINE | *Doctors for Adults*

Medical Knowledge
Self-Assessment
Program® 16

TO EARN *AMA PRA CATEGORY 1 CREDITS*™ YOU MUST:

1. Answer all questions.
2. Score a minimum of 50% correct.
===

TO EARN *FREE* SAME-DAY *AMA PRA CATEGORY 1 CREDITS*™ ONLINE:

1. Answer all of your questions.
2. Go to **mksap.acponline.org** and access the appropriate answer sheet.
3. Transcribe your answers and submit for CME credits.
4. You can also enter your answers directly at **mksap.acponline.org** without first using this answer sheet.

To Submit Your Answer Sheet by Mail or FAX for a $10 Administrative Fee per Answer Sheet:

1. Answer all of your questions and calculate your score.
2. Complete boxes A–F.
3. Complete payment information.
4. Send the answer sheet and payment information to ACP, using the FAX number/address listed below.

COMPLETE FORM BELOW ONLY IF YOU SUBMIT BY MAIL OR FAX

Last Name   First Name |MI

Payment Information. Must remit in US funds, drawn on a US bank.

The processing fee for each paper answer sheet is $10.

☐ Check, made payable to ACP, enclosed

Charge to   ☐ **VISA**   ☐ **MasterCard**   ☐ **AMERICAN EXPRESS**   ☐ **DISCOVER**

Card Number _____

Expiration Date _____ / _____   Security code (3 or 4 digit #s) _____
                      MM   YY

Signature _____

Fax to: 215-351-2799

Mail to:
Member and Customer Service
American College of Physicians
190 N. Independence Mall West
Philadelphia, PA 19106-1572

Questions?
Go to **mskap.acponline.org** or email **custserv@acponline.org**

1 Ⓐ Ⓑ Ⓒ Ⓓ Ⓔ
2 Ⓐ Ⓑ Ⓒ Ⓓ Ⓔ
3 Ⓐ Ⓑ Ⓒ Ⓓ Ⓔ
4 Ⓐ Ⓑ Ⓒ Ⓓ Ⓔ
5 Ⓐ Ⓑ Ⓒ Ⓓ Ⓔ

6 Ⓐ Ⓑ Ⓒ Ⓓ Ⓔ
7 Ⓐ Ⓑ Ⓒ Ⓓ Ⓔ
8 Ⓐ Ⓑ Ⓒ Ⓓ Ⓔ
9 Ⓐ Ⓑ Ⓒ Ⓓ Ⓔ
10 Ⓐ Ⓑ Ⓒ Ⓓ Ⓔ

11 Ⓐ Ⓑ Ⓒ Ⓓ Ⓔ
12 Ⓐ Ⓑ Ⓒ Ⓓ Ⓔ
13 Ⓐ Ⓑ Ⓒ Ⓓ Ⓔ
14 Ⓐ Ⓑ Ⓒ Ⓓ Ⓔ
15 Ⓐ Ⓑ Ⓒ Ⓓ Ⓔ

16 Ⓐ Ⓑ Ⓒ Ⓓ Ⓔ
17 Ⓐ Ⓑ Ⓒ Ⓓ Ⓔ
18 Ⓐ Ⓑ Ⓒ Ⓓ Ⓔ
19 Ⓐ Ⓑ Ⓒ Ⓓ Ⓔ
20 Ⓐ Ⓑ Ⓒ Ⓓ Ⓔ

21 Ⓐ Ⓑ Ⓒ Ⓓ Ⓔ
22 Ⓐ Ⓑ Ⓒ Ⓓ Ⓔ
23 Ⓐ Ⓑ Ⓒ Ⓓ Ⓔ
24 Ⓐ Ⓑ Ⓒ Ⓓ Ⓔ
25 Ⓐ Ⓑ Ⓒ Ⓓ Ⓔ

26 Ⓐ Ⓑ Ⓒ Ⓓ Ⓔ
27 Ⓐ Ⓑ Ⓒ Ⓓ Ⓔ
28 Ⓐ Ⓑ Ⓒ Ⓓ Ⓔ
29 Ⓐ Ⓑ Ⓒ Ⓓ Ⓔ
30 Ⓐ Ⓑ Ⓒ Ⓓ Ⓔ

31 Ⓐ Ⓑ Ⓒ Ⓓ Ⓔ
32 Ⓐ Ⓑ Ⓒ Ⓓ Ⓔ
33 Ⓐ Ⓑ Ⓒ Ⓓ Ⓔ
34 Ⓐ Ⓑ Ⓒ Ⓓ Ⓔ
35 Ⓐ Ⓑ Ⓒ Ⓓ Ⓔ

36 Ⓐ Ⓑ Ⓒ Ⓓ Ⓔ
37 Ⓐ Ⓑ Ⓒ Ⓓ Ⓔ
38 Ⓐ Ⓑ Ⓒ Ⓓ Ⓔ
39 Ⓐ Ⓑ Ⓒ Ⓓ Ⓔ
40 Ⓐ Ⓑ Ⓒ Ⓓ Ⓔ

41 Ⓐ Ⓑ Ⓒ Ⓓ Ⓔ
42 Ⓐ Ⓑ Ⓒ Ⓓ Ⓔ
43 Ⓐ Ⓑ Ⓒ Ⓓ Ⓔ
44 Ⓐ Ⓑ Ⓒ Ⓓ Ⓔ
45 Ⓐ Ⓑ Ⓒ Ⓓ Ⓔ

46 Ⓐ Ⓑ Ⓒ Ⓓ Ⓔ
47 Ⓐ Ⓑ Ⓒ Ⓓ Ⓔ
48 Ⓐ Ⓑ Ⓒ Ⓓ Ⓔ
49 Ⓐ Ⓑ Ⓒ Ⓓ Ⓔ
50 Ⓐ Ⓑ Ⓒ Ⓓ Ⓔ

51 Ⓐ Ⓑ Ⓒ Ⓓ Ⓔ
52 Ⓐ Ⓑ Ⓒ Ⓓ Ⓔ
53 Ⓐ Ⓑ Ⓒ Ⓓ Ⓔ
54 Ⓐ Ⓑ Ⓒ Ⓓ Ⓔ
55 Ⓐ Ⓑ Ⓒ Ⓓ Ⓔ

56 Ⓐ Ⓑ Ⓒ Ⓓ Ⓔ
57 Ⓐ Ⓑ Ⓒ Ⓓ Ⓔ
58 Ⓐ Ⓑ Ⓒ Ⓓ Ⓔ
59 Ⓐ Ⓑ Ⓒ Ⓓ Ⓔ
60 Ⓐ Ⓑ Ⓒ Ⓓ Ⓔ

61 Ⓐ Ⓑ Ⓒ Ⓓ Ⓔ
62 Ⓐ Ⓑ Ⓒ Ⓓ Ⓔ
63 Ⓐ Ⓑ Ⓒ Ⓓ Ⓔ
64 Ⓐ Ⓑ Ⓒ Ⓓ Ⓔ
65 Ⓐ Ⓑ Ⓒ Ⓓ Ⓔ

66 Ⓐ Ⓑ Ⓒ Ⓓ Ⓔ
67 Ⓐ Ⓑ Ⓒ Ⓓ Ⓔ
68 Ⓐ Ⓑ Ⓒ Ⓓ Ⓔ
69 Ⓐ Ⓑ Ⓒ Ⓓ Ⓔ
70 Ⓐ Ⓑ Ⓒ Ⓓ Ⓔ

71 Ⓐ Ⓑ Ⓒ Ⓓ Ⓔ
72 Ⓐ Ⓑ Ⓒ Ⓓ Ⓔ
73 Ⓐ Ⓑ Ⓒ Ⓓ Ⓔ
74 Ⓐ Ⓑ Ⓒ Ⓓ Ⓔ
75 Ⓐ Ⓑ Ⓒ Ⓓ Ⓔ

76 Ⓐ Ⓑ Ⓒ Ⓓ Ⓔ
77 Ⓐ Ⓑ Ⓒ Ⓓ Ⓔ
78 Ⓐ Ⓑ Ⓒ Ⓓ Ⓔ
79 Ⓐ Ⓑ Ⓒ Ⓓ Ⓔ
80 Ⓐ Ⓑ Ⓒ Ⓓ Ⓔ

81 Ⓐ Ⓑ Ⓒ Ⓓ Ⓔ
82 Ⓐ Ⓑ Ⓒ Ⓓ Ⓔ
83 Ⓐ Ⓑ Ⓒ Ⓓ Ⓔ
84 Ⓐ Ⓑ Ⓒ Ⓓ Ⓔ
85 Ⓐ Ⓑ Ⓒ Ⓓ Ⓔ

86 Ⓐ Ⓑ Ⓒ Ⓓ Ⓔ
87 Ⓐ Ⓑ Ⓒ Ⓓ Ⓔ
88 Ⓐ Ⓑ Ⓒ Ⓓ Ⓔ
89 Ⓐ Ⓑ Ⓒ Ⓓ Ⓔ
90 Ⓐ Ⓑ Ⓒ Ⓓ Ⓔ

91 Ⓐ Ⓑ Ⓒ Ⓓ Ⓔ
92 Ⓐ Ⓑ Ⓒ Ⓓ Ⓔ
93 Ⓐ Ⓑ Ⓒ Ⓓ Ⓔ
94 Ⓐ Ⓑ Ⓒ Ⓓ Ⓔ
95 Ⓐ Ⓑ Ⓒ Ⓓ Ⓔ

96 Ⓐ Ⓑ Ⓒ Ⓓ Ⓔ
97 Ⓐ Ⓑ Ⓒ Ⓓ Ⓔ
98 Ⓐ Ⓑ Ⓒ Ⓓ Ⓔ
99 Ⓐ Ⓑ Ⓒ Ⓓ Ⓔ
100 Ⓐ Ⓑ Ⓒ Ⓓ Ⓔ

101 Ⓐ Ⓑ Ⓒ Ⓓ Ⓔ
102 Ⓐ Ⓑ Ⓒ Ⓓ Ⓔ
103 Ⓐ Ⓑ Ⓒ Ⓓ Ⓔ
104 Ⓐ Ⓑ Ⓒ Ⓓ Ⓔ
105 Ⓐ Ⓑ Ⓒ Ⓓ Ⓔ

106 Ⓐ Ⓑ Ⓒ Ⓓ Ⓔ
107 Ⓐ Ⓑ Ⓒ Ⓓ Ⓔ
108 Ⓐ Ⓑ Ⓒ Ⓓ Ⓔ
109 Ⓐ Ⓑ Ⓒ Ⓓ Ⓔ
110 Ⓐ Ⓑ Ⓒ Ⓓ Ⓔ

111 Ⓐ Ⓑ Ⓒ Ⓓ Ⓔ
112 Ⓐ Ⓑ Ⓒ Ⓓ Ⓔ
113 Ⓐ Ⓑ Ⓒ Ⓓ Ⓔ
114 Ⓐ Ⓑ Ⓒ Ⓓ Ⓔ
115 Ⓐ Ⓑ Ⓒ Ⓓ Ⓔ

116 Ⓐ Ⓑ Ⓒ Ⓓ Ⓔ
117 Ⓐ Ⓑ Ⓒ Ⓓ Ⓔ
118 Ⓐ Ⓑ Ⓒ Ⓓ Ⓔ
119 Ⓐ Ⓑ Ⓒ Ⓓ Ⓔ
120 Ⓐ Ⓑ Ⓒ Ⓓ Ⓔ

121 Ⓐ Ⓑ Ⓒ Ⓓ Ⓔ
122 Ⓐ Ⓑ Ⓒ Ⓓ Ⓔ
123 Ⓐ Ⓑ Ⓒ Ⓓ Ⓔ
124 Ⓐ Ⓑ Ⓒ Ⓓ Ⓔ
125 Ⓐ Ⓑ Ⓒ Ⓓ Ⓔ

126 Ⓐ Ⓑ Ⓒ Ⓓ Ⓔ
127 Ⓐ Ⓑ Ⓒ Ⓓ Ⓔ
128 Ⓐ Ⓑ Ⓒ Ⓓ Ⓔ
129 Ⓐ Ⓑ Ⓒ Ⓓ Ⓔ
130 Ⓐ Ⓑ Ⓒ Ⓓ Ⓔ

131 Ⓐ Ⓑ Ⓒ Ⓓ Ⓔ
132 Ⓐ Ⓑ Ⓒ Ⓓ Ⓔ
133 Ⓐ Ⓑ Ⓒ Ⓓ Ⓔ
134 Ⓐ Ⓑ Ⓒ Ⓓ Ⓔ
135 Ⓐ Ⓑ Ⓒ Ⓓ Ⓔ

136 Ⓐ Ⓑ Ⓒ Ⓓ Ⓔ
137 Ⓐ Ⓑ Ⓒ Ⓓ Ⓔ
138 Ⓐ Ⓑ Ⓒ Ⓓ Ⓔ
139 Ⓐ Ⓑ Ⓒ Ⓓ Ⓔ
140 Ⓐ Ⓑ Ⓒ Ⓓ Ⓔ

141 Ⓐ Ⓑ Ⓒ Ⓓ Ⓔ
142 Ⓐ Ⓑ Ⓒ Ⓓ Ⓔ
143 Ⓐ Ⓑ Ⓒ Ⓓ Ⓔ
144 Ⓐ Ⓑ Ⓒ Ⓓ Ⓔ
145 Ⓐ Ⓑ Ⓒ Ⓓ Ⓔ

146 Ⓐ Ⓑ Ⓒ Ⓓ Ⓔ
147 Ⓐ Ⓑ Ⓒ Ⓓ Ⓔ
148 Ⓐ Ⓑ Ⓒ Ⓓ Ⓔ
149 Ⓐ Ⓑ Ⓒ Ⓓ Ⓔ
150 Ⓐ Ⓑ Ⓒ Ⓓ Ⓔ

151 Ⓐ Ⓑ Ⓒ Ⓓ Ⓔ
152 Ⓐ Ⓑ Ⓒ Ⓓ Ⓔ
153 Ⓐ Ⓑ Ⓒ Ⓓ Ⓔ
154 Ⓐ Ⓑ Ⓒ Ⓓ Ⓔ
155 Ⓐ Ⓑ Ⓒ Ⓓ Ⓔ

156 Ⓐ Ⓑ Ⓒ Ⓓ Ⓔ
157 Ⓐ Ⓑ Ⓒ Ⓓ Ⓔ
158 Ⓐ Ⓑ Ⓒ Ⓓ Ⓔ
159 Ⓐ Ⓑ Ⓒ Ⓓ Ⓔ
160 Ⓐ Ⓑ Ⓒ Ⓓ Ⓔ

161 Ⓐ Ⓑ Ⓒ Ⓓ Ⓔ
162 Ⓐ Ⓑ Ⓒ Ⓓ Ⓔ
163 Ⓐ Ⓑ Ⓒ Ⓓ Ⓔ
164 Ⓐ Ⓑ Ⓒ Ⓓ Ⓔ
165 Ⓐ Ⓑ Ⓒ Ⓓ Ⓔ

166 Ⓐ Ⓑ Ⓒ Ⓓ Ⓔ
167 Ⓐ Ⓑ Ⓒ Ⓓ Ⓔ
168 Ⓐ Ⓑ Ⓒ Ⓓ Ⓔ
169 Ⓐ Ⓑ Ⓒ Ⓓ Ⓔ
170 Ⓐ Ⓑ Ⓒ Ⓓ Ⓔ

171 Ⓐ Ⓑ Ⓒ Ⓓ Ⓔ
172 Ⓐ Ⓑ Ⓒ Ⓓ Ⓔ
173 Ⓐ Ⓑ Ⓒ Ⓓ Ⓔ
174 Ⓐ Ⓑ Ⓒ Ⓓ Ⓔ
175 Ⓐ Ⓑ Ⓒ Ⓓ Ⓔ

176 Ⓐ Ⓑ Ⓒ Ⓓ Ⓔ
177 Ⓐ Ⓑ Ⓒ Ⓓ Ⓔ
178 Ⓐ Ⓑ Ⓒ Ⓓ Ⓔ
179 Ⓐ Ⓑ Ⓒ Ⓓ Ⓔ
180 Ⓐ Ⓑ Ⓒ Ⓓ Ⓔ